Pediatric Anesthesia

THE REQUISITES IN ANESTHESIOLOGY

SERIES EDITOR

Roberta L. Hines, M.D.
Chair and Professor
Department of Anesthesiology
Yale University School of Medicine
New Haven, Connecticut

Pediatric Anesthesia

THE REQUISITES IN ANESTHESIOLOGY

Ronald S. Litman, D.O.

Associate Professor of Anesthesiology and Pediatrics
University of Pennsylvania School of Medicine
Attending Anesthesiologist
The Children's Hospital of Philadelphia
Philadelphia, Pennsylvania

ELSEVIER
MOSBY

ELSEVIER
MOSBY

The Curtis Center
170 S Independence Mall W 300E
Philadelphia, Pennsylvania 19106

PEDIATRIC ANESTHESIA: THE REQUISITES IN ANESTHESIOLOGY   ISBN: 0-323-02216-2
Copyright © 2004, Mosby, Inc. All rights reserved.

NOTICE

Anesthesiology is an ever-changing field. Standard safety precautions must be followed, but as new research and clinical experience broaden our knowledge, changes in treatment and drug therapy may become necessary or appropriate. Readers are advised to check the most current product information provided by the manufacturer of each drug to be administered to verify the recommended dose, the method and duration of administration, and contraindications. It is the responsibility of the treating physician, relying on experience and knowledge of the patient, to determine dosages and the best treatment for each individual patient. Neither the publisher nor the editor assume any liability for any injury and/or damage to persons or property arising from this publication.

Library of Congress Cataloging-in-Publication Data

Litman, Ronald S.
    Pediatric anesthesia : the requisites in anesthesia / Ronald S. Litman.—1st ed.
        p. ; cm.
    ISBN 0-323-02216-2
    1. Pediatric anesthesia. 2. Postoperative care. 3. Pediatrics. I. Title.
    [DNLM: 1. Anesthesia—methods—Child. 2. Anesthetics—administration &
    dosage—Child. 3. Pediatrics—methods—Child. 4. Perioperative Care—methods—Child. WO
    440 L776p 2004]
    RD139.L58 2004
    617.9′6798—dc22   2004042572

Acquisitions Editor: Natasha Andjelkovic
Developmental Editor: Anne Snyder
Project Manager: Daniel Clipner

Printed in the United States of America

Last digit is the print number: 9   8   7   6   5   4   3   2   1

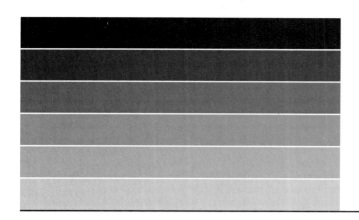

Contributors

Aisling Conran, MD
Assistant Professor of Anesthesia and Critical Care
University of Chicago Hospitals
Chicago, Illinois

Michael J. Fisher, MD
Assistant Professor of Pediatrics
University of Pennsylvania School of Medicine
Division of Oncology
The Children's Hospital of Philadelphia
Philadelphia, Pennsylvania

James W. Huh, MD
Assistant Professor of Anesthesiology and Pediatrics
University of Pennsylvania School of Medicine
Attending Intensivist
The Children's Hospital of Philadelphia
Philadelphia, Pennsylvania

Ronald S. Litman, DO
Associate Professor of Anesthesiology and Pediatrics
University of Pennsylvania School of Medicine
Attending Anesthesiologist
The Children's Hospital of Philadelphia
Philadelphia, Pennsylvania

Deirdre E. Logan, PhD
Psychologist, Pain Treatment Service
Children's Hospital Boston, and
Instructor, Harvard University Medical School
Boston, Massachusetts

Catherine S. Manno, MD
Director, Transfusion Service
Director, Hemophilia Program
Associate Professor of Pediatrics
The Children's Hospital of Philadelphia
Philadelphia, Pennsylvania

Bradley S. Marino, MD, MPP
Assistant Professor of Anesthesiology and Pediatrics
University of Pennsylvania School of Medicine
Attending Intensivist and Cardiologist
Department of Anesthesiology and Critical Care
Medicine
The Children's Hospital of Philadelphia
Philadelphia, Pennsylvania

Lynne G. Maxwell, MD
Associate Professor of Anesthesiology and Pediatrics
University of Pennsylvania, School of Medicine
Attending Anesthesiologist
The Children's Hospital of Philadelphia
Philadelphia, Pennsylvania

Margaret A. Priestley, MD
Assistant Professor of Anesthesiology and
Pediatrics
University of Pennsylvania School of Medicine
Clinical Director, Pediatric Intensive Care Unit
The Children's Hospital of Philadelphia
Philadelphia, Pennsylvania

John B. Rose, MD
Assistant Professor of Anesthesiology and
Pediatrics
University of Pennsylvania, School of Medicine
Associate Anesthesiologist
The Children's Hospital of Philadelphia
Philadelphia, Pennsylvania

Daniel S. Samadi, MD
Clinical Professor of Otolaryngology and Pediatrics
Pediatric Otolaryngology – Head and Neck Surgery
Director of the Cochlear Implant Center
The Joseph M. Sanzari Children's Hospital
Hackensack University Medical Center
Hackensack, New Jersey

Mary C. Theroux, MD
Clinical Associate Professor of Anesthesiology and
Pediatrics
Jefferson University
Attending Anesthesiologist
duPont Hospital for Children
Wilmington, Delaware

Joseph D. Tobias, MD
Vice-Chairman, Department of Anesthesiology
Chief, Division of Pediatric Anesthesiology/Pediatric
Critical Care
Russell and Mary Shelden Chair of Pediatric Intensive
Care Medicine
Professor of Anesthesiology and Pediatrics
University of Missouri
Columbia, Missouri

Monica S. Vavilala, MD
Assistant Professor of Anesthesiology and Pediatrics
University of Washington
Attending Anesthesiologist, Harborview Medical Center
Attending Physician, Emergency Department,
Children's Hospital Regional Medical Center
Seattle, Washington

Athena F. Zuppa, MD
Assistant Professor of Anesthesiology and Pediatrics
University of Pennsylvania School of Medicine
Attending Intensivist
The Children's Hospital of Philadelphia
Philadelphia, Pennsylvania

Preface

Welcome to the magical world of pediatric anesthesia! The art and science of pediatric anesthesia allows the anesthesia practitioner to employ a unique set of psychological, intellectual, and physical skills that are not applicable when caring for adult patients. It is my hope that the reader of this book will discover and develop these unique skills, thereby enhancing the safety of children requiring our services.

This book is written primarily for the anesthesiology resident rotating through his or her core or elective block in pediatric anesthesia. It represents a combination of the educational program in pediatric anesthesia that I created for the residents at the University of Rochester, and the educational curriculum for rotating residents at The Children's Hospital of Philadelphia. It was designed to be used as a stand-alone text for anesthesia residents during their rotation in pediatric anesthesia, and subsequently for preparing for the written and oral boards. If mastered, this information should allow the graduating resident to practice safe pediatric anesthesia in a nonpediatric environment, and will assist the practicing anesthesiologist who is preparing for his or her recertification exam.

The material contained in this book reflects my background as a pediatrician as well as my extensive experience as an adult anesthesiologist. Since most anesthesiology residents do not have experience in either general pediatrics or pediatric anesthesia, these principles are explained on a basic level with special emphasis on the differences between children and adult anesthesia practice. Thus, the material is written with the assumption that the reader possesses a basic fund of knowledge of adult anesthesia. In general, material that is well explained in adult anesthesia textbooks is omitted from this book.

The book is organized into eight main sections, each of which contains one or more chapters. The first section contains chapters on birth transition and pediatric physiology and pharmacology – the type of knowledge easily acquired by pediatric residents but not well known by anesthesiologists. The second section is divided into chapters that represent important coexisting diseases found in children. The next three sections address aspects of preoperative, intraoperative, and postoperative pediatric care. The final several sections comprise pediatric anesthesia subspecialty care – all the various surgical subspecialties, acute and chronic pain management, and essentials of critical care, including pediatric advanced life support (PALS).

The principles covered in this book are based on the scientific basis of clinical practice with an emphasis on maintaining the standard of care. Most chapters contain thought-provoking clinical scenarios. They are designed to be controversial. When the literature does not contain a clear answer to a clinical question, the anesthesiologist must practice according to personal experience and the prevailing standard of care. These cases will help the anesthesiologist determine the best course of action in controversial situations. Some chapters contain "Article To Know" boxes. These sections describe important articles that have shaped the way we practice. Nearly every chapter also contains a section called "Additional Articles To Know" – note that these are *not* called "suggested" readings.

The first edition of any book will subsequently require additions, changes, and other types of fine-tuning in subsequent editions. Readers of this book shouldn't hesitate to make these types of suggestions to the editor: litmanr@email.chop.edu.

Ronald S. Litman, D.O.

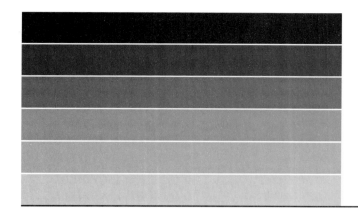

Acknowledgments

This book was written almost entirely on personal time. Thus, it would not have been possible without the love and patience of my wife, Ruth, and my children, Alan and Cory, who endured countless nights and weekends during the extensive writing and editing process that encompassed more than two years.

Many of my residents, fellows, and colleagues reviewed the chapters for accuracy and readibility. Phil Bailey, D.O., reviewed every chapter and contributed many helpful comments and suggestions for improvement. Additional reviewers included Ann Cherie Fox, M.D., Leslie Friskell, M.D., Jeff Goldsmith, M.D., Brian Grace, M.D., Amit Gupta, M.D., Tom Henthorn, M.D., Tuta Ion, M.D., Max Kelz, M.D., Scott Loev, M.D., Maggie Myers, M.D., Hector Nicodemus, M.D., Marnie Robinson M.D., Gordana Stjepanovic M.D., and Albert Telfeian, M.D.

The content of this book has been indirectly influenced by four Chairmen that made a large impact on my career: William T. Speck, M.D., Joel A. Kaplan, M.D., Ronald A. Gabel, M.D., and Denham S. Ward, M.D., Ph.D. Collectively they instilled in me principles of intellectual honesty and a love for reading and interpreting the literature. Additional thanks go to Zeev Kain, M.D. and Roberta L. Hines, M.D. for giving me this opportunity. Allan Ross and Anne Snyder from Elsevier, and Antonella Collaro and Maureen Allen, project managers.

Lastly I would like to thank past, present, and future residents and fellows from the University of Rochester and The Children's Hospital of Philadelphia for your eternal enthusiasm for learning pediatric anesthesia. It is the ultimate motivation for a career in academic practice and education.

Ronald S. Litman

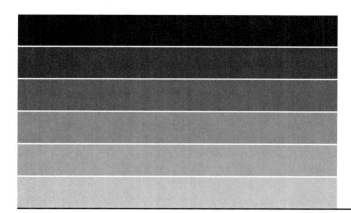

Contents

PART VIII
PEDIATRIC CRITICAL CARE

THE NORMAL PEDIATRIC PATIENT

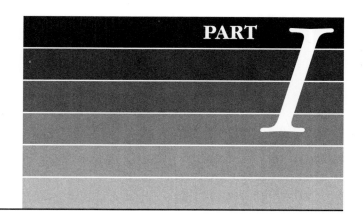

PART

I

CHAPTER 1

Fetal Physiology and Birth Transition

RONALD S. LITMAN

The Fetal Pulmonary System
The Fetal Circulatory System
Cardiopulmonary Changes at Birth
Persistent Pulmonary Hypertension of the Newborn

We begin this journey into pediatric anesthesia by looking at fetal cardiopulmonary physiology and the changes that occur during the birth process. Knowledge of these changes is important for understanding a variety of pathophysiologic conditions of the neonate. For purposes of clarity and consistency, the term "neonate" will henceforth refer to an infant in the first 28 days of life, regardless of the gestational age. The term "infant" will refer to a child in the first year of life. The "gestational" age refers to the number of weeks between conception and birth; the normal term gestational age is between 38 and 42 weeks of pregnancy.

Newborn infants can be classified by their size relative to their gestational age:

- *Appropriate for gestational age* (AGA) describes an infant whose birthweight is between the 10th and 90th percentiles.
- *Small for gestational age* (SGA) describes an infant whose birthweight is below the 10th percentile.
- *Large for gestational age* (LGA) describes an infant whose birthweight is above the 90th percentile.

Intrauterine growth restriction (or *retardation*) (IUGR) is an abnormal pattern of restricted fetal growth for gestational age. An easy way to think of the distinction between IUGR and SGA is that IUGR is a term used by obstetricians to describe a pattern of growth over a period of time, whereas SGA is a term used by pediatricians to describe a single point on a growth curve.

THE FETAL PULMONARY SYSTEM

As the lungs grow and develop during fetal life, they do not function in the capacity of oxygen and carbon dioxide exchange, for this role is carried out by the placenta. Rather, the lungs are fluid-filled organs that grow terminal bronchioles and alveoli in preparation for the air-breathing that is required after birth.

Fetal lung development is divided into four stages of progressive lower airway and alveolar growth (Table 1-1). During the last or saccular stage, the fetal lung finalizes the physiologic processes that will allow respiration in an extrauterine environment. This includes maturation of the alveolar–vascular interface and development of a full complement of surfactant, which will reduce surface tension within the alveoli and prevent their collapse. The fetal airways and alveoli are distended by secreted lung fluid, which becomes a component of the amniotic fluid.

As the peripheral chemoreceptors and the respiratory center of the brain mature, the fetus develops stronger and more regular breathing patterns throughout development. After the 30th week of gestation, the fetus is noted to "practice" breathing at about 60 times per minute, approximately 40% of the time.

THE FETAL CIRCULATORY SYSTEM

The overall goal of fetal circulation is to distribute oxygen, glucose, and other nutrients from the placenta to the developing brain and vital organs (Fig. 1-1), and is outlined in the following steps.

In the placenta, the organ of fetal respiration, fetal blood picks up oxygen and releases carbon dioxide. Fetal-type hemoglobin (Hgb F) is characterized by its leftward shift of the oxyhemoglobin dissociation curve. Therefore, fetal blood has a greater affinity for oxygen than does maternal blood, and oxygen is transferred to fetal hemoglobin in the placenta. Release of oxygen from Hgb F to fetal tissues is facilitated by the relatively increased temperature and lower pH of the fetus, both of which shift the oxyhemoglobin dissociation curve to the right.

Table 1-1 Stages of Fetal Lung Development

Stage	Gestational Weeks	Noteworthy Events
Embryonic	4–7	Initial formation of primitive lung tissue and vascular connections
Pseudoglandular	5–17	Development of a bronchial tree that begins to form lumens
Canalicular	16–26	Alveoli begin to form
		Vascular and lymphatic systems develop alongside the bronchial tree
		Differentiation of type 1 and type 2 pneumocytes with beginning of surfactant production
		Extrauterine life possible at later weeks
Saccular	24th–birth	Peripheral bronchiole branching
		Maturation of surfactant system
		Breathing efforts begin
		Alveoli at birth number 30–50 million
Alveolar	Birth–3 years	Continued alveolar growth to adult level of approximately 500 million
		Reduction of interstitial tissues

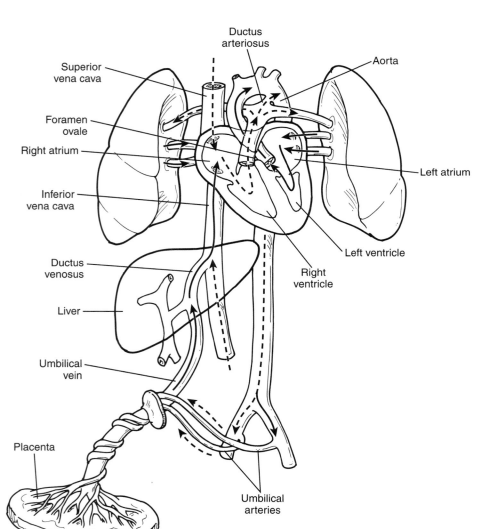

Figure 1-1 Anatomy of the fetal circulation. (Redrawn with permission from Bell C, Kain ZN, Hughes C: *The Pediatric Anesthesia Handbook*, 2nd edn, Mosby, Philadelphia, 1997.)

Oxygenated blood travels to the fetus in a single umbilical vein (contained within the umbilical cord). The maximal Pa_{O_2} in the umbilical vein measures only 30–35 mmHg. The umbilical vein travels through the liver, where approximately half the blood flow joins the hepatic circulation, while the other half bypasses the liver through the *ductus venosus*, a structure present only in fetal life. The ductus venosus carries the oxygenated blood from the umbilical vein into the inferior vena cava (IVC), where it mixes with poorly oxygenated blood from the fetal lower extremities and then travels to the right atrium.

Inside the fetal right atrium the relatively oxygenated blood from the IVC is preferentially directed across the *foramen ovale* and into the left atrium, while deoxygenated blood from the head via the superior vena cava (SVC) is preferentially directed through the tricuspid valve into the right ventricle.

The deoxygenated blood that enters the right ventricle is ejected into the pulmonary artery; but owing to high pulmonary vascular resistance, only a small portion (about 10%) flows into the pulmonary arterial system. The remainder is directed across the *ductus arteriosus* and into the aorta, where it joins aortic blood flow returning to the placenta via the umbilical arteries. The ductus arteriosus usually enters the aorta just proximal to the origin of the left subclavian artery.

The oxygenated blood that has crossed into the left atrium passes through the mitral valve into the left ventricle, and is ejected out from the ascending aorta where it provides oxygen and glucose to the developing brain via the carotid arteries. The Pa_{O_2} is now about 26–28 mmHg, but provides sufficient oxygen for fetal organ growth.

CARDIOPULMONARY CHANGES AT BIRTH

The birth process entails a number of simultaneous and dramatic cardiopulmonary changes that allow fetal transition to extrauterine life. The lung becomes the organ of respiration, and the cardiovascular system undergoes conversion from two parallel circulations to two circulations in series. These changes include the following important processes.

During the newborn's first breaths, air is drawn into the lungs, and lung fluid is absorbed or expelled. Intrathoracic distending pressures are estimated to reach −60 cmH$_2$O, and facilitate opening of fluid-filled alveoli. The pressure required for lung expansion becomes increasingly less negative over several breaths. These initial breaths will establish the residual volume (RV) and functional residual capacity (FRC) of the newborn's lungs, and will facilitate the absorption of lung fluid and the spread of surfactant.

The umbilical cord (containing the umbilical vein and arteries) is severed and clamped, which results in a dramatic increase in systemic vascular resistance (SVR). The umbilical arteries form a portion of the internal iliac and superior vesical arteries, and the ductus venosus (previously supplied by the umbilical vein) will atrophy and form a remnant known as the *ligamentum venosum*.

Pulmonary vascular resistance (PVR) decreases secondary to the establishment of negative intrathoracic pressure during inspiration, the increase in blood Pa_{O_2}, decrease in Pa_{CO_2}, and correction of fetal acidosis. Pulmonary blood flow is established, and arterial blood gas values normalize within the first 24 hours of life (Fig. 1-2).

The combined increase in SVR and decrease in PVR no longer allow blood to flow through the ductus arteriosus. Left atrial pressure increases causing the "flap-valve" foramen ovale to close, thus establishing for the first time a circulation in series.

Over the first several hours of life, the ductus arteriosus functionally closes as a result of constriction of specialized contractile tissue within its arterial wall. This constriction is caused by a number of factors, including

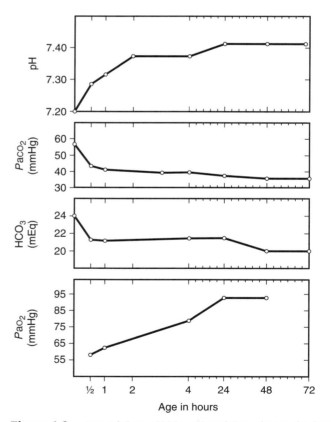

Figure 1-2   Arterial Pa_{CO_2}, HCO$_3$, pH, and Pa_{O_2} during the first hours and days of life. (Redrawn with permission from Klaus MH, Fanaroff AA: *Care of the High Risk Neonate*, 5th edn, WB Saunders, Philadelphia, 2001.)

withdrawal from placenta-derived prostaglandin E_2, an increase in arterial oxygen tension, and a decrease in blood acidosis. Over several weeks the ductus arteriosus becomes anatomically closed; its remnant is called the *ligamentum arteriosum*.

PERSISTENT PULMONARY HYPERTENSION OF THE NEWBORN

During the first several days of life, a number of pathological conditions of the newborn prevent the normal decrease in PVR and closure of the ductus arteriosus. These conditions include processes that cause hypoxemia, hypercarbia, and/or acidosis. Examples include respiratory distress syndrome of the premature infant and meconium aspiration syndrome, as well as hypothermia and congenital heart disease, among others. In the past, this condition was referred to as "persistent fetal circulation" (PFC); it is now referred to as "persistent pulmonary hypertension of the newborn" (PPHN). The lower the gestational age, the more likely that PPHN will occur.

Because of the abnormally high PVR, the fetal pattern of circulation continues: blood flows through the patent ductus arteriosus (PDA) or foramen ovale in a right-to-left direction and hypoxemia worsens, thus creating a vicious cycle that can be overcome only by aggressive therapy for the underlying disorder as well as correction of hypoxemia, hypercarbia, and acidosis. Selective pulmonary vascular dilatation using inhaled nitric oxide is a promising future therapeutic option.

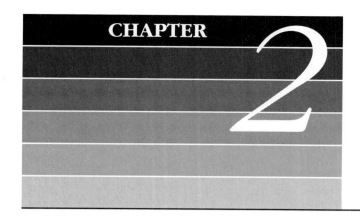

Developmental Physiology and Pharmacology

RONALD S. LITMAN

Developmental physiology encompasses the bodily changes taking place after birth that affect clinical anesthetic management. This chapter covers the basic principles of these changes, including cardiac, respiratory, neurologic, hematologic, and renal physiology. In addition, principles of developmental pharmacology as they pertain to the administration of intravenous and inhalational anesthetic agents are reviewed.

RESPIRATORY PHYSIOLOGY

The normal newborn achieves almost full functionality of the lungs within several hours after birth. The full-term newborn lung contains approximately 50 million alveoli, which proliferate during early childhood until reaching the adult level of approximately 500 million by about age 4 years.

The biochemical and reflex control of ventilation is well developed in the healthy full-term neonate. Periodic breathing is common in full-term newborns, with episodes of central apnea lasting 5 seconds or more.

In healthy infants, these episodes of central apnea are self-limited and are not associated with significant or prolonged bradycardia, as often occurs in preterm infants. In most healthy full-term infants, periodic breathing no longer exists after the first month of life.

Newborns exhibit a relatively normal ventilatory increase in response to inhaled carbon dioxide (CO_2), albeit to a smaller degree. The ventilatory response to hypoxia is characterized by an immediate increase in ventilation that lasts about 1 minute, followed by a decrease in ventilation that lasts about 5 minutes. This differs from older children in whom the initial protective phase of ventilatory stimulation has a substantially longer duration. This phase of ventilatory depression is even more prominent during concomitant hypercarbia, acidosis, or hypothermia.

Newborns demonstrate maladaptive respiratory depression (including apnea) in response to certain provocations that would normally result in stimulation of respiratory function in older infants. These include lung inflation (Hering–Breuer reflex), stimulation of the carina or superior laryngeal nerve, and upper-airway obstruction.

The most important differences in respiratory physiology between children and adults are related to the growth and maturity of the chest wall within the first 2 years of life. These differences directly influence the mechanism by which the functional residual capacity (FRC) is maintained. The newborn infant's FRC is established in the first several breaths after birth. In conscious subjects, it is estimated that the FRC is not significantly different between infants and adults, even though the mechanisms by which FRC is attained are different in these two populations. However, it is this difference that imparts such substantial effects on anesthetic practice.

In neonates and small infants, the orientation of the ribs is more parallel than angled, which predisposes to inefficiency of movement, since the volume of the rib cage is not increased by raising the ribs, as in older children and adults (Fig. 2-1). The infant's chest wall does not become more adult-like until the second year of age, when the child assumes an upright posture, and the effect of gravity causes the ribs to be angled downward. At about the same time, the structure of the ribs becomes less cartilaginous and more bony, conferring an inherent stiffness to the thoracic cavity. This stiffness imparts a tendency for the chest wall to expand outward, at the same time that the lungs tend to collapse inward. These opposing pressures generate the slightly negative intrapleural pressure at the end of exhalation, and serve to maintain FRC.

The chest wall of neonates and small infants has not yet developed its bony frame, so it is highly compliant and tends to collapse inward. As a consequence, young children must maintain a negative intrathoracic pressure by active recruitment of accessory muscles of respiration, such as intercostal muscles. In addition, the adductor muscles of the larynx of the young infant act as an expiratory "valve," serving to restrict exhalation in order to maintain positive end-expiratory pressure, and contribute to the maintenance of the FRC. This is often referred to as "laryngeal braking." Prominent abdominal excursions during normal breathing are common in newborns because of their reliance on diaphragmatic contraction for development of a sufficiently negative intrapleural pressure to initiate inspiration. Neonates may even exhibit small-airway collapse during normal tidal breathing.

These differences explain the marked changes in FRC in infants *after the onset of general anesthesia* that is normally not observed to a great extent in older children and adults. Because of the bony make-up of their rib cage, and noncompliant chest wall, older children and adults tend to maintain FRC when muscle tone is decreased following the administration of sedatives, anesthetics, or neuromuscular blockers. Infants and small children will respond to the administration of these agents by losing the FRC that depends on tonic muscular contraction, and thus rapidly develop hypoxemia. This effect can be overcome by application of continuous positive airway pressure (CPAP) or institution of positive-pressure breathing.

Differences in the anatomy of the infant diaphragm affect respiratory function. Prior to inspiration, the newborn diaphragm is relatively flat. Its anterior insertion onto the internal surface of the rib cage confers a mechanical disadvantage during inspiration when compared with the high-domed structure of the adult diaphragm (see Fig. 2-1). The muscular composition of the newborn's diaphragm is also unique. In contrast to the adult diaphragm, which has a high proportion (50–60%) of slow-twitch, high-oxidative, fatigue-resistant fibers (type 1), the newborn diaphragm is made up of only 10–30% of type 1 fibers. This characteristic predisposes the newborn diaphragm to fatigue, and may contribute to the inherent instability of the chest wall, as well as apnea and respiratory failure in the face of increased ventilatory demands or work of breathing.

The relatively compliant chest wall plays a role in determining the work of breathing, and thus the respiratory rate. Respiratory rates normally range between 30 and 70 breaths per minute in full-term newborns; this declines gradually throughout childhood, and reflects the optimal rate at which work of breathing is minimized.

On a per-kilogram basis, tidal volume is the same for both neonates and adults, and ranges from 7 to 10 mL/kg. Since oxygen consumption is relatively high in neonates and small infants (6–7 mL/kg versus 3 mL/kg for the adult), minute ventilation must be increased to deliver a sufficient amount of oxygen into the lungs (nearly three times that of the adult). As a consequence, small children have a relatively increased ratio of minute volume to FRC. This results in more rapid oxyhemoglobin desaturation during ventilatory depression or apnea.

HEMATOLOGIC PHYSIOLOGY

The hemoglobin concentration at birth is approximately 19 g/dL, of which about 70% is fetal hemoglobin (Hgb F). This relatively high concentration is a consequence of the requirement for an increased oxygen delivery *in utero*, when the oxyhemoglobin dissociation curve is shifted to the left, and oxygen is held tightly by Hgb F. Hgb F is progressively replaced by adult hemoglobin

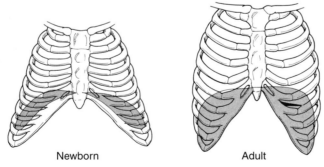

Newborn   Adult

Figure 2-1   Developmental changes of the rib cage and diaphragm from birth to adulthood. Adults can increase lung volume by raising the ribs and contracting the diaphragm. Early in development, the configuration of the rib cage and muscular attachments of the diaphragm place the newborn at a mechanical disadvantage because the ribs are already "raised," and contraction of the diaphragm results in a relatively small increase in thoracic cavity volume. (Reproduced with permission from Devlieger H, Daniels H, Marchal G et al: The diaphragm of the newborn infant: anatomical and ultrasonographic studies, *J Dev Physiol* 16:321–329, 1991.)

Table 2-1   Effect of Age on Coagulation Tests[a]

Test	28–31 Weeks Gestation	30–36 Weeks Gestation	Full-term Newborn	1–10 Years	11–18 Years
Prothrombin time (s)	15.4 (15–17)	13 (11–16)	13 (10–16)	11 (10–12)	11 (10–12)
Partial thromboplastin time (s)	108 (80–168)	54 (28–79)	43 (31–54)	30 (24–36)	32 (26–37)
Bleeding time (min)	?[b]	?[b]	?[b]	7 (3–13)	5 (3–8)

[a] Values are mean (normal range in parentheses).
[b] Unknown.

(Hgb A) during the first year of life. Production of erythropoietin is absent until hemoglobin levels drop to the physiologic nadir of about 9 or 10 g/dL at between 6 and 10 weeks of age. This is often referred to as the "physiologic anemia of infancy." Although this relative anemia may decrease oxygen delivery to the peripheral tissues, it is offset by the increased production of Hgb A and increase in red-cell 2,3-diphosphoglycerate, both of which shift the oxyhemoglobin dissociation curve to the right, and facilitate unloading of oxygen to the peripheral tissues.

Coagulation factors are relatively low at birth and normalize within the first year of life (Table 2-1).

CARDIOVASCULAR PHYSIOLOGY

Substantial cellular and structural changes occur in the heart in the first several months of life. Neonatal cardiac muscle cells contain all the normal structural elements of the adult heart, but are qualitatively and quantitatively different. The pattern of myofilaments is described as chaotic, compared to the long parallel rows of the mature heart. More specifically, the elements of the myocyte that are responsible for contraction are less able to function properly when challenged with a resistive load. Thus, force development is impaired when compared to the adult heart, and cardiac output is relatively less in response to changes in preload and afterload. This makes intuitive sense when one considers that during fetal life the left side of the heart has little responsibility against a low-pressure systemic circuit, but in the postnatal period must adapt to a higher stroke volume and increased wall tension.

The postnatal left ventricle develops into a thicker organ capable of contracting against higher systemic pressures by increasing the size and number of myocytes. In addition, the shape of the myocyte changes from spheroidal to one with more tapered edges, to increase efficiency of contraction. Factors that increase systemic vascular resistance (e.g., acidosis, cold, pain) in the newborn may lead to a decrease in cardiac output.

Therefore, it is possible that intraoperative cardiovascular stability can be enhanced in the newborn by preventing hypothermia and adequately blunting the stress response by titration of opioids. Indeed, studies in newborn cardiac anesthesia have suggested that a primarily opioid-based anesthetic technique is associated with improved postoperative cardiac function.

One of the most important clinical correlations of these morphological differences in the neonate is the decrease in compliance of the left ventricle. The newborn, therefore, is more prone to development of congestive heart failure during periods of fluid overload, as the left ventricle is less able to stretch in response to this increase in stroke volume. Also, because of this stiffness, distension of either ventricle will result in compression and dysfunction of the contralateral ventricle, thus further decreasing cardiac function. Newborns with respiratory disease who require high inspiratory pressures may develop left ventricular dysfunction with right ventricular overload. Perhaps more importantly, the newborn left ventricle is unable to shorten normally, and the heart is less able to increase left ventricular stroke volume during periods of hypovolemia or bradycardia when compared to the adult heart. Thus, episodes of hypovolemia or bradycardia can drastically decrease cardiac output in the neonate, and will endanger end-organ perfusion.

These deficits in neonatal cardiac function are often misinterpreted to mean that the only method with which to increase cardiac output is by increasing the heart rate. However, cardiac output will fail to increase substantially by increasing the heart rate to levels significantly above normal. Volume expansion remains an effective method, albeit possibly less effective than in an older child, to increase blood pressure and cardiac output, especially during periods of hypovolemia.

Sympathetic innervation of the heart and production of catecholamines, which are not fully developed at birth, increase during postnatal maturation. In contrast, the parasympathetic system appears to be fully functional at birth. Thus, neonates and small infants will demonstrate an imbalance, such that seemingly minor stimuli (suctioning of the pharynx) will result in an exaggerated parasympathetic or vagal response that results in bradycardia. For this reason, many pediatric anesthesiologists will routinely administer atropine prior to airway manipulation in small infants.

These structural and physiologic differences explain why neonates and infants under 6 months of age appear to be more sensitive to the depressant effects of volatile anesthetics, especially halothane. Isoflurane, sevoflurane, and desflurane depress myocardial contractility equally, though less than halothane.

The normal heart rate of the newborn ranges from 120 to 160 beats per minute (bpm), although lower rates (e.g., 70 bpm) are frequently observed during sleep, and higher rates (>200 bpm) are common during anxiety or pain. Heart rates tend to decrease with age, and parallel decreases in oxygen consumption. Many children have a noticeable variation in heart rate that varies with respiration (i.e., sinus arrhythmia).

Blood pressure increases gradually throughout childhood (Figs 2-2 and 2-3) and is also dependent on the height of the child such that taller children will demonstrate a higher blood pressure. Blood pressure ranges in

premature infants have been defined (Table 2-2) and will vary depending on the health status of the infant and mother.

In most children, careful auscultation of the heart reveals a soft, vibratory, systolic flow murmur. A heart murmur is not considered normal when it is louder than II/VI or has a diastolic component. Peripheral pulses in children of all ages should be clearly palpable. Absence of femoral pulses may indicate an aortic arch abnormality. Capillary refill in the distal extremities should be brisk (<3 seconds), but may be slightly delayed in the first few hours of life. Distal limb cyanosis (acrocyanosis) is normal in the first few hours of life.

As described in Chapter 1, the fetal heart is characterized by right-sided dominance that gradually abates in the first few months of life as pulmonary pressures decrease toward normal adult values. The normal newborn electrocardiograph (Fig. 2-4) demonstrates a preponderance of right-sided forces with a mean QRS axis of +110 degrees (range +30 to +180 degrees), and decreasing R wave size from leads V1 to V6. T waves are normally inverted in lead AVR and the right-sided precordial leads. This gradually shifts to left-sided dominance during early

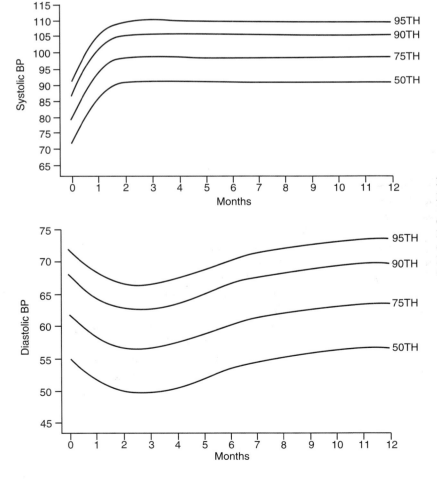

Figure 2-2 Age-specific percentiles of blood pressure measurements in boys, from birth to 12 months of age. Values for girls are slightly lower. (From National Heart, Lung, and Blood Institute, Bethesda, MD: Report of the Second Task Force on Blood Pressure Control in Children, 1987. Reproduced with permission from *Pediatrics* 79:1. Copyright 1987.)

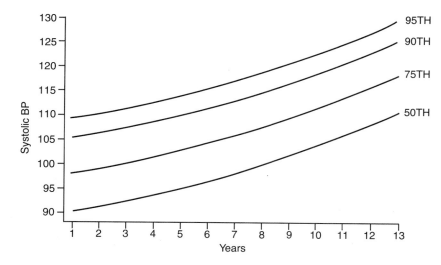

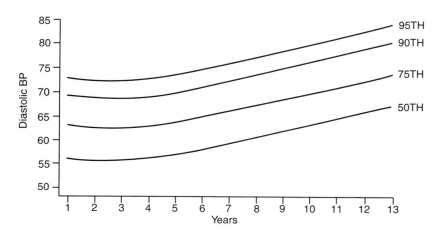

Figure 2-3   Age-specific percentiles for blood pressure measurements in boys, from 1 to 13 years of age. Values for girls are slightly lower. (From National Heart, Lung, and Blood Institute, Bethesda, MD: Report of the Second Task Force on Blood Pressure Control in Children, 1987. Reproduced with permission from *Pediatrics* 79:1. Copyright 1987.)

childhood as the left ventricle hypertrophies to its normal size and the electrocardiograph becomes more like that of an adult.

The newborn cardiac output (about 350 mL/kg/min) falls over the first 2 months of life to about 150 mL/kg/min and then more gradually to the normal adult cardiac output of about 75 mL/kg/min.

RENAL PHYSIOLOGY

By the 36th week of gestation, the formation of nephrons in the kidney is complete. However, the nephrons are small, and the glomerular filtration rate (GFR) is only 25% of adult values at birth. GFR reaches adult levels over the first several weeks of life. Tubular function is also immature – the ability to concentrate and dilute the urine is impaired in the immediate newborn period. The maximal concentrating ability of the full-term newborn is 700 mOsm/L; the adult value of

Table 2-2   Blood Pressure Ranges in Healthy Premature Infants (birthweight 501–2000 g)[a]

Age (days)	Systolic (mmHg)		Diastolic (mmHg)	
	Minimum	Maximum	Minimum	Maximum
1	48±9	63±12	25±7	35±10
2	54±10	63±	30±0	39±8
3	53±9	67±10	31±8	43±8
4	57±10	71±11	32±8	45±10
5	56±9	72±14	33±9	47±12
6	57±9	71±11	32±7	47±10

[a] Values are mean ± standard deviation.
Reproduced with permission from Hegyi T, Anwar M, Carbone MT et al: Blood pressure ranges in premature infants: II. The first week of life, *Pediatrics* 97:336–342, 1996.

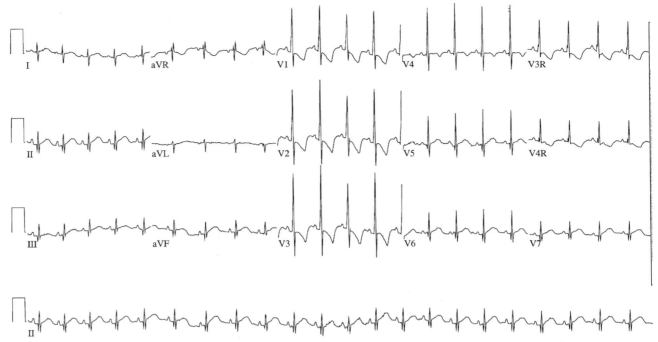

Figure 2-4   The normal newborn electrocardiograph demonstrates a preponderance of right-sided forces as evidenced by a QRS axis greater than 90 degrees, and decreasing R wave size from right to left in the precordial leads. T waves are normally inverted in lead AVR and the right-sided precordial leads.

1200 mOsm/L is attained within the first several months of life. Therefore, intraoperative evaporative fluid losses may result in development of hypernatremia in the neonate.

In newborn infants, daily fluid intake is gradually increased from 80 mL/kg on the first day of life to 150 mL/kg by the third or fourth day of life, and is adjusted based on additional factors, such as extreme prematurity or use of a radiant warmer, in which evaporative losses from the skin are increased. Neonates who are unable to ingest enteral feeds will receive supplementation of electrolytes (sodium, potassium, and calcium) on the second day of life (Table 2-3). Normal daily sodium requirement is 2-3 mEq/kg.

Table 2-3	Normal Newborn Daily Electrolyte Requirements
Electrolyte	**Average Daily Requirement**[a]
Sodium	2-3 mEq/kg
Potassium	1-2 mEq/kg
Calcium[b]	150-200 mg/kg

[a]Adjusted to normal values on a daily basis.
[b]In premature infants under 2000 g.

CENTRAL NERVOUS SYSTEM (CNS) PHYSIOLOGY

The skull and central nervous system undergo a substantial amount of postnatal maturation. At birth, the brain is encased within several pieces of the skull that are separated by strong, fibrous, elastic tissues called "cranial sutures" (Fig. 2-5). The anterior fontanel, located at the junction of the frontal and parietal bones, is formed by the intersection of the metopic, coronal, and sagittal sutures; it normally closes by 20 months of age. The posterior fontanel, located at the junction of the parietal and occipital bones, is formed by the intersection of the lambdoid and sagittal sutures; it usually closes by 3 months of age.

The metabolic demand of the brain increases throughout the first year of life and then decreases gradually throughout childhood. The average cerebral metabolic rate of oxygen consumption ($CMRO_2$) of the child's brain (5.2 mL/min of oxygen per 100 g of brain tissue) is greater than in the adult's brain (3.5 mL/min/100 g) and greater than that of anesthetized newborns and infants (2.3 mL/min/100 g).

Cerebral blood flow (CBF) is closely coupled to the $CMRO_2$. Whereas in adults the CBF is 50–60 mL/min per 100 g of brain tissue, the CBF of premature and term

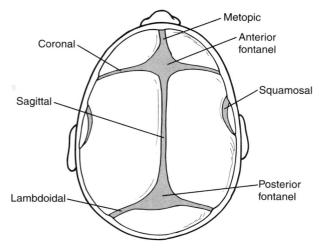

Figure 2-5 Open sutures of the newborn cranium. (Reproduced with permission from Greeley WJ: *Pediatric Anesthesia. Vol VII: Atlas of Anesthesia*, Churchill-Livingstone, Edinburgh, 1999.)

newborns is approximately 40 mL/min/100 g; in older children the CBF may reach 100 mL/min/100 g.

Autoregulation of CBF is based on systemic blood pressure and is thought to occur in newborns, but the limits are unknown. Extrapolation from animal studies indicates an approximate range of 20–80 mmHg, in contrast to the adult whose autoregulatory limits lie between 60 and 150 mmHg.

DEVELOPMENTAL PHARMACOLOGY

The broad subject of pharmacology encompasses the study of *pharmacokinetics*, the body's influence on the drug, and *pharmacodynamics*, the drug's influence on the body. Each of these two components is influenced by age, especially during the first few weeks of life. Thus the major differences in pharmacology between adults and children occur in early life, when the factors of body composition that influence pharmacokinetics and pharmacodynamics are decidedly different. This section will review the ways in which these factors influence the pharmacology of intravenous and inhalational anesthetics in children.

Pharmacokinetics of Intravenous Drugs

The term "pharmacokinetics" describes the physiological processes that alter a drug's disposition after entering the body. Pharmacokinetic processes determine the amount of drug that arrives at the effect site (usually the central nervous system for general anesthetic agents) at a given point in time (i.e. the "effect site" concentration), and the speed at which it arrives. The two general

pharmacokinetic processes of interest are those that determine the rate and amount of drug that initially reaches the effect site, and those that determine the rate and amount of drug that leaves the effect site. These two processes, which are of prime importance to anesthesiologists, are determined by a drug's unique combination of pharmacokinetic parameters: volume of distribution, distribution clearance, protein binding, and elimination clearance (metabolism and excretion). Each of these parameters will be discussed, with an emphasis on the changes that occur during development.

Volume of Distribution

The total (or steady-state) volume of distribution is the *calculated* amount of plasma into which the drug appears to have distributed at some specified interval after intravenous administration. The volume of distribution is not a discrete body compartment, but rather is calculated by dividing the dose administered by the plasma concentration. Put another way, the dose of an intravenously administered drug is determined by multiplying the volume of distribution and the desired effect site concentration:

Dose (mg/kg) = volume of distribution (L/kg)
× desired effect site concentration (mg/L)

The relative percentage of extracellular and total body water is greatest at birth and declines with advancing age during childhood (Fig. 2-6). Since younger children have a relatively greater amount of extracellular body water, and possess adipose stores with a relatively higher ratio

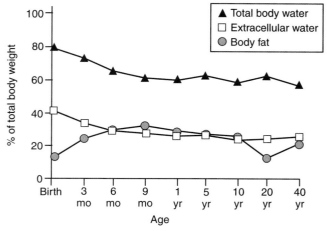

Figure 2-6 Developmental changes in body composition, which influence the apparent volume of distribution for drugs. Infants in the first 6 months of life have markedly expanded total-body water and extracellular water, expressed as a percentage of total bodyweight, compared with older infants and adults. (Reproduced with permission from Kearns GL, Abdel-Rahman SM, Alander SW et al: Developmental pharmacology: drug disposition, action, and therapy in infants and children, *N Engl J Med* 349:1157–1167, 2003.)

of water to lipid than adults, the volume of distribution for water-soluble drugs, such as neuromuscular blockers, will be greater. *A larger volume of distribution will be reflected as a larger loading (bolus) dose to achieve the desired plasma concentration and, if clearance is unchanged, a longer half-life.*

Protein Binding

Parenterally administered medications are bound primarily to two proteins that are manufactured in the liver: albumin and α_1-acid-glycoprotein. Albumin binds weak acids (e.g., aspirin), while α_1-acid-glycoprotein binds weak bases (e.g., local anesthetics). Albumin levels are only slightly reduced in the newborn period but may have some qualitative immaturity. Alpha$_1$-acid-glycoprotein is not fully produced until some time in the first year of life. Therefore, drugs such as local anesthetics that are normally bound to α_1-acid-glycoprotein may have a larger free fraction in the blood of young infants, which predisposes to systemic toxicity.

Metabolism

Most intravenously administered anesthetic-related drugs are lipid soluble and, therefore, are metabolized in the liver or in the bloodstream. In general, children have more rapid clearance of drugs because of the relatively high proportion of blood traversing the liver. However, in neonates, the phase I (cytochrome-dependent) reactions – oxidation, reduction, and hydrolysis – are not fully developed. Therefore, some anesthetic-related drugs that rely on hepatic metabolism for termination of their action (e.g., vecuronium) may last longer than anticipated. These processes are usually fully functional within the first week after birth. However, the activity of some cytochromes, such as CYP3A4 and CYP3A5, which metabolize intravenous midazolam, continue to increase during the first 3 months of life. It appears that chronological age, not postconceptional age, is important for development of these metabolic pathways.

The phase II reactions consist primarily of conjugation with sulfate, acetate, glucuronic acids, and amino acids. These reactions convert the parent drug to a more polar metabolite by introducing or unmasking a functional group (-OH, NH$_2$, -SH). These reactions are limited at birth but mature within the first few weeks of age, and may differ between classes of drugs.

Excretion

Excretion of intravenously administered anesthetic-related drugs is primarily via the kidney. In the first several weeks of life, especially in infants born at less than 34 weeks' gestation, GFR is below normal values, so excretion of drugs may be delayed. After the first several weeks of life, GFR and tubular secretion rise steadily until adult values are reached at 8–12 months of age.

Elimination Clearance

Clearance is the volume of drug removed by metabolism or excretion per unit of time. Like the volume of distribution, it is a calculated value that is obtained by dividing the continuous infusion dose of a drug by the resulting plasma concentration:

$$\text{Clearance}\,(\text{L/kg/h}) = \frac{\text{dose}\,(\text{mg/kg/h})}{\text{plasma concentration}\,(\text{mg/L})}$$

Infants and children tend to have a more rapid clearance of drugs than adults, and for drugs metabolized in the liver, there is an age-dependent increase in plasma clearance up to approximately 10 years of age. The mechanism of this is largely unknown, but it may be related to the fact that the liver receives a proportionately higher fraction of cardiac output in children than in adults.

Pharmacodynamics of Intravenous Anesthetic Agents

Pharmacodynamics refers to the processes that affect the drug's action at a given plasma (or effect site) concentration. Developmental pharmacodynamic differences for most intravenously administered anesthetic agents are not well studied. However, it appears that neonates may be more sensitive to drugs that act in the central nervous system. This may be due, in part, to an age-dependency for passive diffusion into the brain (i.e., an immature blood–brain barrier), and relatively greater central nervous system blood flow in neonates and small infants.

Pharmacokinetics of Inhalational Anesthetics

A variety of pharmacokinetic factors can influence the concentration of inhalational anesthetics in the brain and the speed at which this process occurs (i.e., uptake and distribution). The rate of rise of inhalational anesthesia into the lungs is determined by the delivered concentration of the anesthetic and the minute ventilation of the patient, and is quantitatively described as the alveolar to inspired concentration ratio (F_A/F_I). Compared with adults, children demonstrate a higher minute ventilation per bodyweight and a higher tidal volume to FRC ratio, so the F_A/F_I ratio rises faster during an inhalational induction.

Once in the lungs, uptake of the anesthetic into the bloodstream is determined by the cardiac output, the blood-gas coefficient of the anesthetic agent, and the arterial-to-venous (A-V) concentration difference. All of these factors are influenced by the developmental age of the child.

Cardiac output per bodyweight is relatively higher in children than in adults. A higher cardiac output will tend to slow inhalational induction of anesthesia by removing anesthetic from the alveoli at a more rapid rate.

The blood-gas partition coefficient will determine the speed at which the inhalational anesthetic equilibrates between the alveolar gas and the blood. Although blood-gas partition coefficients have been shown to be lower in small children, it is to an insignificant degree and without clinical importance.

Anesthetic breathed into the alveoli moves into the bloodstream based on the concentration gradient difference between the alveolus and the blood in the pulmonary artery. Therefore, the larger the pulmonary A-V concentration difference, the more rapid the anesthetic will leave the alveoli, and thus the speed of induction is slowed. Upon initial uptake of inhalational anesthetic from the alveoli into the bloodstream, the anesthetic will be distributed to the various body tissues. As anesthetic partial pressures in tissues equilibrate with those in the blood, the concentration of the agent that returns to the lungs in the pulmonary artery increases. Consequently, the A-V difference decreases, which reduces the amount of anesthetic agent that is removed from the alveoli. This increases the partial pressure of the anesthetic agent in the alveolus and speeds loss of consciousness. Children demonstrate a faster decrease in the A-V difference because of their proportionately larger vessel-rich group that equilibrates anesthetic relatively faster than in adults (Table 2-4). As children grow, they increase their content of muscle and fat and take longer to equilibrate inhalational anesthetic.

The combination of these differences in factors that affect uptake and distribution of inhalational anesthetics results in children demonstrating a more rapid induction of inhalational anesthesia when compared with adults.

Pharmacodynamics of Inhalational Agents

The relative potency of inhalational anesthetics, which is quantitatively described as the minimum alveolar concentration (MAC), changes with age (Fig. 2-7). MAC is relatively low for premature infants and gradually increases with age until approximately 6 months of age, after which it tends to decrease with advancing age. The reasons for these changes in anesthetic potency with age are unknown.

Table 2-4	Effect of Age on Body Compartments		
Age Group	Vessel-rich Group	Muscle Group	Fat Group
Newborn	22.0%	38.7%	13.2%
1 year	17.3%	38.7%	25.4%
4 years	16.6%	40.7%	23.4%
8 years	13.2%	44.8%	21.4%
Adult	10.2%	50.0%	22.4%

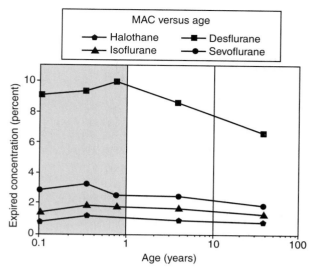

Figure 2-7   Changes in MAC with age. (Reproduced with permission from Miller RD: *Anesthesia*, 5th edn, Churchill-Livingstone, Edinburgh, 2000.)

ARTICLES TO KNOW

Anand KJ, Sippell WG, Aynsley-Green A: Randomised trial of fentanyl anaesthesia in preterm babies undergoing surgery: effects on the stress response. *Lancet* i(8524):62-66, 1987.

Anand KJS, Phil D, Hickey PR: Halothane–morphine compared with high-dose sufentanil for anesthesia and postoperative analgesia in neonatal cardiac surgery. *N Engl J Med* 326:1-9, 1992.

Andrew M, Paes B, Johnston M: Development of the hemostatic system in the neonate and young infant. *Am J Pediatr Hematol Oncol* 12:95, 1990.

Andrew M, Vegh P, Johnston M et al: Maturation of the hemostatic system during childhood. *Blood* 80:1998, 1992.

Baum VC, Palmisano BW: The immature heart and anesthesia. *Anesthesiology* 87:1529-1548, 1997.

de Wildt SN, Kearns GL, Leeder JS, van den Anker JN: Cytochrome P450 3A: ontogeny and drug disposition. *Clin Pharmacokinet* 37:485-505, 1999.

Devlieger H, Daniels H, Marchal G et al: The diaphragm of the newborn infant: anatomical and ultrasonographic studies. *J Dev Physiol* 16:321-329, 1991.

England SJ, Gaultier C, Bryan AC: Chest wall mechanics in the newborn. In Roussos Ch ed: *The Thorax. Pt B: Applied Physiology*, Marcel Dekker, 1541-1556, 1995

Kearns GL, Abdel-Rahman SM, Alander SW et al: Developmental pharmacology: drug disposition, action, and therapy in infants and children. *N Engl J Med* 349:1157-1167, 2003.

Papastamelos C, Panitch HB, England SE, Allen JL: Developmental changes in chest wall compliance in infancy and early childhood. *J Appl Physiol* 78:179-184, 1995.

Rigatto H: Maturation of breathing. *Clin Perinatol* 19:739-755, 1992.

IMPORTANT PEDIATRIC DISEASES

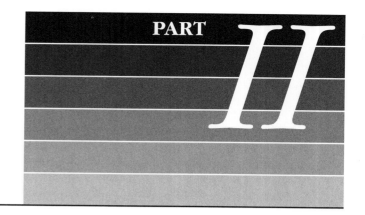

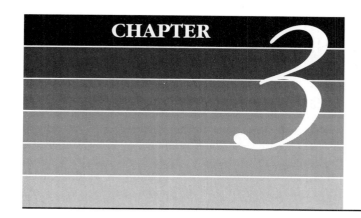

CHAPTER 3

Congenital Heart Disease

AISLING CONRAN
BRADLEY S. MARINO

In the United States each year, 40,000 children are born with congenital heart disease (CHD). Important acyanotic lesions, listed in descending order of frequency, include ventricular septal defect (VSD), atrial septal defect (ASD), persistent ductus arteriosus (PDA), aortic stenosis (AS), coarctation of the aorta (CoA), and complete common atrioventricular canal (CCAVC). Cyanotic defects, in descending order of frequency, include pulmonary stenosis (PS), tetralogy of Fallot (ToF), transposition of the great arteries (TGA), tricuspid atresia (TA), and pulmonary atresia with

intact ventricular septum (PA/IVS). Anesthesiologists should also be familiar with the clinical characteristics of children with hypoplastic left heart syndrome (HLHS) and single-ventricle physiology and palliation. Children with CHD are living longer as a result of earlier palliative or corrective repairs, innovations in interventional catheterization procedures, decreased surgical morbidity, and improvements in anesthetic technique and postoperative intensive care. Many with previously fatal defects are now living well into adulthood.

This chapter offers general information about specific lesions and medical management of children with common forms of CHD. It includes a discussion of the perioperative management of children with CHD for noncardiac procedures.

PATHOPHYSIOLOGY OF CONGENITAL HEART DISEASE

When formulating an anesthetic plan for a child with congenital heart disease, the anesthesiologist should attempt to understand the anatomical defects and how the blood flows through the heart and lungs in each patient. This can often be quite confusing because of the complexity of the lesions and the subsequent repairs. A structured approach that stresses the relative ratios of pulmonary and systemic blood flow, based on the resistance of these vascular beds, is often helpful. An understanding of normal fetal circulation and the transitional circulation (see Chapter 1) is also helpful when considering neonatal heart defects.

Consideration of the following questions may help the anesthesiologist understand the pathophysiology of the child's heart defect.

Is there an obstruction?

Obstructions on the right side of the heart will decrease pulmonary blood flow and cause hypoxemia and cyanosis. Obstructions on the left side of the heart will decrease systemic blood flow and cause tissue hypoperfusion, metabolic acidosis, and shock.

Is there a shunt?

Mixing of the pulmonary and systemic circulations may occur at the level of the atrium or ventricle, or through a patent ductus arteriosus. When blood is primarily shunted from the right to the left side of the heart, effective pulmonary blood flow (deoxygenated blood circulating through the lungs) will be decreased, and significant pulmonary and systemic blood flow mixing will occur, resulting in hypoxemia and cyanosis. When blood is primarily shunted from the left to the right side of the heart, congestive heart failure (CHF) results from volume and pressure overload on either or both ventricles. Pulmonary overcirculation may lead to pulmonary hypertension, which, if left untreated, results in irreversible pulmonary vascular obstructive disease.

When considering shunting, it should be clear whether there is too much or too little pulmonary blood flow. In some cardiac lesions, the answer to this question will be determined not by a shunt or an obstruction, but by the resistance in the pulmonary and systemic circuits. The ratio of pulmonary vascular resistance (PVR) to systemic vascular resistance (SVR) can be affected by a number of processes (see below) and will determine whether the patient has a right-to-left shunt, a left-to-right shunt, or both at different times during the cardiac cycle.

Is there a volume load or pressure load on the heart?

CHF results when a ventricle is overburdened by volume overload or obstruction to forward flow. Volume overload occurs in lesions that produce left-to-right shunts or valve insufficiency. Obstruction occurs in lesions that produce valve or outflow tract stenosis, or abnormal increases in PVR or SVR.

ACYANOTIC CONGENITAL HEART DISEASE

Ventricular Septal Defect

Ventricular septal defect (VSD) is the most common congenital heart defect, accounting for 25% of all congenital cardiac lesions. The five types of ventricular septal defects are:
- Muscular
- Inlet
- Conoseptal hypoplasia
- Conoventricular
- Malalignment.

Muscular VSDs occur in the posterior, apical, or anterior portion of the muscular septum and may be single or multiple. The inlet VSD occurs in the inlet portion of the septum beneath the septal leaflet of the tricuspid valve. The conoseptal hypoplasia VSD is positioned in the outflow tract of the right ventricle beneath the pulmonary valve, and the conoventricular VSD occurs in the membranous portion of the ventricular septum. Malalignment VSDs result from malalignment of the infundibular septum.

When the VSD is large (i.e., nonrestrictive), PVR and SVR determine shunt flow. When the PVR is less than the SVR, the shunt flow is left-to-right. Large defects result in pulmonary hypertension, and over time will increase PVR, whereas small defects do not change PVR. If left untreated, the large VSD may result in pulmonary vascular obstructive disease, and Eisenmenger's syndrome. In some cases of Eisenmenger's syndrome, the VSD shunt may reverse and flow right-to-left.

Clinical symptoms are related to the size of the shunt. A small shunt produces no symptoms, whereas a large shunt without elevated pulmonary vascular resistance results in growth failure, CHF, and increased susceptibility to lower respiratory tract infections. CHF is treated with digoxin, diuretics, and an angiotensin-converting enzyme (ACE) inhibitor. Most small muscular and conoventricular VSDs close without intervention (40% by 3 years, 75% by 10 years), whereas the treatment for large VSDs is surgical closure before pulmonary vascular changes become irreversible. The incidence of postoperative myocardial dysfunction or arrhythmias is greatly increased if the VSD repair is accomplished through a ventriculotomy. Permanent right bundle branch block is common.

Atrial Septal Defect

Atrial septal defects (ASD) account for 7.5% of congenital heart disease. There are three types of ASDs:
- Ostium secundum defect, located in the mid-portion of the atrial septum
- Ostium primum defect, located in the low atrial septum
- Sinus venosus defect, located at the junction of the right atrium and the superior or inferior vena cava.

Most children with an ASD are asymptomatic. Spontaneous closure of small secundum ASDs occurs in the majority of cases in the first year of life. If the atrial defect is large enough, significant left-to-right shunting can occur and will require surgical repair or placement of a device via cardiac catheterization. Ostium primum and sinus venosus ASDs do not close spontaneously and must be addressed surgically. Children are generally asymptomatic after successful ASD repair, and there are no unique anesthetic considerations for noncardiac surgery. Subacute bacterial endocarditis prophylaxis is not recommended for secundum atrial septal defects but is indicated in primum and sinus venosus atrial septal defects.

Common Complete Atrioventricular Canal

Common complete atrioventricular canal consists of an ostium primum ASD and an inlet VSD with lack of septation of the mitral and tricuspid valves (common atrioventricular valve) (Fig. 3-1). It is often seen in children with trisomy 21. In this defect, there is a left-to-right shunt at the atrial and ventricular levels. CHF is seen early in infancy, with tachypnea, dyspnea, and poor feeding. Because of the increase in pulmonary blood flow, pulmonary hypertension and pulmonary vascular disease may develop over time.

Surgical repair for complete common atrioventricular canal is usually performed within the first year of life. Prior to surgical repair, CHF is treated with digoxin, diuretics, and an ACE inhibitor. Complete heart block occurs in 5% of patients undergoing repair, and residual mitral insufficiency is often seen.

Persistent Ductus Arteriosus

In fetal life, the ductus arteriosus is the conduit through which blood bypasses the lungs and travels

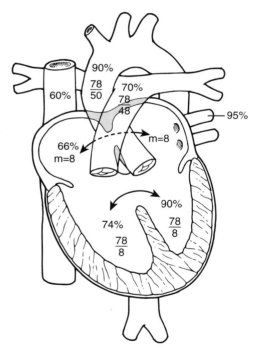

Figure 3-1   Complete common atrioventricular canal. Anatomic and hemodynamic findings include: (a) large atrial and ventricular septal defects; (b) single, atrioventricular valve; (c) pulmonary artery hypertension (due to the large VSD); (d) bidirectional shunting (with mild hypoxemia) at the atrial and ventricular levels when PVR is elevated in the initial neonatal period. With the subsequent fall in PVR, the shunt becomes predominantly left-to-right with symptoms of CHF. The percentages represent the oxygen saturation; blood pressure is represented by mean (*m*) or systolic/diastolic. (Reproduced with permission from Cloherty JP, Stark AR: *Manual of Neonatal Care*, 4th edn, Lippincott-Raven, Philadelphia, 1998.)

from the main pulmonary artery to the descending aorta (see Chapter 1). In the normal newborn, the ductus functionally closes within the first several days of life. Patency of the ductus arteriosus (PDA) is seen most often in prematurely born infants, and represents 7.5% of congenital heart disease.

There are a number of factors that may contribute to a persistent PDA. These include a low oxygen level, high blood P_{CO_2}, acidosis, and persistent pulmonary hypertension of the newborn. These can all occur in conditions of the newborn that cause cardiorespiratory dysfunction, such as respiratory distress syndrome of the premature infant (see Chapter 10). The direction of flow through a large PDA depends on the relative resistances in the pulmonary and systemic circuits. In the nonrestrictive PDA, a left-to-right shunt is present as long as SVR is greater than PVR. Infants with a large PDA and a left-to-right shunt may exhibit signs of pulmonary overcirculation and CHF, which include a widened pulse pressure, a continuous murmur, and an inability to wean ventilatory parameters.

When a PDA is thought to significantly interfere with normal cardiorespiratory function, it requires closure. In the premature neonate, indomethacin is often effective in closing the PDA by decreasing PGE_1 levels. If this is unsuccessful, surgical ligation is performed by thoracotomy or video-assisted thoracoscopic surgery, or coil embolization in the cardiac catheterization laboratory. Infants with a PDA require SBE prophylaxis when undergoing surgical procedures. This risk decreases by 6 months after closure as long as residual flow is absent. There are no additional anesthetic considerations in children with a history of a PDA who are otherwise doing well.

Aortic Stenosis

Congenital aortic stenosis (AS) represents up to 5% of all congenital heart defects (Fig. 3-2). It most commonly occurs at the level of the valve and ranges from very mild to complete atresia as a component of hypoplastic left heart syndrome. The neonate with critical aortic stenosis has ductal-dependent systemic blood flow and may present with circulatory collapse after the ductus closes. Most cases, however, are detected later in childhood by the presence of a murmur.

The level of symptomatology is related to the severity of the stenosis and the ventricular function. The stenotic valve produces a pressure gradient between the left ventricle and the aorta that results in left ventricular hypertrophy and, over time, decreased compliance and ventricular performance.

If intervention is required, relief of the aortic valve gradient may be accomplished by open surgical valvotomy or by balloon valvuloplasty. These treatment modalities may cause progressive aortic regurgitation, which

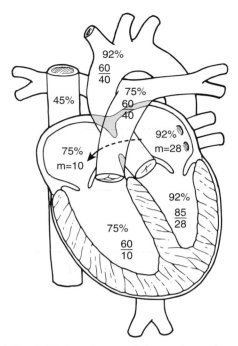

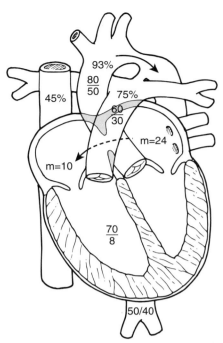

Figure 3-2   Critical aortic stenosis. Anatomic and hemodynamic findings include: (a) morphologically abnormal, stenotic valve; (b) poststenotic dilatation of the ascending aorta; (c) elevated left ventricular end-diastolic pressure and left atrial pressures contributing to pulmonary edema (mild pulmonary venous and arterial desaturation); (d) a left-to-right shunt at the atrial level (note increase in oxygen saturation from the SVC to the right atrium); (e) pulmonary artery hypertension (also secondary to the elevated left atrial pressure); (f) only a modest (25-mmHg) gradient across the valve. The low measured gradient across the aortic valve, despite severe anatomic obstruction, is due to a severely limited cardiac output, as evidenced by the low mixed venous oxygen saturation (45%) in the SVC. The percentages represent the oxygen saturation; blood pressure is represented by mean (*m*) or systolic/diastolic. (Reproduced with permission from Cloherty JP, Stark AR: *Manual of Neonatal Care*, 4th edn, Lippincott-Raven, Philadelphia, 1998.)

Figure 3-3   Coarctation of the aorta in a critically ill neonate with a nearly closed ductus arteriosus. Anatomic and hemodynamic findings include: (a) "juxtaductal" site of the coarctation; (b) bicuspid aortic valve (seen in 80% of patients with coarctation); (c) narrow pulse pressure in the descending aorta and lower body; (d) bidirectional shunt at the ductus arteriosus. As in critical aortic stenosis (see Fig. 3-2), there is an elevated left atrial pressure, pulmonary edema, a left-to-right shunt at the atrial level, pulmonary hypertension, and only a moderate (30-mmHg) gradient across the arch obstruction because of a low cardiac output. The percentages represent the oxygen saturation; blood pressure is represented by mean (*m*) or systolic/diastolic. (Reproduced with permission from Cloherty JP, Stark AR: *Manual of Neonatal Care*, 4th edn, Lippincott-Raven, Philadelphia, 1998.)

may eventually require aortic valve replacement with a mechanical, homograft, or autograft valve. In selected children, a Ross procedure (pulmonary autograft) is performed, in which the child's own pulmonary valve is moved into the aortic position, a right ventricle to pulmonary artery homograft conduit is placed, and the coronary arteries are reimplanted. Residual left ventricular dysfunction may cause CHF and dysrhythmias. AS represents the lesion that is most associated with SBE, so prophylaxis is indicated prior to surgical procedures.

Coarctation of the Aorta

Coarctation of the aorta (CoA) represents approximately 8% of all congenital heart defects. The aortic constriction most often occurs just distal to the take off of the left subclavian artery at the insertion site of the ductus arteriosus (Fig. 3-3). The coarctation results in

mechanical obstruction between the proximal and distal aorta, and increases left ventricular afterload. CHF develops in 10% of cases in infancy. Girls with Turner syndrome (45, XO) have a 15–20% risk of having CoA.

Neonates with critical coarctation have ductal-dependent systemic blood flow and may present with circulatory collapse. PGE₁ is administered to keep the ductus open until definitive therapy is complete. These infants may require inotropic support. More commonly, CoA presents during childhood as a murmur, or hypertension of the upper extremities and decreased lower-extremity pulses. Chronic pressure overload can lead to left ventricular hypertrophy and CHF.

Palliation may be accomplished via balloon dilation angioplasty, stent placement, surgical end-to-end anastomosis, subclavian flap repair, patch repair, or graft placement. Postoperative hypertension is common and may persist throughout childhood. The major risk factor for long-term postoperative hypertension is the duration of preoperative hypertension. Since a bicuspid aortic valve is a common accompanying lesion in patients with CoA (80%), SBE prophylaxis should be given if a murmur is heard on physical exam prior to elective surgery.

CYANOTIC DEFECTS

Hypoplastic Left Heart Syndrome

Hypoplastic left heart syndrome (HLHS) is the second most common congenital cardiac lesion presenting in the first week of life and the most common cause of death from congenital heart disease in the first month of life. In this syndrome, there is hypoplasia of the left ventricle, aortic valve stenosis or atresia, mitral valve stenosis or atresia, and hypoplasia of the ascending aorta with discrete coarctation of the aorta (Fig. 3-4). These lesions reduce or eliminate blood flow through the left side of

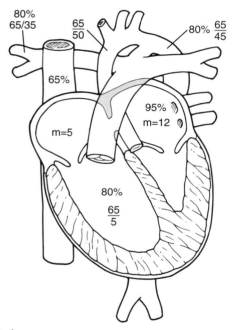

Figure 3-4   Hypoplastic left heart syndrome in a 24-hour-old patient with falling PVR and a nonrestrictive PDA. Anatomic and hemodynamic findings include: (a) atresia or hypoplasia of the left ventricle, mitral, and aortic valves; (b) a diminutive ascending aorta and transverse aortic arch, usually with an associated coarctation; (c) coronary blood flow usually retrograde from the ductus arteriosus through the tiny ascending aorta; (d) systemic arterial oxygen saturation (in room air) of 80%, reflecting relatively balanced systemic and pulmonary blood flows – the pulmonary artery and aortic saturations are equal; (e) pulmonary hypertension secondary to the nonrestrictive ductus arteriosus; (f) minimal left atrial hypertension; (g) normal systemic cardiac output (note SVC oxygen saturation of 65%) and blood pressure (65/45). The percentages represent the oxygen saturation; blood pressure is represented by mean (*m*) or systolic/diastolic. (Reproduced with permission from Cloherty JP, Stark AR: *Manual of Neonatal Care*, 4th edn, Lippincott-Raven, Philadelphia, 1998.)

the heart, causing an obligatory left-to-right shunt at the atrial level and a right-to-left shunt at the ductus arteriosus. Systemic flow is completely ductal dependent, and coronary perfusion is retrograde when aortic atresia or critical aortic stenosis is present. As the ductus closes, neonates with HLHS have severely diminished systemic blood flow and present in shock. They manifest signs of CHF with moderate cyanosis, tachycardia, tachypnea, pulmonary rales (from pulmonary edema), and hepatomegaly. Poor or absent peripheral pulses with poor distal capillary refill are characteristic. PGE_1 should be immediately started and the infant should be prepared for urgent palliative surgery.

Although some institutions proceed directly to heart transplantation, in most centers the palliative treatment approach consists of three separate surgical procedures:

1. Norwood palliation, which is performed in the first week of life, establishes unobstructed systemic blood flow and allows the majority of neonates to survive infancy. The procedure consists of an amalgamation of the pulmonary artery and aorta (*neoaorta*) to provide unobstructed systemic blood flow, an atrial septectomy to create an unobstructed atrial communication, and a modified Blalock–Taussig (BT) shunt (see below) or right ventricle to PA conduit to provide restrictive pulmonary blood flow. This prevents pulmonary vasculature obstructive disease that may result from too much pulmonary blood flow.

2. The second stage is performed at 4–6 months of age and is called a hemi-Fontan or bidirectional Glenn procedure (see below). A superior cavopulmonary connection is created between the superior vena cava (SVC) and the right pulmonary artery, so that blood returning from the head bypasses the right ventricle and flows passively into the pulmonary circulation.

3. The third stage, which is performed at approx 2 yrs of age, is the completion Fontan procedure, in which the inferior vena cava is joined into the superior cavopulmonary circulation. At the completion of this procedure, all venous blood returning to the heart bypasses the right heart and flows passively into the lungs, while the right ventricle now has the responsibility for pumping oxygenated blood returning from the lungs to the body.

The circulatory anatomy that remains in these children is commonly referred to as "Fontan physiology." Blood flow to the lungs becomes completely dependent on the transpulmonary gradient, which is the pressure difference between the Fontan circuit (systemic veins and pulmonary arteries) and the pulmonary venous atrium. Thus, any condition that increases PVR will decrease blood flow through the lungs, and cause hypoxemia if a fenestration is present, and thereby reduce preload to the single ventricle. A number of perioperative factors can decrease pulmonary blood flow (Box 3-1). After a Fontan procedure, patients may develop atrial arrhythmias or complete heart block. As patients with Fontan physiology reach adulthood, the incidence of myocardial failure increases.

Inhalational anesthetics, particularly sevoflurane and isoflurane, decrease SVR by arteriolar and venous dilatation. This decrease in venous return may critically limit pulmonary blood flow by decreasing the transpulmonary gradient (see Box 3-1). In a patient with Fontan physiology, positive-pressure ventilation should be instituted only when necessary as this can also decrease pulmonary blood flow. Positive end-expiratory pressure (PEEP) and elevated mean airway pressures can impede venous return and further decrease pulmonary blood flow. Spontaneous ventilation is preferred in these patients because negative intrathoracic pressure increases the gradient between extrathoracic and intrathoracic pressures and results in increased flow through the pulmonary circulation. Preferred anesthetic techniques in the Fontan patient include use of a facemask or laryngeal mask airway (LMA) with spontaneous ventilation, or a regional technique with IV sedation. However, atelectasis is likely in longer cases, in which controlled ventilation may be the most prudent option, with the goal of immediate tracheal extubation at the completion of the procedure when possible.

Pulmonary Stenosis (PS)

Pulmonary stenosis (PS) represents approximately 8% of all congenital heart defects and occurs primarily at the level of the valve itself, although subvalvular and supravalvular stenosis can occur. It also commonly

---

Box 3-1 Determinants of Pulmonary Blood Flow

Increase Pulmonary Blood Flow

Decreased PVR

Hyperoxia

Alkalosis

Hypertension or increased SVR (e.g., inotropic therapy) in patients with single-ventricle physiology

Low mean airway pressure

Decrease Pulmonary Blood Flow

Increased PVR

Hypoxemia

Acidosis

Hypotension or lowering of SVR (e.g., inhalational anesthetics) in patients with single-ventricle physiology

Positive end-expiratory pressure (PEEP)

---

occurs as a component of other complex congenital heart defects. PS should not be confused with peripheral pulmonic stenosis, which represents a benign condition of the newborn that produces a murmur as a result of the acute angle of bifurcation of the main pulmonary artery. The clinical manifestations of PS will depend on the degree of narrowing. Right ventricular hypertrophy occurs over time as the ventricle attempts to maintain cardiac output. Symptoms of severe PS include CHF and cyanosis if there is a patent foramen ovale or ASD.

Moderate or severe PS (gradient ≥50 mmHg) is treated with balloon valvuloplasty in the cardiac catheterization laboratory. An open surgical repair may be necessary in certain cases. Once dilated or repaired, children with isolated PS are relatively healthy and present no further anesthetic considerations. SBE prophylaxis should be administered for all future surgical procedures.

Tetralogy of Fallot

Tetralogy of Fallot (ToF; Fig. 3-5) is the third most prevalent cyanotic congenital heart lesion during the

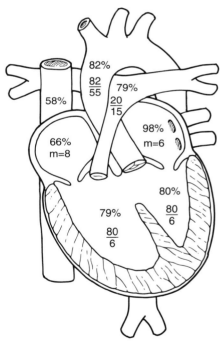

Figure 3-5 Tetralogy of Fallot. Anatomic and hemodynamic findings include: (a) anteriorly displaced infundibular septum, resulting in subpulmonary stenosis, a large VSD and overriding aorta over the muscular septum; (b) hypoplasia of the pulmonary valve, main and branch pulmonary arteries; (c) equal right and left ventricular pressures; (d) a right-to-left shunt at the ventricular level, with a systemic oxygen saturation of 82%. The percentages represent the oxygen saturation; blood pressure is represented by mean (*m*) or systolic/diastolic. (Reproduced with permission from Cloherty JP, Stark AR: *Manual of Neonatal Care*, 4th edn, Lippincott-Raven, Philadelphia, 1998.)

neonatal period, and after the third week of life it becomes the leading cause of cyanosis due to congenital heart disease in childhood. The four defects noted by Fallot include an anterior malalignment VSD, right ventricular outflow tract obstruction, right ventricular hypertrophy, and an "overriding" large ascending aorta.

Children with ToF exhibit a wide variety of lesion severity, depending mainly on the degree of right ventricular outflow tract obstruction. Neonates with ToF become cyanotic from right-to-left shunting across the VSD and decreased pulmonary blood flow. Shunting occurs when the combination of PVR and the resistance created by the right ventricular outflow tract obstruction exceed SVR.

Children with uncorrected ToF may exhibit sudden episodes of intense cyanosis secondary to infundibular "spasm," which worsens right ventricular outflow tract obstruction. Such spells may last minutes to hours, may resolve spontaneously, and may lead to syncope, seizures, progressive hypoxia, acidosis, and death. These spontaneous episodes are commonly called "Tet spells" and can occur at any time in the perioperative setting. The treatment of Tet spells is aimed at diminishing right-to-left shunting by increasing SVR and decreasing PVR (Box 3-2).

Therapy for ToF consists of patch closure of the VSD and relief of the right ventricular outflow tract obstruction, usually within the first 6 months of life. Postoperatively, these infants commonly exhibit some degree of residual pulmonary insufficiency and right bundle-branch block. Ventricular arrhythmias may occur in adolescence when there is severe pulmonary insufficiency and right ventricular dilatation or dysfunction.

D-Transposition of the Great Arteries

D-transposition of the great arteries (TGA) accounts for 5% of congenital heart defects and is the most common form of cyanotic congenital heart disease presenting in the neonatal period. In this defect, the aorta arises anteriorly from the right ventricle, and the pulmonary artery rises posteriorly from the left ventricle (Fig. 3-6). Thus, circulation exists as two separate parallel circuits

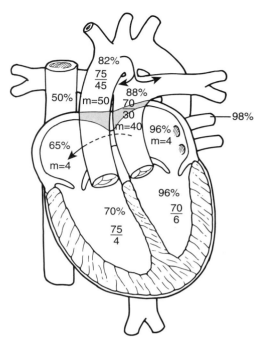

Figure 3-6   D-transposition of the great arteries with an intact ventricular septum, a large PDA (on PGE_1), and an ASD (status after balloon atrial septostomy). Anatomic and hemodynamic findings include: (a) aorta arising from the anatomic right ventricle, and the pulmonary artery from the anatomic left ventricle; (b) "transposition physiology," with a higher oxygen saturation in the pulmonary artery than in the aorta; (c) mixing between the parallel circulations at the atrial (after balloon septostomy) and ductal levels; (d) shunting from the left atrium to the right atrium through the ASD with equalization of atrial pressures; (e) shunting from the aorta to the pulmonary artery through the PDA; (f) pulmonary hypertension due to a large PDA. The percentages represent the oxygen saturation; blood pressure is represented by mean (*m*) or systolic/diastolic. (Reproduced with permission from Cloherty JP, Stark AR: *Manual of Neonatal Care*, 4th edn, Lippincott-Raven, Philadelphia, 1998.)

unless a communication (e.g., PDA, VSD, or patent foramen ovale) exists. Infants with TGA are cyanotic shortly after birth.

Therapy for TGA consists of an arterial switch procedure in the early newborn period, for which survival exceeds 95%. Left ventricular function remains good throughout childhood. Supravalvular pulmonary stenosis is a recognized sequela that may require repeat intervention. Occasionally, children will demonstrate atrial and ventricular tachyarrhythmias. Additional postoperative sequelae are uncommon, but include supravalvular aortic and pulmonary stenosis, and branch pulmonary stenosis.

Tricuspid Atresia (TA)

Tricuspid atresia with normally related great arteries (Fig. 3-7) is a rare defect that consists of complete

---

Box 3-2	Treatment Strategies for "Tet Spells"

IV volume administration
Knee-to-chest position
Liver compression
Phenylephrine 1 µg/kg/dose
Esmolol 100–200 µg/kg/min
Morphine 0.1 mg/kg/dose
Induction of general anesthesia

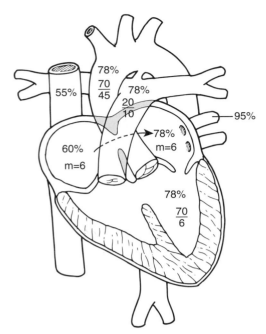

Figure 3-7 Tricuspid atresia with normally related arteries and a small PDA. Anatomic and hemodynamic findings include: (a) atresia of the tricuspid valve; (b) hypoplasia of the right ventricle; (c) restriction to pulmonary blood flow at two levels: a (usually) small VSD and a stenotic pulmonary valve; (d) all systemic venous return must pass through the PFO to reach the left ventricle; (e) complete mixing at the left atrial level, with systemic oxygen saturation of 78% (in room air), suggesting balanced systemic and pulmonary blood flow. The percentages represent the oxygen saturation; blood pressure is represented by mean (*m*) or systolic/diastolic. (Reproduced with permission from Cloherty JP, Stark AR: *Manual of Neonatal Care*, 4th edn, Lippincott-Raven, Philadelphia, 1998.)

absence of the right atrioventricular connection, which leads to severe hypoplasia or absence of the right ventricle. Ninety percent of cases of tricuspid atresia have an associated VSD. In children with TA with normally related great arteries, the VSD allows blood to pass from the left ventricle to the right ventricle and pulmonary arteries. The majority of patients with TA and normally related great arteries also have pulmonary stenosis. In TA, the systemic venous return is shunted from the right atrium to the left atrium through the patent foramen ovale or an ASD; the left atrium and left ventricle handle both systemic and pulmonary venous return. Oxygenated and deoxygenated blood is mixed in the left atrium. Cyanosis is severe in the neonatal period and is proportionally related to the amount of pulmonary blood flow. In 30% of cases, there is transposition of the great arteries, which results in blood passing from the left ventricle through the ventricular septal defect to the right ventricle and the ascending aorta. TA with transposition of the great arteries is often associated with coarctation of the aorta or aortic arch hypoplasia. Unlike tricuspid

atresia with normally related great arteries, it is a cyanotic lesion with ductal-dependent systemic blood flow.

Clinical manifestations of TA and normally related great arteries include progressive cyanosis, poor feeding, and tachypnea that develop in the first 2 weeks of life. PGE_1 should be started to maintain pulmonary flow, and a balloon atrial septostomy is performed if the atrial defect is not adequate. Surgical management for tricuspid atresia involves placing a modified Blalock–Taussig shunt (see below) to maintain pulmonary blood flow. Ultimately, a cavopulmonary anastomosis (hemi-Fontan or bidirectional Glenn; see below) is performed to provide stable pulmonary blood flow. In most centers, a modified Fontan procedure is performed to redirect the inferior vena cava and hepatic vein flow into the pulmonary circulation.

Pulmonic Atresia with Intact Ventricular Septum (PA/IVS)

PA/IVS (Fig. 3-8) is a rare defect consisting of pulmonary valvular and infundibular atresia and varying degrees of right ventricular and tricuspid valve hypoplasia.

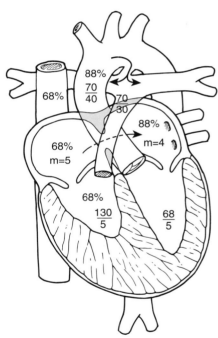

Figure 3-8 Pulmonary atresia with intact ventricular septum in a neonate with a nonrestrictive PDA while receiving PGE_1. Anatomic and hemodynamic findings include: (a) hypertrophied, hypoplastic right ventricle; (b) hypoplastic tricuspid valve and pulmonary annulus; (c) atresia of the pulmonary valve with no antegrade flow; (d) suprasystemic right ventricular pressure; (e) pulmonary blood flow through the PDA; (f) right-to-left shunt at the atrial level with systemic desaturation. The percentages represent the oxygen saturation; blood pressure is represented by mean (*m*) or systolic/diastolic. (Reproduced with permission from Cloherty JP, Stark AR: *Manual of Neonatal Care*, 4th edn, Lippincott-Raven, Philadelphia, 1998.)

There is an obligate atrial shunt from right to left, and pulmonary blood flow is dependent on a patent ductus arteriosus. PA/IVS may also be associated with coronary artery–myocardial sinusoid communications. If the coronaries are right-ventricle dependent, any palliative procedure that decompresses the right ventricle may lead to myocardial infarction and death.

Neonates with PA/IVS are extremely cyanotic and tachypneic shortly after birth. PGE_1 should be started to ensure pulmonary blood flow initially. If the coronary circulation is not right-ventricle dependent (based on a cardiac catheterization procedure), a right ventricle to pulmonary artery conduit or pulmonary valvotomy is performed to provide pulmonary blood flow. A modified Blalock–Taussig shunt is also performed to augment pulmonary blood flow further. If the coronary circulation is RV-dependent, the right ventricle is not decompressed and a modified BT shunt is performed. After modified BT shunt placement, patients with RV-dependent coronary circulation undergo either a Fontan palliation or heart transplantation.

ANESTHETIC MANAGEMENT OF CHILDREN WITH CHD

Anesthesiologists will encounter children with CHD for *elective* noncardiac surgery at one of three stages:
1. *Unpalliated.* The unpalliated cardiac anomaly will generally not cause hemodynamic compromise and may improve with age if the child is still in infancy. Examples of these include small VSDs or mild valvular stenoses. The anesthesiologist may also encounter an infant with unpalliated heart disease who presents with a surgical emergency (e.g., intestinal obstruction). In this situation the child may be waiting for palliative or more definitive surgery, so the anomaly may be more complex (e.g., ToF). In either case, the anesthesiologist must be completely familiar with the anatomic and hemodynamic function of the child's heart and ideally will have discussed the case with the child's pediatrician or pediatric cardiologist prior to surgery.
2. *Partially palliated.* Many children are born with complex lesions that require nondefinitive palliative surgery during the newborn period and complete palliation during or after infancy. An example of this is the staged repair of HLHS. Again, detailed knowledge of the anatomic and functional status of the heart is essential before formulating the anesthetic plan.
3. *Completely palliated.* Children whose congenital heart defects have been fully surgically palliated (Fontan for HLHS, arterial switch procedure for TGA, etc.) may or may not have unique anesthetic considerations. Therefore, the anesthesiologist should be familiar with the common sequelae after repair of that particular defect and should recognize existing noncardiac anomalies that may affect anesthetic management. ASD and PDA are the only congenital lesions that can be truly "corrected."

Preoperative Assessment

The child's diagnosis and current medical condition will determine the preoperative evaluation. The anesthesiologist should attempt to understand the anatomic and hemodynamic function of the child's heart in its present state, and try to piece together an approximate history of the management of the child. Often, the child's cardiologist or pediatrician will provide valuable clinical information and draw a "road map" to help the anesthesiologist understand a complex lesion. All prior diagnostic and therapeutic interventions should be reviewed if relevant to the child's current health. These factors will provide an estimate of the severity of the child's disease. The functional status of the child is largely assessed by determining the child's daily activities and (more specifically) exercise tolerance. In infants, feeding patterns are important indications of normal cardiac function because of the effort involved for coordination of sucking and swallowing. If an infant is unable to finish a feed without tiring, or develops cyanosis, diaphoresis, or respiratory distress during feeding, cardiac reserve is likely reduced. Smaller children with critically limited cardiac output and increasing oxygen consumption will demonstrate failure to thrive or decreased normal activity. Older children may become more sedentary, watching television instead of playing in the backyard. Syncope, palpitations, and chest pain are additional symptoms of cardiac decompensation that are a cause of concern and should be thoroughly investigated prior to elective surgery.

The child's medications should be reviewed. Children with CHD commonly receive diuretics, afterload reduction agents, antiarrhythmics, antiplatelet or anticoagulation drugs, and possibly even inotropic agents or immunosuppressant medications if they have received a heart transplant. All scheduled medications should be taken on the day of surgery, except for diuretics, which are often withheld, depending on the clinical condition of the child.

The preoperative physical exam in children with CHD is focused on cardiorespiratory parameters and determination of changes from baseline. Documentation of preoperative vital signs, including room air Spo_2, is essential to use as a baseline intraoperatively. The cardiac exam will determine the rate and rhythm of the heart, and identify the presence of cyanosis or pallor. Auscultation of the lung field will detect tachypnea or rales, either of which may be indicative of pneumonia or CHF. Observation of the child's breathing pattern will reveal use of accessory muscles of respiration, which may also signal an acute cardiac decompensation. Unlike normal healthy children, the presence of even a mild upper respiratory tract infection virtually always results in cancellation of elective surgery, especially during the winter months when respiratory syncytial virus (RSV) abounds and causes significant morbidity in children with CHD.

The incidence of tracheobronchial anomalies is increased in children with CHD. Tracheal shortening or stenosis may remain unrecognized until the time of general anesthesia. This is especially true in children with trisomy 21. A history of prolonged intubation after surgery for CHD raises the possibility of significant airway abnormalities. On physical exam, inspiratory stridor is an indication of tracheal narrowing due to subglottic stenosis or associated vascular malformations. Associated pulmonary anomalies are rare.

Children with CHD may demonstrate neurologic abnormalities. Strokes from embolic phenomena occur in children with a right-to-left shunt and polycythemia. In addition, during cardiopulmonary bypass, microemboli to the brain can cause "mini-strokes." A stroke at a very young age may not be noticeable as the child grows because of compensation by the developing brain.

There are no specific laboratory tests or diagnostic procedures that are always indicated in children with CHD. Each patient is individually assessed and the appropriate tests ordered. Most commonly, a complete blood count and coagulation tests are indicated. Children with cyanotic CHD compensate for chronic hypoxemia by developing polycythemia, an increased red cell mass over the normal value. Polycythemia is a physiologic mechanism which increases the oxygen-carrying capacity of the blood. When the hematocrit approaches 65%, the increase in blood viscosity interferes with tissue microcirculation, contributes to tissue hypoxia, increases SVR, and predisposes to venous thrombosis and strokes. Conversely, a "normal" or low hematocrit indicates relative anemia, most commonly caused by iron deficiency. Iron-deficient red blood cells are less deformable and independently increase the blood viscosity. Therefore, anemia or polycythemia must be evaluated and corrected prior to elective surgery. This is often done in consultation with the patient's pediatric cardiologist and/or hematologist.

Preoperative electrolyte determination is indicated in children taking diuretics, which can cause a hypochloremic, hypokalemic metabolic alkalosis. Depending on the patient's current clinical condition, an electrocardiogram or echocardiogram might be indicated preoperatively. A chest radiograph is rarely indicated prior to elective surgery.

Preoperative dehydration should be avoided in children with cyanotic CHD and polycythemia. Hydration is especially important for children with ToF, cyanotic patients with polycythemia, and children with Fontan physiology. ToF patients may have a hypercyanotic episode or "Tet spell" when dehydrated. Fontan patients are dependent on venous return for their pulmonary blood flow. Dehydration leads to a decreased central venous pressure and subsequent decreased pulmonary blood flow and poor cardiac output. These patients may benefit from a preoperative admission for overnight hydration. Fasting intervals should be no different for children with CHD than for healthy children (see Chapter 12).

The level of anxiety reflected by the child and/or their parents will factor into the anesthetic plan. The best anxiolytic is the preoperative visit in which the anesthesiologist ascertains the patient's and parent's concerns, discusses the anesthetic plan, and answers questions. If the child is hemodynamically stable and monitored by anesthesia staff, a preoperative anxiolytic is indicated. Oral or intravenous midazolam is used most often. The potential advantages of preoperative sedation in children with CHD include easy separation from parents, less crying, decreased oxygen consumption, and decreased levels of intraoperative anesthetics. Some anesthesiologists fear that even minimal respiratory depression caused by sedatives may cause significant oxyhemoglobin desaturation in children with cyanotic CHD whose resting oxyhemoglobin saturations lie on the steep portion of the hemoglobin dissociation curve. However, several investigations that assessed this risk demonstrated that preoperative anxiolysis resulted in less oxyhemoglobin desaturation during induction of anesthesia.

Subacute Bacterial Endocarditis (SBE) Prophylaxis

SBE can occur in susceptible patients following surgical procedures which result in bacteremia (Box 3-3). The American Heart Association has published guidelines concerning the administration of prophylactic antibiotics to susceptible patients. Pericardial patch closures, primary closures and device closures of ASDs and VSDs should receive SBE prophylaxis for 6 months after repair, or longer if a residual shunt is present. Perioperative antibiotic administration is recommended in "high-risk" and "moderate-risk" patients (Box 3-4). The current recommendations include administration of oral antibiotics 60 minutes prior to surgery or parenteral antibiotics 30 minutes prior to surgery.

Anesthetic Techniques in Children with CHD

All anesthetic agents can cause hemodynamic compromise when given to susceptible patients in certain situations. Inhalation anesthetic agents can alter PVR, SVR, myocardial contractility, heart rhythm, heart rate, and shunt flow. For example, halothane depresses myocardial

Box 3-3 Procedures for which Endocarditis Prophylaxis is Recommended

Respiratory Tract

All mouth, nose, and dental procedures
Tonsillectomy and/or adenoidectomy
Surgical operations that involve respiratory mucosa
Bronchoscopy with a rigid bronchoscope
Nasotracheal intubation

Gastrointestinal Tract

(Prophylaxis recommended for high-risk patients;
   optional for moderate-risk patients)
Sclerotherapy for esophageal varices
Esophageal stricture dilation
Endoscopic retrograde cholangiography with biliary
   obstruction
Biliary tract surgery
Surgical operations that involve intestinal mucosa

Genitourinary Tract

Prostatic surgery
Cystoscopy
Urethral dilation

Reproduced with permission from Dajani AS, Taubert KA, Wilson W et al: Prevention of bacterial endocarditis. *JAMA* 277:1794–1801, 1997.

Box 3-4 Cardiac Conditions Associated with Endocarditis

High-risk Category

Prosthetic cardiac valves, including bioprosthetic and
   homograft valves
Previous bacterial endocarditis
Complex cyanotic congenital heart disease (e.g., single-
   ventricle lesions, TGA, ToF)
Surgically constructed systemic pulmonary shunts or
   conduits

Moderate-risk Category

Most other congenital cardiac malformations (other
   than above)
Acquired valvar dysfunction (e.g., rheumatic heart disease)
Hypertrophic obstructive cardiomyopathy (HOCM)
Mitral valve prolapse with valvar regurgitation and/or
   thickened leaflets

Reproduced with permission from Dajani AS, Taubert KA, Wilson W et al: Prevention of bacterial endocarditis. *JAMA* 277:1794–1801, 1997.

function, alters sinus node function, sensitizes the myocardium to catecholamines, and produces hypotension in normal children. In the presence of CHD, halothane decreases mean arterial pressure (MAP), ejection fraction (EF), and cardiac index, although heart rate is generally maintained. On the other hand, because of its propensity to depress myocardial contractility, halothane is considered to be the agent of choice in patients with a left ventricular outflow tract obstruction, such as hypertrophic obstructive cardiomyopathy (HOCM). Isoflurane produces a drop in SVR in normal patients by vasodilation, which decreases MAP, but less than halothane. Isoflurane slightly increases heart rate and thus tends to maintain cardiac index in children with CHD. Sevoflurane decreases SVR and can decrease LV shortening fraction in children with normal hearts. However, in children with CHD, sevoflurane produces less of a decrease in SVR and LV shortening fraction than halothane, while at the same time maintaining cardiac index and heart rate. Sevoflurane can also produce diastolic dysfunction. Desflurane can cause an adverse cardiovascular reaction by stimulating the sympathetic system. This effect may be decreased by prior administration of fentanyl.

Inhalational induction in children with right-to-left shunts may result in an increased shunt fraction and cyanosis secondary to a decrease in SVR. In this situation, a slow, careful titration of agent is necessary with frequent measurements of blood pressure during induction. Oxyhemoglobin desaturation that is not caused by respiratory difficulty should be attributed to systemic vasodilation and right-to-left shunting, and should be treated with a direct vasoconstrictor such as phenylephrine.

Intracardiac shunts can affect the rate of anesthetic induction. In the presence of a right-to-left shunt, dilution of anesthetic agent in the left ventricle by venous blood that bypasses the lung results in a decreased concentration of agent reaching the brain. This will, theoretically, slow the rate of induction of anesthesia. Conversely, left-to-right shunts may speed induction of anesthesia by rapidly decreasing the arterial-to-venous difference of agent in the lungs (see Chapter 19).

High oxygen concentrations decrease PVR and increase SVR; hypoxemia increases PVR and decreases SVR. These changes may significantly alter pulmonary blood flow by changing the PVR to SVR ratio in the presence of a large, unrestrictive intracardiac shunt. Nitrous oxide produces minimal myocardial depression, and although it is associated with increased PVR in adults, it produces minimal changes in infants with both normal and increased PVR. Nitrous oxide can, however, increase the size of an air embolus.

Because of these deleterious effects of inhalational agents in children with CHD, many pediatric anesthesiologists prefer to induce general anesthesia with intravenous agents. Thiopental and propofol can be administered judiciously, and with consideration of the patient's underlying medical condition. Intravenous induction is theoretically slower in the presence of a left-to-right shunt and faster in children with a right-to-left shunt. These effects are difficult to appreciate clinically.

Ketamine and etomidate may provide greater hemodynamic stability, especially in hypovolemic or dehydrated children. Ketamine's sympathomimetic effects will tend to maintain heart rate, contractility, and SVR. There are theoretical concerns with ketamine's ability to cause increases in pulmonary vascular pressures, especially in patients with Fontan physiology. However, this has not been substantiated in clinical studies performed in children with CHD. Multiple studies have examined the effects of opioids on hemodynamics in children with CHD and have concluded that there exist no cardiodepressant effects if bradycardia is avoided. Similar results have been achieved with benzodiazepine administration in children with CHD.

Regional anesthesia and analgesia can be used in children with CHD with several caveats:

1. The child with longstanding coarctation of the aorta and dilated tortuous intercostal arteries may be at risk for arterial puncture or excessive absorption of local anesthetic during intercostal blockade.
2. Since the lungs may absorb up to 80% of the local anesthetic on first passage, the risk of local anesthetic toxicity is theoretically increased in patients with right-to-left shunts.
3. Vasodilatation resulting from central axis blockade may be hazardous in patients with significant AS or other left-sided obstructive lesions. Vasodilatation may also cause a decrease in oxyhemoglobin saturation in children with a right-to-left shunt. On the other hand, peripheral vasodilatation in patients with polycythemia may have the benefit of improved microcirculatory flow and decreased venous thrombosis.
4. Children with chronic cyanosis are at risk for coagulation abnormalities and should be adequately evaluated prior to initiation of regional anesthesia.

Intraoperative Monitoring

Children with CHD are susceptible to abnormal pulmonary ventilation/perfusion ratios resulting in increased dead space and/or shunt. These abnormalities alter the arterial to end-tidal carbon dioxide ($P_{ET}CO_2$) difference. In children with CHD, $P_{ET}CO_2$ will tend to underestimate P_aCO_2. Clinical studies demonstrate that intraoperative $P_{ET}CO_2$ monitoring can be unreliable in children with CHD.

Although pulse oximetry may have limited accuracy at oxyhemoglobin saturations below 70%, they reliably predict oxyhemoglobin saturations in the range that is normally encountered in children with cyanotic CHD (70–90%). An acute oxyhemoglobin desaturation below 70%, regardless of the accuracy of the pulse oximeter, should warrant immediate evaluation of conditions that cause hypoxemia.

Blood pressure monitoring of children with CHD can easily be obtained with a noninvasive automatic cuff. However, accuracy may depend on arterial tree malformations and previous surgical corrections. For example, a previous modified Blalock–Taussig shunt or left subclavian flap procedure for a coarctation repair can render the blood pressure reading in the respective extremity inaccurate or difficult to obtain. Similarly, in a patient with a left aortic arch and aberrant right subclavian artery, the right radial artery will give similar readings as the left radial artery. Lower-extremity blood pressure readings may be inaccurate in children with coarctation of the aorta prior to repair. An arterial catheter may be required when it is important to closely monitor changes in acid–base status or during procedures associated with wide hemodynamic swings or large volume shifts.

Intravenous lines must be completely de-aired prior to connection in children with CHD who possess a shunt or fenestration. With a right-to-left shunt, an injected air bubble can cross into the systemic circulation and cause a stroke if it passes from the aorta to the brain via a carotid or vertebral artery, or result in other end-organ damage. With a left-to-right shunt, most air bubbles pass into the lungs and are absorbed.

Postoperative Management of Children with CHD

Children with CHD are particularly susceptible to the deleterious effects of hypoventilation and/or mild decreases in oxyhemoglobin saturation. Following tracheal extubation, oxygen should be administered during transport to the postanesthesia care unit (PACU) and gradually weaned based on the patient's clinical condition. Oxygen saturation should be titrated to 85% in patients with single ventricle or stage I physiology for fear of decreasing PVR, increasing pulmonary blood flow, and decreasing systemic blood flow. It is imperative that these children be followed closely in the PACU by an anesthesiologist familiar with their specific cardiac disease. There are no reasons to withhold adequate treatment of pain with opioid agents, and commonly used antiemetics are also well tolerated.

FUNCTIONAL HEART DISEASE IN CHILDREN

Myocarditis

Most cases of myocarditis in North America result from viral infection of the myocardium, predominantly

Article To Know

Warner MA, Linn RJ, O'Leary PW, Schroeder DR: Outcomes of noncardiac surgical procedures in children and adults with congenital heart disease. Mayo Clin Proc 73:728-734, 1998.

There is a paucity of published data that indicate the perioperative risk to children or adults with previously existing CHD when undergoing noncardiac surgery. This article describes a retrospective cohort study of children and adults with CHD less than 50 years of age who underwent noncardiac surgical or diagnostic procedures with anesthesia over a 6-year period (1987–92) at the Mayo Clinic. Risk factors for 30-day perioperative morbidity and mortality were determined. Patients received a general anesthetic, monitored anesthesia care (MAC), or a regional technique. Patients with all types of CHD except minor abnormalities (e.g., bicuspid aortic valve, PFO, mitral valve prolapse without regurgitation) were included for analysis.

Perioperative morbidity included: (1) onset of a new cardiac problem or exacerbation of a previously stable cardiac condition; (2) onset of a new respiratory problem or exacerbation of a previously stable respiratory condition; and (3) onset of a new neurologic deficit.

The authors analyzed 480 procedures in 276 eligible patients. Fifteen patients (5.4%) experienced a perioperative complication during their first noncardiac procedure. Risk factors associated with a perioperative complication included age less than 2 years, presence of cyanosis, use of medication for CHF, procedures scheduled on an inpatient basis, high ASA status, and pulmonary hypertension. The highest rates of complications occurred in patients undergoing respiratory or nervous system procedures. Overall, the complication rate was low (5.4%) for the first noncardiac procedure with an unanticipated admission rate of 1.7% (consistent with group's unexpected admission rate for their entire outpatient surgery patient population).

enteroviruses (coxsackie B virus and echovirus). It is unclear whether myocardial damage from viral myocarditis results from direct viral invasion or an autoimmune antibody response. Depending on the degree of damage to the myocardium, patients may be asymptomatic and the diagnosis may be made only by finding ST- and T-wave changes on an electrocardiogram done for an unrelated reason, whereas others may present with fulminant CHF. Common symptoms include fever, dyspnea, palpitations, and chest pain (usually due to a secondary pericarditis). Signs include tachycardia, evidence of CHF, and S3 ventricular gallop. Therapy for patients with viral myocarditis is supportive to maintain perfusion and oxygenation, and includes pharmacologic management of ventricular arrhythmias, conduction abnormalities, and CHF as indicated. The prognosis depends on the extent of myocardial damage. Anesthetic management for patients with myocarditis will depend entirely on the severity of myocardial depression and should, therefore, be individualized. For obvious reasons, only urgent surgery is performed in these patients.

Dilated Cardiomyopathy

Dilated or congestive cardiomyopathy is characterized by myocardial dysfunction and ventricular dilatation. Although usually an idiopathic disorder in childhood, it can be caused by neuromuscular disease (Duchenne muscular dystrophy) or drug toxicity (anthracyclines). Dilation of the left ventricle results in CHF. An increase in left atrial pressure, pulmonary venous pressure, and pulmonary capillary wedge pressure results in pulmonary edema.

Symptoms include dyspnea, orthopnea, and paroxysmal nocturnal dyspnea. Medical therapy includes inotropic agents and vasodilators to improve myocardial contractility and decrease the afterload on the weakened ventricle. Diuretics decrease preload and hopefully improve cardiac output by moving the dilated ventricle to a more favorable position on the Frank–Starling curve. Antiarrhythmic medications are used to control potentially fatal ventricular arrhythmias. If medical therapy fails, heart transplantation may be necessary.

Hypertrophic Cardiomyopathy

Also known as "idiopathic hypertrophic subaortic stenosis" (IHSS), hypertrophic obstructive cardiomyopathy (HOCM) is an autosomal dominant genetic disorder in which the ventricular septum is thickened, resulting in left ventricular outflow tract obstruction. In the thickened stiff left ventricle, systolic function is well preserved, but diastolic function is compromised. Abnormal motion of the mitral valve results in mitral insufficiency. Symptoms include dyspnea on exertion, chest pain, and syncope.

Therapy includes prevention of fatal ventricular arrhythmias and decreasing the stiffness of the left ventricle with negative inotropic medications, such as calcium-channel blockers, and beta-adrenergic blocking agents. The avoidance of competitive sports is essential because sudden death during exertion is a significant risk. Many pediatric anesthesiologists feel that halothane is the most ideal anesthetic for use in these patients because of its negative inotropic actions.

Case

A 12-year-old boy is scheduled for an urgent repair of a proximal femur fracture after being hit by a car while riding his bicycle. Past medical history reveals that he was born with tricuspid atresia. He underwent a right modified BT shunt in the first days of life, a Glenn shunt at 4 months of age, and a completion Fontan at 18 months. His current medications include furosemide, ASA, and enalapril. He ate a large meal shortly before the accident occurred.

His current vital signs are: blood pressure 90/40 mmHg; heart rate 110/min; respiratory rate 32/min; temperature 36.5°C; SpO_2 96% on room air. Physical exam reveals an alert, anxious, child who is moaning in pain. There is no murmur heard on chest auscultation, and his lung fields are clear. He has full distal-extremity pulses, absence of clubbing, a cut-down scar over the right radial artery, and multiple scars over the dorsal aspects of both hands. His airway exam is otherwise unremarkable.

What is a modified BT shunt? What is a Glenn shunt?

Described in 1945, a Blalock–Taussig (BT) shunt is a palliative procedure that is performed in the newborn period in children with single ventricle anatomy (e.g. HLHS, PA/IVS, TA) to provide pulmonary blood flow. A *modified* BT shunt involves the insertion of a synthetic tube graft between the subclavian artery and the pulmonary artery. A properly sized BT shunt provides enough pulmonary blood flow to maintain oxygen saturation at between 75% and 85%.

The Glenn shunt, first described in 1951, is another method to provide stable pulmonary blood flow. In the bidirectional Glenn shunt the SVC is anastomosed to an *undivided* ipsilateral pulmonary artery to provide blood flow to both lungs. The superior cavopulmonary anastomosis is performed at about 6 months of age to provide stable pulmonary blood flow after PVR has dropped to normal levels.

Is there anything else you want to know before preceding with this case?

Yes – I want to further investigate his cardiac status. I'll ask the patient's family about his current health status, exercise tolerance, recent medication history, and previous cardiology evaluations. From this information, I'll try to estimate his cardiovascular status. I'll also try to ascertain the results of his most recent cardiac catheterization, and obtain a preoperative ECG and chest radiograph. Preoperative lab tests should include a complete blood count, type and crossmatch, and electrolytes since he is taking a diuretic.

The patient's family observes that he has been doing well recently. An echocardiogram performed a year ago revealed "slightly decreased function." There were no anesthetic problems in the past, and the parents do not know the result of his most recent catheterization, which was approximately 2 years ago. However, they have a schematic drawing of their son's heart, which was given to them by the cardiologist (Fig. 3-9). His preoperative ECG reveals sinus rhythm, rate 78, and an increased P-R interval.

Is premedication indicated in this patient?

Yes – both anxiolysis and analgesia are indicated in this patient. An opioid will relieve the patient's pain and may also relieve anxiety. Opioids will maintain hemodynamic stability, but may produce respiratory depression. The risk of respiratory depression increases with addition of a benzodiazepine. SBE prophylaxis is also indicated in the preoperative period (see Boxes 3-3 and 3-4).

What invasive monitoring is indicated for this case?

Placing an arterial line for continuous BP monitoring should be considered in a patient with decreased cardiac function, and when there is the potential for intraoperative blood loss. However, because of the prior cut-down attempts, there may be abnormal radial artery anatomy, and one would have to weigh the benefits and risks of placing it at an alternate site. I would probably attempt radial artery catheterization if the pulses were strong, following induction of general anesthesia.

Following a Fontan procedure, central venous pressure monitoring can be used to estimate intravascular volume, which determines the pulmonary filling pressure. Central venous access also provides large-bore IV access, which may be required for a procedure with potential blood loss in a patient with questionable peripheral IV access routes. On the other hand, because of previous central line placements, the anatomy of the internal jugular and subclavian veins may be aberrant, thereby increasing the risk of complications. Central access in a patient with Fontan physiology carries further risk; if a thrombus develops, it could potentially travel into the pulmonary circulation and obstruct blood flow. Therefore, my first choice would be to attempt to secure adequate peripheral access. If this is not possible, then I would consider central access via the femoral veins after induction of general anesthesia. Central access may be required if there is the potential for significant blood loss and hypovolemia prior to surgery. The use of transesophageal echo can also be considered, to help estimate volume status and ventricular function.

All intravenous access lines should be completely de-aired prior to connection. Air bubbles in the venous system can travel to the left side of the heart and lead to a paradoxical embolus in the cerebral, coronary, mesenteric, or renal circulations.

Case *Cont'd*

How would you induce and maintain general anesthesia in this patient?

A rapid sequence induction is indicated in a patient with a full stomach. After volume loading this patient in the preoperative period, I would choose a modified rapid sequence induction with gentle mask ventilation and cricoid pressure (keeping airway pressure <20 cmH$_2$O) while gradually titrating a hypnotic induction agent. Etomidate is the induction agent of choice in the hypovolemic patient with decreased cardiac function. Thiopental or propofol could be utilized in this modified rapid sequence induction, albeit at a lower dose, and titrated to effect in combination with an opioid. Maintenance of general anesthesia can be achieved with a balanced technique consisting of an inhalational agent (except halothane) and an opioid, and tailored toward tracheal extubation at the completion of the procedure. Unless otherwise indicated, postoperative mechanical ventilation should be avoided in this patient since increased mean airway pressures will impede pulmonary circulation, decrease preload to the systemic ventricle, and decrease cardiac output to the body. Pain relief in this patient is best provided by patient-controlled analgesia with opioids and an adjunctive analgesic such as ketorolac.

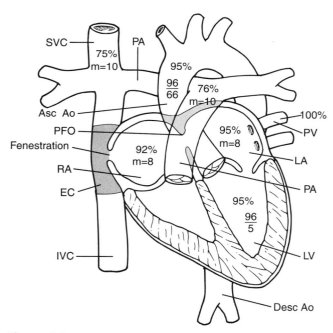

Figure 3-9   Anatomy and pathophysiology of tricuspid atresia with normally placed great arteries after a bidirectional Glenn and Fontan procedure. Blood flows from the SVC and IVC directly to pulmonary arteries and lungs. Blood flow is dependent on the transpulmonary gradient from the pulmonary arteries to the pulmonary venous atrium. The percentages represent the oxygen saturation; blood pressure is represented by mean (*m*) or systolic/diastolic. SVC = superior vena cava; IVC = inferior vena cava; RPA = right pulmonary artery; LPA = left pulmonary artery; PVA = pulmonary venous atrium; EC = extracardiac conduit; RV = (hypoplastic) right ventricle; LV = left ventricle; RA = right atrium; FO = foramen ovale; Asc Ao = ascending aorta; Desc Ao = descending aorta.

Arrhythmias

Arrhythmias in children are much less common than in adults but can be just as life-threatening. They may result from congenital, functional, or acquired structural heart disease; electrolyte disturbances (potassium, calcium, and magnesium); drug toxicity; poisoning; or an acquired systemic disorder. Bradyarrhythmias generally result from impulse formation or atrioventricular conduction abnormalities, whereas tachyarrhythmias result from increased automaticity or a reentrant circuit.

When halothane is used, the most common intraoperative ventricular arrhythmias are premature ventricular beats (PVCs) that are isolated, or occur as bigeminy or trigeminy. The incidence of intraoperative PVCs is increased in the presence of catecholamine release or hypercapnia. When halothane is not used, narrow complex tachyarrhythmias are the most common arrhythmia seen in the perioperative period; the rate is regular and ranges from 150 to 350 beats per minute. In most patients they are idiopathic or related to fever, stress, dehydration, or anemia. In others they are associated with an undiagnosed atrial conduction system abnormality, such as Wolff-Parkinson-White syndrome. If the patient is normotensive, treatment should be instituted with vagal maneuvers, and/or adenosine. If the patient is hemodynamically unstable, then cardioversion is indicated.

ADDITIONAL ARTICLES TO KNOW

Burrows FA: Physiologic dead space, venous admixture, and the arterial to end-tidal carbon dioxide difference in infants and children undergoing cardiac surgery. *Anesthesiology* 70:219-225, 1989.

DeBock TL, Davis PJ, Tome J et al: Effect of premedication on arterial oxygen saturation in children with congenital heart disease. *J Cardiothor Anesth* 4:425-429, 1990.

Fontan F, Kirklin JW, Fernandez G et al: Outcome after a "perfect" Fontan operation. *Circulation* 81:1520-1536, 1990.

Gaca JA, Douglas WI, Barnes SD. Anesthetic implications of the Fontan procedure for single ventricle physiology. *Semin Cardiothorac Vasc Anesth* 5:31-39, 2001.

Goldstein-Dresner MC, Davis PJ, Kretchman E et al: Double-blind comparison of oral transmucosal fentanyl citrate with oral meperidine, diazepam, and atropine as preanesthetic medication in children with congenital heart disease. *Anesthesiology* 74:28-33, 1991.

Hickey PR, Hansen DD, Cramolini GM, Vincent RN, Lang P: Pulmonary and systemic hemodynamic responses to ketamine in infants with normal and elevated PVR. *Anesthesiology* 62:287-293, 1985.

Lebovic S, Reich DL, Steinberg G, Vela FP, Silvay G: Comparison of propofol versus ketamine for anesthesia in pediatric patients undergoing cardiac catheterization. *Anesth Analg* 74:490-494, 1992.

Levine MF, Hartley EJ, Macpherson BA, Burrows FA, Lerman J: Oral midazolam for children with congenital cyanotic heart disease undergoing cardiac surgery: a comparative study. *Can J Anaesth* 40:934-938, 1993.

Morris CD, Reller MD, Menashe VD: Thirty-year incidence of infective endocarditis after surgery for congenital heart defect. *JAMA* 279:599-603, 1998.

Nicolson SC, Dorsey AT, Schreiner MS: Shortened preanesthetic fasting interval in pediatric cardiac surgical patients. *Anesth Analg* 74:694-697, 1992.

Rivenes SM, Lewin MB, Stayer SA et al: Cardiovascular effects of sevoflurane, isoflurane, halothane, and fentanyl–midazolam in children with congenital heart disease. *Anesthesiology* 94:223-229, 2001.

Stow PJ, Burrows FA, Lerman J, Roy WL: Arterial oxygen saturation following premedication in children with cyanotic congenital heart disease. *Can J Anaesth* 35:63-66, 1988.

Tanner, GE, Angers DG, Barash PG et al: Effects of left-to-right, mixed left-to-right, and right-to-left shunts on inhalational anesthetic induction in children: a computer model. *Anesth Analg* 64:101-107, 1985.

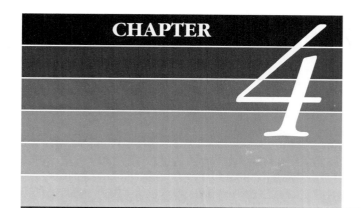

CHAPTER 4

Respiratory Diseases

RONALD S. LITMAN

Respiratory diseases represent the most common systemic illnesses in children, and are likely to influence anesthetic management. This chapter reviews the most common or important upper and lower airway diseases in children.

UPPER AIRWAY DISEASES

Laryngomalacia

Laryngomalacia is the most common laryngeal disorder of the newborn. It is a congenital abnormality of the epiglottis and aryepiglottic folds that allows their inward collapse into the airway during inspiration. This inward collapse results in nearly complete upper airway obstruction that is manifested by audible inspiratory stridor, usually in the few several months of life. The stridor is usually more prominent when the infant is lying supine, crying, or feeding. In most cases it is benign, and will be outgrown during the first year of life. Laryngomalacia is occasionally associated with gastroesophageal reflux and, in rare cases, causes hypoxemia or hypoventilation, and interferes with normal feeding and subsequent growth. Infants in this latter group require definitive diagnosis by direct laryngoscopy under general anesthesia. Rigid bronchoscopy is performed at the same time

to rule out subglottic causes of airway obstruction. Severe laryngomalacia is treated by performing a supra-glottoplasty, in which a CO_2 laser is used to trim the length of the epiglottis and partially sever the aryepiglottic folds to prevent the epiglottis from infolding into the glottic opening during inspiration.

During induction of general anesthesia, infants with laryngomalacia commonly exhibit airway obstruction that is not relieved by placement of an oral airway device. Deepening the anesthetic will often relieve the obstruction because of progressive weakening of the diaphragm and decreasing the strength of inspiration. However, during upper airway obstruction, speed of inhalational induction is slowed. Positive-pressure ventilation is usually easily accomplished in these infants, especially after the onset of neuromuscular blockade.

Obstructive Sleep Apnea

Obstructive sleep apnea (OSA) in children is the result of adenotonsillar hypertrophy, combined with an abnormally small retropharyngeal space, and altered neuromuscular control of upper airway patency during sleep. It mainly occurs in children between the ages of 2 and 4 years, and is especially prevalent in children with obesity and trisomy 21. The clinical manifestations include partial or complete upper airway obstruction during sleep, restless sleep, morning headaches, behavioral disturbances, and daytime somnolence. Severe cases of untreated longstanding OSA can result in chronic hypoxemia, polycythemia, and cor pulmonale. Children with electrocardiographic or radiographic cardiac abnormalities should be referred to a pediatric cardiologist for further evaluation and management.

The most common therapy for pediatric OSA is adenotonsillectomy (see Chapter 29), which alleviates symptoms in most children. Some pediatric anesthesiologists prefer to reduce the dose of the preoperative sedative in children with OSA, for fear of causing life-threatening upper airway obstruction in an unmonitored environment. However, it has been this author's experience that a routine dose of oral midazolam in children with OSA does not cause significant upper airway obstruction.

During induction of general anesthesia, virtually all children with untreated OSA will exhibit partial or complete upper airway obstruction. Insertion of an artificial oral airway device after loss of consciousness will bypass the obstruction and allow easy bag-mask ventilation. In the immediate postoperative period following adenotonsillectomy, the incidence of airway obstruction is higher in children with OSA when compared with those who undergo adenotonsillectomy for recurrent infections. Therefore, children with significant OSA should be hospitalized overnight following the procedure. Even some time after adenotonsillectomy has been performed, a predisposition toward upper airway obstruction during sleep or sedation may persist throughout childhood. Children with OSA are more likely to develop adult-type OSA.

Subglottic Stenosis

Subglottic stenosis is an abnormal narrowing of the extrathoracic trachea below the level of the vocal cords. It may be present at birth (webs, strictures, etc.) or, more commonly, is acquired secondary to chronic inflammation and scarring from the presence of an endotracheal tube. Congenital subglottic stenosis is more common in children with multiple congenital anomalies and in children with trisomy 21.

Acquired subglottic stenosis is the most common acquired anomaly of the larynx in children and the most common abnormality requiring tracheotomy in children younger than 12 months. The chronic presence of an endotracheal tube causes inflammation and scarring, particularly at the level of the cricoid ring, and a restrictive scar is formed. The clinical manifestations of subglottic stenosis include inspiratory stridor during crying or at the time of an upper respiratory tract infection, during which tracheal narrowing increases secondary to edema.

Subglottic stenosis is diagnosed using rigid bronchoscopy under general anesthesia. Positive-pressure ventilation via bag and mask can be difficult when the narrowing is severe. An additional anesthetic implication is the need for an endotracheal tube that is markedly smaller than that predicted for age. Severe cases require treatment with an anterior cricoid split procedure or a more complete tracheal reconstruction (laryngotracheoplasty), and some children require tracheostomy. Following tracheal reconstruction, these children will remain paralyzed and mechanically ventilated for several days while the tracheal tissue heals over the endotracheal tube.

Tracheomalacia

Tracheomalacia is defined as a softening of the tracheal cartilage, which then becomes susceptible to collapse when the intraluminal tracheal pressure is less than the extraluminal tracheal pressure. Thus, airway collapse can occur during forceful coughing or exhalation. Congenital tracheomalacia occurs in infants with a tracheoesophageal fistula and some genetic disorders such as trisomy 21 and the mucopolysaccharidoses. Acquired tracheomalacia occurs in children who required long-term mechanical ventilation during early infancy, and in children with tracheal compression lesions such as a vascular ring.

Clinical manifestations of tracheomalacia include noisy breathing, "barky" cough, wheezing, and respiratory distress (e.g., dyspnea). These symptoms are often exacerbated during a URI (upper respiratory infection). Many children with tracheomalacia are initially thought to be asthmatic until properly diagnosed.

Anesthetic implications for children with tracheomalacia are similar to those for laryngomalacia. Positive-pressure ventilation, especially after administration of a neuromuscular blocker, will characteristically result in the ability to easily open the softened trachea and establish adequate ventilation. Coughing and partial upper airway obstruction will exacerbate tracheal collapse and rapidly lead to hypoxemia. This is particularly difficult to manage during emergence from general anesthesia and after tracheal extubation. Children with severe tracheomalacia may require a "deep extubation" to avoid these complications.

Upper Respiratory Tract Infection (URI)

Viral upper respiratory tract infections (URIs) are frequent in children, especially during the winter months. Typical symptoms include rhinorrhea, congestion, cough, fever, and malaise. Subclinical manifestations may include upper and lower airway edema, increased respiratory tract secretions, pneumonia, and bronchial irritability.

Intraoperative airway complications during general anesthesia seem to be more common in children with a URI. These include coughing, laryngospasm, bronchospasm, and hypoxemia. Infants under 12 months of age tend to have more intraoperative complications than older children, and use of an endotracheal tube as compared with a facemask or laryngeal mask airway (LMA) increases the risk of these complications. Passive exposure to cigarette smoke is an additional risk factor.

In infants and children with a URI, apneic oxygenation is less effective; thus oxyhemoglobin desaturation may occur when, during rapid sequence induction, the child is not receiving positive-pressure ventilation. Use of

Box 4-1   Distinguishing a Viral URI from Allergic Rhinitis

Viral URI	***Allergic Rhinitis***
Purulent rhinorrhea	Clear rhinorrhea
Presence of fever	Absence of fever
Productive cough	Unproductive cough
Other family members ill	No other family members ill
Lower respiratory tract signs (e.g., wheeze, rales, bronchospasm)	History of atopy in patient or family

thiopental for induction of general anesthesia is associated with more airway complications than when propofol is used.

Transient postoperative hypoxemia, postintubation croup, and postoperative pneumonia are more likely to occur in children with a URI. Long-term complications and true outcomes are difficult to define and quantify and may not differ between normal children and those with a current or recent URI.

With these possible complications in mind, when a child presents with a URI, it is intuitive that an elective procedure requiring general anesthesia should be canceled. But, because so many children have a concurrent URI at the time of their scheduled surgery, and long-term negative outcomes have not been demonstrated, this decision process is complex. How, then, should the anesthesiologist decide when to cancel an elective procedure in a child with a URI? First, one should assess the severity of the child's illness. The child with a runny nose without additional findings may be suffering from vasomotor or allergic rhinitis (Box 4-1), which is usually not associated with perioperative airway complications. If it is clear that the illness is viral, one must then identify the factors that are likely to increase perioperative complications (Box 4-2). If any of these risk factors are present, it may be prudent to perform the procedure at a later date when the child is in better health. On the other hand, there are a variety of additional factors that may influence the anesthesiologist's decision to proceed with surgery or cancel the case. The most common reason for proceeding with a case even though risk factors are present is the continuous presence of a URI that will likely continue without surgical intervention. This occurs when children require adenoidectomy or myringotomy to relieve chronic middle ear fluid collections. Nonmedical factors that might sway the anesthesiologist in favor of proceeding with the case are logistical family concerns, such as the parents taking a day off from work, difficulty finding day care, traveling a long distance at a great inconvenience to the family, etc. Since outcomes are not proven to be worse after surgery in children with a URI, these factors may play a role

in the decision of whether or not to proceed. Most children who present with a URI have neither extremely mild symptoms nor severe symptoms. In these children we must use our judgment to determine the proper course of action based on what we believe is best for the child.

To minimize airway irritability, sevoflurane should be chosen for an inhalational induction and propofol for an intravenous induction. Neuromuscular blockade should be administered as rapidly as possible to prevent laryngospasm. Some authors suggest administration of an anticholinergic agent, such as atropine or glycopyrrolate, to attenuate vagally mediated airway complications; however, this remains untested. When feasible, facemask or LMA anesthesia is preferred over endotracheal intubation.

There is no consensus when to schedule elective surgery following an acute URI between (and even within!) children's hospitals. In a 1979 publication that described the development of lower respiratory symptoms during general anesthesia in children with a URI, McGill and colleagues from DC Children's Hospital wrote: "the optimal period of recovery from the URI that should be allowed prior to considering the patient a candidate for an elective surgical procedure has not been defined." More than 20 years later, this is still true. Subclinical pathology, such

Box 4-2   Preoperative Factors Suggesting Cancellation of an Elective Procedure in a Child with a URI

Coexisting medical disease (especially cardiac, pulmonary, or severe neuromuscular disease)
History of prematurity
Lower respiratory tract signs (e.g., wheezing, rales)
High fever (>102°F)
Productive cough
Major airway, abdominal, or thoracic surgery
Parent is worried about proceeding
Surgeon is worried about proceeding (Ha!)

Article to Know

Tait AR, Malviya S, Voepel-Lewis T et al: Risk factors for perioperative adverse respiratory events in children with upper respiratory tract infections. Anesthesiology 95:299-306, 2001.

Many studies have attempted to elucidate risk factors associated with perioperative adverse events in children with URIs who undergo general anesthesia. Most of these are limited by the inconsistent definition of a URI, and the retrospective nature of the data collection. Dr Tait and his colleagues performed a prospective study of children with mild URIs presenting for general anesthesia to determine the incidence of and independent risk factors for perioperative complications.

They enrolled 1078 children between the ages of 1 month and 18 years. The children were divided into three cohorts: active URI (n = 407), URI within 4 weeks (n = 335), and 336 controls. They defined a URI as a minimum of two of the following symptoms: rhinorrhea, sore or scratchy throat, sneezing, nasal congestion, malaise, cough, and fever <38°C, together with confirmation from a parent. Occurrence and severity of respiratory complications were collected prospectively (Table 4-1).

Table 4-1 Scoring System for Each of Six Respiratory Events

	Severity Scores			
	1	**2**	**3**	**4**
Spo_2 (%)	95-100	90-94	80-89	<80
Cough (n)	None	1 or 2	3 or 4	Continuous
Breath-holding (s)	None	<15	15-30	>30
Laryngospasm	None	Partial: repositioned airway	Partial: CPAP required	Complete: muscle relaxant required
Bronchospasm	None	Expiration only	Expiration and inspiration	Difficult to ventilate: treatment required
Secretions	None	Minimal: no suctioning	Moderate: suctioned once	Copious: suctioned more than once

From: Tait, et al: *Anesthesiology* 9:299-306, 2001. Copyright © 2001 American Society of Anesthesiologists. Published by Lippincott Williams & Wilkins.

Children with an active or recent URI had a higher risk of major arterial desaturation, severe coughing, and overall adverse respiratory events than controls without an active or recent URI (Table 4-2). Children who had airway management with an endotracheal tube were also more likely to demonstrate airway complications than those managed with an LMA or facemask. There were no differences in the incidences of laryngospasm or bronchospasm between the three groups. As would be expected, children who underwent airway procedures (e.g., adenotonsillectomy) were more likely to have airway complications. Independent risk factors for respiratory complications in children with active URIs included: copious secretions, presence of an endotracheal tube when the child was below 5 years of age, prematurity (<37 weeks), nasal congestion, paternal smoking, reactive airway disease, and airway surgery. One child with a recent URI required hospitalization for stridor, and two children with active URIs were hospitalized with pneumonia.

Table 4-2 Incidence of Perioperative Adverse Respiratory Events by URI Status (n (%))

	Breath-holding	Laryngospasm		Bronchospasm	Severe Cough	Spo_2 <90%	Adverse Event
URI (n = 407)	124 (30.5)[a,b]	8 (2.0)[c]	9 (2.2)[d]	23 (5.7)	40 (9.8)[a,b]	64 (15.7)[a]	122 (30.0)[a]
Recent URI (n = 335)	78 (23.3)	9 (2.7)[c]	5 (1.5)[d]	9 (2.7)	19 (5.7)	49 (14.7)[a]	81 (24.2)[a]
No URI (n = 336)	60 (17.9)	8 (2.4)[c]	5 (1.5)[d]	11 (3.3)	14 (4.2)	26 (7.8)	60 (17.9)

[a] $p < 0.05$ versus no URI.
[b] $p < 0.05$ versus recent URI.
[c] Laryngospasm requiring positive airway pressure.
[d] Laryngospasm requiring succinylcholine.
From: Tait, et al: *Anesthesiology* 9:299-306, 2001. Copyright © 2001 American Society of Anesthesiologists. Published by Lippincott Williams & Wilkins.

The findings in this study confirm that children with an active URI are at increased risk for respiratory complications, especially when intubated, and during airway surgery. These findings also extend to the child with a recent URI within 4 weeks of the surgical procedure. Knowledge of some of the independent risk factors can assist anesthesiologists who are confronted with the often difficult decision of whether or not to cancel the case in the immediate preoperative period.

as airway edema, atelectasis, and bronchial reactivity may remain for up to several weeks after the symptoms of the acute URI have resolved. Three to four weeks seems to be a reasonable waiting time, but for many children this merely represents the period between successive illnesses.

LOWER AIRWAY DISEASES

The "lower airway" is traditionally thought of as that portion of the respiratory system that is contained within the thoracic cavity. Therefore, lower airway diseases are those that primarily involve the lungs and bronchial system.

Asthma

Asthma is defined as a chronic disease of reversible airway obstruction, and is characterized by bronchial hyperreactivity, inflammation, and mucous secretion. Clinical manifestations of asthma include wheezing, persistent dry cough, and dyspnea on exertion. During an acute exacerbation, marked respiratory distress occurs, which may include chest wall retractions and a prolonged expiratory phase secondary to bronchial obstruction. Recent studies suggest that chronic airway inflammation rather than smooth-muscle contraction is the primary underlying pathophysiologic mechanism, and thus, maintenance treatment regimens have changed accordingly.

Case 1

A 13-month-old male is scheduled for bilateral myringotomy and tube insertions. He has a history of wheezing with colds, for which he takes nebulized albuterol as needed. His last episode of wheezing with a cold was 3 weeks ago.

Is there anything else you would like to know before proceeding with general anesthesia?

I'd like to know more about his respiratory history. Specifically, I'm interested to know whether he ever required an emergency room visit or hospitalization for his asthma. This will give me a better idea of the severity of his illness. I want to know about his recent health, with regard to viral illnesses, and I will ask the parents if he is exposed to cigarette smoke at home. Children exposed to second-hand smoke tend to exhibit more airway complications during general anesthesia.

On physical exam, I'll pay careful attention to the respiratory system. I'll try to detect the presence of wheezing on auscultation of the lungs, and I will examine his chest to detect use of accessory muscles of respiration. Respiratory rate and pulse oximetry values should be normal.

How will you induce and maintain general anesthesia in this child? Is it any different from a child without asthma?

This child will receive premedication with oral midazolam 0.5 mg/kg, and oral acetaminophen 15 mg/kg. He will then undergo induction and maintenance of general anesthesia with sevoflurane by facemask throughout the entire procedure, which should last no longer than 10 minutes. I will administer 20 μg/kg of intranasal fentanyl to provide postoperative analgesia. As long as this child does not demonstrate wheezing, I will not do anything differently than I would for a child without asthma. For example, prophylactic inhaled albuterol will *not* be administered, and no intravenous line is necessary.

During the procedure you detect wheezing through the precordial stethoscope. What will you do?

Wheezing is a sign of bronchospasm but can also be caused by other entities. Initially, I will rule out light anesthesia and upper airway obstruction by deepening the general anesthetic while I reposition the head and neck, and suction out the oropharynx to clear any secretions. Simultaneously, I will examine the chest, feel the ventilation bag and observe the capnographic tracing, all of which can give me clues about efficacy of air entry and expiratory time. Again, I'm trying to differentiate upper from lower airway obstruction. These maneuvers, in combination with deepening the anesthetic using positive-pressure ventilation, will extinguish wheezing in almost all cases without requiring bronchodilator therapy.

How will your treatment differ if the patient is tachypneic and is wheezing in the post-anesthesia care unit (PACU)?

Wheezing in the PACU requires a different treatment strategy from the intraoperative setting. Oxygen supplementation will be administered if the oxyhemoglobin saturation is below 96% on room air. Treatment will consist of nebulized albuterol, 2.5 mg diluted in 3–4 mL of normal saline. In the majority of cases, one treatment is all that is needed for the wheezing to abate, and the child can then be observed and discharged to home if otherwise well. Reasons for hospital admission will include continuing bronchospasm that is not responding to one or two bronchodilator treatments, and a persistent oxygen requirement. Intravenous access will be required for administration of methylprednisolone 2.5 mg/kg. If the child appears to be in pain, I will administer oral oxycodone 0.1 mg/kg.

Case 2

A 4-year-old boy with asthma requires general endotracheal anesthesia for umbilical hernia repair. He is maintained on inhaled steroids, inhaled cromolyn, an orally administered leukotriene antagonist, and occasionally requires nebulized albuterol for acute episodes of wheezing. Two weeks prior to the surgery, he required one week of oral prednisone for an asthma exacerbation that was worse than usual.

Does the recent exacerbation and oral steroid requirement change your approach to the anesthetic management?

There are two ways the history of a recent asthma exacerbation may change my anesthetic management approach. First, I will make sure the child is now in excellent health, and without any wheezing or URI. The procedure is purely elective and should not be performed if the child is still having symptoms of his illness. Second, if his illness has completely abated this child may be a candidate for prophylactic oral steroid therapy for several days prior to the procedure. I will make this determination by speaking with the boy's parents several days prior to the procedure. If he has required previous hospitalization for his asthma, or frequent systemic steroid use in the past, it indicates that his disease is prone to flare-ups. I will ask his pediatrician to see him prior to the scheduled surgery and prescribe oral steroids for several days. This usually consists of prednisone, up to 1 mg/kg daily.

If this child has had frequent asthma recurrences, I will alter my intraoperative management approach by avoiding endotracheal intubation. Most surgeons who perform umbilical hernia repair prefer intraoperative paralysis and there is no reason I can't use a LMA with controlled ventilation during the procedure. I will avoid administration of medications that are associated with histamine release, such as morphine and mivacurium, and I will remind the surgeon to administer local anesthetic into the wound, up to 1 mL/kg of 0.25% bupivacaine or 0.2% ropivacaine.

With a prevalence of approximately 10% (and continually increasing in most urban areas) asthma has become the most common chronic illness in children in the United States. Ninety percent of children with asthma present before the age of 6 years. An exacerbation of asthma may be caused by allergic, environmental, infectious, or emotional stimuli, among others, and can last up to several hours. Some resolve spontaneously, whereas others require aggressive medical therapy.

Anesthesiologists will most commonly encounter children with asthma prior to elective surgery. The majority of these children will have not had a recent exacerbation of wheezing, and may be taking maintenance therapy. Preoperatively, the anesthesiologist should assess the severity and current status of the child's illness by focusing on several aspects related to the disease. Important details of the medical history include the number of emergency room visits during the previous year, number of hospitalizations for asthma exacerbations, previous occurrences of pneumothorax or respiratory arrest, and the current and recent medication history. The parents and child (if old enough) will usually be able to provide a relative estimate of the current severity of their condition.

The physical examination of the child is focused on the respiratory system, looking for clues of ongoing bronchospasm. These include audible wheezes on expiration, a prolonged expiratory time, and use of accessory muscles of respiration. Pulse oximetry measurement should be obtained to determine the child's baseline oxyhemoglobin saturation. A reading less than 96% in room air is a cause for concern and further evaluation.

Based on the history and physical exam findings, the anesthesiologist should estimate whether the child is optimized for elective surgery and whether or not to proceed with an elective anesthetic. For example, mild wheezing may be serious in a child who never wheezes between acute exacerbations, as opposed to the child who continually has a baseline wheeze, who may be considered to be optimized at the time of surgery.

The treatment of asthma consists mainly of bronchodilators and inhaled corticosteroids. Nebulized β_2-agonists (e.g., albuterol, levalbuterol) produce bronchodilatation via stimulation of β_2-receptors on airway smooth muscle. They are administered as daily maintenance agents or on an as-needed basis. Administration of steroids is associated with decreased airway inflammation, decreased mucus secretion, and decreased release of proinflammatory cytokines. Aerosolized steroids (e.g., budesonide) are breathed directly into the lungs and are not associated with systemic side-effects, but are generally not useful during acute exacerbations. Intravenous steroids will begin to decrease airway inflammation within several hours of administration and are an appropriate treatment during an acute exacerbation.

Additional preventative therapies include orally administered leukotriene receptor antagonists (leukotrienes are lipid mediators generated from the metabolism of arachidonic acid, and have been shown to play an important role in the pathogenesis of asthmatic inflammation), and inhaled or oral cromolyn, which prevents episodes of bronchospasm by stabilizing the mast cell membrane and preventing release of inflammatory mediators such as histamine. Theophylline is no longer used as a first-line therapy because of its narrow therapeutic range and questionable efficacy; it is reserved for children in status asthmaticus who fail more conventional therapy. Most recently, magnesium has been described as effective treatment for asthma. The suggested mechanism of action is smooth-muscle relaxation secondary to inhibition of calcium uptake. The current dose recommendation of intravenous magnesium for treating asthma is 25–75 mg/kg over 20 minutes.

The anesthetic management of children with asthma is aimed at preventing an exacerbation of the disease.

Case 3

A 10-year-old female is diagnosed with acute appendicitis and is scheduled for an emergency laparoscopic appendectomy. She has a history of asthma for which she takes maintenance therapy with inhaled steroids, inhaled cromolyn, and a leukotriene antagonist. Three days ago she was treated in the emergency room for an acute asthma attack. She received inhaled albuterol and intravenous methylprednisolone. Some residual wheeze remains, and she states she is not back to her usual state of good health.

How will you approach the anesthetic management of this child?

Since this procedure is urgent, I don't have much time to further optimize this child's asthmatic condition prior to appendectomy. She should receive a nebulized albuterol treatment, either in the emergency room or upon arrival to the OR holding area, and one intravenous dose of methylprednisolone. I will also administer intravenous midazolam as a preoperative anxiolytic. Preoperative intravenous hydration is also important in this child – she has probably had limited oral intake recently, and I want to minimize thickening of her bronchial secretions.

Rapid sequence induction of general anesthesia is indicated in this patient owing to the nature of her abdominal process. It should be tailored so as to minimize the chances of bronchial reactivity following endotracheal intubation. Following an adequate interval of preoxygenation, I will administer glycopyrrolate 0.01 mg/kg, fentanyl 2 μg/kg, lidocaine 1.5 mg/kg, propofol 3 mg/kg, and rocuronium 1.2 mg/kg while an assistant holds cricoid pressure. This combination of medications should provide reliable intubating conditions within 60 seconds. For maintenance of general anesthesia I can use any of the inhalational agents (except for desflurane because of its airway irritating properties), and continue administration of fentanyl as needed.

How will the presence of asthma change your ventilator settings?

Minute ventilation settings should be appropriate for this child's age and weight. However, asthmatic patients with a significant degree of airway obstruction will require a longer than usual expiratory time, and a slower ventilatory rate to allow for complete alveolar emptying. In the worse-case scenario, asthmatic patients can develop air trapping, which can lead to tension pneumothorax. However, this rarely occurs in patients who do not exhibit severe airway obstruction at the time of institution of mechanical ventilation. I would choose a pressure ventilation mode over a volume ventilation mode to minimize abrupt increases in peak inspiratory pressures should bronchospasm occur. It is primarily a matter of personal preference and whether one desires to trigger a ventilator alarm if the peak inspiratory pressure is above a predefined setting, or if the delivered tidal volume is below a predefined limit.

During the procedure, you detect wheezing by auscultation, the capnograph changes to an up-sloping shape, and the delivered tidal volume decreases, all of which indicate the onset of bronchospasm. What will you do?

The likelihood of asthmatic-related bronchospasm in this patient is high, but I will initially rule out other obvious causes such as right main stem bronchial intubation (which often happens when a patient is placed in the Trendelenburg position), and excess secretions in the endotracheal tube. I will increase the concentration of the inhalational agent (within hemodynamic limits), and increase the inhaled oxygen concentration if necessary. If none of these rapidly reverse the wheeze, I will administer inhaled albuterol through the endotracheal tube. The most practical way of doing this intraoperatively is by using a metered-dose inhaler that is connected to the anesthesia breathing circuit between the inspiratory limb and patient Y-piece. This can be performed by inserting the bronchodilator canister into a 60-mL syringe barrel and using the plunger to actuate the medication (Fig. 4-1), or by directly inserting the canister into the breathing circuit using a specialized adapter (Fig. 4-2). Access into the circuit is attained through a removable cap, through which the spray is actuated just prior to a positive-pressure breath. In practice, however, a very low percentage of the bronchodilator actually reaches the lungs because it adheres to the circuit and endotracheal tube. The smaller the diameter of the endotracheal tube, the less actuated medication will actually reach the lungs. Therefore, multiple administrations of albuterol are delivered (usually between 10 and 20) until bronchospasm is relieved, or until the patient develops tachycardia from absorption of the adrenergic agonist.

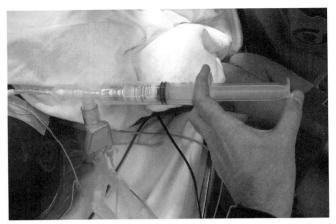

Figure 4-1 The albuterol inhaler can be inserted into a 60-mL syringe and actuated into the anesthesia breathing circuit by pressing on the plunger.

The most common intraoperative cause of bronchospasm in asthmatic children is tracheal stimulation during insertion of an endotracheal tube. Tracheal intubation should be avoided if at all possible in favor of facemask or LMA anesthesia. If tracheal intubation is required, airway reflexes should be suppressed by attaining a sufficiently deep level of general anesthesia prior to endotracheal tube insertion. All inhaled anesthetic agents will accomplish this goal as well as providing some degree of direct bronchodilation, although most pediatric anesthesiologists would not include desflurane in this category because of its irritative effects on the upper and lower airways. Adult studies demonstrate that intravenous induction of general anesthesia with propofol is associated with less bronchospasm than thiopental

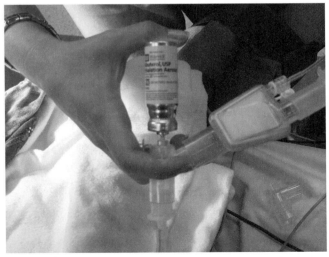

Figure 4-2 The albuterol inhaler can be inserted into an actuator device that is inserted in-line into the anesthesia breathing circuit.

or etomidate. Ketamine is frequently used in asthmatic patients because of its ability to cause bronchodilation by releasing endogenous adrenergic agonists, but there appears to be no advantage over propofol. The use of an opioid or a neuromuscular blocker that causes histamine release (e.g., morphine, mivacurium) is generally avoided; however, there are no data to substantiate this practice. Another theoretical practice is the use of edrophonium instead of neostigmine, which may possess greater tendency to cause bronchoconstriction.

Regional anesthesia is encouraged in patients with asthma. Blunting of the sympathetic response as a result of central regional blockade is not likely to initiate or exacerbate bronchospasm in an asthmatic child since there is no direct adrenergic innervation to human airway smooth muscle.

Bronchiolitis

Bronchiolitis is an acute viral infection of the lower airways that primarily affects children below the age of 2 years. The most common etiologic agent is respiratory syncytial virus (RSV), although most respiratory viruses have been associated with the clinical syndrome of bronchiolitis. Clinical manifestations include wheezing during or after a URI prodrome and varying degrees of respiratory distress. Some infants will exhibit hypoxemia and require oxygen supplementation, bronchodilator therapy, and hospital admission. Children with preexisting bronchopulmonary dysplasia (BPD) or cyanotic congenital heart disease are particularly prone to respiratory failure during an episode of bronchiolitis.

Treatment of bronchiolitis is mainly supportive; endotracheal intubation and mechanical ventilation may be required in children with respiratory failure. Ribavirin is an inhaled antiviral agent, but has equivocal efficacy, and is reserved for children with serious coexisting medical diseases. A history of bronchiolitis during infancy is associated with a higher risk of asthma or wheezing in older children during a URI.

Cystic Fibrosis

Cystic fibrosis (CF) is an autosomal recessive disease that affects approximately 1 in 3000 Caucasian children, and is much less frequent in other racial populations. The basic defect in CF is altered electrolyte secretion and distribution across epithelial membranes. Its major clinical consequences include progressive chronic lung disease, pancreatic destruction with intestinal malabsorption, and progressive liver damage later in life. The lung disease often begins in early childhood and is characterized by increased volume and viscosity of secretions that result in small airway blockage, atelectasis, bronchospasm, pneumothoraces, and frequent

Table 4-3   Classification of Severity of Meconium Aspiration Syndrome (MAS)

Type of MAS	Therapy Required
Mild	<40% oxygen therapy for <48 hours
Moderate	>40% oxygen therapy for >48 hours
Severe	Requirement for mechanical ventilation

antibiotic-resistant bacterial infections. Nasal polyp formation and sinus infections are common. Bronchiectasis develops later in life: occasional bouts of hemoptysis may lead to significant anemia.

Over the past several decades, medical management of this disease has improved significantly, and patients often live well into adulthood. Treatment strategies include chest physical therapy, exercise, and frequent coughing to mobilize secretions. Bronchodilators and anti-inflammatory medications decrease airway reactivity. Bacterial pneumonia requires aggressive antibiotic therapy. Nebulized dornase (Pulmozyme) can be administered to break down thick DNA complexes that are present in mucus due to cell destruction and bacterial infection. Normal growth can often be achieved with pancreatic enzyme replacement, fat-soluble vitamin supplements, and high-calorie high-protein diets.

Common reasons that children with CF require surgery include meconium ileus in the newborn period, nasal polypectomy, and endoscopic sinus surgery. Older or more severely ill children may require anesthesia for placement of indwelling central line access, or gastrostomy tube insertion. Preoperative evaluation of pulmonary function is essential; possible studies include chest radiography, pulmonary function tests, and arterial blood gas analysis. Optimization of infection control and physiotherapy for secretion clearance are priorities, and are coordinated with the child's pulmonologist.

The anesthetic technique of choice for children with CF is controversial. Some advocate use of ketamine because of its minimal effects on ventilatory function; however, others cite ketamine's ability to increase airway secretions, which may worsen respiratory function in patients with CF. Fluid management is also controversial – some pediatric anesthesiologists prefer a liberal fluid strategy to decrease viscosity of bronchial secretions while others advocate minimization of fluids to decrease airway secretions at the expense of increased viscosity. It seems that avoidance of either overhydration or dehydration is the most prudent course of action.

In children with significant pulmonary disease and poor nutritional status, placement of an endotracheal tube and application of mechanical ventilation often entails postoperative transfer to the ICU and the difficult decision-making process concerning the timing and appropriateness of tracheal extubation. Postoperative management should be proactively planned in conjunction with the intensive care physicians, and with the input of the patient and family.

Meconium Aspiration Syndrome

Fetal hypoxia triggers the passage of meconium into the amniotic fluid, which is then swallowed into the oropharynx and aspirated into the trachea and lungs prior to or at the time of birth. Passage of thin meconium in a vigorous, otherwise well neonate can result in mild meconium aspiration syndrome (MAS; Table 4-3). The passage of thick meconium in an asphyxiated newborn can result in moderate or severe MAS. Moderate or severe MAS occurs when aspirated meconium causes bronchial obstruction and pneumonitis, which leads to ventilation/perfusion mismatch and hypoxemia. The presence of meconium in the amniotic fluid warrants aggressive suctioning of the fetal mouth and pharynx prior to delivery, and attempted tracheal suctioning prior to the newborn taking its first breaths. However, when a substantial amount of thick meconium has been aspirated by an asphyxiated infant, peripartum suctioning does not prevent severe MAS.

Hypoxemia and acidosis increase pulmonary vascular resistance and lead to persistent pulmonary hypertension of the newborn (PPHN) (see Chapter 1). Treatment includes optimization of mechanical ventilation and possible institution of extracorporeal membrane oxygenation (ECMO) until lung function returns to normal and PPHN is resolved.

ADDITIONAL ARTICLES TO KNOW

Cohen MM, Cameron CB: Should you cancel the operation when a child has an upper respiratory tract infection? *Anesth Analg* 72:282–288, 1991.

DeSoto H, Patel RI, Soliman IE, Hannallah RS: Changes in oxygen saturation following general anesthesia in children with upper respiratory infection signs and symptoms undergoing otolaryngological procedures. *Anesthesiology* 68:276–279, 1988.

Habre W, Matsumoto I, Sly PD: Propofol or halothane anaesthesia for children with asthma: effects on respiratory mechanics. *Br J Anaesth* 77:739–743, 1996.

Kinouchi K, Tanigami H, Tashiro C et al: Duration of apnea in anesthetized infants and children required for desaturation of hemoglobin to 95%. The influence of upper respiratory infection. *Anesthesiology* 77:1105–1107, 1992.

McGill WA, Coveler LA, Epstein BS: Subacute upper respiratory infection in small children. *Anesth Analg* 58:331–333, 1979.

Schreiner MS, O'Hara I, Markakis DA, Politis GD: Do children who experience laryngospasm have an increased risk of upper respiratory tract infection? *Anesthesiology* 85:475–480, 1997.

Tait AR, Pandit UA, Voepel-Lewis T, Munro HM, Malviya S: Use of the laryngeal mask airway in children with upper respiratory tract infections: a comparison with endotracheal intubation. *Anesth Analg* 86:706–711, 1998.

Warner DO, Warner MA, Barnes RD et al: Perioperative respiratory complications in patients with asthma. *Anesthesiology* 85:460–467, 1997.

Willliams OA, Hills R, Goddard JM: Pulmonary collapse during anaesthesia in children with respiratory tract symptoms. *Anaesthesia* 47:411–413, 1992.

CHAPTER 5

Neurologic and Neuromuscular Diseases

RONALD S. LITMAN
MARY C. THEROUX

Neurologic and neuromuscular disorders represent a substantial percentage of pediatric coexisting disease, and are associated with the need for a variety of surgical procedures during childhood. Cerebral palsy and seizure disorders are very common in the pediatric population, and thus anesthesiologists should be familiar with their clinical characteristics and the pharmacologic agents used for their treatment. Although less common, myopathies are associated with significant morbidity in children, and are noteworthy because of their association with malignant hyperthermia and the potentially catastrophic hyperkalemic response to administration of succinylcholine.

CEREBRAL PALSY

Cerebral palsy (CP) is defined as a static motor encephalopathy. It encompasses a collection of motor system disorders caused by perinatal or early childhood neurological insult (Table 5-1). The incidence of CP in the United States is approximately 0.7 per 1000 live births and is rising. The contribution of very low birthweight infants to this population of children is significant: approximately 52,000 very low birthweight infants (<1500 g) are born annually. These infants make up more than 25% of the children diagnosed with CP.

Children with CP exhibit a wide variety of clinical manifestations that range from mild (e.g., slight lower-extremity spasticity and normal cognitive function) to severe (e.g., spastic quadriplegia and profound mental retardation).

Respiratory system dysfunction usually parallels the overall severity of the disease. Bulbar motor dysfunction causes a loss of normal airway protective mechanisms (cough, gag, etc.) and leads to chronic pulmonary aspiration, recurrent pneumonia, development of reactive airway disease, and parenchymal lung damage. Consequently, children with severe CP will often exhibit a reduced functional residual capacity and lower than normal oxygen saturation. Bulbar dysfunction also causes gastroesophageal symptoms that include gastroesophageal reflux and an inability to swallow oropharyngeal secretions. Gastrostomy tubes are often placed during infancy to optimize nutritional status.

Infants born prematurely may develop areas of brain ischemia secondary to cerebral hemorrhages in the early newborn period. The area of infarction is termed "periventricular leukomalacia" (white matter atrophy surrounding the ventricles) and is associated with development of varying degrees of limb spasticity. Chronic absence of motor input results in progressive development of limb contractures during childhood that worsen with age.

Baclofen, a gamma amino butyric acid (GABA) agonist, reduces pain associated with muscle spasms and slows development of contractures. Most children receive it orally; however, intrathecal administration is possible for severe cases. Side-effects of baclofen include urinary retention and leg weakness, which usually abate when the dose is reduced. Abrupt withdrawal from oral or intrathecal baclofen may cause seizures, hallucinations, disorientation, and dyskinesias. Overdose of baclofen is associated with depressed consciousness and hypotension.

Botulinum toxin is also used to treat spasticity associated with CP. While the child is sedated, it is injected into contracted muscles and produces a functional denervation of the muscle by preventing release of acetylcholine from the presynaptic motor end-plate. This results in a temporary reduction in muscle tone that may

Table 5-1 Types of Cerebral Palsy

Type	Anatomical Location of Pathology	Symptoms
Spastic (most common: 70%)	Cerebrum	Quadriplegia, diplegia, and hemiplegia. The number of extremities affected and the degree of spasticity correlate with level of intelligence.
Dyskinetic	Basal ganglia; associated with kernicterus (severe hyperbilirubinemia in the newborn period).	Dystonia (twisting position of torso), athetosis (purposeless movements of extremities), and chorea (quick, jerky proximal movements of extremities); seizures.
Ataxic	Cerebellum	Tremor, loss of balance and speech.
Mixed	Cerebrum and cerebellum	Spasticity and athetoid movements.

last for months. There are no significant side-effects from its use or known interactions of botulinum toxin with anesthetic agents.

Seizures are present in about 30% of patients with cerebral palsy. Anticonvulsants should be continued until the morning of surgery and reinstituted as quickly as possible during the postoperative period. When it is not feasible to continue oral or gastrostomy anticonvulsant administration, rectal (e.g., phenytoin, valproic acid, and carbamazepine) and intravenous (e.g., phenytoin, valproic acid, and phenobarbital) options are possible. If the surgical procedure causes significant blood loss, anticonvulsant levels should be checked postoperatively, and doses should be adjusted to reestablish optimal levels.

Children with CP are often subjected to numerous surgical interventions during childhood. Orthopedic procedures are the most common and include scoliosis repair, and a variety of limb procedures to improve range of motion and decrease progression of contractures. Dorsal rhizotomy may be required to control painful lower limb spasticity. Nissen fundoplication is performed to control chronic gastroesophageal reflux and may include a feeding gastrostomy. This is now performed by laparoscopy in many centers.

Preoperative assessment includes defining and optimizing all systemic medical illnesses. Concurrent upper respiratory infections are poorly tolerated and exacerbate preexisting respiratory disease. Preoperative anxiolysis should be administered to children who are not cognitively impaired. Some children with CP are prone to upper airway obstruction when consciousness is depressed and should be closely monitored after the administration of the premedication. Administration of an anticholinergic agent may decrease pooling of oropharyngeal secretions.

There are no special considerations when choosing an agent for induction or maintenance of general anesthesia. If a gastrostomy tube is present, the stomach should be evacuated prior to induction of general anesthesia. Because of malformation of facial structures, mask ventilation may be difficult, but endotracheal intubation should be straightforward. Presence of gastroesophageal reflux and increased oropharyngeal secretions may encourage the anesthesiologist to rapidly secure the airway using an intravenous induction agent. Children with cerebral palsy demonstrate increased sensitivity to succinylcholine but do not exhibit excessive potassium release after its use. Nevertheless, succinylcholine should be used only to treat life-threatening airway emergencies. Nondepolarizing muscle relaxants are less potent and have a relatively shorter duration of action in children with CP. This may be related to chronic anticonvulsant administration or underlying spasticity.

Sevoflurane and halothane are relatively more potent (i.e., lower minimum alveolar concentration; MAC) in children with CP. Increased sensitivity to narcotics is present in all but mild forms of cerebral palsy. Doses should be reduced, and greater vigilance at the time of extubation is necessary to ensure the child's ability to maintain a patent upper airway. Hypothermia is a common intraoperative problem in children with CP. Impaired temperature regulation is caused by hypothalamic dysfunction and the patient's absence of muscle and subcutaneous fat.

Postoperative regional analgesia may benefit children with CP who have difficulty communicating the severity of their pain. Addition of epidural clonidine may help reduce postoperative lower-limb spasticity. Oral diazepam 0.2–0.3 mg/kg is used as an adjuvant to help alleviate muscles spasms.

SEIZURE DISORDERS

Seizures are clinical manifestations of a variety of disorders. Febrile seizures represent the most common type of seizure disorder in the pediatric population (5%). Idiopathic epilepsy, which is primarily seen in older children, is much less common, with an estimated incidence of approximately 0.6% of the population.

Trauma, hypoxia, and infection are the primary causes of seizures in infants. Additional causes of seizures in children include metabolic disease, hypoglycemia, electrolyte and metabolic abnormalities, toxic ingestions, and congenital or developmental defects. However, in up to 50% of seizure disorders, the etiology remains unknown.

The currently accepted international classification of epileptic seizures divides these disorders into two broad categories: partial and generalized (Box 5-1). *Partial seizures* are those in which the initial clinical and electroencephalographic (EEG) changes indicate activation of a system of neurons limited to part of one cerebral hemisphere. When consciousness is not impaired, it is labeled a *simple* partial seizure and indicates a unilateral cerebral event. When consciousness is impaired, it is called a *complex* partial seizure and indicates a bilateral cerebral event. Partial seizures can consist of a variety of manifestations that includes motor, sensory, autonomic, or psychic phenomena. With partial seizures, there is usually no specific postictal state. Partial seizures can also exhibit progression to generalized seizure activity.

There are four basic types of *generalized* seizures:
- Absence seizures are also called "petit mal" seizures. They consist of staring spells during which the patient is not responsive, and last usually only a few seconds.
- Myoclonic seizures consist of brief twitching muscle activity that is uncoordinated. There are two types of myoclonic seizures: *epileptic* are those that originate

from cortical or subcortical tissues; *nonepileptic* myoclonus originates from the brainstem or spinal cord and is due to loss of cortical inhibition or impaired function of spinal interneurons.
- Tonic–clonic seizures are those with which most people are familiar. They consist of an initial tonic contraction phase, during which it is common for patients to become apneic and cyanotic from the tonic rigidity of the thoracic cavity. This is followed by the clonic, repetitive twitching phase, where breathing resumes but can be shallow and irregular.
- Atonic seizures are characterized by a state of immobility and unresponsiveness.

Infantile spasms (West syndrome) consist of the triad of unique "salaam-like" seizure movements, arrest of psychomotor development, and a characteristic EEG pattern called "hypsarrhythmia." The onset peaks between 4 and 7 months of age and almost always occurs before 12 months. It can be associated with a known underlying neurological disorder, or can be idiopathic, and is associated with a poor neurodevelopmental outcome. Lennox–Gastaut syndrome consists of different types of seizures which occur frequently and are difficult to control. It usually manifests itself in the 3- to 5-year age group, and is associated with severe mental retardation. Both infantile spasms and Lennox–Gastaut syndrome are notoriously difficult to control with anticonvulsant agents.

There are a variety of treatment regimens that are individualized for each child and the particular type of seizure disorder (Table 5-2). Anesthesiologists should be familiar with the clinical indications and major side-effects of the most commonly used anticonvulsants.

Anesthetic concerns for children with seizure disorders will depend on coexisting morbidities and will be individualized depending on the mental status of the child. If necessary, children who require strict pharmacologic control of their seizure disorder should have their oral anticonvulsants converted to the intravenous forms (or equivalent medications if intravenous forms are not available) during the preanesthetic fasting interval and during the postoperative period if oral intake is not possible. In most cases preanesthetic anticonvulsant levels are not necessary.

Most anesthetic and analgesic agents can be safely administered to children with seizure disorders. A possible exception is multiple doses of meperidine because its metabolite, normeperidine, possesses proconvulsant properties. Nitrous oxide, sevoflurane, methohexital, etomidate, and all opioids have been anecdotally associated with seizure-like movements in both healthy and epileptic patients, without serious sequelae. In most of these cases these movements were likely a benign form of myoclonus. Virtually all general anesthetic agents are anticonvulsants in doses associated with loss of consciousness.

Box 5-1   International Classification of Epileptic Seizures

Partial Seizures

Simple partial (intact consciousness)
    Motor
    Sensory
    Autonomic
    Psychic
    Complex partial (impaired consciousness)

Generalized Seizures

Absence
Tonic
Clonic
Tonic–clonic
Myoclonic
Atonic

Unclassified Seizures

Infantile spasms (West syndrome)
Lennox–Gastaut syndrome

Reproduced with permission from Marino BS, Snead KL, McMillan JA eds: *Blueprints in Pediatrics*, 3rd edn, Blackwell Science Inc., Malden, MA, 2003.

Table 5-2 Indications for and Side-effects of Anticonvulsants

Medication	Indications	Side-effects/Toxicity
Conventional Drugs		
Carbamazepine (Tegretol)	Partial, tonic–clonic	Diplopia, nausea and vomiting, ataxia, leukopenia, thrombocytopenia
Ethosuximide (Zarontin)	Absence	Rash, anorexia, leukopenia, aplastic anemia
Phenobarbital (Luminal)	Tonic–clonic, partial	Hyperactivity, sedation, nystagmus, ataxia
Phenytoin (Dilantin)	Tonic–clonic, partial	Rash, nystagmus, ataxia, drug-induced lupus, gingival hyperplasia, anemia, leukopenia, polyneuropathy
Valproic acid (Depakene, Depakote)	Tonic–clonic, partial, absence	Hepatotoxicity, nausea and vomiting, abdominal pain, weight loss, weight gain, anemia, leukopenia, thrombocytopenia
Recently Developed Drugs		
Gabapentin (Neurontin)	Partial	Somnolence, dizziness, ataxia, fatigue
Lamotrigine (Lamictal)	Tonic–clonic, partial, absence, Lennox–Gastaut syndrome	Dizziness, ataxia, blurred or double vision, nausea, vomiting, and rash. A few cases of Stevens–Johnson syndrome reported.
Levetiracetam (Keppra)	Partial	Somnolence, asthenia, dizziness
Tiagabine (Gabitril)	Partial	Dizziness, somnolence, and tremor. May make absence epilepsy worse
Topiramate (Topamax)	Tonic–clonic, partial, Lennox–Gastaut syndrome, infantile spasms	Somnolence, fatigue, weight loss, nervousness

Reproduced with permission from Marino BS, Snead KL, McMillan JA eds: *Blueprints in Pediatrics*, 3rd edn, Blackwell Science Inc., Malden, MA, 2003.

Higher doses and shorter dosing intervals of neuromuscular blockers are required in patients taking anticonvulsant medications. The precise mechanism of this phenomenon has not been elucidated. However, this resistance is not as prominent for those neuromuscular blockers that are metabolized in the plasma (i.e., atracurium, mivacurium), so it may be related to a pharmacokinetic effect based in the liver. There is also some data and clinical experience indicating that anticonvulsants may cause some resistance to opioids. Although definitive data are lacking, it does not appear that general anesthesia impacts the subsequent frequency or severity of seizures postoperatively.

NEUROMUSCULAR DISEASES

Neuromuscular diseases can be broadly divided into disorders of the muscle, and disorders of neuromuscular transmission (Box 5-2). Muscle diseases can be further categorized into developmental myopathies, muscular dystrophies, and metabolic myopathies. Disorders of neuromuscular transmission can be further categorized into diseases of the neuromuscular junction and anterior horn cell diseases. This list is extensive and only the most common and most important in pediatric anesthesia will be reviewed here.

Muscle diseases, or *myopathies*, are characterized by muscle weakness and atrophy. Many children are symptomatic at birth, while others are normal in early infancy

Box 5-2 Classification of Neuromuscular Diseases of Childhood

Muscle Diseases

Developmental
  Nemaline rod myopathy
  Central core myopathy
  Myotubular myopathy
Muscular dystrophies
  Duchenne muscular dystrophy
  Becker muscular dystrophy
  Myotonic dystrophy
  Limb-girdle muscular dystrophy
  Facioscapulohumeral muscular dystrophy
  Congenital muscular dystrophy
Metabolic myopathies
  Potassium-related periodic paralysis
  Glycogenoses
  Mitochondrial myopathies
  Lipid myopathies

Diseases of Neuromuscular Transmission

Neuromuscular junction disorders
  Myasthenia gravis
  Organophosphate poisoning
  Botulism
  Tick paralysis
Anterior horn cell diseases
  Spinal muscular atrophies (SMA)
  Poliomyelitis

only to develop weakness in the first few years of life. The myopathies are of interest to anesthesiologists for two major reasons. First, some are associated with an increased risk of malignant hyperthermia (see Chapter 21); and second, all are associated with development of life-threatening hyperkalemia after administration of succinylcholine (see Chapter 19). Children with myopathies often require multiple surgical procedures throughout childhood. These include a muscle biopsy as a component of the diagnostic work-up, insertion of a gastrostomy or tracheostomy as weakness worsens, and a variety of orthopedic procedures for alleviation of contractures and scoliosis.

As with neurological diseases, anesthetic considerations for children with muscle diseases will largely depend on the medical condition of the child, as there is a wide spectrum of affliction, even between children with the same diagnosis. Even though central core myopathy is one of the only diseases genetically linked to malignant hyperthermia, most pediatric anesthesiologists will perform a nontriggering anesthetic technique for all children with myopathies. Use of nondepolarizing muscle relaxants will depend on the baseline strength of the child. Careful titration of the neuromuscular blocker based on train-of-four monitoring is recommended. Children with muscle weakness are at increased risk for requiring postoperative mechanical ventilation, and thus, this possibility should be proactively addressed with the parents and child if appropriate.

Developmental Myopathies

The developmental myopathies consist of a heterogeneous group of congenital myopathies that are mostly nonprogressive, although some patients show slow clinical deterioration. Most of these conditions are hereditary; others are sporadic. These include nemaline rod myopathy, central core myopathy (CCM), and myotubular myopathy. CCM is an autosomal dominant disease characterized by hypotonia and proximal weakness at birth. Unlike other muscle diseases, there appears to be a predisposition of CCM patients to malignant hyperthermia susceptibility in the form of a genetic linkage to the ryanodine receptor on chromosome 19. However, the literature is conflicting, and the subject of myopathies and susceptibility to malignant hyperthermia continues to evolve.

Muscular Dystrophies

Although the muscular dystrophies are a group of unrelated disorders, there are four obligatory criteria that distinguish them from other neuromuscular diseases:
(1) It is a primary myopathy.
(2) It has a genetic basis.

(3) The course is progressive.
(4) Degeneration and death of muscle fibers occur at some stage in the disease.

Duchenne-type muscular dystrophy (DMD) is an X-linked recessive disease that, although present at birth, usually presents in early childhood as weakness and motor delay. Additional clinical manifestations include pseudohypertrophy of the calves and markedly elevated baseline creatine phosphokinase (CPK). Since weakness is greatest in the proximal muscle groups, the child must rise from the sitting position in two steps: first leaning on the hypertrophied calves and then pushing the trunk up with the arms. This is referred to as Gower's sign, and is nearly pathognomonic for one of the muscular dystrophies. Eventually, progressive and severe muscle atrophy and weakness cause loss of the ability to ambulate. The most serious aspects of DMD include a progressive cardiomyopathy and respiratory failure secondary to ventilatory pump failure. Cognitive abnormalities are usually mild. Most children become wheelchair-bound early in the second decade, with death before age 30 from either respiratory failure or cardiomyopathy.

Although no definitive genetic link to malignant hyperthermia has been found, most pediatric anesthesiologists consider these children to be MH-susceptible based on anecdotal reports, and will perform a nontriggering technique. However, as stated above for CCM, definitive proof of association between myopathies and MH susceptibility is lacking. Use of inhalational agents, albeit for a relatively short period of time, appears to be safe when intravenous access is not available.

A less severe (yet debilitating) related disease is the Becker-type muscular dystrophy. Similar features to DMD include calf pseudohypertrophy, cardiomyopathy, and elevated serum levels of CPK. However, the onset of weakness in Becker-type dystrophy is later in life than with DMD, and death often occurs at a later age than with DMD. The anesthetic considerations are identical to those for DMD.

Myotonic dystrophy is an autosomal dominant muscular dystrophy that is characterized by the persistent contracture of both striated and smooth muscle after its stimulation. Myotonia refers to the slow relaxation of a contracted muscle and is observed in children over the age of 5 years. All muscle tissues in every organ system are affected, leading to widespread disease that begins mildly in the neonatal period but progresses throughout childhood. Additional clinical manifestations include cardiac, respiratory, and gastrointestinal dysfunction, endocrinopathies, immunologic deficiencies, cataracts, dysmorphic facies, intellectual impairment, and other neurologic abnormalities. Succinylcholine and cholinesterase inhibitors will exacerbate the myotonia.

Case

An 11-month-old female is scheduled for a diagnostic muscle biopsy and open gastrostomy tube insertion. She has a history of hypotonia, developmental delay, and failure to thrive secondary to poor feeding effort. Chromosomal analysis is normal, and her physicians suspect she may have a mitochondrial myopathy.

What is a mitochondrial myopathy? Is it associated with unique considerations for administration of general anesthesia?

A mitochondrial myopathy is a type of genetic disease that is encompassed within a broad category of entities whose origin is a defect in mitochondrial function, and thus interfere with normal adenosine triphosphate (ATP) production. Although mitochondrial defects can affect almost every organ system, those organs with high metabolic rates – such as the heart, brain, and skeletal muscle – are particularly vulnerable. ATP depletion results in accumulation of lactate, a byproduct of anaerobic metabolism. Clinical manifestations include abnormalities of the heart (e.g., cardiomyopathy, conduction defects), skeletal muscle (e.g., atrophy, weakness), and central nervous system (e.g., seizures, encephalopathy, peripheral neuropathies, ophthalmologic manifestations), among many others. Examples of mitochondrial diseases include chronic progressive external ophthalmoplegia, Kearns–Sayre syndrome, Leigh's disease, Leber's hereditary optic neuropathy (LHON), mitochondrial myopathy, and myoclonic epilepsy with lactic acidosis and stroke-like episodes (MELAS syndrome). Treatment options are limited, and primarily supportive. Carnitine may lessen muscle weakness and fatigue in some children, and does not interact with anesthetic agents.

Preanesthetic assessment of a child with a suspected or confirmed mitochondrial disease includes evaluation of comorbidities – in particular, cardiac, respiratory, hepatic, and renal function. Premedication should be tailored to the individual patient; respiratory depressants should be avoided in children with weak ventilatory drive. The overall goal of anesthetic management is avoidance of metabolic stressors, such as hypoxemia and hypoglycemia, which may potentially exacerbate lactic acidosis. Clear glucose-containing liquids should be administered 2 hours prior to the anticipated induction of anesthesia. All anesthetic agents have been used safely in patients with mitochondrial diseases, although prolonged use of propofol should be avoided because of its association with lactic acidosis in the critical care setting. Neuromuscular blockers should be carefully titrated to maintain one or two twitches on train-of-four monitoring, as patients with myopathies may demonstrate a unique sensitivity to these drugs. Steroidal neuromuscular blockers, which depend on adequate liver function for metabolism and termination of action, should probably be avoided.

Should this patient be considered malignant hyperthermia (MH)-susceptible?

There is no definitive genetic link between mitochondrial disease and MH susceptibility. In the presence of muscle atrophy, elective use of succinylcholine is contraindicated, as it may cause life-threatening hyperkalemia. Inhalational agents have been used safely in patients with mitochondrial diseases.

How would you induce and maintain general anesthesia? Is a muscle relaxant necessary?

Induction and maintenance of general anesthesia will be routine: inhaled sevoflurane and N$_2$O for induction of anesthesia, or an intravenous induction agent if the child has intravenous access. Since this child has preexisting hypotonia, I don't expect that he will be able to adequately ventilate and oxygenate using a spontaneous ventilation technique. Therefore, I will likely use controlled ventilation, using either a laryngeal mask airway (LMA) or an endotracheal tube. Depending on the severity of the child's hypotonia, I may choose to omit neuromuscular blockade from the induction regimen, since there are no surgical requirements for paralysis.

What are appropriate extubation criteria for this patient?

Extubation criteria for patients with hypotonia or developmental delay are ill-defined. The three criteria that are used in healthy children are: (1) sufficient muscle strength to maintain upper airway patency; (2) a regular respiratory pattern; and (3) wakefulness (e.g., spontaneous eye opening, following commands). The child in this case may demonstrate abnormalities for one or more of these criteria. Tracheal extubation will therefore become incumbent on the child attaining their preoperative or baseline parameters.

Spinal Muscle Atrophy

Spinal muscle atrophy (SMA) is an inherited autosomal recessive disorder characterized by anterior horn cell degeneration and is found as three clinical syndromes. Type 1 is called Werdnig–Hoffman disease and is the most severe beginning in early infancy. It is characterized by significant muscle weakness and atrophy, except for diaphragmatic sparing which occurs later in life. Type 2 presents at between 6 and 12 months of age and has a more prolonged, slightly milder course. Type 3 is the least debilitating and is called Kugelberg–Welander disease. Cognitive abilities remain unaffected in all forms of the illness. Life-expectancies vary with the severity of the disease; death occurs from repeated aspiration or lung infections.

ARTICLES TO KNOW

Brenn BR, Brislin RP, Rose JB: Epidural analgesia in children with cerebral palsy. *Can J Anaesth* 45:1156–1161, 1998.

Choudhry DK, Brenn BR: Bispectral index monitoring: a comparison between normal children and children with quadriplegic cerebral palsy. *Anesth Analg* 95:1582–1585, 2002.

Keyes MA, Van de Wiele BV, Stead SW: Mitochondrial myopathies: an unusual cause of hypotonia in infants and children. *Paediatr Anaesth* 6:329–335, 1996.

Theroux MC, Brandom B, Zagnoev M et al: Dose response of succinylcholine at the adductor pollicis in anesthetized children with cerebral palsy during propofol and nitrous oxide anesthesia. *Anesth Analg* 79:761–765, 1994.

Theroux MC, Akins RE, Barone C et al: Neuromuscular junctions in cerebral palsy: presence of extrajunctional acetylcholine receptors. *Anesthesiology* 96:330–335, 2002.

Wallace JJ, Perndt H, Skinner M: Anaesthesia and mitochondrial disease. *Paediatr Anaesth* 8:249–254, 1998.

CHAPTER 6

Gastrointestinal Diseases

RONALD S. LITMAN

Gastroesophageal Reflux
Inflammatory Bowel Disease
Neonatal Hyperbilirubinemia
Chronic Liver Disease

Most serious gastrointestinal diseases in children are surgical in nature and are discussed in detail in Chapter 28. In this chapter common pediatric medical diseases of the digestive tract are reviewed. These include gastroesophageal reflux, inflammatory bowel disease, neonatal hyperbilirubinemia, and chronic liver disease.

GASTROESOPHAGEAL REFLUX

In gastroesophageal reflux (GER), the lower esophageal sphincter is incompetent and the child regurgitates recently ingested meals. It is very common in the first year of life, especially in children born prematurely, and is commonly seen in children with respiratory disorders such as asthma and bronchopulmonary dysplasia. Children with GER related to neuromuscular disorders, such as cerebral palsy, will continue to reflux throughout childhood. Because of weakened airway protective mechanisms, these children will demonstrate chronic pulmonary aspiration that results in repeated episodes of pneumonitis and chronic hypoxemia. Some children will have undergone a Nissen fundoplication, a surgical "tightening" of the lower esophageal sphincter, to prevent chronic GER.

Many anesthesiologists assume that children with GER are at risk for pulmonary aspiration on induction of anesthesia, and will therefore opt for a rapid sequence induction. But in order to do so, an IV catheter must be placed preoperatively, which is not a routine procedure in most pediatric centers. This practice also obligates the placement of an endotracheal tube instead of facemask or LMA anesthesia. However, no data exist to justify this practice. Studies that assessed residual gastric volumes

after a normal preanesthetic fast have demonstrated no differences between children with GER and normal controls. This author's opinion is that GER occurs only when there is food in the stomach of susceptible children, and when these children are fasted normally, gastric volumes at induction of anesthesia are low and do not pose an increased risk for pulmonary aspiration.

There are additional valid reasons for not performing a rapid sequence induction of general anesthesia in children with GER. Firstly, the performance of cricoid pressure reflexively decreases lower esophageal pressure, thus promoting passive regurgitation of gastric contents. Second, paralysis or relaxation of the cricopharyngeus muscle (a striated skeletal muscle) that forms the upper esophageal sphincter may allow passively regurgitated gastric contents to reach the larynx. Lastly, acid reflux into the lower third of the esophagus reflexively causes an increase in upper esophageal sphincter tone, which would not occur in the presence of neuromuscular blockade.

INFLAMMATORY BOWEL DISEASE

Inflammatory bowel disease (IBD) primarily consists of Crohn's disease and ulcerative colitis (UC). Crohn's disease is a chronic inflammatory bowel disease that is seen in older children and young adults. Clinical manifestations include diarrhea, abdominal pain, rectal bleeding, anal fistulas, anemia, and weight loss. Extraintestinal manifestations include joint pain and swelling, growth failure and delayed puberty. Therapy includes administration of 5-aminosalicylic acid (5-ASA) preparations (e.g., sulfasalazine, olsalazine, mesalamine), steroids, immunosuppressants, and anti-inflammatory cytokines (e.g., interleukins).

Ulcerative colitis is characterized by intermittent bouts of inflammation of the large intestine that are manifest clinically as abdominal cramping, diarrhea, and bloody stools. Associated systemic findings include anorexia, weight loss, low-grade fever, and mild anemia. Severe cases of colitis can result in hypoalbuminemia and toxic megacolon. Approximately 20% of cases of UC present during childhood. As with Crohn's disease, the primary therapeutic options are anti-inflammatory therapy with 5-ASA preparations, steroids, and immuno-suppressants.

Children with IBD are subjected to repeated colono-scopies during the course of their disease, for which general anesthesia or deep sedation is required. In Crohn's disease, surgery is indicated when medical therapy has failed or when microperforations have resulted in abscesses, strictures, and obstruction. Intestinal or colonic resections are palliative but not curative. In UC, surgery is indicated for intractable colitis and toxic megacolon with peritonitis, or to prevent or treat malignancy. Since UC is confined to the large intestine, colectomy is considered curative.

There are no unique anesthetic considerations for children with IBD. Epidural analgesia is indicated for postoperative analgesia in selected patients. Anecdotal (and unproven) data indicate that these children require higher than usual amounts of opioids. This may be related to tolerance from intermittent or chronic opioid use.

NEONATAL HYPERBILIRUBINEMIA

In the first week of life, unconjugated (indirect) hyperbilirubinemia occurs because of the breakdown of fetal erythrocytes in combination with low activity of glucuronyl transferase, the enzyme responsible for conjugation of bilirubin to glucuronic acid. It is manifested clinically as jaundice of the skin and sclera, and is most prominent after the third day of life, in prematurely born infants, and in term breast-fed infants. Concomitant medical disorders that cause hemolysis and contribute to hyperbilirubinemia in an additive fashion include hemolytic disease of the newborn, spherocytosis, G-6-PD deficiency, and the presence of a cephalohematoma.

Treatment is indicated when serum bilirubin levels rise excessively. The potential for neurotoxicity of the developing brain (kernicterus) is historically associated with bilirubin levels greater than 20 mg/dL in full-term infants. Prematurity, hypoxemia, acidosis, and hypothermia increase the likelihood of kernicterus in the presence of hyperbilirubinemia. Phototherapy is the primary

initial treatment; exchange transfusions are required in accelerated cases. Bilirubin values that trigger phototherapy or exchange transfusion vary widely between institutions.

CHRONIC LIVER DISEASE

Chronic liver disease in children is most commonly associated with congenital biliary atresia for which a Kasai procedure (see Chapter 28) or a liver transplant is required. Other possible causes include α_1-antitrypsin deficiency, cystic fibrosis, tyrosinemia, and Wilson's disease, among others. Clinical manifestations will depend on the remaining degree of liver function and will include ascites, portal hypertension (with esophageal varices), and coagulopathy. Respiratory insufficiency in children with advanced liver disease is caused by loss of functional residual capacity (FRC) from the mass effect of ascites or hepatomegaly, and creation of intrapulmonary shunts (hepatopulmonary syndrome). Fulminant hepatic failure is associated with encephalopathy and increased intracranial pressure (see Chapter 38).

Principles of anesthetic management are centered on avoidance of medications that are metabolized in the liver (e.g., steroidal neuromuscular blockers) and will have an abnormally increased duration of action. All inhalational agents except for halothane demonstrate minimal liver metabolism and reduced hepatic blood flow to a similar extent. Because of halothane's extensive metabolism (20%), and its association with halothane hepatitis, it is relatively contraindicated in children with preexisting liver disease.

ARTICLES TO KNOW

American Academy of Pediatrics practice parameter: Management of hyperbilirubinemia in the healthy term newborn. *Pediatrics* 94:558–565, 1994.

Cuffari C, Darbari A: Inflammatory bowel disease in the pediatric and adolescent patient. *Gastroenterol Clin N Am* 31:275–291, 2002.

Gesink-van der Veer BJ, Burm AG, Vletter AA, Bovill JG: Influence of Crohn's disease on the pharmacokinetics and pharmacodynamics of alfentanil. *Br J Anaesth* 71:827–834, 1993.

Meunier JF, Goujard E, Dubousset AM, Samii K, Mazoit JX: Pharmacokinetics of bupivacaine after continuous epidural infusion in infants with and without biliary atresia. *Anesthesiology* 95:87–95, 2001.

CHAPTER 7

Hematologic Diseases

RONALD S. LITMAN

CATHERINE S. MANNO

This chapter covers the two main classes of hematologic diseases that are common in children: inherited coagulation disorders such as von Willebrand disease and hemophilia, and the hemoglobinopathies, including sickle cell disease and thalassemia. Leukemia is discussed in the chapter on oncological diseases (Chapter 8).

INHERITED COAGULATION DISORDERS

Hemophilia

The hemophilias are a group of X-linked inherited bleeding disorders in which there is insufficient production of functional coagulation factor VIII or factor IX. The best known is hemophilia A, which results from a deficiency of factor VIII and occurs in approximately 1 per 10,000 males. Hemophilia B, which results from a deficiency of factor IX, occurs in 1 per 25,000 males. Some female carriers produce low concentrations of these factors, which can predispose to excessive bleeding. Clinically, adequate clotting usually occurs with 30% of normal factor levels.

In hemophilia, formation of the platelet plug (primary hemostasis) is normal; however, stabilization of the plug by fibrin (secondary hemostasis) is defective because an insufficient amount of factor VIII or IX causes a delay in the production of thrombin, which is necessary for the conversion of fibrinogen to fibrin. Diagnosis is confirmed by family history, or by demonstration of a prolonged partial thromboplastin time (PTT) plus low functional concentrations of factor VIII or factor IX.

The clinical manifestations of hemophilia A and B are indistinguishable. The severity of each disorder is determined by the degree of factor deficiency (Table 7-1). Mild hemophilia may go undiagnosed for many years, whereas severe hemophilia manifests during early infancy as a result of a traumatic delivery or bleeding after circumcision. The remainder of children are asymptomatic until they begin to crawl or walk. Severe hemophilia is characterized by spontaneous or traumatic hemorrhages, which can be subcutaneous, intramuscular, or within joints (hemarthroses). Hemarthroses are exquisitely painful, and result in synovial inflammation, chronic scarring, and disability.

Hemophilia is treated by administration of the appropriate coagulation factor. Currently, these factors are produced by recombinant technology and are not associated with infectious complications. However, prior to the 1990s, coagulation factor replacements were derived from pooled plasma, which contained viral contaminants such as human immunodeficiency virus (HIV) and those causing hepatitis. Between 1979 and 1984, 80% of US patients with hemophilia who received plasma-derived factor products became HIV seropositive. HIV infection is the most common cause of death in older patients with hemophilia.

In the United States, the majority of children with hemophilia are treated with prophylactic therapy, which consists of factor administration at regular intervals to prevent spontaneous bleeds. A minority of severe hemophiliacs are administered factor only during acute bleeding episodes. In general, for mild to moderate bleeding episodes, such as hemarthroses, coagulation factor activity should be raised to 40% of normal. For life-threatening

Table 7-1   Classification and Symptoms of Hemophilia

Concentration of Factor (VIII or IX)	Classification	Clinical Manifestations
<0.01 IU/mL (<1% of normal)	Severe	Spontaneous joint and muscle bleeding; bleeding after injuries, accidents and surgery
0.01–0.05 IU/mL (1–5% of normal)	Moderate	Bleeding into joints and muscles after minor injuries; excessive bleeding after surgery and dental extractions
>0.05–0.40 IU/mL (5–40% of normal)	Mild	No spontaneous bleeding; bleeding after surgery, dental extractions and accidents

Reproduced with permission from Bolton-Maggs PH, Pasi KJ: Haemophilias A and B, *Lancet* 361(9371):1801–1809, 2003.

bleeding, such as during major trauma or surgery, coagulation factor activity is raised to 80–100% of normal. The recommended perioperative treatment strategy will vary depending on the type of surgical procedure, and the relative risks and complications of postoperative bleeding. For example, following joint surgery, 100% correction is continued into the postoperative period because bleeding into the joint is a critical complication (Box 7-1). Following tonsillectomy, 100% correction is continued until the eschar has fallen off (approximately 8 days).

Factor doses are calculated as follows:

Dose of factor VIII (units)
= desired rise in % factor activity × weight (kg) × 2

Dose of *plasma-derived* factor IX (units)
= desired rise in % factor activity × weight (kg) × 1

Box 7-1   Example of Perioperative Hemophilia Management for Elbow Synovectomy

1. Administer factor to 100% correction 15–30 minutes prior to the start of surgery.
2. Administer factor to 100% correction immediately postoperatively (approximately two-thirds of initial dose).
3. Administer factor to 50% correction (half of initial dose) 6 hours after the initial postoperative dose and continue every 6 hours for 24 hours, then every 8 hours for an additional 24 hours.
4. Continue to administer factor to 50% correction every 12 hours until hospital discharge.
5. After discharge to home, administer factor to 50% correction every 12 hours for 10 days; then administer factor to 100% correction once a day for 4 days; then resume normal prophylactic regimen.

Reproduced with permission from Montgomery RR, Gill JC, Scott JP: Hemophilia and von Willebrand disease. In Nathan DG, Orkin SH eds: *Hematology of Infancy and Childhood*, 5th edn, WB Saunders, Philadelphia, 1998.

Dose of *recombinant* factor IX (units)
= desired rise in % factor activity × weight (kg) × 1.4

Desmopressin acetate (DDAVP), a synthetic vasopressin analogue, causes release of factor VIII from endothelial cells, and has also been used effectively for prevention or treatment of bleeding episodes associated with mild hemophilia A. A trial administration to demonstrate that a rise in factor VIII levels occurs in a particular individual is recommended before using DDAVP in the perioperative setting.

Up to 50% of patients with hemophilia A and 3–5% of patients with hemophilia B develop an immune response to the administered coagulation factors, with development of IgG antibodies against factor VIII or IX. These antibodies are called "inhibitors" and significantly complicate therapy by preventing the normal response to coagulation factor administration.

Von Willebrand Disease

Present in up to 1% of the population, von Willebrand disease (vWD) is the most common hereditary bleeding disorder. It results from a deficiency of von Willebrand factor (vWF), a glycoprotein synthesized by endothelial cells and megakaryocytes. vWF is involved with primary hemostasis by acting as an adhesive bridge between the platelets and damaged subendothelium at the site of vascular injury. It is involved with secondary hemostasis by functioning as the carrier protein for factor VIII.

There are multiple forms of vWD:

- *Type 1* (>85% of cases) is associated with quantitative reductions in all multimeric sizes of vWF. There is a wide variation of clinical manifestations, even for members of the same family. Children with type 1 vWD may be asymptomatic, or may have a history of frequent nosebleeds, mucosal bleeding, and easy bruising. A history of excessive bleeding during menses, or after mucosal surgery such as tonsillectomy or wisdom tooth extraction, is common. These patients are usually responsive to treatment with DDAVP.

- *Type 2* is associated with quantitative and qualitative abnormalities of vWF, and accounts for 10% of cases. There are various forms of type 2 vWD, depending on the mode of inheritance and the particular structural abnormality. Some forms are associated with thrombocytopenia. In general, these patients are not responsive to DDAVP therapy, so they require replacement of vWF.
- *Type 3* is the rarest and most severe form that is associated with major bleeding (similar to moderate hemophilia) requiring treatment with vWF-containing concentrates. Patients have little or no functional vWF.

Laboratory screening may reveal a prolonged bleeding time (>9 minutes) and a prolonged partial thromboplastin time (PTT), but in many children screening coagulation testing is normal. More directed tests for vWD include a quantitative assay for vWF antigen, vWF (ristocetin cofactor) activity, plasma factor VIII activity, determination of vWF structure, and a platelet count (decreased in type 2B vWD).

Replacement of vWF can be accomplished using plasma-derived factor VIII concentrates that retain vWF activity (e.g., Humate-P). Most commonly, however, children with type 1 vWD are pretreated 30 minutes prior to surgery with intravenous DDAVP, 0.3 µg/kg, which induces endothelial cells to release intracellular stores of the highest-molecular-weight vWF multimers. Additional doses can be administered 12 hours postoperatively, and the next morning after surgery. In the case of tonsillectomy, an additional dose is administered 8 days postoperatively, when the eschar is expected to fall off. DDAVP is not used in patients with type 2 or type 3 vWD. In these patients, plasma-derived factor VIII concentrate with vWF is administered preoperatively and for 1 week postoperatively in tonsillectomy patients. Careful consideration should be given to the indications for mucous membrane surgery in children with types 2B or 3 vWD and surgery avoided if possible.

HEMOGLOBINOPATHIES

The understanding of hemoglobinopathies requires knowledge of the structure and function of the hemoglobin molecule. All normal forms of hemoglobin contain a tetramer consisting of two α polypeptide (globin) chains and two non-α chains. The non-α chains vary by the stage of maturation. For example, fetal hemoglobin (hemoglobin F) is composed of two α chains and two γ chains, whereas adult hemoglobin (hemoglobin A) consists of two α and two β chains. Each globin chain binds one heme group. A heme group consists of a porphyrin ring and a ferrous atom that binds to an oxygen molecule.

Sickle Cell Disease

Sickle cell disease, which occurs in approximately 1 in 650 (0.15%) African Americans, is an autosomal recessive disorder that results when an S-type β globin gene is inherited from each parent. This results in the formation of hemoglobin that contains a valine-for-glutamine substitution in position 6 of the β globin chain. Under conditions of deoxygenation, the altered hemoglobin assumes an abnormal sickled shape and aggregates, which predisposes the cells to abnormal motility characteristics and hemolysis. Specifically, the sickled red cell membrane becomes more permeable to sodium, potassium, magnesium, and calcium ions, and the sickled shape of the red cell more easily adheres to capillary endothelium resulting in occlusion of small capillaries. Formation of sickled cells is promoted by hypoxemia, acidosis, hypothermia, dehydration, and hypotension, thus leading to reduction of perfusion in the peripheral tissues.

The heterozygous state, in which a child inherits a single affected β globin gene, is called "sickle cell trait" and is found in approximately 8% of African Americans. It does not cause anemia or red cell fragility. Rarely, an individual with sickle trait will exhibit painless hematuria and the inability to properly concentrate the urine (isosthenuria).

Clinical Syndromes in Sickle Cell Disease

Children with sickle cell disease exhibit a number of clinical syndromes, all of which are caused by aggregation of sickled red cells in small vessels, or hemolysis and decreased survival of abnormal red cells.

Painful vaso-occlusive crises are the hallmarks of sickle cell disease during childhood. Pain results from vascular occlusion and resultant ischemia, and can be seen in bony or soft tissues. Precipitating factors include infection, fever, cold exposure, dehydration, venous stasis, and acidosis. Dactylitis, or hand–foot syndrome, is painful swelling of the dorsal surface of the hands and feet caused by vaso-occlusion of the metacarpal and metatarsal bones. It is often the initial clinical manifestation of sickle cell disease in the first year of life. Older children typically develop pain crises in the long bones of the arms, legs, vertebral column, and sternum. Pain episodes typically last up to a week and may warrant hospitalization for administration of nonsteroidal anti-inflammatory drugs (NSAIDs), opioid analgesics, and rarely regional analgesia.

Hemolytic anemia becomes apparent at approximately 4–6 months of age when the percentage of hemoglobin F diminishes and that of hemoglobin S rises. The anemia of sickle cell disease is chronic and well-compensated, and does not require red cell transfusion except during life-threatening complications such as aplastic crises, splenic sequestration, acute chest syndrome, or in preparation for major surgery. The hemolytic anemia is responsible for development of gallstone formation and cholecystitis.

Splenic sequestration of sickled red blood cells typically occurs at between 6 months and 2 years of age. It can lead to splenomegaly, acute exacerbation of anemia, and possibly hypovolemic shock. Splenic dysfunction occurs from repeated episodes of splenic infarction during childhood and results in susceptibility to sepsis from encapsulated organisms such as *Streptococcus pneumoniae* and *Haemophilus influenzae*. Children with sickle cell disease routinely receive vaccination against these organisms as well as daily penicillin prophylaxis.

Aplastic crises are typically caused by temporary cessation of red blood cell production in the bone marrow, and are most often associated with parvovirus B-19 infection. Symptomatic anemia is treated with hospitalization and red cell transfusion.

Acute chest syndrome is a vaso-occlusive crisis within the lungs precipitated by pulmonary infection and infarction. Patients present with severe chest pain, fever, respiratory distress, new pulmonary infiltrates, and hypoxia. Oxygen, analgesia, antibiotics, and red cell transfusion are used to maximize respiratory function and minimize further pulmonary damage. Pulmonary complications account for a large proportion of morbidity and mortality in patients with sickle cell disease.

During childhood, a substantial number of children with sickle cell disease will develop reactive airway disease and progressive pulmonary dysfunction. Up to 40% of adult patients develop moderate to severe pulmonary hypertension, which is associated with an increased mortality rate.

Stroke is caused by vaso-occlusion of the middle-sized cerebral vessels. Patients present with mental status changes, seizures, and focal paralysis (e.g., hemiparesis). Children who have had a stroke are placed on a chronic red cell transfusion protocol to maintain a hemoglobin S below 30% and minimize the risk of future strokes. Recently, the use of transcranial Doppler imaging, which measures the velocity of cerebral blood flow, has allowed clinicians to detect which children are at risk for a first stroke. These children then receive prophylactic red cell transfusions, although the optimal duration of transfusion in such children is unknown.

Additional complications of sickle cell disease include priapism (in boys older than 6 years of age), retinopathy, leg ulcers, and progressive renal failure. By adolescence the effects of chronic myocardial microvascular obstruction and anemia result in ventricular hypertrophy. Microvascular obstruction of the intestinal circulation results in abdominal crises that manifest as signs and symptoms of an acute abdomen.

Treatment

Principles of treatment of sickle cell crises include volume support, administration of antimicrobial agents, prevention or reversal of anemia, hypothermia, hypoperfusion, acidosis, and pulmonary dysfunction. Hydration decreases blood viscosity and helps prevent capillary stasis. Red cell transfusion is an important aspect of sickle cell treatment because it increases the amount of hemoglobin A, while reducing the proportion of the patient's own hemoglobin S, which is responsible for sickling. Red cell transfusions are targeted to a hemoglobin level of 10–12 g/dL; higher hemoglobin levels will unnecessarily increase blood viscosity. Exchange transfusion to reduce the hemoglobin S level to less than 30% is used in the context of life-threatening vaso-occlusive episodes such as stroke and acute chest syndrome accompanied by hypoxemia that does not resolve with simple red cell transfusion.

Perianesthetic Management of Children with Sickle Cell Disease

Historically, patients with sickle cell anemia have not fared well in the perioperative period. Perioperative development of hypoxemia, hypotension, hypothermia, hypovolemia, and acidosis is associated with exacerbation of vaso-occlusive events, and should be avoided in these patients. Preoperatively, all medical problems should be optimized prior to elective surgery. Except for extremely short and minor procedures, red cells should be administered to achieve a hemoglobin level of 10 g/dL. During general anesthesia, all measures are taken to avoid hypothermia and hypovolemia. Mild hypoxemia or acidosis will precipitate a vaso-occlusive crisis and should be prevented or, upon occurrence, rapidly reversed. The use of a tourniquet during limb surgery is discouraged because of the possibility of precipitating distal limb hypoxia, hypothermia, and acidosis; however, poor outcomes after tourniquet use in these patients have not been systematically proven. When appropriate, regional analgesic techniques are recommended for management of postoperative pain to reduce acute painful crises, to enhance respiratory function, and to minimize opioid use in the postoperative period. Postoperative mortality is often related to development of severe acute chest syndrome.

Thalassemia

The thalassemias encompass a group of inherited disorders of hemoglobin synthesis that involve decreased or defective synthesis of one or more globin chains. Thalassemias are named after the affected globin chain, with α and β thalassemia being the most common and clinically important types. When one globin chain is ineffectively produced, the unaffected chains are overproduced, causing red cell abnormalities that lead to immature red cell destruction and a subsequent microcytic, hypochromic, hemolytic anemia.

Vichinsky EP, Haberkern CM, Neumayr L et al: A comparison of conservative and aggressive transfusion regimens in the perioperative management of sickle cell disease. N Engl J Med 333:206-213, 1995.

The high incidence of perioperative complications in patients with sickle cell disease is thought to be related to the relative percentage of hemoglobin S. Various types of preoperative transfusion regimens have been recommended to lower the percentage of hemoglobin S to less than 30-50%. Simple transfusion of red cells to a predetermined hemoglobin level is a conservative approach that will decrease hemoglobin S and increase hemoglobin A while correcting the underlying anemia. A more aggressive approach is exchange transfusion, which purposely removes hemoglobin S while simultaneously transfusing hemoglobin A, in an attempt to decrease the hemoglobin S concentration below a predetermined level. However, exchange transfusion requires the administration of a greater amount of transfused blood, and is associated with more complications than simple transfusion. Furthermore, it is unknown whether the incidence of vaso-occlusive crises is related to the relative percentage of hemoglobin S, or the total hemoglobin A level.

A multicenter study was designed to compare these two perioperative transfusion approaches in adults and children with sickle cell disease scheduled for elective surgery. Eligible patients were randomly assigned to either (1) an *aggressive* transfusion regimen, with goals of a hemoglobin level of approximately 10 g/dL plus a hemoglobin S level below 30%, or (2) a *conservative* transfusion regimen, in which the goal was to achieve a hemoglobin level of approximately 10 g/dL regardless of the percentage of hemoglobin S. The outcome variables of interest were perioperative sickle-related complications. Approximately 300 patients were recruited for each group.

To achieve the goals of the assigned regimens, most patients assigned to the aggressive group (57%) required an exchange transfusion to decrease the percentage of hemoglobin S. Patients assigned to the conservative transfusion regimen had a mean hemoglobin S concentration of 59%. There was no significant difference in major perioperative complications between groups (Table 7-2). The most frequent postoperative major complication was acute chest syndrome, which occurred in 10% of patients in both groups. Development of acute chest syndrome was associated with a history of pulmonary disease, and a higher surgical risk category. Patients in the aggressive regimen group were more likely to develop new alloantibodies because they received a greater number of transfusions.

As a result of this study, pediatric hematologists no longer require sickle cell patients to achieve a certain hemoglobin S concentration prior to elective surgery. Rather, these patients are admitted to the hospital preoperatively for intravenous hydration, and receive red cell transfusions to increase their hemoglobin level to approximately 10 g/dL. The types of surgical procedures for which preoperative transfusion is required remains unknown. At The Children's Hospital of Philadelphia, all children with sickle cell disease are transfused preoperatively except when undergoing extremely minor or short procedures (e.g., myringotomy and tube insertion).

Table 7-2   Comparison of Serious or Life-threatening Complications

	Percentage of Operations	
Complication	Aggressive Transfusion Therapy (exchange transfusion) (n = 303)	Conservative Transfusion Therapy (RBC transfusion to hemoglobin of 10 g/dL) (n = 301)
Before, during, or soon after surgery		
Miscellaneous intraoperative event	19	20
Acute chest syndrome	11	10
Fever or infection	7	7
Miscellaneous postoperative event	6	5
Painful crisis	5	7
Neurologic event	1	1
Renal complication	1	<1
Death	1	0
Any complication	31	35
After surgery		
Acute chest syndrome	10	10
Fever or infection	7	5
Miscellaneous postoperative event	6	5
Painful crisis	4	7
Neurologic event	1	<1
Renal complication	1	<1
Death	1	0
Any complication	21	22

Reproduced with permission from Vichinsky EP et al: *N Engl J Med* 333:206-213, 1995.

Alpha Thalassemias

Alpha thalassemia major is the homozygous form of the disease that results in the absence of all four α globin chains. This condition results in the fetal overproduction of γ globin chains (hemoglobin Bart's) that are incapable of releasing oxygen to the tissues. Severe fetal anemia (hydrops fetalis) develops and is not compatible with postnatal life.

Alpha thalassemia intermedia (hemoglobin H disease) results when three globin chains are absent. Hemoglobin H is the β-4 tetramer that forms as a result of decreased α globin production and relative overproduction of β globin chains. It is characterized by moderately severe anemia, splenomegaly, jaundice, and bone changes that are caused by marrow expansion from increased red cell production.

Alpha thalassemia trait (alpha thalassemia minor) is the heterozygous form of the disease that results in the absence of two globin chains. It is present in approximately 3% of African Americans, and manifests as a mild microcytic anemia (rarely less than 9 g/dL) that is often confused with mild iron deficiency.

Silent-carrier alpha thalassemia is characterized by the absence of only one globin chain. The hemoglobin concentration and red cell indices are normal.

Beta Thalassemias

Thalassemia major (Cooley's anemia) is the homozygous form of the disease characterized by the absence of β globin chains. These children develop a severe hemolytic anemia and splenomegaly during the first year of life. If the condition is left untreated, bone marrow hyperplasia and extramedullary hematopoiesis produce characteristic features such as tower skull, frontal bossing, maxillary hypertrophy with prominent cheekbones, and an overbite. In the absence of blood transfusions, death occurs within the first few years of life owing to progressive congestive heart failure. A typical treatment regimen will consist of 10–20 mL/kg of leukodepleted red blood cells every 3–5 weeks to maintain the hemoglobin above 10 g/dL. Transfusion therapy prevents the clinical manifestations of the anemia but requires concomitant chelation therapy to reverse transfusional overload. These children may require splenectomy during childhood if more than 200–250 mL/kg per year of transfused red cells are required to maintain a hemoglobin level of 10 g/dL.

Thalassemia intermedia represents a compound heterozygous state, and results in a moderate anemia that does not usually require regular blood transfusions. These patients usually present later in childhood, and may develop clinical manifestations of chronic anemia as seen in thalassemia major. Transfusion therapy is reserved for acute illnesses.

Beta thalassemia trait is caused by the absence of one β chain, and is characterized by an asymptomatic mild microcytic anemia with a hemoglobin level rarely less than 9 g/dL.

Silent-carrier beta thalassemia is also asymptomatic with the possibility of mildly abnormal red cell indices.

ADDITIONAL ARTICLES TO KNOW

Bolton-Maggs PH, Pasi KJ: Haemophilias A and B. *Lancet* 361(9371):1801–1809, 2003.

Cameron CB, Kobrinsky N: Perioperative management of patients with Von Willebrand's disease. *Can J Anaesth* 37:341–347, 1990.

Haberkern CM, Neumayr LD, Orringer EP et al: Cholecystectomy in sickle cell anemia patients: perioperative outcome of 364 cases from the National Preoperative Transfusion Study. *Blood* 89:1533–1542, 1997.

Koshy M, Weiner SJ, Miller ST et al: Surgery and anesthesia in sickle cell disease: Cooperative Study of Sickle Cell Diseases. *Blood* 86:3676–3684, 1995.

Vichinsky EP, Neumayr LD, Haberkern C et al: The perioperative complication rate of orthopedic surgery in sickle cell disease: report of the National Sickle Cell Surgery Study Group. *Am J Hematol* 62:129–138, 1999.

Waldron P, Pegelow C, Neumayr L et al: Tonsillectomy, adenoidectomy, and myringotomy in sickle cell disease: perioperative morbidity. *J Pediatr Hematol/Oncol* 21:129–135, 1999.

CHAPTER 8

Oncologic Diseases

MICHAEL J. FISHER

BRADLEY S. MARINO

RONALD S. LITMAN

Oncologic diseases are common in the pediatric population and account for a substantial proportion of general anesthetics performed in this age group. This chapter reviews the clinical features of common oncologic disorders in children, and the adverse effects of chemotherapy that impact on anesthetic management. Anesthetic considerations for the child with an anterior mediastinal mass are emphasized because of the contribution of this condition to anesthetic morbidity and mortality.

COMMON ONCOLOGIC DISORDERS

Leukemia

The leukemias, which result from malignant transformation of hematopoietic cells, are the most common malignancies of childhood (Table 8-1). Leukemias are subdivided into acute and chronic types. Acute leukemias account for 97% of all childhood leukemias and are subdivided into acute lymphocytic leukemia (ALL) and acute myelogenous leukemia (AML). Chronic leukemias account for 3% of childhood leukemias and are always nonlymphocytic. ALL, the most common pediatric neoplasm, accounts for 80% of all childhood acute leukemia. The incidence of ALL peaks between the ages of 3 and 5 years.

Clinical manifestations of the leukemias are similar and consist primarily of lethargy, malaise, fever, and signs of bone marrow failure such as pallor, ecchymoses, or petechiae. Bone or joint pain related to marrow infiltration from tumor cells is also a common presenting symptom. Initial laboratory findings usually include signs related to bone marrow dysfunction, such as anemia, neutropenia, and thrombocytopenia.

Table 8-1 Distribution of Childhood Cancer by Diagnosis

Type of Cancer	Total Pediatric Malignancies Annually (%)
ALL	23.3
CNS	20.7
Neuroblastoma	7.3
Non-Hodgkin's disease	6.3
Wilms tumor	6.1
Hodgkin's disease	5.0
AML	4.2
Rhabdomyosarcoma	3.4
Retinoblastoma	2.9
Osteosarcoma	2.6
Ewing's sarcoma	2.1
Other	16.1

ALL, acute lymphocytic leukemia; AML, acute myelogenous leukemia; CNS, central nervous system
Adapted with permission from Gurney JG, Severson RK, Davis S, Robinson LL: Incidence of cancer in children in the United States: sex-, race-, and 1-year age-specific rates by histologic subtype. *Cancer* 75:2186, 1995.

The treatment strategy for leukemia is to treat the complications of the disease at presentation, to treat the leukemia, and to manage the complications of treatment. ALL therapy is usually instituted in three distinct phases, each with specific objectives:

1. *Induction* of remission generally lasts 4 weeks, during which the most number of tumor cells are killed.
2. The *consolidation* phase consists of additional intensified treatment plus intrathecal chemotherapy and, if central nervous system disease is present, cranial radiation.
3. The objectives of *maintenance therapy* (usually 2–3 years) are to continue the remission achieved in the previous two phases and to provide additional cytoreduction to cure the leukemia.

Chemotherapy is discontinued when the patient has remained in remission throughout the course of maintenance therapy. A small percentage (<10%) of children with standard risk ALL who successfully complete the maintenance phase will have a recurrence of their leukemia.

Chemotherapy for AML is more intensive than for ALL and results in significant myelosuppression. The prognosis for AML is worse than that for ALL, but it varies between subtypes. With chemotherapy alone, a cure is achieved in fewer than 50% of patients with AML. Up to two-thirds of patients with AML can be cured by addition of bone marrow transplantation.

Central Nervous System Tumors

Central nervous system (CNS) tumors are the most common solid tumors in children and are second to leukemia in overall incidence of malignant diseases (see Table 8-1). In contrast to adults, brain tumors in children are located predominantly infratentorial in the cerebellum and brainstem. Childhood brain tumors are usually low-grade astrocytomas or malignant neoplasms such as medulloblastoma or high-grade glioma. Infratentorial tumors may present with signs of increased intracranial pressure (headache, nausea, emesis, lethargy, impaired upward gaze), nystagmus, difficulty walking, new deficits of balance, or cranial nerve deficits. Children with supratentorial tumors commonly present with signs of increased intracranial pressure, seizures, hemiparesis, or visual-field deficits. The treatment regimen depends on the size and location of the tumor (Table 8-2).

Lymphoma

Lymphomas are the third most common malignancy in childhood (see Table 8-1). Approximately 60% of pediatric lymphomas consist of non-Hodgkin's lymphoma, and the remainder is Hodgkin's disease.

Table 8-2	Treatment Approaches for Childhood CNS Tumors
Treatment	**Goals**
Surgery	Establish diagnosis
	Debulk/resect tumor
	Treat increased ICP (ventricular shunt may be required)
Radiation	Control residual disease
	Control tumor dissemination
	Cure
Chemotherapy	Adjuvant therapy for malignant tumors
	Minimize radiation exposure
	Delay/obviate need for radiation
Immunotherapy	Adjuvant therapy for malignant tumors
	Scavenger for minimal residual disease
Molecularly targeted therapy	Downregulation of abnormal growth factor receptor pathway

Adapted with permission from Pizzo PA, Poplack DG eds: *Principles and Practice of Pediatric Oncology*, 3rd edn, Lippincott-Raven, Philadelphia, 1997.

Non-Hodgkin's Lymphoma

Non-Hodgkin's lymphoma (NHL) encompasses a heterogeneous group of diseases caused by neoplastic proliferation of immature lymphoid cells, which, unlike the malignant lymphoid cells of ALL, accumulate outside the bone marrow. Just as the immune system can be divided into T and B cell compartments, NHL falls into T and B cell categories. Histopathologic subtypes in childhood NHL include lymphoblastic (usually T cell), 30%; undifferentiated small cell (B cell), 50%; and large cell (T, B, or indeterminate cell origin), 20%. Undifferentiated small cell NHL is subdivided into Burkitt's and non-Burkitt's types. Most cases of NHL in children are diffuse and highly malignant. Distant noncontiguous metastases to the CNS and bone marrow are common. The abdomen is the most common site of initial manifestations of B cell NHL, whereas the anterior mediastinum is the primary site for T cell NHL. Initial clinical manifestations may include fever, weight loss, and other nonspecific constitutional symptoms. Gastrointestinal involvement can result in rapid abdominal enlargement, pain, or ascites; intestinal obstruction occurs when the lymphoma serves as the lead point for an intussusception. Anterior mediastinal masses are associated with pleural effusions, airway compromise, and superior vena cava syndrome (see below).

NHL is treated using an aggressive multidrug regimen similar to that used for ALL. Induction produces remission in 90% of affected children, and maintenance chemotherapy, including intrathecal prophylaxis, reduces the incidence of relapse. Patients with localized disease have a significantly better survival rate than patients with disseminated disease.

Hodgkin's Disease

Hodgkin's disease accounts for 5% of all childhood cancer (see Table 8-1). Histopathologic subtypes are similar to those in adults: 40–60% nodular sclerosis, 10–20% lymphocyte predominance, 20–40% mixed cellularity, and 10% lymphocyte depletion. Its incidence has a bimodal distribution with peaks occurring at 15–30 years of age and after the age of 50 years. The most common presentation is painless, firm lymphadenopathy involving either the supraclavicular or cervical nodes. Two-thirds of patients will also have mediastinal lymphadenopathy. Fever, night sweats, and weight loss occur in 30% of children.

Four stages of Hodgkin's disease are described (Box 8-1), and for any given stage, patients are further subdivided into "A" or "B" subgroups depending on the absence (A) or presence (B) of systemic symptoms (e.g., weight loss, fever, or night sweats). Definitive staging sometimes requires exploratory laparotomy, but is not indicated unless therapy will be influenced by the findings.

Most pediatric treatment protocols consist of multiagent chemotherapy, which may be combined with low-dose radiation therapy. The addition of radiation improves disease-free survival in children with bulky disease and "B" subgroup symptoms. Prognosis varies from a 90–95% cure of stage I disease to a 70% cure of stage IV disease. As in adults, lymphocyte predominance is most favorable and lymphocyte depletion least favorable.

Box 8-1 Staging of Hodgkin's Disease

Stage I

Involvement of a single lymph node region or a single extralymphatic organ

Stage II

Involvement of two or more lymph node regions on the same side of the diaphragm, or localized involvement of an extralymphatic organ and one or more lymph node regions on the same side of the diaphragm

Stage III

Involvement of lymph node regions on both sides of the diaphragm

This may be accompanied by localized involvement of an extralymphatic organ or site, involvement of the spleen, or both

Stage IV

Disseminated involvement of the liver, bone marrow, lungs, or other nonlymph node sites.

Neuroblastoma

Neuroblastoma accounts for 7% of all childhood cancers and, in children, is the most common solid tumor outside the central nervous system (see Table 8-1). A neuroblastoma is a malignancy of the primitive neural crest cells that form the adrenal medulla and the paraspinal sympathetic ganglia. Abdominal tumors account for 70% of cases, one-third of which arise from the retroperitoneal sympathetic ganglia and two-thirds from the adrenal medulla itself. Thoracic masses, accounting for 20% of the tumors, tend to arise from paraspinal ganglia in the posterior mediastinum. Neuroblastoma of the neck occurs in 5% of cases and often involves the cervical sympathetic ganglion.

The clinical manifestations are extremely variable and depend on the location and spread of the tumor. Abdominal pain and systemic hypertension occur if the mass compresses the renal vasculature. Hypertension can also result from tumor secretion of catecholamines. Respiratory distress is the primary symptom seen in thoracic neuroblastoma tumors. Thoracic or abdominal tumors may invade the epidural space posteriorly in a dumbbell fashion, and cause back pain and symptoms of spinal cord compression. Children with neuroblastoma may be volume depleted secondary to chronic hypertension or diarrhea resulting from tumor production of vasoactive intestinal peptides. Metastatic sequelae include bone marrow failure, liver infiltration, periorbital infiltration, and distant lymph node enlargement.

The treatment of neuroblastoma consists of surgery and subsequent chemotherapy; the type of treatment depends primarily on the tumor staging and risk classification. Radiation after surgery is used to treat residual local disease and selected metastatic foci. Bone marrow transplantation is often the best therapy for high-risk disease. Prognosis is dependent on age, stage, and histological and molecular characteristics.

Wilms Tumor

Wilms tumor, a cancer of embryonal renal cells, accounts for 6% of all childhood cancers (see Table 8-1), and predominantly occurs in the first 5 years of life. Wilms tumor occurs frequently in the setting of additional genitourinary tract anomalies. Most children are diagnosed after incidental detection of an asymptomatic abdominal mass. Associated findings include microscopic or gross hematuria, and hypertension. Hypertension may occur from renin secretion by tumor cells or compression of the renal vasculature by the tumor. Local extension of the tumor often involves the renal vein and inferior vena cava, with occasional extension cephalad to the level of the right atrium. The lung is the most common site of distant metastases.

Unilateral Wilms tumors are treated with immediate surgical resection of the affected kidney followed by chemotherapy. Radiotherapy is added for high-stage disease. When the tumor is bilateral, presurgical chemotherapy is performed to shrink the tumors in an attempt to salvage some renal function, after which local tumor excision is attempted. Tumors with favorable histology, such as classic nephroblastoma, have a better than 90% overall survival rate. Tumors with unfavorable histology, such as anaplastic or sarcomatous variants, have a 12% cumulative survival rate.

Bone Tumors

Primary malignant bone tumors account for 4% of childhood cancer (see Table 8-1) and consist primarily of Ewing's sarcoma and osteogenic sarcoma.

Ewing's Sarcoma

Ewing's sarcoma, an undifferentiated sarcoma that arises primarily in bone, occurs mostly in adolescents. The most common presenting symptoms include pain and swelling at the site of the tumor. The most commonly involved sites are the femur (20%), pelvis (20%), fibula (12%), humerus (10%), and tibia (10%). Systemic manifestations are more common with metastases and include fever, weight loss, and fatigue.

Treatment consists of radiation, chemotherapy, and surgery to provide local control of the primary tumor. If the tumor affects an expendable bone (proximal fibula, rib, or clavicle), complete surgical excision may be indicated. Most patients with Ewing's sarcoma have micrometastatic disease at the time of diagnosis, and as a result, chemotherapy is needed to reduce the size of the primary tumor, treat metastases seen at diagnosis, and prevent potential future metastases. The prognosis is excellent for patients with distal-extremity nonmetastatic tumors. Children with metastatic disease at diagnosis or tumors of the pelvic bones or proximal femur have less favorable outcomes.

Osteogenic Sarcoma

Osteogenic sarcoma (or osteosarcoma), a malignant tumor of the bone-producing osteoblasts, arises in the medullary cavity or the periosteum. The primary tumor is usually located at the metaphyseal portion of bones associated with maximum growth velocity (e.g., distal femur, proximal tibia, and proximal humerus) and occurs mostly during early adolescence. Similar to Ewing's sarcoma, pain and localized swelling are the most common presenting complaints; but in contrast to Ewing's sarcoma, systemic manifestations are rare. At diagnosis, 20% of patients have clinically detectable metastatic disease and most of the remaining patients have microscopic metastatic disease. When feasible, limb-salvage surgical procedures are performed to limit resection to the tumor-bearing portion of the bone. Neoadjuvant and postoperative chemotherapy increases disease-free survival to greater than 70%.

CHEMOTHERAPEUTIC AGENTS

A variety of classes of chemotherapeutic agents are used in children, depending on the particular type of malignancy and its progression. All chemotherapeutic agents have adverse effects (Table 8-3). In particular, the anthracyclines – doxorubicin (Adriamycin) and daunorubicin – are associated with cardiac toxic effects. Atrial and ventricular conduction disturbances may occur acutely, and left ventricular failure may occur in chronically treated children. Heart failure is associated with a cumulative dose in excess of $300 \, mg/m^2$, age under 4 years, the use of additional chemotherapeutic agents, and mediastinal irradiation. Children who receive these drugs are assessed by serial echocardiography prior to initiation of treatment and at regular intervals during treatment. Other significant chemotherapy toxicities include pulmonary toxicity with bleomycin and renal toxicity with cisplatin. The preanesthetic evaluation should include a review of all chemotherapeutic agents used, as well as the results of toxicity studies, such as serial echocardiograms.

MISCELLANEOUS PROBLEMS IN CHILDREN WITH CANCER

Bone Marrow Dysfunction

Bone marrow dysfunction is a common occurrence in children with cancer, as a result of the tumor's effect on the bone marrow, or as an effect of chemotherapeutic agents. The presence of mild to moderate anemia is not normally hazardous to otherwise healthy children, but it may pose a threat to oxygen delivery when chemotherapy-induced cardiac toxicity is also present. Clinically significant thrombocytopenia is usually considered to be a platelet count <50,000 and should be corrected prior to major surgery. Thrombocytopenia is considered a contraindication to central regional anesthesia or peripheral nerve blocks in the area of large blood vessels. Neutropenic children should be considered to be at increased risk for infection. Anesthesiologists should take extreme care to perform procedures and handle intravenous lines with meticulous sterile technique in these children.

Anterior Mediastinal Mass

An anterior mediastinal mass may be present in children with several different types of tumors, especially T-cell ALL, NHL, Hodgkin's disease, neuroblastoma, and intrathoracic germ cell tumors. These masses may be

Table 8-3   Indications and Adverse Effects of Common Childhood Chemotherapeutic Agents

Chemotherapeutic Agent	Indications	Adverse Effects
Anthracyclines Daunorubicin, doxorubicin, idarubicin, mitoxantrone	Acute leukemia, NHL, bone tumors, Wilms tumor, neuroblastoma, Hodgkin's disease	Cardiomyopathy, cardiac arrhythmias, myelosuppression, mucositis
Alkylating Agents Busulfan, cyclophosphamide, melphalan, thiotepa, ifosfamide	NHL, neuroblastoma, Hodgkin's disease, ALL, sarcoma, bone tumors	Bone marrow suppression, pulmonary fibrosis, hemorrhagic cystitis, SIADH, cardiotoxicity, Fanconi syndrome, renal failure, secondary malignancy
Antimetabolites Methotrexate, fluorouracil, cytarabine, 6-MP (6-mercaptopurine), 6-TG (6-thioguanine)	NHL, osteosarcoma, ALL	Renal insufficiency, mucositis, hepatitis, myelosuppression, cerebellar dysfunction, pulmonary toxicity, conjunctivitis
Plant products Vinblastine, vincristine, VP-16 (etoposide)	ALL, Wilms tumor, Hodgkin's disease, germ cell tumor, neuroblastoma, sarcoma	Bone marrow suppression, peripheral neuropathy, autonomic neuropathy, allergic reaction, secondary malignancy
Bleomycin	Germ cell tumors, Hodgkin's disease	Restrictive pulmonary disease caused by interstitial pneumonitis and fibrosis
Platinum compounds Cisplatin, carboplatin	Germ cell tumors, neuroblastoma, bone tumors, medulloblastoma	Bone marrow suppression, seizures, hypomagnesemia, nephrotoxicity, ototoxicity
Nitrosoureas Carmustine, lomustine	Intracranial tumors	Pulmonary fibrosis, renal failure
L-asparaginase	ALL	Coagulopathy, hepatitis, pancreatitis, allergic reactions
Actinomycin D (dactinomycin)	Wilms tumor, rhabdomyosarcoma, Ewing's sarcoma	Coagulopathy, liver failure, mucositis

ALL, acute lymphocytic leukemia; NHL, non-Hodgkin's lymphoma; SIADH, syndrome of inappropriate antidiuretic hormone secretion.
Modified with permission from Selvin BL: Cancer chemotherapy: implications for the anesthesiologist. *Anesth Analg* 60:425-434, 1981.

Article To Know

Ferrari LR, Bedford RF: General anesthesia prior to treatment of anterior mediastinal masses in pediatric cancer patients. Anesthesiology 72:991-995, 1990.

Drs Ferrari and Bedford describe their successful anesthetic protocol for managing children with known anterior mediastinal masses, in whom general anesthesia was required to facilitate tissue diagnosis. They report the anesthetic technique used on 44 children who required general anesthesia for lymph node biopsy or tumor debulking. Nine of these 44 children were symptomatic preoperatively. In children under 6 years of age, the anesthetic technique initially consisted of intravenous ketamine 1-2 mg/kg, prior to mask anesthesia with halothane. Older children were managed solely with halothane mask anesthesia. If positive-pressure ventilation was easily accomplished, neuromuscular blockade was administered. In children in whom positive-pressure ventilation was not easily accomplished, spontaneous ventilation was maintained and tracheal intubation was performed without neuromuscular blockade.

Two of the 9 patients who were symptomatic preoperatively demonstrated airway difficulties during induction of general anesthesia. In both cases, airway obstruction developed following administration of muscle paralysis, and in both cases, ventilation was easily accomplished after localizing the obstruction with a rigid bronchoscope and advancing the endotracheal tube past the site of obstruction. Two additional patients developed airway obstruction following tracheal intubation. One of these children required maintenance of spontaneous ventilation, and the other developed airway obstruction when placed supine, which was then relieved when the sitting position was resumed.

Because of their apparent success, Drs Ferrari and Bedford emphasized that the benefits of obtaining an accurate tissue diagnosis to facilitate the most appropriate treatment regimen outweigh the potential risks of performing a general anesthetic on a child with a mediastinal mass.

sufficiently large as to cause tracheal and/or bronchial compression that leads to airway obstruction. Great vessel or atrial compression may lead to obstruction of blood flow into (superior vena cava syndrome) or out of the heart. In severe cases, the patency of the lower airway and great vessels is precariously maintained by the negative intrathoracic pressure generated by spontaneous ventilation. Induction of general anesthesia or neuromuscular blockade causes loss of negative intrathoracic pressure as a result of weakening of the chest wall muscles, and is associated with life-threatening airway obstruction and great vessel compression. This obstruction cannot always be alleviated by administration of positive-pressure ventilation.

Any child with a history of a newly diagnosed or chronic malignancy known to be associated with anterior mediastinal mass should be evaluated prior to anesthesia. An anterior mediastinal mass should also be considered in otherwise healthy children who present for cervical lymph node biopsy with a potential diagnosis of lymphoma. Typical symptoms of an anterior mediastinal mass include gradual worsening of dyspnea, cough, or stridor, especially when supine. These children will often reveal that they have recently begun to sleep in the lateral or prone position, although they may not know the reason. Children with more advanced tumors may have begun to sleep in the upright or semierect position. *However, cases of life-threatening airway obstruction or death during induction of general anesthesia have occurred in children without classic symptomatology.*

When a mediastinal mass is suspected, a diagnostic evaluation is indicated. Chest radiography may reveal a widened mediastinum, but CT or MRI is better suited for demonstrating the extent of spread of the mediastinal mass and the severity of tracheal compression. Echocardiography is indicated to evaluate the severity of great vessel compression. Since tumor growth is often rapid, these studies should be performed immediately prior to any planned procedure requiring general anesthesia or sedation.

Because of the risk of life-threatening airway obstruction during loss of spontaneous ventilation, chemotherapy and/or radiation should be used to decrease the size of the mediastinal mass prior to elective procedures requiring sedation or general anesthesia. However, in many instances, the tissue diagnosis is not known; thus, sedation or general anesthesia is required to facilitate a biopsy of the mass or other accessible lymph node prior to initiating treatment because radiation or chemotherapy may distort tissue histology.

The principles of anesthetizing children with an anterior mediastinal mass are similar to those of the difficult airway secondary to upper-airway obstruction (see Chapter 18) and are based on maintenance of negative intrathoracic pressure provided by continuous spontaneous

---

Box 8-2 Principles for Anesthetizing a Child with an Anterior Mediastinal Mass

Preoperative Issues

- Attempt tissue diagnosis of peripheral lymph nodes without the use of sedation or general anesthesia.
- If a tissue diagnosis has already been obtained, attempt to reduce the size of the mediastinal mass using chemotherapy and/or radiation before proceeding with an elective procedure that requires sedation or general anesthesia.
- Use radiologic techniques to evaluate the size and location of the mass, and the extent of tracheal compression. It has been suggested that a greater than 50% compression of the trachea is associated with airway obstruction during induction of general anesthesia.
- A rigid bronchoscope and a physician with expertise in its use should be immediately available prior to and during induction of general anesthesia (some centers advocate the availability of cardiopulmonary bypass).

Intraoperative Management

- Induction of general anesthesia should be performed while maintaining spontaneous ventilation. Continuous positive airway pressure may help maintain upper-airway patency and preserve function residual capacity (FRC).
- Some children may require induction of anesthesia in the sitting or semisitting position.
- Tracheal intubation should be accomplished during deep anesthesia and spontaneous ventilation. It is preferable to avoid neuromuscular blockers for fear of losing airway muscle tone and exacerbating airway obstruction.

Management of Airway Obstruction

In the event of airway obstruction during induction of general anesthesia, the standard algorithm for alleviating upper airway obstruction should be applied (see Chapter 18). In the event that ventilation cannot be accomplished despite proper placement of an endotracheal tube in the trachea, the following steps should be performed:

1. Attempt to push the endotracheal tube distally past the tracheal obstruction or into the right main bronchus. If the endotracheal tube cannot be advanced past the obstruction, rigid bronchoscopy should be performed.
2. Alleviate gravity-induced compression of the trachea or great vessels by placing the patient into the sitting, lateral, or prone position.
3. If the above measures are unsuccessful in restoring oxygenation or circulation, consider immediate institution of cardiopulmonary bypass.

Article To Know

Keon TP: Death on induction of anesthesia for cervical node biopsy. Anesthesiology 55:471–472, 1981.

Prior to this report, the airway compression effects of anterior mediastinal masses were well described. But Tom Keon, at The Children's Hospital of Philadelphia, was the first to report a child with an anterior mediastinal mass who died during induction of general anesthesia from the *hemodynamic* effects of the mass. The child had a known mediastinal mass and presented for cervical lymph node biopsy to establish a definitive diagnosis. His preoperative symptoms included dyspnea that worsened when supine, and an episode of cyanosis and loss of consciousness while straining during a bowel movement. Induction of anesthesia was accomplished using halothane and maintenance of spontaneous ventilation with the child in the sitting position. During induction, the child became cyanotic, progressed to full cardiac arrest, and could not be resuscitated, despite seemingly adequate ventilation. Autopsy revealed a large malignant lymphoma that completely enveloped the heart and pericardium, with additional infiltration of the pulmonary artery.

For similar patients, Dr Keon recommended that children with evidence of cardiac involvement should receive only local anesthesia for obtaining a diagnostic tissue biopsy.

ventilation (Box 8-2). However, there are several important differences. Children with mediastinal masses with tracheal compression may require induction of anesthesia in the sitting or semisitting position to avoid gravity-induced tracheal compression by the mass. Prior to induction of anesthesia, intravenous access should be obtained in a vein of the lower extremity, so as to avoid problems with superior vena cava obstruction.

Furthermore, in the event of life-threatening airway obstruction, there are several unique maneuvers that may alleviate the obstruction caused by the mass (see Box 8-2). These include advancing the endotracheal tube (or rigid bronchoscope) distal to the site of the tracheal obstruction, placing the patient in a position other than supine, and possibly instituting emergency cardiopulmonary bypass.

Case

A 17-year-old female was recently diagnosed with Hodgkin's disease based on a biopsy of a new neck mass. She is scheduled for insertion of a permanent indwelling central venous catheter to facilitate administration of chemotherapy.

Is there anything else you would like to know prior to proceeding with administration of general anesthesia?

Patients with newly diagnosed Hodgkin's disease are very likely to have an anterior mediastinal mass. I will perform a detailed history and physical exam looking for evidence of extrinsic airway compression, and review all radiological studies of the chest and neck.

The patient states that she has had progressive dyspnea over the past several weeks while lying down, forcing her to sleep in the semisitting position. Physical exam reveals mild inspiratory stridor and use of accessory muscles of respiration when upright. Review of the chest CT reveals an anterior mediastinal mass that is compressing the distal trachea. Should the case be canceled?

Absolutely – this case should be canceled. Insertion of a central venous catheter to facilitate chemotherapy is an elective procedure. The patient can continue to receive chemotherapy through a peripheral intravenous catheter or temporary percutaneous central venous catheter, and/or radiation until the mediastinal mass has decreased in size and is no longer compressing the trachea.

After 5 days' prednisone and radiation therapy, the patient is markedly improved. She is now able to sit upright without stridor or dyspnea, but is still unable to lie supine without coughing. The surgeon has rebooked the case. How will you induce general anesthesia in this patient?

Although this patient has responded to initial therapy and is markedly improved, she still has symptoms of airway compression, and is at risk for further airway compression upon induction of general anesthesia. Therefore I will again cancel this case. She can continue to receive intravenous chemotherapy via an indwelling peripheral line. This elective case should not be performed until the patient is completely free of any symptoms related to airway compression, which is then confirmed by follow-up CT of the chest.

Tumor Lysis Syndrome

Tumor lysis syndrome describes a constellation of metabolic abnormalities resulting from spontaneous or treatment-induced tumor necrosis, and is generally seen in tumors with high growth rates such as T-cell ALL or Burkitt's lymphoma. Acute lysis of tumor cells results in the rapid release of intracellular contents into the circulation. This leads to hyperphosphatemia, hyperkalemia, and hyperuricemia. Hyperkalemia can cause cardiac arrhythmias. Phosphate, especially at high serum levels, binds to calcium, resulting in precipitation of calcium phosphate in renal tubules, hypocalcemia, and tetany. Purines are processed to uric acid, and hyperuricemia can result in precipitation of uric acid in renal tubules with subsequent renal failure. Management of tumor lysis syndrome includes vigorous hydration, urine alkalinization, uric acid reduction with allopurinol, diuretic therapy, and phosphate reduction. The risk for tumor lysis is greatest during the first 5 days of chemotherapy.

Infection

Neutropenia that results from administration of chemotherapeutic agents predisposes to the development of bacterial and fungal infections, especially at the site of indwelling central venous catheters. Neutropenic patients presenting with fever of unknown origin are hospitalized, cultured, and placed on broad-spectrum antibiotics. Surgical removal of an indwelling central venous catheter may be necessary.

ADDITIONAL ARTICLES TO KNOW

Culshaw V, Yule M, Lawson R: Considerations for anaesthesia in children with haematological malignancy undergoing short procedures. *Paediatr Anaesth* 13:375–383, 2003.

Prakash UBS, Abel MD, Hubmayr RD: Mediastinal mass and tracheal obstruction during general anesthesia. *Mayo Clin Proc* 63:1004–1011, 1988.

Shamberger RC, Holzman RS, Griscom NT, Tarbell NJ, Weinstein HJ: CT quantitation of tracheal cross-sectional area as a guide to the surgical and anesthetic management of children with anterior mediastinal masses. *J Pediatr Surg* 26:138–142, 1991.

Viswanathan S, Campbell CE, Cork RC: Asymptomatic undetected mediastinal mass: a death during ambulatory anesthesia. *J Clin Anesth* 7:151–155, 1995.

CHAPTER 9

Genetic and Inherited Diseases

RONALD S. LITMAN

MARY C. THEROUX

This chapter covers a variety of common genetic syndromes and other inherited diseases that impact upon the practice of pediatric anesthesiology but that are not covered in other chapters. These include trisomy 21 (Down syndrome), the various phakomatoses, dwarfism, and the mucopolysaccharidoses.

TRISOMY 21 (DOWN SYNDROME)

With an incidence of 1 in 800 live births, trisomy 21 is one of the more common genetic diseases in children, and the most common cause of mental retardation associated with genetic disease. These children are characterized by their distinctive facial appearance (Fig. 9-1) and varying degrees of developmental delay.

Surgical intervention is required for a number of disease entities that are common in children with trisomy 21 (Table 9-1). Furthermore, a number of associated congenital anomalies may cause unique anesthetic-related challenges.

Preoperative evaluation is focused on delineation of associated comorbidities. Many children with trisomy 21 are only mildly mentally retarded and will benefit from a full explanation of the perioperative processes. An anxiolytic premedication such as oral midazolam should be ordered unless there are serious concerns about upper-airway obstruction in children with sleep apnea syndrome. Older children with trisomy 21 tend to have a large body-mass index (BMI) which, along with developmental delay, may present as a preoperative behavioral management problem. Administration of intramuscular ketamine 2–3 mg/kg is often required to facilitate parental separation and facilitate mask induction of anesthesia or intravenous line placement.

Airway Abnormalities

Children with trisomy 21 have inherently smaller upper airways. Upper-airway obstruction during inhalation induction of general anesthesia is common and is probably caused by a combination of a large tongue, large adenoidal and tonsillar tissue, an abnormally small pharynx, and hypotonia of the pharyngeal dilator muscles. Almost always, placement of an oral airway device provides satisfactory relief of this obstruction.

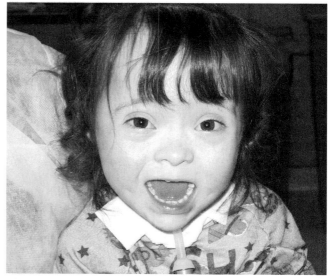

Figure 9-1   The distinctive facies of Down syndrome.

Table 9-1	Common Medical Diseases and Surgical Procedures in Children with Trisomy 21
Medical Disease	**Surgical Procedure**
Leukemia	Lumbar puncture, bone marrow aspiration and biopsy
Eustachian tube dysfunction and chronic middle ear infections	Myringotomy and tube insertion, tympanomastoidectomy
Sleep apnea	Tonsillectomy and adenoidectomy
Poor dentition	Dental rehabilitation
Congenital heart disease	Cardiac surgery
Hirschsprung's disease	Neonatal colostomy and pull-through procedure during infancy
Imperforate anus	Neonatal colostomy and definitive repair during infancy
Duodenal atresia	Exploratory laparotomy in the newborn period

Children with trisomy 21 have an increased incidence of congenital subglottic stenosis and an abnormally short trachea, which are more likely if there is associated congenital heart disease. Therefore, whenever tracheal intubation is performed, one should ensure that the endotracheal tube is not too large, and that the endotracheal tube is normally positioned above the carina (see Chapter 17).

Lower-airway anomalies are also common in children with trisomy 21. These include tracheomalacia and bronchomalacia, which predispose to intrathoracic tracheal and bronchial collapse during forced expiration, and extrathoracic tracheal collapse during forced inspiration.

Atlantoaxial Instability

One of the most important anesthetic considerations in children with trisomy 21 is the possible presence of atlantoaxial instability (AAI). Children with trisomy 21 tend to have generalized ligamental laxity, which includes the transverse ligament that holds the dens of the axis (C2) in place against the posterior surface of the anterior arch of the atlas (C1). Normally this ligament holds the dens tightly against the anterior arch of the atlas to facilitate rotatory neck motion, and maintains cervical stability during flexion, extension, and side-bending of the neck. However, when the ligament is lax, the dens may separate from the anterior arch of the atlas and compress the spinal cord. The severity of AAI can be evaluated using flexion and extension lateral radiographic views of the cervical spine. Spinal cord compression is possible when the distance between the anterior surface of the dens and the posterior surface of the anterior arch of the atlas is greater than 5 mm.

There have been a number of cases of children with trisomy 21 who, upon awakening from general anesthesia or sedation, exhibited new signs and symptoms of spinal cord damage. This spinal cord damage was presumed to be secondary to excessive neck movement during the anesthetic or surgical procedure. In the 1980s the American Academy of Pediatrics recommended that children with trisomy 21 be screened for AAI with serial cervical radiographs, especially prior to participating in physical activities. However, subsequent research has demonstrated that radiographs are not sufficiently sensitive nor specific for diagnosing AAI, nor predictive of those children who go on to develop signs of spinal cord compression. Therefore, children with trisomy 21 do not require precautionary cervical spine radiographs prior to elective procedures requiring general anesthesia, unless the child demonstrates signs or symptoms of spinal cord compression, in which case subspecialist consultation is warranted. Nevertheless, all children with trisomy 21, once anesthetized, should be treated as if they are at risk for AAI. The head and neck should be kept in as neutral a position as clinically feasible, and it should be documented in the anesthesia record that these safety precautions were observed. During myringotomy and tube placement, the child's entire body can be turned along with the neck while the tubes are being placed; during tonsillectomy, the OR table can be placed in an exaggerated Trendelenburg position instead of extreme neck extension.

Congenital Heart Disease

Approximately 40% of children born with trisomy 21 have clinically significant congenital heart disease. Common lesions include endocardial cushion defects, ventricular septal defects, and Tetralogy of Fallot. Pulmonary hypertension is common in these children, and may even occur in the absence of apparent heart disease. Optimization of cardiac status is essential prior to elective surgery, and prophylaxis against infective endocarditis may be necessary.

Miscellaneous Problems

Additional reported medical problems in children with trisomy 21 that do not often impact on anesthetic management include immunodeficiency, hypothyroidism, an increased incidence of leukemia, early Alzheimer disease, epilepsy, and a shortened average life-expectancy. An unusually exaggerated response to atropine has been reported but has not been clinically substantiated.

PHAKOMATOSES

The phakomatoses encompass a group of inherited neuroectodermal diseases, several of which are important in pediatric anesthesia because they are associated with lesions that require surgical intervention, and may predispose to anesthetic-related complications. This section will review neurofibromatosis, tuberous sclerosis, Sturge–Weber syndrome, and Klippel–Trenaunay–Weber syndrome.

The two most common types of neurofibromatosis (NF) in children are type 1, von Recklinghausen disease, and type 2, bilateral acoustic neurofibromatosis. The clinical presentation of type 1 disease is extremely variable and may include multiple café-au-lait spots, nodular neurofibromas in the skin, upper airway, and nervous system, Lisch nodules (iris lesions), optic gliomas, bony dysplasias, central nervous system (CNS) tumors of the brain or spine that cause neurologic symptoms (e.g., seizures, increased intracranial pressure) or lead to kyphoscoliosis, and variable degrees of developmental delay or mental retardation. Patients with NF type 2 may demonstrate hearing loss and vestibular disorientation. Neurofibromas, meningiomas, schwannomas, and astrocytomas are also associated with NF type 2. Surgical debulking is indicated when hearing becomes substantially impaired.

Children with NF require general anesthesia for a variety of reasons, the most common being surveillance magnetic resonance imaging (MRI) of the head to detect CNS tumors (e.g., optic glioma) or to monitor the growth or recurrence of a known tumor. There are few discrete anesthetic risks in these children, and there are few data in the anesthesia literature to indicate any type of unique anesthetic management. In rare cases, patients with NF type 1 will demonstrate hypertension caused by either renal artery stenosis or a pheochromocytoma. Laryngeal involvement with a tumor that impedes airflow has been reported but is also rare.

Tuberous sclerosis is a progressive, multisystemic disorder characterized by angiofibromas of the face, mental retardation (with hyperactivity), seizures, tuberous nodules in the brain, rhabdomyomas of the heart, a variety of congenital heart disease defects, renal cysts and tumors, and bone and lung cysts. As with NF type 1, these children most often present for MRI examination under general anesthesia. If the child is severely retarded, and is not amenable to routine mask or intravenous induction, intramuscular ketamine is a useful alternative. If cardiac tumors are present, a recent echocardiogram is indicated to confirm their anatomical location and effect on cardiovascular physiology.

Sturge–Weber syndrome (encephalofacial angiomatosis) is a progressive neurologic disorder associated with unilateral capillary hemangiomas (port-wine stains) of the face over the area innervated by the first division of the trigeminal nerve (V_1). They may also rarely involve CNS structures with accompanying neurologic symptoms such as mental retardation, seizures, and visual impairment. These children commonly undergo laser removal of the hemangioma, which often requires several treatments over time.

Klippel–Trenaunay–Weber syndrome consists of unilateral vascular malformations of the lower limbs causing hypertrophy or atrophy of the affected limb. Rarely, these children may have hematuria, anemia, thrombocytopenia, or high-output congestive heart failure.

DWARFISM (OSTEOCHONDRODYSTROPHY)

Short stature is a relative term that refers to individuals more than two standard deviations below the average height for a person of the same age and gender. Children with severe short stature are generally divided into two categories:

1. Those with proportionate growth and a normal ratio of trunk length to limb length.
2. Those with disproportionate development characterized by short limbs or short trunk that in many cases are deformed.

The latter group are referred to as "dwarfs" (Table 9-2). Achondroplasia is the most common form of dwarfism, with an incidence of 1.5 per 10,000 live births.

Table 9-2	Classification of Disproportionate Short Stature
Defects of tubular bone growth (Identifiable at birth)	Achondroplasia
	Camptomelic dysplasia
	Chondrodysplasia punctata
	Diastrophic dysplasia
	Metatrophic dysplasia
	Chondroectodermal dysplasia
	Asphyxiating thoracic dysplasia
	Spondyloepiphyseal dysplasia congenita
	Kniest dysplasia
	Mesomelic dysplasia
	Acromesomelic dysplasia
Defects of tubular bone growth (Identifiable in later life)	Metaphyseal chondroplasia
	Spondylometaphyseal dysplasia
	Pseudoachondroplastic dysplasia
	Spondyloepiphyseal dysplasia tarda
Abnormal density of cortical diaphyseal structure or metaphyseal modeling	Osteogenesis imperfecta
Primary metabolic abnormality of calcium or phosphorous	Hypophosphatemic rickets
	Hypophosphatasia
Primary metabolic abnormality of complex carbohydrates	Mucopolysaccharidosis
	Mannosidosis
	Fucosidosis

Reproduced with permission from Berkowitz ID, Raja SN, Bender KS, Kopits SE: Dwarfs: pathophysiology and anesthetic implications. *Anesthesiology* 73:739–759, 1990.

Significant anesthetic concerns in dwarfs include abnormalities of the cervical spine, cardiopulmonary system, neuromuscular and skeletal systems, and a hyperthermic response to general anesthesia.

Cervical spine abnormalities include odontoid hypoplasia and atlantoaxial instability. These abnormalities may cause restriction of cervical spine motion, and predisposition to spinal cord damage with extremes of neck movement during general anesthesia. Endotracheal intubation and ventilatory management is often difficult in dwarfs with cervical spine immobility.

The most important pulmonary abnormality in the dwarf syndromes is thoracic dystrophy, which predisposes to inefficient ventilation and is frequently associated with recurrent chest infections, chronic hypoxemia, pulmonary hypertension, and cor pulmonale. Tracheal stenosis and absence of tracheal cartilage may also be present. In the 'thanatophoric' dwarf, severe asphyxiating thoracic dystrophy is incompatible with life – these children are aborted *in utero* or die shortly after birth. Severe sleep apnea results from upper-airway obstruction due to anatomic abnormalities and generalized hypotonia. Central apnea in dwarfs is caused by stenosis of the foramen magnum, which causes compression of the distal medulla and upper cervical spinal cord at the craniovertebral junction. In severely affected patients, avoidance of preoperative sedation and preoperative administration of an antisialagogue may be indicated.

Cardiac valvular lesions and cardiomyopathy are common in many different types of dwarf syndromes, such as the mucopolysaccharidoses.

Neurological dysfunction includes hydrocephalus and compressive spinal cord and nerve root syndromes. Macrocephaly is caused by accelerated head growth but is not associated with elevated intracranial pressure. Kyphoscoliosis, lumbar lordosis, and a stenotic spinal canal may impede effective neuraxial regional anesthesia techniques.

Several forms of dwarfism, particularly osteogenesis imperfecta, are associated with development of hyperthermia during general anesthesia. The etiology is unknown, and no association with malignant hyperthermia has been established. The elevated temperature is not associated with muscle cell injury or with metabolic or respiratory acidosis. Temperature should be monitored carefully in these patients to attain normothermia. Hyperthermia accompanied by hypercapnia that does not respond to an increase in minute ventilation is

Table 9-3   Clinical Manifestations of Mucopolysaccharidoses

Syndrome	Clinical Manifestations			
	Cardiovascular	Pulmonary	CNS	Musculoskeletal
Hurler (Type I)	Coronary artery narrowing, myocardial stiffening, valve and endocardial thickening	Enlarged tongue, frequent upper respiratory tract infections, restrictive pulmonary disease secondary to kyphoscoliosis	Mental retardation, developmental delay, hydrocephalus with increased intracranial pressure, macrocephaly, conductive hearing loss	Joint stiffness, cervical spine immobility and/or instability
Hunter (Type II)	Valvular dysfunction, myocardial thickening, coronary artery narrowing, myocardial infarction	Short neck, thick tongue, upper-airway obstruction	Mental retardation, hyperactivity, hydrocephalus with increased intracranial pressure, seizures	Joint stiffness, cervical spine immobility and/or instability
Sanfilippo (Type III)	None	Frequent upper respiratory tract infections	Developmental delay, hyperactivity, mental retardation, bulbar dysfunction with ataxia, dementia, seizures	Short stature, same as Hurlers and Hunters but milder forms
Morquio (Type IV)	Valvular lesions, aortic regurgitation	Short neck, midface hypoplasia	Normal intelligence	Atlantoaxial instability with possible spinal cord compression, kyphoscoliosis
Maroteaux–Lamy (Type VI)	Aortic stenosis, mitral insufficiency	Restrictive lung disease secondary to kyphoscoliosis	Normal intelligence, hydrocephalus with increased intracranial pressure	Atlantoaxial instability with possible spinal cord compression, decreased joint mobility

suggestive of malignant hyperthermia; it warrants blood gas analysis to detect metabolic acidosis (see Chapter 21).

MUCOPOLYSACCHARIDOSES

The mucopolysaccharidoses are lysosomal storage disorders that are characterized by the accumulation of acid mucopolysaccharides (heparan, keratan, and dermatan sulfates) in the connective tissue throughout the body (Table 9-3). Accumulation of these substances causes progressive skeletal and soft tissue deformities throughout childhood and is associated with early death secondary to cardiopulmonary dysfunction. The most important anesthetic-related considerations include difficult airway management due to anatomical abnormalities and cervical spine instability. Because of soft tissue infiltration of the upper airway and frequent adenotonsillar hypertrophy, these patients can prove difficult to ventilate as well as intubate, and a laryngeal mask airway may be indispensable during anesthetic management. Difficult ventilation can also present following tracheal extubation at the completion of the procedure. Patients with Morquio's syndrome (type IV) can have atlantoaxial instability with spinal cord compression. Therefore, these patients need thorough preoperative evaluation and screening for subtle neurologic signs of spinal cord compression, and appropriate radiological assessment.

ARTICLES TO KNOW

Aboussouan LS, O'Donovan PB, Moodie DS, Gragg LA, Stoller JK: Hypoplastic trachea in Down's syndrome. *Am Rev Respir Dis* 147:72–75, 1993.

Berkowitz ID, Raja SN, Bender KS, Kopits SE: Dwarfs: pathophysiology and anesthetic implications. *Anesthesiology* 73:739–759, 1990.

Jacobs IN, Gray RF, Todd W: Upper airway obstruction in children with Down syndrome. *Arch Otolaryngol Head Neck Surg* 122:945–950, 1996.

Litman RS, Perkins FM: Atlanto-axial subluxation after tympanomastoidectomy in a child with trisomy-21. *Otolaryngol Head Neck Surg* 110:584–586, 1994.

Litman RS, Zerngast BA, Perkins FM: Preoperative evaluation of the cervical spine in children with trisomy-21: results of a questionnaire study. *Pediatr Anesth* 5:355–361, 1995.

Miller R, Gray SD, Cotton RT, Myer CM, Netterville J: Subglottic stenosis and Down syndrome. *Am J Otolaryngol* 11:274–277, 1990.

Mitchell V, Howard R, Facer E: Down's syndrome and anaesthesia. *Pediatr Anesth* 5:379–384, 1995.

Msall ME, Reese ME, DiGaudio K et al: Symptomatic atlantoaxial instability associated with medical and rehabilitative procedures in children with Down syndrome. *Pediatrics* 85(Suppl):447–449, 1990.

Risser WL, Anderson SJ, Bolduc SP et al: Atlantoaxial instability in Down syndrome: subject review. *Pediatrics* 96:151–154, 1995.

CHAPTER 10

The Premature Infant

RONALD S. LITMAN

In the last several decades, the incidence of prematurity in the United States has remained relatively constant at approximately 10%. Maternal risk factors for prematurity include absence of prenatal care, low socioeconomic status, tobacco abuse, poor nutrition, and genitourinary tract infections, to name only a few. Despite relatively constant rates of prematurity, perinatal mortality rates have decreased to approximately 9 in 1000 live births, due primarily to the advent of surfactant replacement therapy.

Despite improvements in morbidity and mortality, prematurity remains an independent risk factor for increased mortality during childhood. Singleton infants born between 34 and 36 completed weeks of gestation have a three-fold risk of dying in the first year of life when compared to term infants. Those born between 32 and 33 completed weeks of gestation have an almost seven-fold risk of dying in the first year of life.

This chapter reviews the most common medical problems seen in premature infants. These include respiratory distress syndrome (hyaline membrane disease), apnea of prematurity, anemia of prematurity, patent ductus arteriosus, intraventricular hemorrhage, and hypoglycemia. When appropriate, anesthetic implications of these disorders will be included.

DEFINITIONS

It is useful to review some common definitions. The *premature* infant is often defined as a viable newborn delivered after the twentieth completed week of gestation, and before full term, with an arbitrary weight of 500–2499 g at birth. The *preterm* infant is born at any time before the thirty-seventh completed week (259 days) of gestation (although most clinicians usually consider infants born any time in the thirty-seventh week to be full term). *Low birthweight* (LBW) is defined as less than 2500 g at birth. *Very low birthweight* (VLBW) is defined as less than 1500 g at birth. *Extremely low birthweight* (ELBW) is defined as less than 1000 g at birth.

RESPIRATORY DISTRESS SYNDROME

Premature infants are born with a deficiency of alveolar type 2 pneumocytes, which are responsible for surfactant production. Surfactant is mainly comprised of phosphatidylcholine, which lowers surface tension inside the alveoli, thus preventing alveolar collapse. Type 2 pneumocytes begin to appear in the fetus at about 22 weeks' gestation, and surfactant is primarily produced during the second trimester of pregnancy. Fifty percent of surfactant is produced by the twenty-eighth week of gestation, and production is usually complete by 36 weeks.

Surfactant deficiency is associated with a clinical syndrome of pulmonary insufficiency known as respiratory distress syndrome (RDS), formerly termed "hyaline membrane disease" (HMD). The incidence and severity of RDS are inversely correlated with gestational age; it affects approximately one-half of infants born between 28 and 32 weeks' gestation, and is rare in infants born after the thirty-fifth week of gestation. Conditions that decrease surfactant production and increase the incidence of RDS include perinatal asphyxia, maternal diabetes, multiple pregnancies, cesarean section delivery, precipitous delivery, cold stress, and a history of affected siblings. Prenatal factors that increase fetal stress and, therefore, increase surfactant production and lower the risk of RDS include pregnancy-associated hypertension, maternal opiate addiction, prolonged rupture of the membranes, and antenatal administration of corticosteroids.

Absence or deficiency of surfactant leads to widespread atelectasis, decreased lung compliance, and loss of functional residual capacity (FRC) (Fig. 10-1). This correlates with the clinical manifestations of RDS that usually appear shortly after birth, and include tachypnea, nasal flaring, audible grunting, chest wall retractions, and use of accessory muscles of respiration. Severely affected infants with substantial ventilation-to-perfusion mismatch will demonstrate cyanosis and respiratory failure. Blood gas analysis will usually reveal hypoxemia, hypercarbia, and metabolic acidosis. The classic finding on chest radiography in infants with RDS is a bilateral diffuse "ground glass" appearance and multiple air bronchograms (Fig. 10-2). On occasion, these radiographic findings may not develop until the second day of life.

Treatment of RDS initially includes supplemental oxygen to achieve a target Pao_2 between 55 and 70 mmHg. Although treatment regimens vary by institution, continuous positive airway pressure (CPAP), up to 10 cmH₂O, is added if this oxygen tension cannot be achieved with inspired oxygen concentrations less than 60%. Institution of mechanical ventilation is indicated if the infant on CPAP cannot maintain an arterial oxygen tension above 50 mmHg while breathing inspired

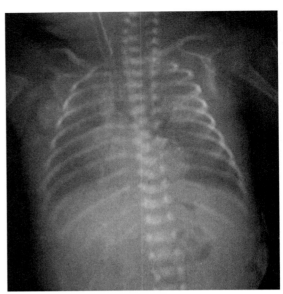

Figure 10-2 The chest radiograph of an infant with RDS demonstrates a bilateral diffuse "ground glass" appearance and multiple air bronchograms.

concentrations of oxygen up to 100%. Additional indications for mechanical ventilation include persistent pH less than 7.2, and central apnea that is unresponsive to pharmacologic therapy.

Since oxygen toxicity and pulmonary barotrauma/volutrauma are thought to be responsible for the development of neonatal chronic lung disease, the goals of mechanical ventilation in the infant with RDS are to achieve relative normoxemia ($Pao_2 > 50$ mmHg) and mild (permissive) hypercapnia ($Paco_2$ in the range 45–60 mmHg) while minimizing the concentration of inspired oxygen and the level of artificially maintained lung pressures. A modest amount of positive end-expiratory pressure (PEEP) is used (3–5 cmH₂O) and ventilatory settings are weaned aggressively as the infant improves.

The majority of infants with RDS who require mechanical ventilation are placed on conventional ventilators that deliver continuous breathing cycles, usually at a rate between 30 and 50 breaths per minute. Infants who are unresponsive to conventional ventilation may be switched to high-frequency jet ventilation (HFJV), which can attain respiratory rates of 150–600 breaths/min, or an oscillating type ventilator which can deliver 300–1800 breaths/min. The main advantage of these unconventional ventilators is the ability to decrease mean airway pressure and tidal volumes while maintaining the ability to oxygenate and eliminate carbon dioxide.

In prematurely born infants at risk of developing RDS (<28 weeks' gestation), artificial surfactant is administered into the lungs via the trachea shortly after delivery. Additional doses can be administered at regular intervals

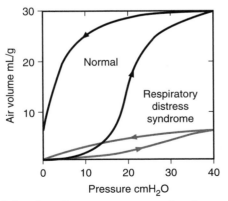

Figure 10-1 Compliance curves comparing the normal newborn lung with the lung of a prematurely born infant with RDS. The RDS lung requires a much greater amount of pressure per volume to achieve lung expansion. (Redrawn with permission from Klaus MH, Fanaroff AA: *Care of the High Risk Neonate*, 5th edn, WB Saunders, Philadelphia, 2001.)

if respiratory distress persists. Infants born later than 28 weeks of gestation receive surfactant therapy if they develop clinical signs of RDS. Exogenously administered surfactant has been shown to decrease RDS-related morbidity and mortality.

Intraoperative Ventilator Management

In infants with RDS, intraoperative ventilator management using the anesthesia machine can be challenging. Attempts to duplicate preoperative settings often result in hypoxemia and/or hypercarbia. This is partly due to differences in ventilatory equipment, anesthetic-related changes in chest wall and lung compliance, and surgical conditions that affect the efficiency of ventilation. The primary goal of intraoperative ventilation in premature infants is avoidance of hypoxemia ($Pa_{O_2} < 50$, or $Sp_{O_2} < 87\%$). Secondary goals include avoidance of high inspired oxygen concentration and high mean airway pressures.

Pressure-limited ventilation will assure that airway obstruction does not result in peak airway pressures (PIP) that may cause pneumothorax. The "right" amount of PIP is that pressure that adequately provides lung expansion as evidenced by the degree of chest wall rise. This can be rapidly achieved by manually ventilating the intubated infant, and noting the PIP that is associated with adequate chest rise and maintenance of normoxemia. Unless chest wall excursions are excessive, increases in PIP can be used to treat intraoperative hypoxemia and/or hypercarbia. During abdominal or thoracic surgery, where lung and chest wall compliance are changing minute-by-minute, experienced pediatric anesthesiologists will manually ventilate the infant, and constantly adjust inspiratory pressures while viewing the operative field and "feeling" changes in compliance.

PEEP is used in infants with RDS to maintain alveolar patency, increase and stabilize FRC, and decrease ventilation–perfusion mismatch. Preoperative levels of PEEP should be maintained intraoperatively. Increasing PEEP may increase Pa_{O_2}, but may also increase Pa_{CO_2} (secondary to decreased tidal volume) and interfere with venous return, which affects cardiac output in very small infants. In infants with RDS, excess PEEP may also have a deleterious effect on lung compliance.

In general, respiratory rates between 30 and 50 breaths per minute are adequate for small infants with RDS. Increasing the respiratory rate will increase alveolar ventilation and decrease Pa_{CO_2} without affecting Pa_{O_2} if the inspiratory/expiratory ratio remains the same.

Inspiratory-to-expiratory (I/E) ratios in infants with RDS range from 1:1 to 1:3. Increasing the inspiratory component will facilitate opening of atelectatic areas, with a resultant increase in Pa_{O_2}. However, increasing the inspiratory time may substantially increase mean airway pressure, with the potential for barotrauma. Furthermore, a shortened expiratory time may cause air-trapping and predispose to interstitial emphysema and pneumothorax. Carbon dioxide elimination is not usually affected by changing the I/E ratio.

Outcome of RDS

In most cases, the severity of RDS reaches a peak in 3–5 days and is followed by a gradual improvement provided the infant is not burdened by additional medical problems. In severe cases, ventilatory therapy may be associated with the development of interstitial emphysema, pneumothorax, pulmonary hemorrhage, and death. Infants who survive severe RDS are likely to develop neonatal chronic lung disease (see Chapter 11).

APNEA OF PREMATURITY

Apnea is commonly defined as a cessation of breathing for greater than 20 seconds, or less if accompanied by bradycardia (heart rate 30 beats/min less than baseline) or hypoxemia ($Sp_{O_2} < 90\%$). Apnea is extremely common in premature infants, with an incidence that increases with decreasing gestational age. Up to 90% of infants with birthweights less than 1500 g exhibit some form of apnea. Apnea of prematurity usually resolves by the fifty-second week following conception.

Apnea is classified as *central* (lack of respiratory effort) or *obstructive* (lack of airflow in the presence of respiratory effort). Most apneic events in prematurely born infants are *mixed* (some combination of central and obstructive apnea).

Apnea of prematurity is likely caused by neuronal immaturity of the respiratory control center in the brainstem and the peripheral chemoreceptors. Vital organ blood flow decreases significantly during bradycardic events in these infants. However, the association of apnea of prematurity with long-term neurodevelopmental outcomes is not clearly defined.

Acute episodes of apnea are treated initially with tactile stimulation and simple airway maneuvers to relieve upper-airway obstruction (e.g., chin lift or jaw thrust). Bag–mask positive-pressure breathing is required if breathing does not resume spontaneously or if hypoxemia continues. Infants with recurrent apneic episodes are placed on prophylactic stimulant therapy consisting of theophylline or caffeine. Nasal CPAP treatment or mechanical ventilation is used as a last resort in infants who continue to demonstrate life-threatening apneic events despite pharmacologic therapy.

PATENT DUCTUS ARTERIOSUS

A patent ductus arteriosus (PDA) is a common finding in preterm infants with respiratory disease (see Chapter 3). In normal newborns, the ductus arteriosus closes within the first few days of life. This process is initiated by the normal increase in blood oxygen tension and decreased levels of circulating maternal prostaglandins. The incidence of a PDA in premature infants is inversely related to birthweight and gestational age. Virtually all shunting through a PDA in a preterm infant is left-to-right, and only in larger infants is persistent pulmonary hypertension with right-to-left shunting across a PDA an issue. In premature infants, a PDA is associated with the development of intraventricular hemorrhage, necrotizing enterocolitis, oliguria, and increased pulmonary disease.

A symptomatic PDA may be closed in the early newborn period by pharmacologic therapy using indomethacin or by surgical ligation. Side-effects of indomethacin include platelet and renal dysfunction. The American Heart Association recommends that infants with a history of a PDA should receive procedure-associated subacute bacterial endocarditis (SBE) prophylaxis for 6 months following artificial closure.

ANEMIA OF PREMATURITY

Anemia in premature infants is often more severe and protracted than the physiologic anemia of infancy. This "anemia of prematurity" is most commonly attributed to decreased production of erythropoietin, decreased erythrocyte production, decreased erythrocyte lifespan, and frequent blood sampling. Its incidence increases with decreasing gestational age. Up to 95% of infants weighing less than 1000 g receive a red cell transfusion at some time during their hospitalization. Anemia of prematurity has been implicated as a cause of apnea of prematurity, poor feeding, inadequate weight gain, persistent tachycardia, and unexplained persistent metabolic acidosis.

Treatment of anemia of prematurity is transfusion of red cells. However, there is not a universal agreement as to the proper indications for treatment. Triggering hemoglobin levels vary between centers and range between 10 and 14 g/dL, depending on the concurrent illness of the infant. Some centers administer recombinant human erythropoietin (EPO) and iron to these infants. Most centers agree that the infant's hemoglobin level should be greater than 10 g/dL prior to any surgical procedure. In older infants recovering from prematurity, lower hemoglobin levels (7–10 g/dL) are tolerated in the absence of symptoms, as well as a reticulocyte count that demonstrates active production of red blood cells.

INTRAVENTRICULAR HEMORRHAGE

Intraventricular hemorrhage (IVH) describes a condition almost exclusively seen in premature infants that involves spontaneous bleeding into and around the lateral ventricles of the brain. The bleeding originates in the subependymal germinal matrix, an area surrounding the lateral ventricles that contains fragile blood vessels in the premature brain. This fragility is no longer seen in most infants born at term.

The incidence of IVH increases with decreasing birthweight; it occurs in up to 70% of infants with a birthweight less than 750 g, and most cases occur between birth and the third day of life. Additional predisposing factors include RDS, hypoxic–ischemic injury, and episodes of acute blood pressure fluctuation accompanied by rapid increases or decreases in cerebral blood flow, such as might be observed during endotracheal intubation without administration of a sedative or anesthetic agent. Rapid infusion of a hyperosmolar solution, such as sodium bicarbonate, has also been shown experimentally to induce IVH in the premature brain.

IVH is typically classified into four stages of relative severity, based on ultrasound examination of the brain (Table 10-1). Higher grades of bleed correlate with worse clinical symptoms and neurodevelopmental outcome.

Clinical manifestations of IVH include signs of abrupt neurological changes in the first several days of life, such as hypotonia, apnea, seizures, loss of the sucking reflex, and a bulging anterior fontanelle. More severe cases are manifest as unexplained anemia or hypovolemic shock.

IVH into or beyond the lateral ventricles may result in an obliterative arachnoiditis that causes blockage of cerebral spinal fluid (CSF) resorption and/or blockage of CSF flow at the Aqueduct of Sylvius. This leads to a communicating hydrocephalus which often necessitates ventriculoperitoneal shunt placement early in life.

Table 10-1	Grading of IVH Based on Ultrasound Exam
Grade	**Severity**
I	Bleeding confined to the periventricular germinal matrix
II	Bleeding into the lateral ventricle without ventricular dilatation
III	A substantial amount of bleeding into the lateral ventricle that causes ventricular dilatation
IV	Bleeding that extends into the brain parenchyma

Bleeding into the brain parenchyma causes areas of hemorrhagic infarction and leads to the development of periventricular leukomalacia (PVL). PVL, which consists of cavitary cysts in the white matter surrounding the ventricles, is thought to be the single strongest predictor of cerebral palsy later in life. PVL may develop in patients without prior history of IVH or parenchymal hemorrhage.

RETINOPATHY OF PREMATURITY

Retinopathy of prematurity (ROP), formerly called "retrolental fibroplasia" (RLF), is a disease of the premature infant that is associated with immature development of the retinal vasculature. ROP occurs when the retinal vessels become vasoconstricted before their full maturation and growth into the periphery of the retina. New abnormal vessels proliferate in the area of devascularization and are characterized by their propensity for abnormal growth, hemorrhage, and edema, all which may lead to retinal scarring and loss of vision.

Risk factors for development of ROP include low gestational age, low birthweight, prolonged oxygen exposure, mechanical ventilation, and comorbidities. The precise concentration of inspired oxygen or Pao_2 that results in retinal vessel vasoconstriction is unknown and probably varies between patients. There are even reports of cyanotic infants who have developed ROP!

The incidence of ROP has declined in mildly premature infants because of the recognition of hyperoxia as a major contributing factor. However, the overall incidence of ROP has remained steady because of improved care and survival of extremely premature infants. Most infants with mild to moderate disease will attain normal vision without treatment; advanced disease is treated by laser therapy or retinal cryotherapy to prevent retinal detachment and vision loss.

Does oxygen administered during general anesthesia cause or exacerbate ROP? Although scattered reports implicate oxygen administration during general anesthesia as a contributing factor, this does not support withholding oxygen in fear of causing or exacerbating ROP. Intraoperatively, the oxygen saturation (Spo_2) should be maintained in the low to mid 90's (%) in extremely premature infants. In the presence of anemia, this concentration should be increased. If unsure, the anesthesiologist should always err on the side of keeping the O_2 saturation too high, rather than too low, because of the known devastating effects of hypoxemia.

HYPOGLYCEMIA

Glucose is a crucial substrate for proper brain growth and development. *In utero*, glucose is maternally derived by transfer through the placenta. After birth, the newborn infant brain receives glucose by exogenous sources or endogenous gluconeogenesis from glycogen stores. However, glycogen is accumulated in the fetal liver mostly during the third trimester of pregnancy. Therefore, premature infants are at risk for developing hypoglycemia. This risk is also increased in infants with intrauterine growth retardation, infants of diabetic mothers, and infants suffering from hypothermia, respiratory distress, polycythemia, or perinatal asphyxia.

The definition of hypoglycemia has been a subject of debate. Currently, neonatologists advocate treatment of blood glucose levels <50 mg/dL, or more if there are symptoms. Symptoms of hypoglycemia include tremors (or jitteriness), cyanosis, neonatal convulsions (e.g., eye-rolling, limpness), apnea, high-pitched or weak cry, or refusal to eat.

The major consequence of prolonged hypoglycemia in the newborn period is a severe neurodevelopmental deficit. Therefore, hypoglycemia should be treated aggressively. Premature newborns who are not expected to receive glucose by enteral feedings are administered 10% dextrose intravenously, with a target glucose infusion rate of 8 mg/kg/min by the second day of life. Symptomatic hypoglycemia is treated with intravenous bolus dosing of 10% dextrose (2–4 mL/kg) until the symptoms resolve and the blood glucose has risen above normal levels. Rebound hypoglycemia commonly occurs; therefore, these infants are placed on a continuous glucose infusion, and blood glucose levels are monitored frequently.

Premature infants who present for surgical procedures under general anesthesia will be receiving glucose solutions in the immediate preoperative period. Since the stress response that accompanies the onset of surgery usually results in an elevation of blood glucose, many pediatric anesthesiologists will reduce the rate of the maintenance glucose infusion by 50% or more at the beginning of the surgical procedure. Subsequent intraoperative glucose measurements are usually performed on an hourly basis.

ARTICLES TO KNOW

Flynn JT, Bancalari E, Snyder ES et al: Cohort study of transcutaneous oxygen tension and the incidence and severity of retinopathy of prematurity. *N Engl J Med* 326:1050–1080, 1992.

Fowlie PW, Davis PG: Prophylactic intravenous indomethacin for preventing mortality and morbidity in preterm infants. Cochrane Neonatal Group. *Cochrane Database of Systematic Reviews* 1, 2003.

Lloyd J, Askie L, Smith J, Tarnow-Mordi W: Supplemental oxygen for the treatment of prethreshold retinopathy of prematurity. Cochrane Neonatal Group. *Cochrane Database of Systematic Reviews* 1, 2003.

Perlman JM, Volpe JJ: Episodes of apnea and bradycardia in the preterm newborn: impact on cerebral circulation. *Pediatrics* 76:333–338, 1985.

Soll RF: Synthetic surfactant for respiratory distress syndrome in preterm infants. Cochrane Neonatal Group. *Cochrane Database of Systematic Reviews* 1, 2003.

Steer PA, Henderson-Smart DJ: Caffeine versus theophylline for apnea in preterm infants. Cochrane Neonatal Group. *Cochrane Database of Systematic Reviews* 1, 2003.

Wheeler AS, Sadri S, DeVore JS, David-Mian Z, Latyshevsky H: Intracranial hemorrhage following intravenous administration of sodium bicarbonate or saline solution in the newborn lamb asphyxiated in utero. *Anesthesiology* 51:517–521, 1979.

Woodgate PG, Davies MW: Permissive hypercapnia for the prevention of morbidity and mortality in mechanically ventilated newborn infants. Cochrane Neonatal Group. *Cochrane Database of Systematic Reviews* 1, 2003.

CHAPTER 11

The Formerly Premature Infant

RONALD S. LITMAN

With the advent of surfactant therapy, and the generalized improvement in care of extremely premature infants, mortality from medical problems of prematurity has decreased substantially. As a consequence, anesthesiologists are exposed to an increasing number of infants who were born prematurely. This chapter reviews the most important medical problems of former premature infants that are of importance to anesthesiologists – those related to the respiratory system. These include chronic neonatal respiratory disease (bronchopulmonary dysplasia), laryngeal and tracheal injury, and persistent respiratory center immaturity that manifests as postoperative apnea following general anesthesia.

BRONCHOPULMONARY DYSPLASIA

Bronchopulmonary dysplasia (BPD) describes the clinical, radiographic, and pathologic sequelae of respiratory distress syndrome (RDS), and is classified as mild, moderate, or severe (Table 11-1). It is the leading cause of chronic lung disease during infancy, occurring in up to 36% of infants born prematurely who require early mechanical ventilation. The risk of developing BPD increases with decreasing birthweight and younger gestational age. BPD has also been termed "chronic neonatal lung disease" and "chronic lung disease of prematurity," but it is more precisely characterized as one of many causes of "chronic lung disease of infancy" (CLDI). Additional causes of CLDI include pneumonia/sepsis, meconium aspiration pneumonitis, pulmonary hypoplasia, persistent pulmonary hypertension (see Chapter 1),

apnea of prematurity (see Chapter 10), and any other systemic disease that affects lung function.

Various factors have been implicated in the pathogenesis of BPD. These include oxygen toxicity, barotrauma/volutrauma from prolonged mechanical ventilation, fluid overload, a persistent ductus arteriosus (PDA), congenital or nosocomial infection, and genetic predisposition, among others. No one factor appears to be primarily responsible and the etiology is likely to be multifactorial. Some authors have suggested that BPD is likely the end result of the reparative process of the lung after therapy for RDS as well as the arrest of lung growth during the neonatal period.

The clinical manifestations of the classic, more severe form of BPD include tachypnea, rales, bronchospasm, and a persistent requirement for supplemental oxygen. Carbon dioxide retention is a prominent finding and is presumably due to increased deadspace ventilation. Radiographic abnormalities include hyperinflation, bleb formation, and interstitial densities. The underlying pathologic findings include pulmonary fibrosis, necrotizing bronchiolitis, peribronchial smooth muscle hypertrophy, and widespread inflammatory changes in the distal bronchioles and alveoli.

Infants with severe BPD may demonstrate episodes of sudden, severe bronchospasm and cyanosis following agitation or physical stimulation ("BPD spell"), which is thought to be caused by nearly complete tracheal collapse as a result of underlying tracheomalacia, a common complication of prolonged mechanical ventilation. These episodes are treated with sedation or calming of the infant combined with application of continuous positive airway pressure (CPAP) or positive pressure ventilation in the event of unremitting hypoxemia.

Throughout the past several decades the clinical nature of BPD has evolved into a milder form ("new BPD") than seen in the past. This is primarily associated with an increased survival rate of extremely premature

Table 11-1   Classification and Diagnostic Criteria for Bronchopulmonary Dysplasia

	Gestational Age	
Classification	**<32 Weeks**	**≥32 Weeks**
Mild BPD	Breathing room air at 36 weeks postmenstrual age[a] or hospital discharge, whichever comes first	Breathing room air by 56 days postnatal age or discharge, whichever comes first
Moderate BPD	Need for <30% oxygen at 36 weeks postmenstrual age[a] or discharge, whichever comes first	Need for <30% oxygen at 56 days postnatal age or discharge, whichever comes first
Severe BPD	Need for ≥30% oxygen and/or positive pressure, at 36 weeks postmenstrual age[a] or discharge, whichever comes first	Need for ≥30% oxygen and/or positive pressure at 56 days postnatal age or discharge, whichever comes first

[a] Postmenstrual age is the postconceptional age (PCA) + 2 weeks.
Reproduced with permission from Jobe JH, Bancalari E: Bronchopulmonary dysplasia. *Am J Respir Crit Care Med* 163:1723-1729, 2001.

infants, and increased recognition of the role of oxygen toxicity and barotrauma/volutrauma in causing BPD. The newer, milder form of BPD is characterized by a minimal oxygen requirement in early life, although ventilatory therapy may be required for persistent central apnea. As the infant with mild BPD grows, there is a comparatively less bronchospastic component than with the more severe form.

With all forms of BPD, the ventilatory treatment is a two-pronged approach. First, the inspired fractional concentration of oxygen is minimized to prevent further oxygen toxicity. Second, "atelectrauma" is minimized by increasing PEEP (maximum 10 cmH$_2$O), which maintains functional residual capacity (FRC) and reduces the relative amount of chronically underventilated atelectatic areas of the lung.

Pharmacologic therapy includes diuretics, inhaled bronchodilators, theophylline, caffeine, and short courses of inhaled or oral steroids. Long-term treatment with diuretics results in hypokalemia, hypochloremia, and increased serum bicarbonate. Additional supportive therapy includes optimization of nutrition, fluid restriction, and aggressive treatment of infectious processes.

The vast majority of infants with BPD will regain normal lung function by 12 months of age. However, many will continue to demonstrate periodic episodes of bronchospasm, especially during upper respiratory tract infections. In severe cases, this predisposition can last into adolescence. Infants who develop the newer, milder form of BPD tend to be more premature and therefore more likely to suffer from an arrest in alveolar development. Long-term pulmonary function in these infants is unknown.

Anesthetic Management of Infants with BPD

Preoperative assessment of infants with BPD is focused on optimization of their respiratory status, with particular regard for treating underlying bronchoconstriction. Infants with severe BPD who are likely to develop bronchospasm and cyanosis during physical stimulation should receive an anxiolytic premedication. Principles of management of general anesthesia in these infants centers on the avoidance of endotracheal intubation. Whenever feasible, a laryngeal mask airway (LMA) is preferred. If endotracheal intubation is performed, a "deep extubation" may be warranted to avoid bronchospasm. In abdominal procedures, a regional analgesic technique is indicated for adequate postoperative pain control, as well as to avoid chest wall splinting and to preserve the ability to cough without pain. In infants with BPD, there are insufficient data with which to predict the incidence of intraoperative or postoperative pulmonary complications.

LARYNGEAL AND TRACHEAL INJURY

Premature infants who required prolonged endotracheal intubation and mechanical ventilation are prone to develop injury to the laryngeal and tracheal tissues, which results in scarring and upper-airway narrowing. Subglottic stenosis, a fibrotic narrowing usually located at the level of the cricoid cartilage, occurs in up to 15% of infants who survive prolonged mechanical ventilation in the neonatal period. When anesthetized, these infants will require an unexpectedly smaller diameter endotracheal tube. Following extubation, they may develop stridor as a result of further tracheal narrowing from acute subglottic edema. Therefore, the endotracheal tube should permit an air leak below 30 cmH$_2$O to help prevent excessive swelling of the subglottic mucosa.

Tracheal and bronchial injury that occurs during repeated deep suctioning techniques may result in lower-airway narrowing and granuloma formation. Tracheobronchomalacia may occur in up to 50% of premature infants with CLDI. It is thought to be partially responsible for tracheal collapse that manifests as wheezing or cyanosis during "BPD spells."

POSTOPERATIVE APNEA

Formerly premature infants who are growing and otherwise doing well will often demonstrate central apnea following administration of general anesthesia for elective surgical procedures, such as an inguinal herniorrhaphy. These episodes of postoperative apnea may be accompanied by bradycardia and may require bag–mask assisted ventilation to relieve the hypoxemia. The cause of this phenomenon is unknown, but it is probably related to the effects of general anesthetic agents on the immature respiratory control center in the brainstem.

Article To Know

Coté CJ, Zaslavsky A, Downes J et al: Postoperative apnea in former preterm infants after inguinal herniorrhaphy: a combined analysis. Anesthesiology 82:809-822, 1995.

Individually published studies that determine risk factors for postoperative apnea in former premature infants are unconvincing because of their retrospective nature or the relatively small number of patients studied. Therefore, in an attempt to determine true risk factors for postoperative apnea, Charlie Coté, at Children's Memorial Hospital in Chicago, obtained the original data from eight prospective studies that examined risk factors for postoperative apnea in former premature infants undergoing inguinal herniorrhaphy, and performed a reanalysis with the larger dataset. Dr Coté analyzed data from 255 patients from four institutions, and determined the influence of the following patient- or anesthetic-related factors on the incidence of development of postoperative apnea: a history of respiratory distress syndrome, BPD, apnea of prematurity, previous necrotizing enterocolitis, ongoing apnea at the time of surgery, use of narcotics or long-acting muscle relaxants, anemia (hematocrit level <30%), gestational age, and postconception age (PCA). Of these, only two, lower gestational age and lower PCA, were directly correlated with the risk of postoperative apnea (Fig. 11-1). Additional risk factors included ongoing apnea at home and presence of anemia, particularly in infants greater than 43 weeks PCA.

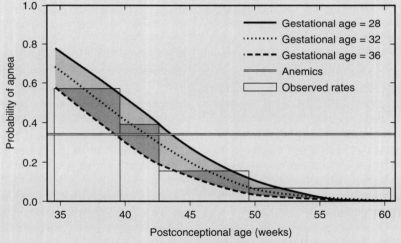

Figure 11-1   Influence of gestational age and PCA on risk of postoperative apnea in former premature infants. The risk of apnea is inversely related to the gestational age and PCA. The risk of anemia is represented by the horizontal double line, which is not altered by the gestational age or PCA. The shaded boxes represent the overall rates of apnea for infants within that gestational age range. (Redrawn with permission from Coté CJ et al: *Anesthesiology* 82:809-822, 1995.)

Coté's reanalysis showed that the risk for apnea does not decrease to below 1% with 95% statistical confidence until infants with a gestational age of 32-35 weeks reached a PCA of 56 weeks, and infants with a gestational age of 35 weeks or more reached a PCA of 54 weeks. He suggested that premature infants less than 55 weeks PCA are at sufficient risk to warrant overnight hospitalization and monitoring. The length of the required hospital stay is unknown; however, most pediatric institutions require monitoring for at least 12 apnea-free hours with a cardiopulmonary monitor (pulse oximetry and electrocardiography).

Both retrospective and prospective studies have been performed in an attempt to delineate the types of patients at risk for postoperative apnea. Characteristics of premature infants that are likely to develop postoperative apnea include low gestational age, low postconceptional age (PCA), preoperative apnea of prematurity, and anemia (usually defined as a hemoglobin level <10 g/dL). The PCA at which postoperative apnea will not occur is unknown; however, there are no reports of postoperative apnea in infants aged greater than 60 weeks PCA. The true risk for an individual patient is indeterminate and is likely a continuum based on the infant's gestational and chronological age, and coexisting medical conditions.

Strategies for Prevention of Postoperative Apnea

There are three main anesthetic strategies for preventing postoperative apnea in susceptible infants:
1. Performing a regional anesthetic instead of a general anesthetic
2. Perioperative administration of intravenous caffeine
3. Selection of general anesthetic agents or opioids that are characterized by their limited duration of action.

Spinal anesthesia for premature infants was popularized in 1984 by Chris Abajian from the University of Vermont (see Chapter 20). Since publication of that report, numerous additional publications have examined the benefits and risks of spinal or epidural anesthesia in this patient population for lower abdominal or groin procedures. Most reported series confirm that spinal or epidural anesthesia is associated with a lower incidence (but not complete absence) of postoperative apnea, provided additional systemic sedative agents are avoided. Comparative studies have not been performed with individual sedative agents; however, it appears that when systemic sedatives are administered intraoperatively to treat pain or agitation, the risk of postoperative apnea increases to a level similar to that after general anesthesia. This has been confirmed for ketamine as well. Therefore, infants at risk of postoperative apnea who receive regional anesthesia with sedative supplementation should receive the same postoperative apnea monitoring as that used after administration of general anesthesia. There is currently a debate in the pediatric anesthesia community concerning the appropriate level of postoperative monitoring in infants receiving regional anesthesia without sedative supplementation. Although some centers routinely discharge these infants on the day of surgery, the majority of pediatric centers require overnight monitoring.

The second strategy is perioperative administration of caffeine base, 10 mg/kg. Caffeine is a respiratory stimulant that, when administered during induction of general anesthesia, decreases the incidence of postoperative apnea, bradycardia, and hypoxemia in susceptible infants. Anesthesiologists caring for infants at risk of postoperative apnea should proactively consult with their center's neonatologists and develop a treatment plan for the administration of perioperative caffeine. At The Children's Hospital of Philadelphia, many of these susceptible infants will already be receiving caffeine as part of their prophylactic management of apnea of prematurity, so additional perioperative administration is not required. In formerly premature infants who present for elective surgery after discharge from the hospital, caffeine is administered on a case-by-case basis, after assessment of the risk factors and discussion with the infant's neonatologist.

Almost all studies on risk of postoperative apnea following general anesthesia were performed prior to the advent of short-acting anesthetic agents, such as sevoflurane, desflurane, and remifentanil. It is theoretically possible that use of these newer agents of limited duration will result in a decreased incidence of postoperative apnea, so they should be used in susceptible infants when available. However, definitive data on the association of postoperative apnea with use of these agents is lacking.

ADDITIONAL ARTICLES TO KNOW

Statement on the care of the child with chronic lung disease of infancy and childhood. *Am J Respir Crit Care Med* 168:356-396, 2003.

Cox RG, Goresky GV: Life-threatening apnea following spinal anesthesia in former premature infants. *Anesthesiology* 73: 345-347, 1990.

Jobe AH, Bancalari E: Bronchopulmonary dysplasia. *Am J Respir Crit Care Med* 163:1723-1729, 2001.

Kramer MS, Demissie K, Yang H et al: The contribution of mild and moderate preterm birth to infant mortality. Fetal and Infant Health Study Group of the Canadian Perinatal Surveillance System. *JAMA* 284:843-849, 2000.

Krane EJ, Haberkern CM, Jacobson LE: Postoperative apnea, bradycardia, and oxygen desaturation in formerly premature infants: prospective comparison of spinal and general anesthesia. *Anesth Analg* 80:7-13, 1995.

Kurth CD, Lebard SE: Association of postoperative apnea, airway obstruction, and hypoxemia in former premature infants. *Anesthesiology* 75:22-26, 1991.

Kurth CD, Spitzer AR, Broennle AM, Downes JJ: Postoperative apnea in preterm infants. *Anesthesiology* 66:483-488, 1987.

Sartorelli KH, Abajian JC, Kreutz JM, Vane DW: Improved outcome utilizing spinal anesthesia in high-risk infants. *J Pediatr Surg* 27:1022-1025, 1992.

Shenkman Z, Hoppenstein D, Litmanowitz I et al: Spinal anesthesia in 62 premature, former-premature or young infants: technical aspects and pitfalls. *Can J Anaesth* 49:262-269, 2002.

Steward DJ: Preterm infants are more prone to complications following minor surgery than are term infants. *Anesthesiology* 56:304-306, 1982.

Welborn LG, Hannallah RS, Fink R, Ruttimann UE, Hicks JM: High-dose caffeine suppresses postoperative apnea in former preterm infants. *Anesthesiology* 71:347-349, 1989.

Welborn LG, Hannallah RS, Luban NLC, Fink R, Ruttimann UE: Anemia and postoperative apnea in former preterm infants. *Anesthesiology* 74:1003-1006, 1991.

Welborn LG, Rice LJ, Hannallah RS et al: Postoperative apnea in former preterm infants: prospective comparison of spinal and general anesthesia. *Anesthesiology* 72:838-842, 1990.

William JM, Stoddart PA, Williams SA, Wolf AR: Post-operative recovery after inguinal herniotomy in ex-premature infants: comparison between sevoflurane and spinal anaesthesia. *Br J Anaesth* 86:366-371, 2001.

PREOPERATIVE ASSESSMENT

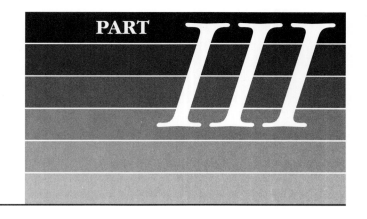

PART

III

Preanesthetic Preparation of the Pediatric Patient

RONALD S. LITMAN

Prior to the day of surgery, preanesthetic preparation of pediatric patients involves the appropriate choice of laboratory tests that will influence anesthetic management, the assignment of a preoperative fasting interval, and a focused history and physical exam that may influence anesthetic management (although this may occur on the day of surgery). On the day of surgery, the history and physical exam are updated, and the anesthesiologist then must focus on alleviating stress and anxiety of the patient and family (Box 12-1).

PREOPERATIVE LABORATORY TESTING

Hemoglobin determination is probably the most commonly performed preoperative blood test in children.

Each center varies with regard to its requirement for preoperative hemoglobin testing in healthy children. Some children's hospitals mandate routine preoperative hemoglobin testing in selected infants under 12 months. Furthermore, each has policies concerning the minimum hemoglobin level for performance of elective surgery on small infants. For example, at The Children's Hospital of Philadelphia, infants below the arbitrary age of 6 months require a hemoglobin level above 10 g/dL to proceed with elective surgery. Unfortunately, there are little or no data to guide current recommendations for obtaining preoperative hemoglobin values in this age range. Healthy children over the age of 12 months do not require preoperative hemoglobin testing. Additional blood tests, radiographs, and urinalysis are not obtained in healthy pediatric patients prior to most surgical procedures. These studies are determined solely by the medical condition of the patient and the nature of the surgical procedure.

Collection of a preoperative type-and-screen or type-and-crossmatch to prepare for a potential blood transfusion will depend on the nature of the surgery and the expected blood loss. In general, if a blood sample is sent to the blood bank because of a possible anticipated transfusion, a hemoglobin value should also be obtained. Coagulation studies are not routinely performed except when there is a history of a potential bleeding disorder in the child or among his or her first-degree relatives. Many otolaryngology surgeons, however, will require these tests prior to elective tonsillectomy.

PREOPERATIVE FASTING

Multiple studies in the pediatric physiology literature have demonstrated that clear liquids are rapidly emptied from the stomach, regardless of chronological or gestational age. Children of all age groups who ingest clear fluids 2 hours prior to induction of anesthesia have a similar

---

Box 12-1   The Eleven Ps

The approach to the preoperative assessment of children should be structured with regard to specific tasks that include reviewing the anesthetic considerations for the child's medical condition and surgical procedure, and developing a perioperative plan. A convenient and comprehensive method to remember this structure is to use a system I call the Eleven Ps. These are divided into preoperative, intraoperative, and postoperative considerations. Preoperative considerations are described in this chapter and include assessment of the patient, and decisions concerning premedication, preoperative fasting, and preoperative laboratory tests. In addition, the preoperative period is the time when intraoperative and postoperative concerns are contemplated, and management plans devised.

- *Patient:* An assessment of the patient includes the history, physical exam, obtaining the old chart to review previous anesthetics, and research into the anesthetic implications of any coexisting medical conditions.
- *Procedure:* The anesthesiologist must be familiar with the general aspects of the surgical procedure and the way in which these will affect anesthetic management.
- *Premedication:* Optimal choice of premedication is ordered.
- *Preoperative fasting:* Fasting orders are written. Parents of healthy children are encouraged to offer their child unlimited clear liquids 2 hours prior to the scheduled surgical time.
- *Preoperative labs:* Appropriate tests are chosen depending on the medical condition of the patient and the nature of the surgery.
- *Perioperative monitoring:* Additional monitors are obtained if dictated by the medical condition of the patient or the nature of the surgery.
- *Perioperative fluids:* Appropriate IV fluids are chosen depending on the age and medical condition of the child, and nature of the surgery.
- *Positioning:* Preparations are made to enhance patient safety when using a position other than supine.
- *Plan:* An anesthetic plan for induction, maintenance, and emergence from general anesthesia is formulated based on a combination of the above factors.
- *Pain:* Plans are formulated for intraoperative and postoperative analgesic requirements. This often includes a regional anesthesia technique.
- *Postoperative:* Considerations are given for possible postoperative concerns and complications depending on the medical condition of the patient and the nature of the surgery. Plans are made for possible ICU admission and ventilatory management if necessary.

---

gastric volume and pH as those fasted for longer periods. Shorter fasting intervals have not been studied. Practically speaking, there would be no obvious advantage to allowing ingestion of clear liquids less than 2 hours prior to surgery. Maintaining a 2-hour interval will allow for flexibility in OR scheduling if a case is canceled and if a child needs to be advanced to an earlier time slot in the schedule. There is no known association between the volume and pH of gastric contents and the risk of pulmonary aspiration.

Clear liquids generally consist of any fluid that can easily be seen through. Exceptions include cola soda and black coffee, which are allowable. The presence of fat or particulate matter such as pulp from orange juice will delay gastric emptying. Opinion is mixed on whether or not gelatin (Jell-O) should be considered a clear liquid. Most anesthesiologists have witnessed the clump of gelatinized substance that is present in the vomitus of children who recently ingested Jell-O, and therefore do not include it among the substances that qualify as a clear liquid.

Not only should children be allowed to drink clear liquids 2 hours before induction of anesthesia, they should be actively encouraged to do so. Parents should awaken their small child before an early morning arrival and encourage the ingestion of clear liquids. Advantages to this practice include an increased gastric pH, decreased risk of hypovolemia and hypoglycemia at the time of induction of anesthesia, decreased irritability of the child, and increased parental satisfaction. It has been demonstrated that prolonged preoperative fasting is associated with a greater decrease in blood pressure in infants during halothane administration.

There is no consensus as to the maximal amount of clears that can be ingested. Some studies have used a certain amount by weight, some have limited the amount to 8 ounces, and others have allowed unlimited amounts. Nevertheless, the amount of clear fluids ingested 2 hours prior to surgery does not seem to influence subsequent gastric volumes. Therefore, an unlimited amount should be allowed within the prescribed time frame.

Breast-fed infants can be allowed to nurse up until 3–4 hours prior to surgery. Breast milk contains a large amount of fat, and empties slower from the stomach than clear liquids. However, there is some evidence that breast milk has a faster gastric emptying time than some infant formulas. Furthermore, many breast-fed infants will not be able to drink other types of liquids from a bottle. Since pulmonary aspiration is extremely rare in healthy infants, the advantages of allowing a relatively short fasting interval for breast milk probably outweigh the disadvantages.

Infant formula is completely emptied from the stomach within 4 hours in most children. When compared to infants allowed clear liquids up to 2 hours before surgery, infants who ingest formula 4 hours prior to surgery have similar values for gastric volume and pH. Therefore, infants should be allowed to ingest formula up to 4 hours prior to surgery.

Gastric emptying of solids is more difficult to study in pediatric patients. Most institutions allow solids until 6–8 hours prior to surgery, and will allow a light breakfast for those children whose surgery is scheduled in the late afternoon.

The current preoperative fasting guidelines at The Children's Hospital of Philadelphia (Box 12-2) are a result of a compilation of a large amount of circumstantial evidence based on surrogate outcome variables – residual gastric volume and gastric pH. Since the severity of pulmonary aspiration is directly related to larger volumes and lower pH of the aspirate, anesthesiologists naturally prefer as empty a stomach as possible at the time of induction of anesthesia. However, the occurrence of the most important clinical outcome variable – pulmonary aspiration – has not been definitively associated with

---

Box 12-2 Preoperative Fasting Guidelines at The Children's Hospital of Philadelphia[a]

Clear liquids: until 2 hours prior to surgery
Breast milk: until 3 hours prior to surgery
Formula:
Infants <6 months – until 4 hours prior to surgery
Infants >6: until 6 hours prior to surgery
Non-human milk and solids: until 8 hours prior to surgery[b]

[a]For those with disorders that can affect digestion, such as gastroesophageal reflux, diabetes, and recent trauma, more prolonged fasting recommendations may apply.
[b]Healthy patients scheduled for surgery after 1300h are permitted to eat one of the following before 0700h: a single slice of dry toast (no butter, jam, peanut butter, or cream cheese, etc.) *or* up to one cup of dry, plain Cheerios (no milk or yogurt). Having toast or plain Cheerios before 0700h may limit flexibility in the event of patient cancellation since anesthesia and surgery cannot in most situations start until 6 hours after eating these foods. To maximize a child's chances of safely moving ahead in the surgical schedule, we recommend no solids after midnight and clear liquids up until 2 hours prior to surgery.

---

these surrogate outcome variables. Pulmonary aspiration of gastric contents is more closely linked with other factors such as emergency surgery, multiple intubation attempts, absence of neuromuscular blockade during intubation attempts, and the underlying medical condition of the patient.

Article To Know

Schreiner MS, Triebwasser A, Keon TP: Ingestion of liquids compared with preoperative fasting in pediatric outpatients. Anesthesiology 72:593-597, 1990.

It was not until 1990 that Mark Schreiner and his colleagues at The Children's Hospital of Philadelphia published this landmark article that confirmed the safety of shortened preoperative fasting in children. They compared gastric fluid volume and pH in two randomly selected groups of 121 healthy children between 1 and 18 years of age. The control group received standard fasting orders which consisted of unlimited clear liquids up until 6 hours (≤5 years of age) or 8 hours (>5 years) prior to the scheduled time of surgery. The study group was allowed 8 ounces of a clear liquid up to 2 hours prior to the scheduled time of surgery. The important results are presented in the table below.

	Study Group	Control Group	*P*-value
Gastric volume (mL/kg) (mean ± SD)	0.44 ± 0.51	0.57 ± 0.51	0.12
Gastric volume >0.4 mL/kg	23/48 (48%)	39/67 (58%)	0.77
Gastric pH <2.5	34/35 (97%)	44/48 (92%)	0.47

Reproduced with permission from Schreiner et al: *Anesthesiology* 72:593-597, 1990.

Using parental questionnaires, the investigators determined that children in the study group were significantly less irritable compared with children in the control group, and the parents of the children in the study group were significantly more satisfied. This study was one of the first to demonstrate that shortened preoperative fasts were no less safe than prolonged fasting, by the surrogate outcome measures of gastric volume and pH. Numerous additional studies have since confirmed these findings and extended the same results to infants younger than 12 months.

Children with a Potentially "Full Stomach"

Preoperative administration of pharmacologic agents effectively reduces gastric volume and increases gastric pH in children at the time of induction of anesthesia. These include H_2 receptor antagonists such as cimetidine, ranitidine, and famotidine, and prokinetic agents such as metoclopramide. Various regimens of each have been shown to decrease gastric volume and increase gastric pH in children. None, however, has been associated with a decreased risk of pulmonary aspiration, or decreased severity of aspiration pneumonitis. Therefore, the practice of administering these medications to children is not routine in most pediatric centers.

PREOPERATIVE HISTORY

The preoperative history in children should focus on concurrent medical diseases and their treatment, currently administered medications, previous allergic reactions, previous administration of anesthetics, and family history of problems with anesthesia. A variety of concurrent medical diseases may influence the anesthetic technique. Few concurrent medications influence the anesthetic technique. Examples include anticonvulsants, which tend to shorten the duration of action of the aminosteroidal neuromuscular blockers. The history should elicit problems with previous anesthetics. Anesthetic complications that recur include airway obstruction, postoperative nausea and vomiting, and severity of postoperative pain. If an anesthesia record is accessible, it must be thoroughly reviewed. Finally, the history of anesthetic problems in the family is focused on detecting adverse reactions that may have represented malignant hyperthermia or unexpected prolonged paralysis that may represent familial pseudocholinesterase deficiency.

When anesthetizing a neonate, the preoperative history should also focus on the medical histories of the parents and the course of pregnancy and delivery. A variety of maternal medical conditions during pregnancy affect the newborn (Table 12-1). Furthermore, many different medications administered during pregnancy may potentially affect the health of the newborn (Table 12-2).

A history of an allergy to a medication is common in children presenting for surgery. All children who require insertion of tympanostomy tubes have been exposed to at least one type of antibiotic. Many of these children report development of a rash after administration of antibiotics with a penicillin, cephalosporin, or sulfa base. Children do not routinely undergo further diagnostic testing to determine the cause of the rash. Therefore, the anesthesia practitioner has no accurate way of determining the true allergic status of the child, other than by history, or report

Table 12-1 Maternal Medical Conditions and their Effects on the Newborn	
Maternal Medical Condition	**Effect on Newborn**
Diabetes	Increased incidence of congenital anomalies, hypoglycemia, macrosomia, polycythemia, cardiomyopathy, hypocalcemia, immature lung disease, hypomagnesemia, hyperbilirubinemia
Oligohydramnios	Renal anomalies, fetal distress, growth retardation
Polyhydramnios	Tracheoesophageal fistula
Low α-fetoprotein levels	Trisomy 21 (Down syndrome)
Rh sensitization	Hydrops fetalis, or mild forms of hemolytic anemia
Antepartum bleeding	Anemia, hypovolemia
Premature membrane rupture	Neonatal infection, sepsis
Meconium-stained amniotic fluid	Interstitial pneumonitis
Systemic lupus erythematosus (SLE)	Congenital third-degree heart block
Myasthenia gravis	Neonatal myasthenia
Poor fetal heart rate tracing: late decelerations, poor beat-to-beat variability	Neonatal metabolic acidosis and effects from hypoxia
Preeclampsia	Neonatal neutropenia and thrombocytopenia
Graves' disease	Hypothyroidism or hyperthyroidism
Chorioamnionitis	Neonatal infection, sepsis

Reproduced with permission from Klaus MH, Fanaroff AA eds: *Care of the High Risk Neonate*, 5th edn, WB Saunders, Philadelphia, 2001.

from the parent. Research studies have consistently shown that history of a drug allergy does not accurately predict positive skin testing. In many cases, more detailed questioning of the parent reveals that the reaction was truly not allergic in nature. For example, a parent may report that their child is allergic to morphine because it caused the child to experience somnolence or itching.

Anesthesiologists must take an allergic history seriously, for the very reason that we rarely, if ever, have firm indications for any type of medication, especially antibiotics. In other words, we always have other viable alternatives, although they may not necessarily be cost-effective. On the other hand, the indiscriminant use of more powerful antibiotics (e.g., vancomycin for Gram-positive cocci prophylaxis) leads to the development of antibiotic resistance. One of the most common examples of this is the child who presents with a history of an amoxicillin-related rash, and now requires surgical prophylaxis with cefazolin. The skin-testing literature suggests that the cross-reactivity between (true) penicillin and cephalosporin allergies is approximately 10%.

Table 12-2	Maternal Medications and their Effects on the Newborn
Medication	**Effect on Newborn**
Aspirin and other NSAIDs	Hemorrhage, pulmonary artery hypertension
Opioids	Neonatal depression, or abstinence syndrome if chronic maternal usage
Cephalosporins	Hyperbilirubinemia
Sulfonamides	Hyperbilirubinemia
Anticonvulsants	Congenital anomalies
Warfarin (coumadin)	Congenital anomalies, developmental delay, seizures
Antithyroid medications	Hypothyroidism
Beta-blockers	Neonatal bradycardia, hypoglycemia
Cocaine	Congenital anomalies, placental abruption
Magnesium sulfate	Respiratory depression, hypotonia, sensitivity to neuromuscular blockers
Ritodrine	Neonatal hypoglycemia
Terbutaline	Neonatal hypoglycemia
Alcohol	Fetal alcohol syndrome: dysmorphic facies, growth retardation, developmental delay
Tobacco	Prematurity, IUGR, placental abruption and previa
Lithium	Cardiac anomalies
Isotretinoin	Micrognathia, cardiac and CNS anomalies
ACE inhibitors	Hypotension, oliguria

ACE, angiotensin-converting enzyme; CNS, central nervous system; IUGR, intrauterine growth retardation; NSAID, nonsteroidal anti-inflammatory drug. Reproduced with permission from Klaus MH, Fanaroff AA eds: *Care of the High Risk Neonate*, 5th edn, WB Saunders, Philadelphia, 2001.

When the penicillin allergy is based on history alone, the incidence is much less, and when reactions occur, they are rarely life-threatening. Although there is some room for flexibility, such as the child with mild allergic manifestations to penicillin who may then receive a cephalosporin, there are also some firm absolutes:

1. Never administer a medication for which a child has a history of a true allergy to that same medication.
2. There is no role for desensitization, or test dosing, in the perioperative setting. If the case arises whereby the surgeon insists on a particular medication for which the child has claimed an allergy, consultation with a specialist in immunology or allergy is then indicated.

PREOPERATIVE PHYSICAL EXAM

The focus of the preoperative physical exam is on the cardiovascular system, respiratory system, neurologic

Table 12-3	Key Elements of the Preanesthetic Physical Exam in Children
Observation	**Implications**
General	
Hypotonia or hypertonia	Neurologic or metabolic disease
Cyanosis	Cardiac disease, sepsis
Pallor	Anemia, poor cardiac output
Cardiovascular	
Abnormal murmur	Congenital heart disease
Abnormal or absent pulses	Coarctation of the aorta, poor cardiac output
Respiratory	
Tachypnea, abnormal lung sounds (e.g., wheezing, rales, rhonchi), use of accessory muscles of respiration, grunting	All are nonspecific findings in a variety of respiratory or cardiac disorders
Head and Neck	
Abnormal craniofacial formation (e.g., micrognathia), limited mouth opening and jaw mobility, limited neck mobility	All are indicators of possible difficulty with ventilation or intubation

function, and other indicators of normal function (Table 12-3). These include evaluation for anemia, hypovolemia, and bleeding tendencies, among others. Normal findings on physical exam will vary with age in pediatric patients.

Examination of the cardiovascular system begins with a measurement of vital signs such as heart rate and blood pressure. Normal values for heart rate and blood pressure vary with age, gender, weight, and height (see Chapter 1). Many active and irritable infants will not cooperate with a preoperative physical exam and thus blood pressure measurements are unreliable, and probably irrelevant in otherwise healthy children. Auscultation of the heart should be performed to ascertain the presence of normal heart sounds and absence of unexpected abnormal murmurs.

One of the most vexing issues in pediatric anesthesia is the approach to the child with a heart murmur on preoperative physical exam. The parents should be queried as to whether or not the murmur has been previously detected by any of the child's medical caretakers, and if there was any previous cardiac evaluation. If the murmur was previously detected, the anesthesiologist should determine its cause. In the vast majority of cases, the parent will acknowledge that the murmur has been deemed to be a normal flow murmur. If the murmur has not been previously detected, the anesthesiologist is confronted with a situation whereby he or she must decide rather quickly whether or not to continue with the anesthetic or cancel the case pending cardiology consultation to determine the cause of the murmur. The vast majority of murmurs in otherwise healthy children can be classified as normal flow murmurs. These are not louder than II/VI, are usually vibratory in nature, and occur in systole over the pulmonary or mitral areas of the chest wall. Cardiology consultation should be obtained if these characteristics are not present, or if there are other findings relevant to the cardiovascular system on history or physical exam (Box 12-3).

Important elements of the respiratory system include the upper and lower airways. Facial structure and mandibular mobility should be examined for clues to a possible difficult ventilation or difficult tracheal intubation. Loose teeth should be suspected in children between 5 and 10 years of age. The anesthesiologist should manually remove an extremely loose tooth after induction of anesthesia as a precaution against its unintentional removal during airway manipulation and dislodgment into the bronchial tree. The lungs should be auscultated to ensure normal respiratory rate and breath sounds. Children with a history of reactive airway disease and those with a concurrent upper respiratory tract infection should be assessed for expiratory wheezing. Room air pulse oximetry should be performed; a value less than 96% should warrant an investigation of respiratory related abnormalities. In general, respiratory rates greater than 44 breaths per minute are considered abnormal, except in otherwise healthy neonates and small infants, in whom normal breathing rates can occasionally reach 70 breaths per minute.

Additional elements of the physical exam will be largely dependent on the preexisting medical condition of the child and the nature of the surgery. For example, a focused neurologic exam is indicated prior to any neurologic or orthopedic surgery, and in children with neuromuscular diseases.

PSYCHOLOGICAL PREPARATION OF THE CHILD

The preoperative period is often a stressful and anxiety-provoking phase for the child and his or her family. It is not unusual for the parents to be frightened and to project their fears and anxiety on the child, thereby unintentionally contributing to the child's fear and stress. Anesthesiologists must recognize these interactions and play a proactive role in preventing or treating the entire family's concerns. As pediatricians often treat the parents more than the child, the pediatric anesthesiologist also often assumes a role as a "family practitioner." It is extremely useful for the anesthesiologist to establish rapport with the child, which will then reassure the parents. More than anything, parents (and hospital staff!) will observe the anesthesiologist to ensure that he or she interacts well with the child and tries to relate on the child's level. A very common complaint from parents and nurses is that although the anesthesiologist was very thorough in preoperative discussion with the parents, he or she did not attempt to interact with the child.

One of the most important considerations in pediatric anesthesia is an understanding of age-appropriate behaviors in response to external situations. Once these are recognized, anesthesiologists are able to tailor individual therapy to children and their parents (Table 12-4).

The most important outcome variables related to preoperative distress in children are postoperative behavioral disorders. These include, but are not limited to, sleep disturbances (e.g., nightmares), feeding difficulties, apathy, withdrawal, increased level of separation anxiety, aggression toward authority, fear of subsequent medical procedures and hospital visits, and regressive behaviors such as bed wetting. Although these disturbances are primarily present within the first two postoperative weeks, in some children they may last for many months. Much has been made of this issue in the recent literature, but the concept is not new. In 1953, Eckenhoff demonstrated that personality changes in children occurred and were associated with younger age and unsatisfactory inductions.

Dr Zeev Kain and his colleagues at Yale University School of Medicine comprehensively evaluated the characteristics of children with postoperative behavioral disorders and potential interventions. Children with a high level of preoperative anxiety were found to be at highest risk for these maladaptive behaviors, as were children who underwent "stormy" inductions. Furthermore, children with an extremely high level of preoperative anxiety

---

Box 12-3   Reasons to Obtain Cardiology Consultation for a Previously Undetected Heart Murmur

History

Poor exercise tolerance (or feeding intolerance in an infant)
Patient was supposed to have a cardiology evaluation but it was never done
Congenital heart disease in immediate family
Cyanotic episodes

Physical Exam

Murmur present in diastole
Grade III or louder
Absent or abnormal peripheral pulses
Cyanosis, pallor, or poor capillary refill

Table 12-4	Age-specific Anxieties of Pediatric Patients
Age	**Specific Type of Perioperative Anxiety**
0–6 months	Maximum stress for parents
	Minimum stress for infants: not old enough to be frightened of strangers or to remember unpleasant events
6 months to 4 years	Maximal fear of separation
	Not able to understand processes and explanations
	Significant postoperative emotional upset and behavioral regression
4–8 years	Begins to understand processes and explanations
	Fear of separation remains
	Concerned about body integrity
8 years to adolescence	Tolerates separation well
	Understands processes and explanations
	May fear waking up during surgery or not waking up at all
Adolescent	Developing sexual characteristics and thus fears loss of dignity
	Fear of unknown

Reproduced with permission from Barash PG, Cullen BF, Stoelting RK eds: *Clinical Anesthesia*, 4th edn, Lippincott Williams & Wilkins, Philadelphia, 2003.

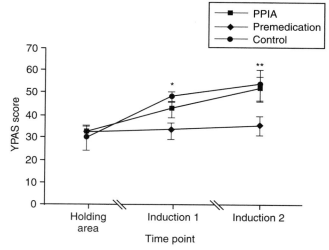

Figure 12-1   Anxiety of the child during the perioperative period. Anxiety of the premedication group was significantly lower during both induction 1 ($*P = 0.0171$) and induction 2 ($**P = 0.0176$). Induction 1 = entrance to the operating room; induction 2 = introduction of the anesthesia mask to the child; mYPAS = Yale Preoperative Anxiety Scale. (Reproduced with permission from Kain ZN, Mayes LC, Wang SM, Caramico LA, Hofstadter MB: Parental presence during induction of anesthesia versus sedative premedication: which intervention is more effective? *Anesthesiology* 89:1147–1156, 1998.)

had higher excitement scores on arrival to the postanesthesia care unit.

Many different modalities have been utilized in an attempt to decrease fear and anxiety in patients and their families. Behavioral interventions include preoperative informational materials that consist of discussions, tours, written literature, and videotapes. In some institutions, personnel from the Child Life department assume an active role in development of these programs and coordinate their efforts with anesthesia personnel. Some centers allow parents to accompany their child into the OR during induction of anesthesia in an attempt to allay anxiety. In carefully performed and controlled studies, however, these aforementioned interventions do not fare much better than placebo in decreasing the incidence of postoperative behavioral disturbances. Premedication with an anxiolytic drug such as midazolam is the only proven intervention to decrease these undesirable outcomes (Fig. 12-1).

Dr Chris Abajian at the University of Vermont has popularized the use of simple magic tricks for allaying preoperative anxiety in children. We have adopted many of these in our own practice to the delight of the patients, families, and our coworkers. The easiest and most basic is to use is the Fun Magic Coloring Book, in which the magician is easily able to turn a normal-appearing coloring book into a fully colored one with the flip of a page.

To date, outcome studies using magic as a preoperative anxiolytic technique have not been performed.

PSYCHOLOGICAL PREPARATION OF THE PARENTS

Allaying Parental Anxiety

One of the most important preoperative jobs of the pediatric anesthesiologist is to attempt to allay anxiety in the parents and other family members. During the preoperative visit the anesthesiologist, while talking to the parents, should initiate contact and communication with the child. It does not matter if the child is too young to understand, or is too premedicated to remember any events. The parents will key in on the anesthesiologist's manner and how he or she relates to the child. Verbal cues such as smiling at the child, or asking the child simple questions, will reassure the parents that their son or daughter is in good hands. This practice will establish confidence and minimize parental anxiety.

Discussing Risks of Pediatric Anesthesia

A controversial issue in pediatric anesthesia is the extent to which the anesthesiologist should reveal the risks of anesthesia to the parents. Will this discussion increase or decrease parental (or child) anxiety? Should the anesthesiologist discuss the risk of death? What risks are appropriate to reveal? The answers to these questions are not easily found, and may partly depend on the informed consent laws of the state in which one practices. Studies universally demonstrate that anxiety is decreased with more information, even though that information may allude to more harmful risks. For example, in a questionnaire study, most parents whose anesthesiologist mentioned the risk of death indicated they were satisfied to hear about this rare risk. Many parents whose anesthesiologist did not specifically mention the risk of death indicated that it should have been mentioned.

This author's practice is to allude to the potentially harmful, yet rare, risks of anesthesia without increasing anxiety by stressing the overall safety of the procedure. One such dialog to the parents of a healthy child for elective surgery is as follows: "I don't expect any risks or complications. Of course, we can never say 'never,' but the risk of a life-threatening complication is extremely rare. Overall the anesthesia is extremely safe, and my job is to make sure it stays that way."

Allowing Parents into the OR

The time of induction of anesthesia represents an enormously frightening time for both patients and parents. Many centers have promulgated a culture of allowing a parent to accompany their child into the OR during induction of general anesthesia. This has paralleled a trend to allow family members into other previously forbidden places where medical procedures are occurring, such as the emergency room or the ICU. Parents assert that they possess a right to be with their child during any and all phases of their child's hospitalization. Studies have clearly shown that parental presence does not alter the acute behavioral distress of the child, nor does it alter outcomes such as negative postoperative behaviors. Furthermore, many parents are terrified as they observe the placing of a mask over their child's face, watching their child become limp as consciousness is lost, and the occasional episode of upper airway obstruction that may occur. Yet when queried, parents who have been with their child in the OR during induction universally feel that they have done the right thing for their child and are more satisfied than if they didn't participate. If a decision is made to allow a parent into the OR during induction, the anesthesiologist should fully explain the events that will occur during induction. Three major points should be addressed:

1. There should be an explanation of the nature of the procedure and the possible effects on the child (excitation, limpness, airway obstruction, etc.).
2. The parent must agree to leave immediately at any time when requested by an OR staff member.

3. The parent must agree to leave immediately once the child has lost consciousness. One of the surgical team members or another OR staff member should accompany the parent from the OR to the parents' waiting area.

Some institutions will ask a parent to sign a written agreement to these terms, as well as a waiver of liability should the parent suffer an injury secondary to fainting or other adverse event.

PHARMACOLOGIC PREPARATION OF THE CHILD

Premedication of pediatric patients prior to induction of anesthesia can accomplish several goals, the primary one being anxiolysis, with a subsequent decrease in the incidence of postoperative negative behaviors. Other indications include preinduction of anesthesia, pain relief, drying of secretions prior to airway manipulation, vagolysis, and decreasing the risk for pulmonary aspiration of gastric contents. Preoperative sedation may be administered via any route, the most common being oral administration since the vast majority of children do not have an existing intravenous catheter. Rectal premedication is acceptable in toddlers, and in some centers the nasal route is preferred for midazolam. Few centers in the United States administer intramuscular premedication, or place intravenous catheters preoperatively.

A ground-breaking study on premedication in children was reported in 1959. Drs Bachman and Freeman, at The Children's Hospital of Philadelphia, successfully used intramuscular injections of various combinations of morphine, atropine, scopolamine, and pentobarbital. Children who received premedication exhibited improved ease of induction, reduced airway secretions, and less emergence delirium. In 1989, Susan Nicolson and her colleagues at The Children's Hospital of Philadelphia challenged the necessity of intramuscular injections by reporting their positive experience with an oral premedication. This latter study marked the beginning of a new era of oral premedication, and an end to painful intramuscular injections in children.

There are various options for treatment of preoperative anxiety. None, however, are ideal – each has drawbacks. Basic principles of pharmacologic treatment of patients dictate that a drug should be administered to target its specific action, and not one of its side-effects. In other words, anxiety should be treated with an anxiolytic; pain should be treated with an analgesic, and so on. Therefore, it is generally unwise to treat anxiety using the sedative effects of an opioid. Unless there are no other options, a drug should not be used for its side-effects. For these reasons, it is best to treat preoperative anxiety with a medication that is specifically designed as an anxiolytic. The benzodiazepines best fit this indication. Common options include midazolam, the most commonly administered premedication, and diazepam. In general, children above the age of 9 or 10 months will benefit from preoperative anxiolysis. Yet, some studies report that only 25% of children under 3 years of age are treated for preoperative anxiety. However, there is mounting evidence that preoperative anxiolysis can affect true patient outcomes in the form of decreased postoperative behavioral disturbances.

Midazolam

Oral Midazolam

Oral midazolam is the most common preoperative anxiolytic for children. This is because it possesses most of the properties of the ideal premedication (Box 12-4). The one exception is that it leaves a very bitter aftertaste when administered orally, even as a specially formulated oral syrup. Many children will attempt to spit it out of their mouth if it is not swallowed rapidly. After oral administration, the commercially available midazolam syrup is rapidly absorbed from the stomach. The absolute bioavailability of midazolam averages 36%, within a variable and large range (9–71%). This large range in bioavailability is consistent with most oral medications administered to children. In a large study, the plasma concentration/time curves of midazolam and its α-hydroxy metabolite were highly variable, and independent of the age of the child and the dose administered (Fig. 12-2).

Caution should be observed in children who are receiving erythromycin, since it can prolong the duration of action of midazolam via cytochrome P-450 inhibition. In children who are currently receiving erythromycin, the midazolam dose should be reduced by at least 50%.

Clinical sedative effects are seen within 5–10 minutes of oral midazolam administration, and appear to peak 15–30 minutes after administration. By 45 minutes, its sedative effects have dissipated in most children.

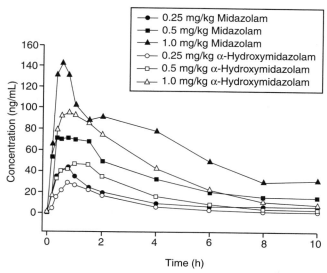

Figure 12-2 Plasma concentration/time curves of midazolam and its major metabolite α-hydroxymidazolam after oral administration in children aged 6 months to 16 years. (Reproduced with permission from Reed MD, Rodarte A, Blumer JL et al: The single-dose pharmacokinetics of midazolam and its primary metabolite in pediatric patients after oral and intravenous administration. *J Clin Pharmacol* 41:1359–1369, 2001.)

Pharmacodynamic studies indicate that sedation level is directly correlated with plasma concentration of midazolam. Plasma midazolam concentrations greater than 50 ng/mL are associated with adequate preoperative sedation. However, plasma concentrations of midazolam are not associated with anxiety scores at the time of mask induction of anesthesia.

The sedative effect of midazolam is best described as inebriation rather than sleepiness. Most children are happy, and will lose their balance. Therefore, after administration, children should be confined to a bed or in the confines of their parent's arms, and be directly observed at all times by medical personnel. Clinically important cardiorespiratory side-effects are not observed in healthy children. Dysphoria may occur in some children. Anterograde amnesia is a favorable clinical effect following most doses of oral midazolam and may be responsible for the decrease in postoperative behavioral disturbances.

Most anesthesiologists find that an oral dose of 0.5–0.7 mg/kg results in the best clinical efficacy. However, recent pharmacodynamic studies suggest that a dose as low as 0.25 mg/kg results in reliable preoperative anxiolysis. There are no data to indicate the most appropriate maximum dose, but most anesthesiologists use between 10 and 20 mg.

Studies are conflicting, but some evidence indicates that midazolam premedication results in longer times to discharge postoperatively following surgeries of relatively short duration. Nevertheless, its preoperative advantages outweigh this disadvantage.

Box 12-4 Desirable Characteristics of a Preoperative Anxiolytic

Effective and reliable anxiolysis and sedation
Amnesia of preoperative events
Facilitates induction of anesthesia
Short latency period to onset of action
Minimal respiratory and cardiovascular effects
Easy to administer (for patient and staff)
Short duration of action
Lowers intraoperative anesthetic requirements
Blocks unwanted autonomic (vagal) reflexes
Prevents excessive airway secretions

Nasal Midazolam

Nasal administration of midazolam can be accomplished in the form of nose drops or a nasal spray. The required dose (0.2–0.3 mg/kg) is lower than with oral administration and its reliability in producing anxiolysis is excellent. However, its administration is associated with an unpleasant burning of the nasal cavity and most children are quite upset following its use. In addition, plasma concentrations of midazolam are generally higher after nasal administration when compared to the oral route. Respiratory depression has been reported on occasion following nasal administration. For these reasons, the nasal route of administration is used infrequently by pediatric anesthesiologists.

Intravenous Midazolam

The intravenous form of midazolam is used when children present with an indwelling intravenous catheter prior to surgery. Since the intravenous form of midazolam is water-soluble, there is little pain on injection. Pharmacokinetic studies indicate a β-elimination half-life of less than 2 hours in children. The half-life of both midazolam and its major metabolite tend to increase with advancing age during childhood. The onset of intravenously administered midazolam is 2–3 minutes and the peak sedative effect is shortly thereafter. The duration of action varies between 2 and 6 hours, with most of the sedative effect dissipating within 30 minutes of a single dose. A standard intravenous dose of intravenous midazolam is 0.05 mg/kg, which can then be titrated to effect, depending on the clinical situation.

Rectal Midazolam

Rectal administration of midazolam in doses of 0.5–1.0 mg/kg effectively produces preoperative anxiolysis equivalent to that seen with nasal or oral administration. There is no specific rectal formulation – the intravenous formulation is most often used and can be diluted with water for injection into the rectal cavity. Children 3 years of age and less are most amenable to this route of administration. The child should be placed prone and the midazolam administered via a lubricated red rubber catheter. Once administered, the buttocks should be held closed for several minutes to prevent immediate egress of the midazolam solution (a struggling and uncooperative child will immediately push out much of the injectate). A small amount of air can also be injected via the catheter to help advance the remaining midazolam solution into the rectal cavity.

Diazepam

Since the advent of midazolam, diazepam has not been used routinely for premedication of children. This is primarily due to its relatively long onset of action and greater duration of action. Diazepam may be indicated for children or adolescents who require anxiolysis prior to approximately 1 hour before surgery. It can be administered orally at a dose of 0.3 mg/kg. It should not be given intravenously because of the extreme pain associated with intravenous injection.

Clonidine

Clonidine, an α$_2$-adrenergic agonist, has been used as an orally administered sedative premedication in children. In doses between 2 and 4 μg/kg, oral clonidine will produce adequate sedation and anxiolysis prior to induction of general anesthesia. A distinct advantage of clonidine is its ability to decrease intraoperative anesthetic requirements. However, the onset of action of oral clonidine is greater than 90 minutes, so it may not be suitable for use in the ambulatory setting where children are not often present in the facility prior to this time. Furthermore, when compared with oral midazolam for children undergoing tonsillectomy, clonidine is less effective as an anxiolytic at the times of separation of the child from the caretaker and of induction of anesthesia. An additional disadvantage of clonidine is its ability to blunt the heart rate response to administration of atropine. For these reasons, clonidine is not used routinely as a premedication in children.

Ketamine

Ketamine is gaining popularity as a premedication in children, in both the oral and rectal forms. At a dose of 5 mg/kg, it reliably produces a state of sedation and disassociation within 20 minutes of its administration. Larger doses have been associated with more reliable anxiolysis at the expense of longer postoperative times to awakening and discharge home. Advantages of its use include a low incidence of respiratory depression, and a possible decrease in intraoperative anesthetic requirements. It also possesses analgesic and amnestic properties. Disadvantages include an increased incidence of oral and airway secretions, an increased incidence of postoperative emesis, and a possible association with adverse psychologic reactions such as delirium, dysphoria, nightmares, and hallucinations. These latter effects have not been observed when ketamine has been used as a premedication. To date, studies have not demonstrated any clear advantages of ketamine over midazolam as a premedication in children. However, it may be a useful substitute in children known to exhibit dysphoric reactions to midazolam, or as an additive to midazolam in children who may be in pain, or difficult to calm.

Intramuscular ketamine is used when children are unusually combative and refuse all attempts at medical attention, including refusal to ingest an oral premedication.

It is most often used in developmentally delayed adolescents, who are unable to understand their circumstances and who may be difficult to physically restrain. To reduce the overall volume of the amount injected, the concentrated form of ketamine (100 mg/mL) should be used. Doses range from 2 to 6 mg/kg. Larger doses will result in greater reliability of anxiolysis and disassociation at the expense of longer times to emergence from general anesthesia, especially for surgeries of relatively short duration. This author prefers a lower dose with the modest goal of obtaining sufficient sedation to facilitate intravenous catheter insertion. Varying amounts of midazolam may be added to the injectate to attenuate possible postoperative psychologic disturbances. Some anesthesiologists will include atropine in the injectate in an attempt to reduce airway secretions.

Methohexital

Rectal administration of methohexital is an effective premedication in children. The powdered drug is dissolved in water to make a 10% solution, and administered at doses of 20–30 mg/kg. After its administration, most children will fall into a deep sleep within 15–20 minutes. Pharmacokinetic studies have demonstrated peak plasma concentrations between 10 and 15 minutes after administration, and a terminal half-life of 1-2 hours. Some children will attain a relatively deep level of unconsciousness after administration of rectal methohexital. Therefore, these children should be closely supervised by medical personnel after its administration. Respiratory depression is occasionally observed. Seizures have also been reported. Other complications include hiccoughs, defecation, and lack of sufficient efficacy, which is probably related to the inconsistent vascular absorption because of stool in the rectal vault.

Fentanyl Orulet

The fentanyl orulet, formally known as oral transmucosal fentanyl citrate (OTFC), is essentially a "lollipop" form of drug administration that has been marketed for its natural appeal to children. Moreover, it does not possess the unpleasant aftertaste associated with the oral formulation of midazolam. Since fentanyl is relatively lipophilic, it readily crosses into the bloodstream across the mucosal barrier of the oral cavity. Peak blood levels are usually achieved within 15–30 minutes after onset of sucking. If chewed or swallowed, it will lose its efficacy, as the bioavailability is then decreased. Pharmacokinetic studies in children indicate a wide variability in times to peak plasma concentration. The dose most often associated with adequate sedation is 10–20 µg/kg. Although its use is associated with significant sedation, its anxiolytic effects are limited and are generally not as effective as

with midazolam. Furthermore, it causes bothersome facial pruritus in many children, respiratory depression in a minority of children, and an increased incidence of postoperative nausea and vomiting. For these reasons, the fentanyl orulet remains unpopular for premedication in children, unless the child is suffering from ongoing pain, and does not have available intravenous access. The major drawback to the use of an opioid as a premedication is that, unless the child is in pain, then we are relying on its side-effects, rather than its intended use. In general, when one uses a medication for its side-effects, its efficacy is less predictable.

Anticholinergics

In the past, anticholinergic drugs such as atropine and glycopyrrolate were routinely administered to children in the preoperative period. The major indication was to prevent undesirable episodes of bradycardia associated with administration of halothane or succinylcholine. An additional indication was to prevent vagally induced bradycardia during airway manipulation in neonates and small infants. Since halothane and succinylcholine are no longer routinely used in children, anticholinergic premedication is no longer routinely administered. However, many pediatric anesthesiologists may include intravenous atropine at the beginning of induction of anesthesia when using succinylcholine for full-stomach precautions, or when anesthetizing neonates. One disadvantage to the use of atropine is its ability to cross the blood–brain barrier and cause nonspecific anticholinergic central effects. These are manifested in infants in the postoperative period as irritability and crying for up to several hours. An additional theoretical disadvantage of atropine is its propensity to lower esophageal pressure within 2 minutes of its administration. This may increase the risk of passive regurgitation of gastric contents into the esophagus.

ADDITIONAL ARTICLES TO KNOW

Cook-Sather SD, Harris KA, Chiavacci R, Gallagher PR, Schreiner MS: A liberalized fasting guideline for formula-fed infants does not increase average gastric fluid volume before elective surgery. *Anesth Analg* 96:965-969, 2003.

Cote CJ, Cohen IT, Suresh S et al: A comparison of three doses of a commercially prepared oral midazolam syrup in children. *Anesth Analg* 94:37-43, 2002.

Freeman A, Bachman L: Pediatric anesthesia: an evaluation of preoperative medication. *Anesth Analg* 38:429-437, 1959.

Friesen RH, Wurl JL, Friesen RM: Duration of preoperative fast correlates with arterial blood pressure response to halothane in infants. *Anesth Analg* 95:1572-1576, 2002.

Hackmann T, Steward DJ, Sheps SB: Anemia in pediatric day-surgery patients: prevalence and detection. *Anesthesiology* 75:27-31, 1991.

Kain ZN, Mayes LC, O'Connor TZ et al: Preoperative anxiety in children: predictors and outcomes. *Arch Pediatr Adolesc Med* 150:1238-1245, 1997.

Kain ZN, Wang S-M, Mayes LC et al: Distress during the induction of anesthesia and postoperative behavioral outcomes. *Anesth Analg* 88:1042-1047, 1999.

Litman RS, Perkins FM, Dawson SC: Parental knowledge and attitudes toward discussing the risk of death from anesthesia. *Anesth Analg* 77:256-260, 1993.

Litman RS, Wu CL, Quinlivan JK: Gastric volume and pH in infants fed clear liquids and breast milk prior to surgery. *Anesth Analg* 79:482-485, 1994.

Marshall J, Rodarte A, Blumer J et al: Pediatric pharmacodynamics of midazolam oral syrup. Pediatric Pharmacology Research Unit Network. *J Clin Pharmacol* 40:578-589, 2000.

Nicolson SC, Betts EK, Jobes DR et al: Comparison of oral and intramuscular preanesthetic medication for pediatric inpatient surgery. *Anesthesiology* 71:8-10, 1989.

O'Connor ME, Drasner K: Preoperative laboratory testing of children undergoing elective surgery. *Anesth Analg* 70:176-180, 1990.

Reed MD, Rodarte A, Blumer JL et al: The single-dose pharmacokinetics of midazolam and its primary metabolite in pediatric patients after oral and intravenous administration. *J Clin Pharmacol* 41:1359-1369, 2001.

Roy WL, Lerman J, McIntyre BG: Is preoperative haemoglobin testing justified in children undergoing minor elective surgery? *Can J Anaesth* 38:700-703, 1991.

INTRAOPERATIVE MANAGEMENT

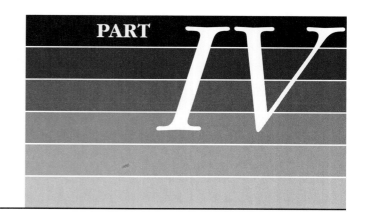

Pediatric Breathing Circuits

RONALD S. LITMAN

Of all the types of anesthesia equipment, breathing circuits for children are the most different from those for adults. Therefore, they are a continual source of controversy and investigation. These differences are most pronounced for neonates and young infants, whose unique anatomic and physiologic characteristics warrant different equipment from adults. Even though we use these on a daily basis, anesthesiologists don't normally think about the "physiology" of the different types of breathing circuits (unless required under the duress of a written board exam). Thus, details of these differences are difficult to learn, and more importantly, to retain in one's mind during a typical anesthesia case.

This chapter reviews types of available anesthesia breathing circuits, with an emphasis on the differences between children and adults. To aid in learning about the differences in breathing circuits, they will be presented here in an order based on the number of valves in the circuit, from zero to 3. The two-valved circuit, which is essentially closed-circuit anesthesia (circle system with the pop-off valve completely closed), will not be covered because closed-circuit anesthesia is rarely utilized in pediatric anesthesia and only by a talented few in the anesthesia community (that does not include this author). Airway humidification will also be reviewed.

CIRCUITS WITHOUT VALVES

A circuit without valves is commonly referred to as an "open" circuit. The ether open-drop technique is the classically-described example. In the author's institution

we use open systems on a daily basis in the form of T-pieces, especially for patients in the postanesthesia care unit (PACU) or when transporting patients between locations within the hospital. Another name for the T-piece is a Mapleson E system (see below).

The T-piece was developed and described by Ayre in the middle of the twentieth century. It consists of:
- An inspiratory limb through which oxygenated air, and possibly anesthetic agents, are delivered
- A connection to the patient
- An expiratory limb for egress of expired air and to act as a reservoir for rebreathing air that contains oxygen (Fig. 13-1).

Since there are no valves in the circuit, inspired air may be derived from either the inspiratory or expiratory limb. However, rebreathing of expired CO_2 can be prevented if the fresh gas flow (FGF) is approximately twice the minute ventilation and if the volume of the expiratory limb is limited to one-third the tidal volume. During the patient's expiratory pause, the fresh gas flow will flush the expired air from the expiratory limb of the circuit.

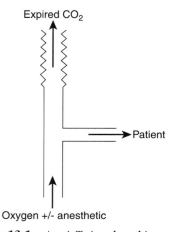

Figure 13-1 Ayre's T-piece breathing system.

Box 13-1 Open Circuit Manipulations

Measures to Increase Pao₂

Increase F₁O₂ (usually at the blender)
Increase fresh gas flow to reduce the amount of entrained room air inspired from the reservoir tubing
Increase length of the reservoir tubing to increase the capacity for storage of oxygenated air

Measures to Decrease Paco₂ (by decreasing the likelihood of rebreathing CO₂)

Increase fresh gas flow to wash out any expired air (containing CO₂) from the reservoir tubing
Decrease length of the reservoir tubing to minimize the amount of expired air it contains (this measure will decrease F₁O₂).

When using the open T-piece system, there are a number of parameters that can be manipulated to increase the Pao_2 or decrease the $Paco_2$ (Box 13-1).

Advantages of open circuits are simplicity and portability. Disadvantages include the inability to precisely control the level of delivered oxygen or anesthetic agent, environmental pollution with anesthetic gases, and the inability to deliver positive-pressure ventilation.

CIRCUITS WITH ONE VALVE

Valved systems are a result of the need for controlled ventilation. Gordon Jackson-Rees, a pediatric anesthesiologist from Liverpool, England, is credited with altering Ayre's T-piece to administer positive-pressure ventilation by adding a double-ended bag (with openings at each end) to the reservoir tubing (expiratory limb). An adjustable expiratory valve is placed at the end of the bag and can be manually adjusted to regulate the amount of delivered inspiratory pressure and positive end-expiratory pressure (PEEP) during controlled ventilation (Fig. 13-2). Positive-pressure ventilation is achieved by partially closing the valve while simultaneously squeezing the bag. When the valve is completely open, the circuit functions identically to a T-piece and can be used during spontaneous ventilation. Partially closing the valve during spontaneous ventilation provides an adjustable method for delivering continuous positive airway pressure (CPAP). The Jackson-Rees circuit (also called a modified Mapleson E circuit or a modified Ayres T-piece) is most commonly used during transport between the operating room and the PACU, or other areas of the hospital. During transport, it allows the anesthesiologist to easily switch between spontaneous and controlled ventilation depending on the clinical status of the patient.

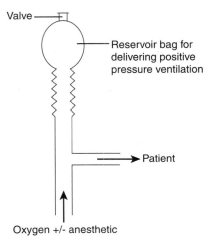

Figure 13-2 Jackson-Rees' modification of Ayre's T-piece for delivering positive-pressure ventilation (modified Mapleson E circuit). An adjustable expiratory valve is placed at the end of the bag and can be manually adjusted to regulate the amount of delivered inspiratory pressure and positive end-expiratory pressure (PEEP) during controlled ventilation, and continuous positive airway pressure (CPAP) during spontaneous ventilation.

In 1954, Mapleson categorized several one-valved circuits based on their "anatomy" and "physiology," which are determined by the locations of the fresh gas inflow, release valve, reservoir bag, and size of the corrugated tubing (Fig. 13-3). The Mapleson A circuit functions best when used during spontaneous ventilation, whereas the Mapleson D circuit is most efficacious when used during controlled ventilation. The Mapleson B and C circuits provide no advantages and so are not in use today. Each system has the potential for rebreathing CO₂, depending on the respiratory rate, fresh gas flow, tidal volume, and inspiratory-to-expiratory time ratio of the patient. However, if the FGF is sufficiently high (two to three times the minute ventilation), rebreathing of CO₂ will not occur. Thus, these are commonly referred to as "non-rebreathing" circuits. Disadvantages to the use of these circuits include loss of heat and humidity, and wastage of anesthetic gases. Therefore, in the OR environment, these systems are largely of historical interest, as most pediatric centers in the United States have abandoned their use in favor of the circle system (see below). Mapleson A and D circuits, however, are still occasionally used in non-OR settings, and for transporting patients between locations within the hospital.

Bain Circuit

The Bain circuit is a modified Mapleson D circuit that is ideally suited for pediatric patients. Its physiology is the same as that of the Mapleson D, but its anatomy is different, in that the inspiratory (fresh gas) limb is contained within the expiratory limb in a coaxial relationship (Fig. 13-4).

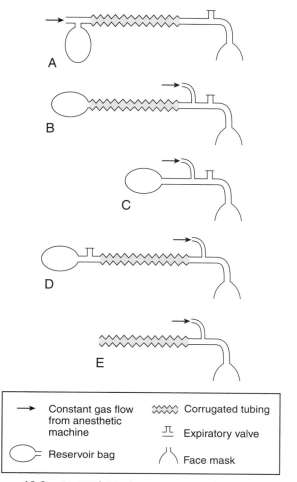

Figure 13-3   In 1954, Mapleson categorized several different one-valved circuits based on their anatomy and physiology, which is determined by the locations of the fresh gas inflow, release valve, reservoir bag, and size of the corrugated tubing. These systems are not widely used in the United States. (Reproduced with permission from Mapleson WW: The elimination of breathing in various semiclosed anaesthetic systems. *Br J Anaesth* 26:323–332, 1954.)

Its major advantage is its lightweight streamlined circuitry. Its coaxial design was originally purported to increase the temperature and humidity of the inspired gas but this has not been demonstrated in clinical use. A disadvantage is that a crack, leak, kink, or other

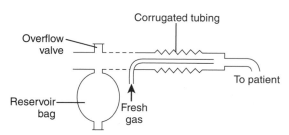

Figure 13-4   The Bain circuit is a coaxial modification of the Mapleson D.

abnormality of the internal inspiratory tubing can remain undetected and cause a decrease in the delivered oxygen concentration and unintentional rebreathing of CO_2.

CIRCUITS WITH THREE VALVES

Circuits with three valves are commonly referred to as semiclosed circle systems and are included in the circuitry of all modern anesthesia machines. The three valves are the pop-off valve, the one-way inspiratory valve, and the one-way expiratory valve. The major distinguishing characteristic of this type of circuit is the presence of a canister containing a CO_2-absorbent material (e.g., soda lime) that prevents rebreathing of CO_2 while allowing rebreathing of the inhaled gases. This reduces cost and OR pollution, and conserves heat and humidity.

The use of three-valved circle systems in pediatric anesthesia was slow to evolve. Pediatric anesthesiologists preferred simple, one-valved circuits because of the small compression volume, the ability to prevent rebreathing of CO_2, and the lack of one-way valves, which may increase the work of breathing in neonates and small infants. However, in the second half of the twentieth century, improvements in technology decreased the airway resistance (and thus work of breathing) caused by the CO_2 canister and the heavy inspiratory and expiratory valves. In addition, smaller, low-compliance tubing was developed for use in pediatric patients to facilitate changes in alveolar gas concentrations relative to the smaller tidal volumes. Ventilators became more sophisticated so that spontaneous ventilation in pediatrics was rarely used. Therefore, in the 1990s, most children's hospitals in the United States discontinued using Mapleson rebreathing circuits in favor of circle systems.

AIRWAY HUMIDIFICATION

Humidification of gases within the anesthesia breathing circuit is thought to prevent respiratory tract damage and promote maintenance of body temperature by decreasing evaporative losses. There are several ways to increase the relative humidity of the breathing circuit. The use of low fresh gas flows will facilitate the rebreathing of gases that are already humidified and have previously passed through the respiratory system and the CO_2 absorber. Low FGFs are possible only when using a circle system, as high FGFs are required to prevent rebreathing when using the Mapleson circuits.

Humidification devices that are added to the anesthesia breathing circuit are classified as passive or active. A passive device is a heat and moisture exchanger (HME), which contains a fine mesh that humidifies the inspired gases by condensation. In most patients, these devices are equal in efficacy to active humidification devices for preventing hypothermia, but at much lower cost. An active device is a hot-water humidifier that is inserted into the anesthesia breathing circuit to add heat and moisture to the gases within the circuit. These devices are reserved for use in small neonates and patients with hypothermia who do not respond to more conservative measures. Nevertheless, despite concerns for adequate humidification of anesthetic gases, there are no data to indicate optimum humidification levels within the anesthesia breathing circuit.

ARTICLES TO KNOW

Ayre P: The T-piece technique. *Br J Anaesth* 28:520, 1956.

Bain JA, Spoerel WE: A streamlined anaesthetic system. *Can Anaesth Soc J* 19:426, 1972.

Bissonnette B, Sessler DI, LaFlamme P: Passive and active inspired gas humidification in infants and children. *Anesthesiology* 71:350-354, 1989.

Carson KD: Humidification during anesthesia. *Resp Care Clin N Am* 4:281-299, 1998.

Peterson BD: Heated humidifiers: structure and function. *Resp Care Clin N Am* 4:243-259, 1998.

Rose DK, Froese AB: The regulation of $Paco_2$ during controlled ventilation of children with a T-piece. *Can Anaesth Soc J* 26:104, 1979.

Stevenson GW, Tobin M, Horn B et al: An adult system versus a Bain system: comparative ability to deliver minute ventilation to an infant lung model with pressure-limited ventilation. *Anesth Analg* 88:527-530, 1999.

CHAPTER 14

Monitoring in Pediatric Anesthesia

RONALD S. LITMAN

Pulse Oximetry
Capnography
Electrocardiography
Blood Pressure Monitoring
Precordial or Esophageal Stethoscope

In pediatric anesthesia, four essential patient monitors are used for virtually every case (unless unusual circumstances preclude their use). They include pulse oximetry, capnography, electrocardiography (ECG), and blood pressure measurement. These monitors are components of the Basic Monitoring Standards of the American Society of Anesthesiologists (www.asahq.org/PublicationsAndServices/standards/02.html#2). Continuous auscultation via a precordial or esophageal stethoscope is strongly encouraged but not mandatory. Temperature monitoring (see Chapter 15) is indicated in all cases except those in which hypothermia or hyperthermia is deemed quite unlikely (e.g., myringotomy and tubes). Train-of-four nerve monitoring is recommended during use of a neuromuscular blocker (see Chapter 19). This chapter reviews the basic characteristics of these monitors, with an emphasis on the unique differences between adults and children.

PULSE OXIMETRY

Pulse oximetry provides an estimate of the oxyhemoglobin saturation. It serves as an early warning signal of impending or actual hypoxemia, often prior to the onset of cyanosis, and frequently reminds anesthesiologists of the alarming rapidity with which infants develop hypoxemia. During rapid changes in oxygen saturation the value represented on the pulse oximeter lags behind the true oxyhemoglobin saturation, such that the recognition of hypoxemia may be delayed. In general, central probe locations (e.g., buccal) will have less of a delay

than an upper extremity, which will have less of a delay than a lower extremity. Conversely, the reestablishment of normoxemia may be associated with a persistently low pulse oximetry value for up to 30 seconds or more.

Most oximetry manufacturers claim a maximum error between 2% and 4% when the true oxyhemoglobin saturation is greater than 70%. Below this value, the precision of the pulse oximeter decreases, and differs between manufacturers. Fetal hemoglobin, which is found in neonates and young infants, does not affect the accuracy of the pulse oximeter.

There are no outcome studies that demonstrate a proven benefit from the use of pulse oximetry. However, anesthesiologist-blinded studies have demonstrated that the use of pulse oximetry results in fewer episodes of hypoxemia and an earlier recognition of hypoxemia. Therefore, pulse oximetry has evolved into a standard monitor during pediatric anesthesia and will never be subjected to rigorous outcome studies with a true control group (i.e., an anesthetic without a pulse oximeter).

Although the use of pulse oximetry in pediatric patients is associated with a relatively high rate of false-positive alarms, all alarms must be taken seriously until proven otherwise. When the oximeter detects a low oxyhemoglobin saturation, the anesthesiologist should immediately turn his or her attention to the adequacy of ventilation by simultaneously evaluating air entry, quality of the capnographic tracing (see later), and the quality of the pulse oximeter signal. In infants and small children, surgical personnel often unknowingly compress the oximeter probe by leaning on the hands or feet. This author prefers to put the oximeter probe on the upper extremity, which can be positioned above the head, when feasible. The audible tone on the oximeter should never be turned off since most anesthesiologists become accustomed to listening to the oxyhemoglobin saturation and becoming aware of a decrease in pitch, rather than continuously visualizing the numeric value.

CAPNOGRAPHY

Prior to 1998, capnography was considered a standard monitor by the ASA for the purpose of confirming the initial placement and continuous presence of an endotracheal tube. This section of the ASA monitoring standards was updated in 1998, and now indicates that capnography should be used to confirm adequate ventilation during airway management without an endotracheal tube (i.e., during laryngeal mask airway, facemask, or natural airway anesthesia). Specifically, these guidelines now state:

"Continual monitoring for the presence of expired carbon dioxide shall be performed unless invalidated by the nature of the patient, procedure or equipment. ...Continual end-tidal carbon dioxide analysis, in use from the time of endotracheal tube/laryngeal mask placement, until extubation/removal or initiating transfer to a postoperative care location, shall be performed using a quantitative method such as capnography, capnometry or mass spectroscopy."

As in adults, capnography in pediatric anesthesia is used to confirm placement of an endotracheal tube in the correct tracheal position, and to continuously assess the adequacy of ventilation. Capnography also provides information about the respiratory rate, breathing pattern, and endotracheal tube patency, and indirectly about the degree of neuromuscular blockade. In pediatric patients, an abnormal increase in end-tidal carbon dioxide ($P_{ET}CO_2$) most commonly signifies hypoventilation, but rarely may also indicate the presence of increased carbon dioxide production as occurs with temperature elevation, or as an early sign of malignant hyperthermia. Conversely, an abnormally low end-tidal CO_2 may indicate an increase in dead-space or suggest a state of low pulmonary perfusion. Sudden absence of the capnographic tracing indicates a breathing circuit disconnection, and the abnormal presence of inspired CO_2 signifies the presence of a faulty unidirectional valve, an exhausted CO_2 absorber or, when a semi-open circuit is being used, rebreathing secondary to an insufficient fresh gas flow.

Capnography use in small children (<12 kg) has several drawbacks owing to the relatively large ratio of dead-space to tidal volume. Therefore, sampling proximal to the endotracheal tube often underestimates the true end-tidal CO_2. It is possible to measure end-tidal CO_2 within the distal portion of the endotracheal tube using a device that resembles a thin straw, which is anchored to a breathing circuit extension piece by a Luer-lock mechanism (Fig. 14-1). Although the use of this device is associated with a more precise end-tidal CO_2 value (Fig. 14-2), it may cause obstruction of a small endotracheal tube, or its sampling lumen may be blocked by secretions.

Although mainstream capnography may provide the most accurate reading, it adds bulk and dead-space to the circuit, both of which are undesirable when anesthetizing small infants. Therefore, side-stream capnography is most often employed for pediatric patients. Disadvantages of side-stream capnography in pediatric patients include the slow response time and, with some devices, a relatively large sampling volume. Recent innovations in capnography technology have allowed a sampling rate as low as 30 mL/min ("microstream technology").

The capnographic tracing of small infants is often characterized by a lack of an apparent alveolar plateau. This is usually a result of a higher respiratory rate, an excessively high sampling flow for the volume of CO_2 produced, excessive dead-space in the breathing circuit, or an excessive leak around an uncuffed endotracheal tube.

ELECTROCARDIOGRAPHY

In pediatric anesthesia, the electrocardiogram (ECG) is most useful for diagnosing intraoperative rate-related

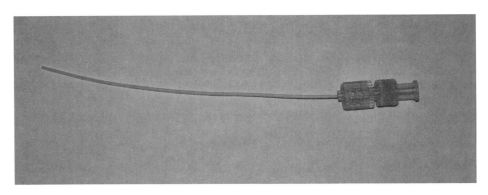

Figure 14-1 It is possible to measure end-tidal CO_2 within the distal portion of the endotracheal tube using a device that resembles a thin straw, which is anchored to a breathing circuit extension piece by a Luer-lock mechanism.

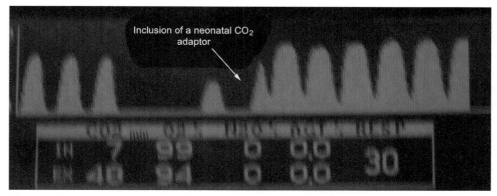

Figure 14-2   An actual tracing of a neonatal capnograph in which a distal sampling adaptor was inserted. Note the higher and more accurate CO_2 value obtained with more distal end-tidal CO_2 sampling.

arrhythmias, the two most common of which are bradycardia and supraventricular tachycardia (SVT). The ECG is much less prone to movement-related artifact than is the pulse oximeter. In small infants, hypoxemia-related bradycardia will often occur prior to the pulse oximeter signaling oxyhemoglobin desaturation. Conversely, resolution of hypoxemia is heralded by the transition from bradycardia to normal sinus rhythm. Premature ventricular contractions (PVCs) are commonly observed when halothane is used as the general anesthetic agent, especially during periods of hypercapnia and/or catecholamine release. More details about the electrical rhythm of the pediatric heart are given in Chapter 2.

BLOOD PRESSURE MONITORING

Nearly all pediatric surgical facilities in the United States are equipped with automated oscillometric blood pressure devices. Oscillometric measurement of systolic blood pressure usually correlates well with the Riva Rocci mercury column method, but it tends to underestimate the diastolic component in children. In most routine cases, measurement of blood pressure should be performed every 3-5 minutes throughout the period of general anesthesia. In children the blood pressure cuff is most commonly placed on the upper arm, but it can alternatively be placed on the forearm, thigh, or calf. However, there is inconsistent correlation of measurements obtained between upper and lower limbs.

The width of the blood pressure cuff should cover approximately two-thirds the total length of the upper arm (or other extremity portion to which it is applied). Too small a cuff is associated with falsely elevated blood pressure values, and too large a cuff is associated with falsely lowered blood pressure values.

PRECORDIAL OR ESOPHAGEAL STETHOSCOPE

Although not an essential monitor (by ASA standards), many pediatric anesthesiologists find that the precordial (or esophageal) stethoscope is indispensable during pediatric anesthesia. It is useful during all phases of general anesthesia, as well as during transport of the child between hospital locations. Continuous auscultation allows the anesthesiologist to immediately detect changes in the rate and character of heart and breath sounds, and it is often the first warning of a physiological alteration during pediatric anesthesia (e.g., right main bronchial intubation, wheezing). During administration of halothane, the character of the heart sounds is often used to judge the depth of anesthesia. During ligation of a patent ductus arteriosus (PDA), a precordial stethoscope can help the surgeon identify the correct structure since clamping the ductus will result in a disappearance of the murmur.

The precordial stethoscope is placed to the left of the sternum in the 3rd or 4th intercostal space. An esophageal stethoscope is placed in the mid-esophagus in intubated children. The proper method for accurate placement of the esophageal stethoscope is to listen while simultaneously advancing the device and placing it at the level where the heart and lung sounds are maximal. In small infants, unintentional placement of the esophageal stethoscope into the stomach can occur easily.

ARTICLES TO KNOW

Badgwell JM, McLeod ME, Lerman J, Creighton RE: End-tidal P_{CO_2} measurements sampled at the distal and proximal ends of the endotracheal tube in infants and children. *Anesth Analg* 66:959-964, 1987.

Badgwell JM, Kleinman SE, Heavner JE: Respiratory frequency and artifact affect the capnographic baseline in infants. *Anesth Analg* 77:708–712, 1993.

Cote CJ, Goldstein EA, Cote MA, Hoaglin DC, Ryan JF: Single-blind study of pulse oximetry in children. *Anesthesiology* 68:184–188, 1988.

Cote CJ, Rolf N, Liu NMP et al: Single-blind study of combined pulse oximetry and capnography in children. *Anesthesiology* 74:980–987, 1991.

Kong AS, Brennan L, Bingham R, Morgan-Hughes J: Audit of induction of anaesthesia in neonates and small infants using pulse oximetry. *Anaesthesia* 47:896–899, 1992.

Reynolds LM, Nicolson SC, Steven JM et al: Influences of sensor site location on pulse oximetry kinetics in children. *Anesth Analg* 76:751–754, 1993.

CHAPTER 15

Temperature Regulation

RONALD S. LITMAN

This chapter reviews the importance of thermoregulation and temperature monitoring in anesthetized children. It addresses the significance of keeping children normothermic, and will help the novice understand why pediatric anesthesiologists become apoplectic when faced with the possibility that the small infant they are caring for may become hypothermic. The chapter also covers the management of postoperative fever, a common cause of concern in children.

NORMAL TEMPERATURE PHYSIOLOGY IN CHILDREN

Body temperature is a result of the balance between heat production by the major organs and heat loss to the environment. There is no standard for normal body temperature; individuals exhibit different temperatures, which will be influenced by the time of day, activity, etc. Like adults, children's bodies contain different compartments that normally exhibit different levels of temperature. The core compartment is composed of the major organs and deep body tissues. The peripheral compartment is composed largely of the extremities. There normally exists a temperature gradient between the core and peripheral compartments that is largely maintained by peripheral vasoconstriction. When vasodilation occurs, during general or regional anesthesia, there is mixing of heat between the core and the peripheral compartments. This normally results in an overall decrease in core temperature. This phenomenon is commonly observed following induction of general anesthesia.

Being a homeotherm, when an infant is placed in a cooler than normal environment, he or she will consume oxygen and expend caloric energy to maintain a normal body temperature. The neutral thermal environment (NTE) is defined as the environmental temperature range that is most consistent with a normal body temperature with the most minimal metabolic heat production, measured as oxygen consumption. The clinical correlate of this is that if a small infant with lung disease has a preexisting defect in transfer of oxygen into the bloodstream and excretion of carbon dioxide, he or she is more likely to suffer from cellular hypoxemia during hypothermia (i.e., when the infant's oxygen consumption and metabolic rate are increased). Indeed, studies have documented differences in infant survival rates that depended on the temperature in the incubator. In one study, with an increase in incubator temperature from 85°F to 89°F, there was an accompanying 15% increase in survival.

Generally, the smaller and younger the infant, the higher the environmental temperature required to achieve the NTE. Graphs and tables are published that list the temperature required to maintain infants in the NTE based on weight and gestational age. For example, for newborns weighing between 1 kg and 3 kg, this temperature can exceed 85°F (29.4°C). The anesthesiologist caring for small infants should attempt to replicate these conditions in the operating room, in the area immediately surrounding the infant. For a naked infant lying supine on an open platform, it is estimated that the abdominal skin temperature should be between 36.5°C and 37°C to approximate the conditions required to be in the NTE.

Within a narrow environmental temperature range (i.e., the NTE) the human infant's oxygen consumption is lowest, meaning that it is expending the minimal amount of energy to maintain normothermia (Fig. 15-1). If this environmental temperature is lowered slightly (point "A" in Fig. 15-1), the infant is able to use its compensatory mechanisms (vasoconstriction, brown fat oxidation) to maintain normothermia. However, once this thermoregulatory range is exceeded (at the lower limit in the figure point "B") the infant's thermal protective mechanisms can no longer sustain normothermia and its core temperature will begin to drop. Eventually, oxygen consumption will also begin to decrease because of impairment of the temperature regulation center. Just because an infant's temperature is relatively normal does not mean that it is still residing in the NTE. In fact, its thermal protective mechanisms may be quite active and on the verge of failing to maintain normothermia. When the infant's body temperature begins to fall, it is an indication that the thermal stress has been so severe that its normal thermal compensatory mechanisms are being overpowered. Furthermore, the presence of either hypoxemia or hypoglycemia impairs the metabolic response to hypothermia, resulting in a more dramatic decrease in body temperature.

The human infant is born with a well-developed temperature regulating system. However, small infants are prone to hypothermia in cold environments and hyperthermia in overly warm environments mainly because of their relatively large surface area-to-volume ratio. The body surface area-to-volume ratio of a tiny premature infant is three to five times higher than an adult's, and the heat loss per unit body mass is about four times that of the adult. Because of less subcutaneous fat (i.e., less insulation), the range of the environmental temperature in which the infant is able to maintain normothermia is severely limited when compared to the adult. For example, in a naked pediatric anesthesiologist, the lower limit of this control range is approximately 0°C (32°F) whereas for the full-term infant it is 20–23°C (68–73.4°F). Therefore, the temperature within the infant's immediate surrounding area in the OR should be maintained at a minimum of approximately 75°F. Since subcutaneous fat is formed mainly in the third trimester of gestation, infants born prematurely are even more at risk for poikilothermic-type behavior.

NORMAL COMPENSATION FOR HYPOTHERMIA

When body temperature begins to vary just slightly away (about ± 0.2°C) from the physiologic set-point, involuntary compensatory mechanisms will attempt to return the body's temperature back to normal. There are a number of these compensatory mechanisms. Those that are most important in small children and that are most different from adults will be reviewed.

Behavioral Mechanisms

When most of us feel cold, we instinctively seek a warmer location, or voluntarily increase our muscle activity to generate heat, or even put on more layers of clothing. The small infant does not have the capability to do any of these (although it is often heard in the ICU that babies will instinctively situate themselves toward the warmest part of the isolette).

Shivering

Adults and older children have the capability to shiver – the high-intensity involuntary rhythmic muscle activity that is probably the most significant means by which adults produce heat. Young children do not have the capability of efficient shivering. Once anesthetized (without muscle paralysis) efficient shivering in adults is greatly attenuated until the process of awakening.

Nonshivering Thermogenesis

Nonshivering thermogenesis describes a cold-induced increase in oxygen consumption and heat production

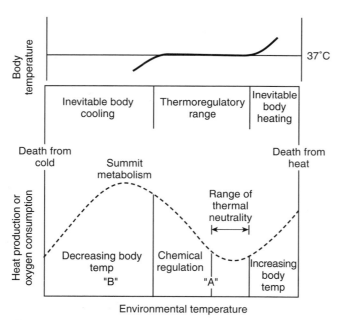

Figure 15-1   Heat production (or oxygen consumption) as a product of body temperature. (Reproduced with permission from Klaus MH, Fanaroff AA: *Care of the High Risk Neonate*, 5th edn, WB Saunders, Philadelphia, 2001.)

that is not inhibited by muscle relaxants. In small infants, nonshivering thermogenesis is probably the most important means of heat production in a cool environment. The thermogenic effector organ – brown fat – is the most significant contributor to nonshivering thermogenesis in the small infant. In the human infant, brown fat accounts for 2–6% of total bodyweight and is located in the abdominal cavity surrounding the kidneys and adrenal glands, in the mediastinum, and between the scapulae. As opposed to the more abundant white fat, brown fat cells are rich in mitochondria, contain a dense capillary network, and are richly innervated with sympathetic nerve endings. When norepinephrine release is stimulated by sympathetic activity, triglycerides are hydrolyzed to free fatty acids and glycerol, with heat production resulting from enhanced oxygen consumption. Immediately after an infant is exposed to a cold stimulus the metabolic rate begins to increase, even before core body temperature decreases. Even a mild cold stimulus such as unheated preoxygenation can trigger the onset of an increase in metabolic heat production. In infants exposed to a cold environment, nonshivering thermogenesis is capable of doubling the metabolic rate. However, the drop in temperature required to initiate nonshivering thermogenesis is unknown. In one study of infants anesthetized with propofol and fentanyl, there was a lack of nonshivering thermogenesis with a temperature drop of 2°C.

Thermoregulatory Vasoconstriction

Thermoregulatory vasoconstriction occurs in the peripheral compartments in response to cold receptors on the skin. It serves to limit heat loss to the environment. In children undergoing abdominal surgery with isoflurane anesthesia, thermoregulatory vasoconstriction is attenuated by an average of about 2.5°C less than the unanesthetized state (Fig. 15-2). This is similar to the values found in anesthetized adults. A similar study using halothane as the maintenance agent demonstrated a higher temperature at which thermoregulatory vasoconstriction was triggered (about 1–2°C difference in triggering threshold). These values are higher than for adults anesthetized with halothane.

COMPLICATIONS OF HYPOTHERMIA IN THE SMALL INFANT

Other than the direct depressant effects of hypothermia on cerebral and cardiovascular function, hypothermia sets into motion a variety of physiological compensation mechanisms that increase oxygen consumption and may ultimately adversely affect normal physiology (Fig. 15-3). Cooling results in release of norepinephrine. This, along with the direct effects of hypothermia, results in

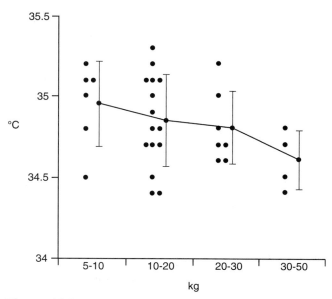

Figure 15-2 The central thermoregulatory threshold in 32 healthy children and infants undergoing abdominal surgery. Although there was a trend towards increased threshold temperatures in smaller patients, differences between the groups were not statistically significant. (Reproduced with permission from Bissonnette B, Sessler DI: Thermoregulatory threshold in infants and children anesthetized with isoflurane and caudal bupivacaine. *Anesthesiology* 73:1114–1118, 1990.)

widespread vasoconstriction. Peripheral vasoconstriction may restrict oxygen delivery to tissues and cause cellular hypoxia manifested as a metabolic acidosis. Pulmonary vasoconstriction will increase pulmonary arterial pressures, and cause increased susceptibility to right-to-left shunting at the atrial level through a patent foramen ovale and through a patent ductus arteriosus. This will in turn cause additional peripheral tissue hypoxia.

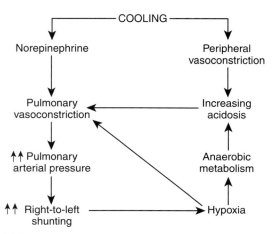

Figure 15-3 Vicious cycle that develops when a neonate is hypothermic. (Reproduced with permission from Klaus MH, Fanaroff AA: *Care of the High Risk Neonate*, 5th edn, WB Saunders, Philadelphia, 2001.)

Mild hypothermia (34–36°C) in healthy infants and children during peripheral procedures probably does not result in adverse effects, and does not influence postoperative recovery indices. Postoperative shivering is uncommon in children. In one audit of 376 children, the incidence of postoperative shivering was 14.4%, and was associated with age >10 years, inhalation induction of anesthesia, use of atropine, use of opioids, duration of anesthesia >40 minutes, and perioperative decrease in body temperature.

HEAT LOSS DURING ANESTHESIA

After induction of general anesthesia, an initial decrease in core temperature results from the redistribution of heat from the core to the periphery. This is largely caused by a combination of direct vasodilation by the anesthetic agents and an anesthetic-induced inhibition of thermoregulatory vasoconstriction that occurs at a lower than normal core temperature. In children the administration of general anesthesia blunts the ability of the central nervous system to trigger compensatory vasoconstriction by approximately 2.5°C, as compared with approximately 0.2°C in the unanesthetized state. This threshold is similar to that of adults. Since infants and small children have a relatively greater proportion of their body mass contained in the core compartment, they may, at least initially, lose proportionately less heat because of redistribution of core heat to the periphery. Their relatively small extremities will not absorb as much heat from the core compared to an adult.

Following this initial decrease in core temperature from redistribution, infants will likely continue to lose heat to the environment at a faster pace than older children and adults. This is mainly caused by their relatively large surface area-to-volume ratio, paucity of subcutaneous fat, immature epidermal barrier, and limited capacity for metabolic heat production. In addition, there is a relatively greater contribution to body cooling from unwarmed intravenous solutions and sterile irrigating solutions.

Mechanisms of Heat Loss to the Environment

Radiation is the process by which heat is lost from the child to any colder surrounding structures (e.g., walls in the OR) by the transfer of photons, and is not influenced by the temperature of the surrounding air. Radiation normally accounts for the greatest percentage of heat lost during anesthesia. During transport of a neonate to and from the operating room, heat lost through radiation can be decreased by use of a double-shelled incubator, or another type of barrier between the infant and the surrounding incubator walls, such as a blanket.

Conduction refers to the direct transfer of heat between contiguous structures. Examples include loss of heat from the child to the operating room table, or the hypothermic effect of infusion of cool intravenous fluids. Because of the relatively larger surface area-to-volume ratio of infants, conduction may influence heat loss more than in older children or adults. Heat lost by conduction is reduced by using a warming mattress underneath the child, increasing the ambient temperature in the operating room, use of a forced warm air blanket on nonsurgical areas of the body, and warming infused intravenous fluids and sterile prep solutions.

Convection is the loss of heat by the movement of air flowing past the surface of the skin. Heat lost through convection is minimized by ensuring that exposed parts of the child are covered as much as possible.

Evaporation describes the loss of heat by the energy depleted when water is dissipated from exposed surfaces of the body, such as the skin, visceral organs, and respiratory epithelium. Evaporative heat loss is minimized by humidification of inspired gases, covering exposed skin surfaces, and using warmed sterile prep solutions.

Prevention and Treatment of Perioperative Hypothermia

Preoperative warming of the extremities is perhaps the most effective method for prevention of the initial decrease in temperature due to redistribution. However, this is not practical in most children. Therefore, more effective means must be utilized to prevent large decreases in temperature. Every attempt should be made to achieve cutaneous warming by covering all exposed areas with sheets or blankets. This will significantly decrease radiant, convective, and evaporative heat loss. Many institutions utilize radiant warmers, which are kept over the infant during induction of anesthesia and placement of lines and monitors. These devices may help prevent heat loss via evaporation and conduction of heat to the surrounding cold air. Airway humidification can prevent evaporation. There are two methods with which to humidify the airway. The simplest is by using a heat and moisture exchanger (HME) to passively trap the patient's own heat and moisture within the airway. The second is the placement of an active humidification device within the anesthesia breathing circuit. This device can both prevent heat loss and add heat to the child's body via the respiratory tract. However, its use is probably not warranted for peripheral surgery of relatively short duration. In a study of 20 infants weighing between 5 kg and 30 kg who were randomized to receive active humidification, passive humidification, or none, there was good correlation between humidification and core body temperature, but no difference between active and passive humidification.

Heated water-filled mattresses are routinely used to prevent conductive heat loss from the infant to the OR table and to transfer heat to the infant. However, its safe temperature range is narrow – below 35°C infants may lose heat to the mattress, and above 38°C there is the possibility of overheating and burns. It is most effective in infants weighing less than 10 kg. All infusions and sterile scrubbing and preparation solutions should also be appropriately warmed to prevent conductive heat loss within and around the child's body. The flow of warm air across a child's skin produced by forced-air warming blankets prevents heat loss to the environment and may even effectively warm patients via radiant shielding and convection. Of all devices, these are one of the most effective and should be used in all cases where hypothermia is possible.

Lastly, one of the most effective methods for prevention of hypothermia in small children is warming the OR environment. Eventually, the walls of the OR will also become warmed with consequent decrease in loss of radiant heat. One must be sensitive, however, to the comfort of the surgeons and nurses under the hot operating lights. Therefore, the OR should be maintained warm, but then, once the child is covered with blankets and a forced-air warming blanket, the air temperature can be turned down for comfort, after ensuring that the child's core temperature is in the satisfactory range.

Where Temperature Should be Measured

Most studies demonstrate that axillary temperature measurement is as efficacious as tympanic, nasopharyngeal, or esophageal sites. However, when hypothermia is possible, true representations of core temperature are preferred, such as distal esophageal, rectal, and nasopharyngeal locations. Tympanic membrane temperatures are also reliable but fear of injuring the tympanic membrane dissuades most anesthesiologists from choosing this route. When using distal esophageal temperature monitoring in neonates and small infants during a laparotomy, one must ensure that the tip of the temperature probe has not entered the stomach – falsely elevated readings can result from warming of the stomach if directly exposed to the heat of the overhead lights or warm irrigation solution. Disposable skin temperature devices are generally not considered to be useful in the perioperative environment where diagnosis of temperature alteration is clinically important.

Regional Anesthesia

Regional anesthesia may also contribute to onset and maintenance of hypothermia by vasodilation within the affected extremities and subsequent redistribution of heat from the core component. Furthermore, inhibition of peripheral sympathetic tone may prevent thermoregulatory vasoconstriction and inhibit heat production by utilization of brown fat. However, few studies in children have been performed to assess the influence of regional anesthesia on intraoperative temperature regulation. A study in children anesthetized with halothane demonstrated that caudal anesthesia with bupivacaine had no effect on the threshold for thermoregulatory vasoconstriction.

PERIOPERATIVE HYPERTHERMIA

Intraoperative hyperthermia is probably less common than hypothermia, yet it occurs regularly in children. It is associated with peripheral or head/neck procedures where there is minimal heat or fluid loss and warming maneuvers are being used. Examples include ear/nose/throat (ENT) and dental surgeries as well as procedures on the distal limbs. For these types of procedures, it is usually sufficient to use a blanket that covers the child's body, and perhaps a warming blanket underneath the child on the OR table. Use of a forced warm blanket in these situations will usually contribute to hyperthermia.

Although relatively common, postoperative fever (generally defined as a core body temperature greater than 37.5°C) in children is a consistent cause of concern. Surgeons worry about wound infections and anesthesiologists worry about postoperative signs of malignant hyperthermia. The fact is, however, that postoperative fever is extremely common in children, and is rarely due to either wound infection or malignant hyperthermia. The precise cause of postoperative fever is unknown, but it is theorized to be a transient adjustment of the body temperature "set-point" as a response to the surgical stress. An audit of 150 consecutive pediatric urologic patients revealed that 74% aged less than 1 year and 28% aged greater than 4 years exhibited postoperative fever, none of whom was otherwise clinically ill. Similar incidences have been reported in the pediatric orthopedic, plastic, and tonsillectomy populations. A study that examined fever patterns in 150 children following inguinal hernia repair demonstrated that one-third of the children had a fever of greater than 37.5°C on the evening of the surgery. No studies in any particular surgical specialty indicate that fever is a marker of a serious clinical entity.

When asked to evaluate a child with postoperative fever, the anesthesiologist should review the anesthetic and surgical events as a prelude to determining the cause. Obvious signs of surgical infection (e.g., redness or exudate at the surgical site) should be sought. The child should be evaluated for concomitant upper respiratory tract illness or middle ear infection that may have been present preoperatively. Abnormal lung sounds should prompt investigation of possible lower respiratory tract infection. If the child is ill-appearing, intravenous hydration should be continued

Article To Know

Goudsouzian NG, Morris RH, Ryan JF: Effects of a warming blanket on the maintenance of body temperatures in anesthetized infants and children. Anesthesiology 39:351-353, 1973.

In this classic article from 1973, Dr Goudsouzian and his colleagues from the Massachusetts General Hospital set out to evaluate the usefulness of a warming blanket placed underneath infants and children above 18 months of age during general anesthesia. The warming blanket was set to a temperature of 40°C and the patients were randomized to the warming blanket group or a control group. Lower esophageal temperatures were recorded every 15 minutes following induction of general anesthesia. When measurements on 25 children were collected, the authors plotted their results on a scatter diagram and observed an obvious difference between children less than or greater than 0.5 m² in surface area. The two groups were then separated and their temperatures throughout the case were graphed separately.

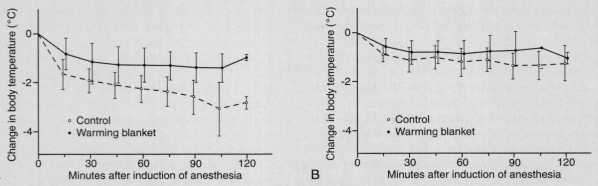

Figure 15-4   Changes in esophageal temperature (mean ± SD) in infants and children: patients with **(A)** <0.5 m² and **(B)** >0.5 m² of body surface area. (Reproduced with permission from Goudsouzian NG et al: *Anesthesiology* 39:351-353, 1973.)

Fig. 15-4A represents 13 children <0.5 m² in surface area, in which 7 were placed on warming blankets. There is an obvious difference in esophageal temperature throughout the case. This difference does not exist in the children >0.5 m² in surface area (Fig. 15-4B). The authors postulated that the results are due to smaller infants having a greater ratio of surface area to volume, and thus able to reap greater benefits from the warming blanket, which prevented conductive heat loss to the operating table. In general, children less than 0.5 m² in surface area weigh less than 10 kg.

and the child evaluated for overnight hospital admission. Malignant hyperthermia is extremely rare in this setting. One possible clue that a malignant hyperthermia episode might be occurring is a child demonstrating a large minute ventilation that is out of proportion to the child's clinical status.

ADDITIONAL ARTICLES TO KNOW

Anand VT, Phillipps JJ, Allen D, Joynson DH, Fielder HM: A study of postoperative fever following paediatric tonsillectomy. *Clin Otolaryngol* 24:360-364, 1999.

Bissonnette B, Sessler DI: Passive or active inspired gas humidification increases thermal steady-state temperatures in anesthetized infants. *Anesth Analg* 69:783-787, 1989.

Bissonnette B, Sessler DI: Thermoregulatory threshold in infants and children anesthetized with isoflurane and caudal bupivacaine. *Anesthesiology* 73:1114-1118, 1990.

Bissonnette B, Sessler DI: Thermoregulatory thresholds for vasoconstriction in pediatric patients anesthetized with

halothane or halothane and caudal bupivacaine. *Anesthesiology* 76:387-392, 1992.

Bissonnette B, Sessler DI: Mild hypothermia does not impair postanesthetic recovery in infants and children. *Anesth Analg* 76:168-172, 1993.

Bissonnette B, Sessler DI, LaFlamme P: Intraoperative temperature monitoring sites in infants and children and the effect of inspired gas warming on esophageal temperature. *Anesth Analg* 69:192-196, 1989.

Frank SM, Kluger MJ, Kunkel SL: Elevated thermostatic setpoint in postoperative patients. *Anesthesiology* 93:1426-1431, 2000.

Kenan S, Liebergall M, Simchen E, Porat S: Fever following orthopedic operations in children. *J Pediatr Orthop* 6:139-142, 1986.

Merjanian RB, Kiriakos CR, Dorey FJ, Apel DM, Oppenheim WL: Normal postoperative febrile response in the pediatric orthopaedic population. *J Pediatr Orthop* 18:497-501, 1998.

Nilsson K: Maintenance and monitoring of body temperature in infants and children. *Paediatr Anaesth* 1:13-20, 1991.

CHAPTER 16

Fluid and Blood Administration

RONALD S. LITMAN

A variety of intravenous fluids are routinely administered to children in the perioperative period. Indications include preoperative deficit replacement, ongoing maintenance requirements, fluid loss replacement, and treatment of anemia and hypovolemia. This chapter reviews the use of these fluid and blood products in pediatric patients.

NORMAL FLUID REQUIREMENTS

Water Requirements

Normal water maintenance rates in children are based on studies that have demonstrated a direct association between metabolic rate and water requirements. In general, water requirements on a per-kilogram basis increase with decreasing size of the child. This is secondary to the higher metabolic rate with decreasing size, as well as the relatively greater evaporative loss from body surfaces in smaller children because of a higher ratio of body surface area to weight. Prematurely born infants have an even greater rate of evaporative loss due to thinner, more permeable, vascularized skin. In general, the amount of evaporative water loss per kilogram is inversely proportional to the gestational age.

In a landmark paper published in 1957, Holliday and Segar developed an easily remembered formula for calculating caloric requirements of the "average" hospitalized child (>2 weeks of age) based on bodyweight (Table 16-1). They also demonstrated that the water requirement in milliliters was equal to the total energy expended (i.e., 1000 mL of water is required for every 1000 kcal expended). Thus, the formula for caloric requirements can easily be used to calculate daily water requirements using the "4–2–1 rule" (Table 16-2). The immature kidney of the neonate lacks the ability to excrete free water, so infants in the first several weeks of life will require less daily water (Table 16-3).

Subsequent studies during pediatric surgery demonstrated that intraoperative caloric and fluid requirements are less than those calculated by Holliday and Segar. Nevertheless, for the vast majority of healthy children undergoing surgery, these formulae will consistently prevent intraoperative fluid and electrolyte abnormalities.

Table 16-1	Daily Caloric Requirements in Children (based on bodyweight)
Bodyweight (kg)	**Daily Requirement**
0–10	100 kcal/kg
11–20	1000 kcal + 50 kcal/kg for each kg over 10 kg
21–70	1500 kcal + 20 kcal/kg for each kg over 20 kg

Table 16-2	Maintenance Fluid Requirements in Children: the "4-2-1 Rule"	
Bodyweight (kg)	**Maintenance Rate**	
0–10	4 mL/kg/h	
11–20	40 mL + 2 mL/kg/h for each kg over 10 kg	
21–70	60 mL + 1 mL/kg/h for each kg over 20 kg	

Table 16-4	Electrolytes Contained in 1 Liter of Lactated Ringers Solution[a]
Electrolyte	**Amount**
Sodium	130 mEq
Potassium	4 mEq
Calcium	3 mEq
Chloride	109 mEq
Lactate	28 mEq

[a] Not including ions for adjusting pH.

Electrolyte Requirements

For each 100 calories metabolized in 24 hours, the average child requires 3 mEq of sodium, 2 mEq of potassium, and 2 mEq of chloride. These recommendations are based on the approximate electrolyte concentration of breast and cow milk, and the resulting normal urine osmolality after milk ingestion. In most healthy children, these electrolyte requirements will be met by administering a solution of 0.2% sodium chloride with 20 mEq of added KCl per liter at the normal maintenance rate.

In the perioperative period, it is necessary to replace surgical losses in addition to providing maintenance fluids and electrolytes. Therefore, in the author's institution we commonly use solutions that contain a greater percentage of sodium. This better approximates the fluid that is associated with losses during surgery, and avoids hyponatremia that would result from large infusions of a hypotonic fluid, especially in the face of an increase in antidiuretic hormone release caused by the stress of surgery. Lactated Ringers solution meets these needs for the majority of surgical procedures in children (Table 16-4). Normal saline (sodium = 154 mEq/L) can also be used, and is often preferred when replacing large amounts of isotonic fluid, since Lactated Ringers is relatively hypotonic.

Table 16-3	Water Requirements of Newborns		
	Water Requirement (mL/kg/24 h) by Age		
Birthweight (g)	**1–2 days**	**3–7 days**	**7–30 days**
<750	100–250	150–300	120–180
750–1000	80–150	100–150	120–180
1000–1500	60–100	80–150	120–180
>1500	60–80	100–150	120–180

Reproduced with permission from Alexander DC, Robin B: Neonatology. In Siberry GK, Iannone R eds: *The Harriet Lane Handbook*, 15th edn, Mosby, St Louis, 2000.

INTRAOPERATIVE FLUID REQUIREMENTS

Intraoperative fluid administration is required to meet the body's needs for ongoing losses secondary to metabolism, as well as water and electrolyte losses caused by medical and/or surgical conditions. Additional fluid deficits are incurred during preoperative fasting and intraoperative evaporation and third-spacing.

Deficit Replacement

Normally, children presenting for elective surgical procedures have incurred a fluid deficit during the preoperative fasting interval. Although in many instances clear liquids may be allowed up to 2 hours prior to the scheduled procedure time, many children have fasted for a longer time. Most pediatric anesthesiologists feel that this deficit should be replaced with isotonic fluid to compensate for anesthetic-induced vasodilatation and unexpected intraoperative or postoperative fluid and blood loss. Preoperative fasting deficits are calculated by multiplying the hourly maintenance rate by the number of hours the child fasted. Traditionally, 50% of this deficit is replaced in the first hour of intravenous hydration and 25% in each of the next 2 hours. For relatively short, minor surgeries, a volume of 4 mL/kg of isotonic solution has been suggested as an appropriate replacement volume that covers the preoperative deficit and intraoperative maintenance requirements.

Children presenting for emergency surgery may have increased fluid losses secondary to fever, vomiting, edema, and blood loss. Therefore, these children should receive earlier and more aggressive volume replacement, until establishment of normal urine production (1–2 mL/kg/h). However, it has been recently shown that aggressive fluid deficit replacement is associated with a decrease in core body temperature.

Glucose Administration

Because of the normal hyperglycemic response to surgery, healthy children over about 1 year of age do not require addition of glucose to intraoperative mainte- nance fluids. Most pediatric anesthesiologists prefer to add glucose to the maintenance fluids of infants weigh- ing less than 10 kg, as hypoglycemia may occur after a prolonged fast. Additional populations of children prone to intraoperative hypoglycemia include those with certain types of metabolic diseases (e.g., inborn errors of metabolism) and malnutrition. A 2% dextrose solution appears to provide the best balance between the risk of hypoglycemia (approximately 1 in 100 fasted infants) and hyperglycemia, which may cause an osmotic diuresis. This solution is not routinely available but can easily be made by adding 2 g of dextrose to 100 mL of Lactated Ringers or normal saline solution.

Hospitalized neonates, especially those born prema- turely, will often be receiving increased amounts of glu- cose to compensate for limited glycogen reserves. Because most of these patients will demonstrate a hyper- glycemic response to the stress of surgery, this author's practice is to initially administer the same solution at half its original rate, check blood glucose values hourly, and readjust the rate if necessary. Normal saline or Lactated Ringers solution is then used to replace any deficit or intraoperative isotonic fluid loss.

Children who received clonidine premedication or neuraxial blockade prior to the surgical incision may not develop the intraoperative hyperglycemic stress response. These patients should receive a maintenance fluid that contains dextrose or should undergo intraop- erative blood glucose monitoring at regular intervals.

Replacement of Intraoperative Fluid Losses

In addition to insensible losses and ongoing metabolic needs, fluid is lost intraoperatively as a result of evapora- tion from exposed tissues, "third-spacing," and surgical blood loss. Third-spacing is the transfer of relatively iso- tonic fluid from the extracellular volume space to a non- functional interstitial compartment, and is triggered by surgical trauma, infection, burns, and other mechanisms of tissue injury. The amount of volume lost to the third space can be estimated based on experience with the particular type of surgery, observation of the surgical field, and the clinical response to volume replacement.

Insensible fluid losses during minor procedures will average less than 3 mL/kg/h. This value will increase based on the location and extent of the surgical injury. For example, a neonate undergoing an exploratory laparo- tomy for necrotizing enterocolitis and gangrenous bowel may require 50–100 mL/kg/h to maintain euvolemia. Most thoracic and neurosurgical procedures require 5–10 mL/kg/h.

Intraoperative fluid losses are replaced with an iso- tonic, non-glucose-containing solution such as Lactated Ringers or normal saline. When using crystalloid to replace surgical blood loss, three times as much crystal- loid solution should be administered as the amount of estimated blood lost. End-points of intraoperative volume replacement include an appropriate blood pressure and heart rate, and adequate tissue perfusion as evidenced by a urine output of 1–2 mL/kg/h.

Massive amounts of replacement with each solution carry unique disadvantages. Because of its slightly hypo- tonic nature, large amounts of administered Lactated Ringers solution are associated with a decreased serum osmolality and development of edema. Large amounts of administered normal saline are associated with develop- ment of dilutional or hyperchloremic acidosis.

Albumin

Albumin preparations are manufactured by pooling plasma from multiple donors. In the perioperative setting, it may be administered for volume expansion or maintenance of the plasma colloid oncotic pressure. It is supplied as a 5% isotonic solution, as well as 20% and 25% hypertonic solutions. These preparations are processed by heating at 60°C for 10 hours or more, and are not associated with transmission of viral diseases.

Administration of albumin may be considered in com- bination with a crystalloid solution when a child has lost more than 50% of his or her circulating blood volume. Doses vary from 5 mL/kg to >20 mL/kg, depending on the clinical situation. Although albumin will maintain the colloid osmotic pressure and serum albumin concentra- tion for a longer duration than crystalloid solutions, there are no proven benefits to its use. In addition, large amounts of administered albumin are associated with development of hypernatremia.

BLOOD PRODUCT ADMINISTRATION

A variety of blood products are available for transfu- sion, depending on the clinical situation. The most com- monly administered blood products in the perioperative setting are packed red blood cells, fresh frozen plasma, and platelets. The indications for administration of each of these products, as well as principles for their use in children, will be discussed.

Red Blood Cells

Since whole blood is rarely available without advanced notice, red blood cell concentrates are almost exclusively administered to correct anemia in pediatric surgical patients. In general, there are few differences between children and adults with regard to the indications for peri- operative red blood cell (RBC) administration (Box 16-1). The primary objective of red cell administration is to enhance oxygen delivery to the peripheral circulation.

Box 16-1   Guidelines for Perioperative RBC Transfusion in Children

Emergency surgical procedure in a patient with significant preoperative anemia (hemoglobin <7 g/dL)
Hemoglobin <8 g/dL in children with signs and symptoms of anemia, or while on chemotherapy/radiotherapy, or if the patient has a chronic congenital or acquired symptomatic anemia
Acute blood loss with hypovolemia not responsive to other therapy
Hematocrit <40% in children with severe pulmonary disease

Reproduced with permission from Roseff SD, Luban NL, Manno CS: Guidelines for assessing appropriateness of pediatric transfusion, *Transfusion* 42:1398–1413, 2002.

A secondary objective is to maintain the circulating blood volume. Preoperative red cell transfusion prior to an elective surgical procedure is rarely justified. Although the incidence of postoperative apnea in premature infants is decreased when the hemoglobin level is >10 g/dL, red cell transfusion is not indicated with mild anemia (7–10 g/dL), provided adequate postoperative monitoring in an intensive care setting is available.

In children without preoperative anemia, intraoperative red cell administration is often based on attainment of the *maximum allowable blood loss* (MABL):

$$MABL = weight\ (kg) \times estimated\ blood\ volume\ (EBV) \times \frac{H_0 - H_1}{H_a}$$

where H_0 is the child's original hematocrit, H_1 is the lowest acceptable hematocrit, and H_a is the average hematocrit, $(H_0 + H_1)/2$.

The lowest acceptable hematocrit, H_1, is determined prior to the onset of the surgical procedure and is based on the health of the child and the clinical situation. The estimated blood volume is calculated based on the patient's age and size (Table 16-5).

Red blood cells should be transfused with an endpoint of achieving an improvement of clinical symptoms.

Table 16-5   Estimated Pediatric Blood Volumes (EBVs)

Age	Estimated Blood Volume (mL/kg)
Premature infant	90–100
Full-term newborn	80–90
Infant 3 months to 1 year	70–80
Child >1 year of age	70

Most preparations of red cell concentrates have a hematocrit between 55% and 75%, depending on the storage solution. On average, 10 mL/kg of packed red blood cells will increase the hemoglobin by 1–2 g/dL. Most pediatric transfusions range between 5 and 15 mL/kg. Larger volumes will be required during periods of hypovolemic shock.

There are several types of preservative solutions that will prolong the shelf-life of red blood cells to 42 days. Each contains a variable amount of adenine, citrate, dextrose, and phosphate. Some contain mannitol. As the duration of blood storage increases, the amount of extracellular potassium increases, the pH decreases, and red cell levels of 2,3-diphosphoglycerate decrease. Furthermore, there are concerns about the potential for hepatic toxicity with adenine, and renal toxicity with mannitol. For most small children, these aforementioned complications are unlikely when red blood cells are administered for small volume (≤15 mL/kg) transfusions. However, in the case of massive transfusion, whole blood (hematocrit approximately 35%) or relatively fresh red blood cell concentrates (<5 days old) with a hematocrit of 50–60% should be used. Since blood banking procedures differ between institutions, anesthesiologists should be familiar with their hospital's specific storage procedures for children.

Massive Transfusion

Massive transfusion is defined as the acute administration of one or more blood volumes. Complications of massive transfusion in pediatric patients include dilutional thrombocytopenia, disseminated intravascular coagulation, hypothermia, metabolic acidosis, hyperkalemia, hyperglycemia, hypocalcemia, and volume overload.

In the emergent transfusion situation, where type O blood is administered prior to an appropriate type and crossmatch, it is inadvisable to switch to the patient's correct blood type after a certain amount of type O blood has been administered. However, there are no national standards that define the amount or duration of transfusion necessary that mandates continuation with type O blood in patients that are type A, B, or AB. This decision is based on local standards, the supply of type O blood, and the amount of plasma in the unit of packed red blood cells after filtration from whole blood.

Fresh Frozen Plasma

Fresh frozen plasma (FFP) is administered to correct bleeding secondary to a documented or presumed coagulation factor deficiency. There are no practical laboratory studies that definitely indicate the need for FFP in the perioperative period. Rather, its use is guided by clinical evidence of nonsurgical bleeding, a high probability of clotting factor deficiency, or a prolonged coagulation time.

The most common perioperative cause of coagulation factor deficiency is dilutional, as a result of massive transfusion of crystalloid or red blood cells. FFP is not indicated for volume expansion without coagulation abnormalities.

The dose of FFP will depend on the desired correction of coagulation factor activity. In general, the minimum blood activity level of coagulation factors for physiological hemostatic effects is approximately 25% of the normal level. The appropriate dose of FFP that will raise the level of coagulation factors to 25% can be determined by first calculating the plasma volume:

$$\text{Plasma volume (mL/kg)} = [\text{Total blood volume (mL/kg)} \times (1 - \text{hematocrit})]$$

For an average child with a hematocrit of 43%:

$$\text{Plasma volume} = [70\,\text{mL/kg} \times (1 - 0.43)] = 40\,\text{mL/kg}$$

If we assume that the administered FFP contains 100% level of coagulation factors, then the volume administered to achieve 25% activity will be 25% × 40 mL/kg (10 mL/kg). One unit of FFP contains approximately 80 mL, so a 20-kg child will require 200 mL (2.5 units) of FFP.

FFP contains a relatively large amount of citrate, so if administered rapidly (>1 mL/kg/min) it may cause a transient decrease in ionized calcium and decrease in arterial blood pressure (Fig. 16-1). In most children, the hypocalcemia is transient because the citrate is metabolized rapidly. However, children with a limited ability to mobilize calcium (e.g., neonates) or a decreased ability to metabolize citrate (e.g., liver failure) may require exogenous calcium administration. FFP is not subjected to inactivation of infectious pathogens, and thus, may transmit infectious diseases.

Platelets

Intraoperative thrombocytopenia is usually dilutional as a result of massive blood transfusion but may result from an underlying illness such as necrotizing enterocolitis, malignancy, or disseminated intravascular coagulopathy (DIC). General indications for the administration of platelets to children include a platelet count $<50 \times 10^9$/L, or $<100 \times 10^9$/L in the presence of active bleeding. Critically ill premature infants are at risk for intracranial hemorrhage, so they should receive platelets when the platelet count is $<100 \times 10^9$/L, even in the absence of active bleeding.

Approximately 5-10 mL/kg from either a random donor or an apheresis unit should result in a rise in platelet count of $50-100 \times 10^9$/L. This is approximately equivalent to 0.1 units of platelets per kilogram of bodyweight. Less of an increase in the platelet count will be observed in the presence of sepsis or a consumptive coagulopathy.

Leukoreduction

At the present time, nearly all blood banks in the United States are performing leukoreduction of all cellular blood components. The goals of leukoreduction are to remove white blood cell (WBC)-associated infectious agents (e.g., cytomegalovirus) and to protect against human leukocyte antigen (HLA) sensitization. It may also

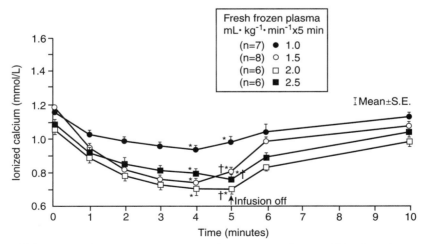

Figure 16-1 Hypocalcemia may accompany administration of citrated blood products, such as FFP or citrated whole blood. Within 5 minutes after administering FFP at rates exceeding 1.0 mL/kg/min, severely burned children will develop hypocalcemia. *$P < 0.001$; †$P < 0.0021$ compared with baseline. (Reproduced with permisssion from Coté CJ, Drop LJ, Hoaglin DC et al: Ionized hypocalcemia after fresh frozen plasma administration to thermally injured children: effects of infusion rate, duration, and treatment with calcium chloride, *Anesth Analg* 67:152, 1988.)

decrease the incidence of febrile nonhemolytic transfusion reactions, and alter the immunomodulation that occurs after transfusion of cellular blood components. Leukoreduction removes approximately 99% of WBCs; fewer than 5×10^6 WBCs should remain in the blood product.

Irradiation

Gamma irradiation of cellular blood components destroys the proliferative capacity of WBCs and is used to prevent transfusion-associated graft-vs-host disease (TAGVHD). TAGVHD occurs when transfused lymphocytes engraft and proliferate in the transfusion recipient's bone marrow, and is fatal in over 50% of patients.

Irradiated blood should be administered to immunocompromised children and those with normal immunity who share an HLA haplotype with the donor (i.e., first- or second-degree relatives), which would enable the donor lymphocytes to engraft without being initially destroyed by the recipient. Determination of irradiation is usually institution-specific with regard to the types of patients that are considered immunocompromised (Box 16-2).

Irradiation limits the shelf life of red cell concentrates to 28 days (after the irradiation) by accelerating storage abnormalities. When red cell concentrates are irradiated, the potassium level rises rapidly after 3 days of storage, and can reach 7 mEq/L after 2 weeks of storage. Therefore, hyperkalemia may occur during rapid and/ or massive transfusion of irradiated blood, and when transfusing premature infants or children with renal failure.

Complications of Blood Product Administration

Complications from blood product administration range from mild febrile reactions to fatal hemolytic reactions. Although the general public is usually most concerned

---

Box 16-2   Criteria for Using Irradiated Blood Products

Patient with decreased cellular immunity
Premature infant
Fetus receiving transfusion *in utero*
Bone marrow transplant recipient
Patient receiving chemotherapy that results in severe immune suppression
Critically ill child
Donated blood from a first- or second-degree relative

---

about the risk of viral infection from transfusions, the leading causes of transfusion-related mortality include acute hemolysis due to ABO incompatibility (usually a result of human error), bacterial contamination, and transfusion-related acute lung injury (TRALI).

ABO Incompatibility

Despite all safeguards, human error accounts for an ABO-incompatible transfusion in up to 1 in 6000 transfusions, and causes approximately 25 deaths per year in the United States. In fact, ABO errors cause more transfusion-related deaths than transmission of HIV from blood products. Many centers are now requiring two separate sample specimens before releasing type-specific blood. A variety of methods to prevent these human errors are being investigated, including strategies to convert type A or B donor blood into type O blood by altering the molecular structure of the red blood cells.

Bacterial Contamination

Because of the improved detection of viral agents in the blood supply, the risk of infection from bacterial contamination may now exceed that from viral agents. Bacterial infection is most commonly seen following platelet transfusion compared with red blood cells or FFP. Recipients of components containing Gram-negative organisms are at highest risk for transfusion-related death.

Transfusion Related Acute Lung Injury (TRALI)

TRALI is characterized by the development of dyspnea, cyanosis, hypotension, fever, and chills, along with radiologic findings of bilateral pulmonary edema. These findings are usually apparent within several hours following a blood transfusion, and often progress to hypoxemic respiratory failure with an approximate 6% mortality. The treatment is largely supportive.

TRALI is most often associated with transfusion of whole blood, packed red blood cells, and FFP, with an incidence of 0.014–0.02% per unit transfused. TRALI is thought to result from the sequestration of WBCs in the pulmonary microvasculature, which leads to increased vascular permeability and pulmonary edema. The underlying etiology is not precisely known, but it is likely to be related to the presence of antibodies against granulocyte or HLA antigens in the transfusion donor or recipient.

Viral Infection

Viral infection remains a serious, albeit less frequent complication from blood transfusion in children. Recent adaptation of nucleic acid technology (NAT) screening has increased the sensitivity of detecting certain infectious agents in donor blood (e.g., HIV, hepatitis C) and subsequently decreased the risk of transmission to its

Table 16-6	Approximate Risk of Viral Transmission from Red Cell Transfusion[a]
Virus	**Risk per Unit of Blood Transfused**
HIV	1 in 1,800,000
Hepatitis C	1 in 1,600,000
Hepatitis B[b]	1 in 220,000

[a] West Nile Virus infection has been reported but the incidence is unknown. NAT testing for West Nile Virus in blood products is under way.

[b] NAT is not currently being used.

lowest value in history (Table 16-6). This is because NAT tests for the virus as opposed to previous methods that tested the host's response to the viral infection.

An infectious complication with unique considerations for neonates and infants is cytomegalovirus (CMV). CMV resides in the WBCs of many healthy blood donors and can be transmitted through transfusion of cellular blood components. CMV infection in older, immunocompetent children is usually associated with a mild, transient systemic illness. However, CMV infection in neonates or immunocompromised children is associated with a severe systemic illness and may be fatal. Therefore, CMV screening is essential when transfusing these susceptible children. Anesthesiologists caring for children should be familiar with their own institution's guidelines for patients who should receive CMV-seronegative blood products.

CMV in donor blood can be removed by leukodepletion (see above) or detected by serologic methods. Which of these two methods is the most appropriate screening method is unknown, and will be institution-dependent. High-risk patients should receive blood products that are both leukodepleted and CMV-seronegative. However, despite these precautions, CMV transmission may still occur owing to false-negative serologic testing, or a higher-than-anticipated residual number of leukocytes following leukodepletion.

ARTICLES TO KNOW

Busch MP, Kleinman SH, Nemo GJ: Current and emerging infectious risks of blood transfusions. *JAMA* 289:959–962, 2003.

Cote CJ, Liu LM, Szyfelbein SK et al: Changes in serial platelet counts following massive blood transfusion in pediatric patients. *Anesthesiology* 62:197, 1985.

Ezri T, Szmuk P, Weisenberg M et al: The effects of hydration on core temperature in pediatric surgical patients. *Anesthesiology* 98:838–841, 2003.

Fergusson D, Hebert PC, Lee SK et al: Clinical outcomes following institution of universal leukoreduction of blood transfusions for premature infants. *JAMA* 289:1950–1956, 2003.

Hebert PC, Fergusson D, Blajchman MA et al: Clinical outcomes following institution of the Canadian universal leukoreduction program for red blood cell transfusions. *JAMA* 289:1941–1949, 2003.

Holliday MA, Segar WE: The maintenance need for water in parenteral fluid therapy. *Pediatrics* 19:823–832, 1957.

Holliday MA, Segar WE, Friedman A: Reducing errors in fluid therapy management. *Pediatrics* 111:424–425, 2003.

Hume HA, Limoges P: Perioperative blood transfusion therapy in pediatric patients. *Am J Ther* 9:396–405, 2002.

Lindahl SGE: Energy expenditure and fluid and electrolyte requirements in anesthetized infants and children. *Anesthesiology* 69:377–382, 1988.

Moritz ML, Ayus JC: Prevention of hospital-acquired hyponatremia: a case for using isotonic saline. *Pediatrics* 111:227–230, 2003.

Roseff SD, Luban NL, Manno CS: Guidelines for assessing appropriateness of pediatric transfusion. *Transfusion* 42:1398–1413, 2002.

Welborn LG, McGill WA, Hannallah RS et al: Perioperative blood glucose concentrations in pediatric outpatients. *Anesthesiology* 65:543–547, 1986.

Welborn LG, Hannallah RS, McGill WA, Ruttimann UE, Hicks JM: Glucose concentrations for routine intravenous infusion in pediatric outpatient surgery. *Anesthesiology* 67:427–430, 1987.

Welborn LG, Norden JM, Seiden N et al: Effect of minimizing preoperative fasting on perioperative blood glucose homeostasis in children. *Pediatr Anesth* 3:167–171, 1993.

Pediatric Airway Management

RONALD S. LITMAN

Airway management is one of the most important aspects of pediatric anesthesia because of its inextricable relationship to the most important complication – the development of hypoxemia. This importance is further exemplified by the inherent differences in pediatric airway management when compared with adults. This chapter reviews the basics of pediatric airway management, with an emphasis on the differences between children and adults. The anatomy of the pediatric airway is reviewed, followed by a discussion of pediatric airway management techniques. Pediatric airway complications are discussed, including laryngospasm, pulmonary aspiration, and negative-pressure (postobstructive) pulmonary edema.

PEDIATRIC UPPER AIRWAY ANATOMY

The approach to airway management of infants and young children is influenced by developmental differences in head and neck anatomy. These differences include:

1. A larger occiput, which influences head and neck positioning during airway management, such that neck flexion is not required to attain the "sniffing" position
2. The presence of hypertrophied tonsil and adenoid tissue, which causes rapid development of upper-airway obstruction after administration of general anesthesia
3. A more cephalad larynx (C2–C3) than in the adult (C4–C5), which renders it more easily visualized using a straight, rather than a curved laryngoscope (Fig. 17-1)
4. A narrower and shorter epiglottis which is angled into the lumen of the airway, making it difficult to displace anteriorly during laryngoscopy.

In paralyzed children, the cricoid cartilage is the narrowest portion of the upper airway because of its inability to distend in a similar manner as the vocal cords. Therefore, an endotracheal tube that easily passes through the vocal cords may compress tracheal mucosa at the level of the cricoid cartilage and predispose to inflammation, edema, and subsequent scarring and stenosis. Although the infant tongue is relatively larger in proportion to the oral cavity when compared with the adult, MRI studies of the upper airway during general anesthesia have demonstrated that, as in adults, upper-airway obstruction occurs primarily at the levels of the soft palate and epiglottis, and rarely by the tongue.

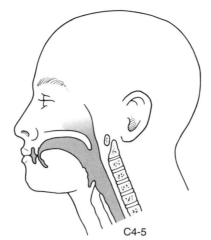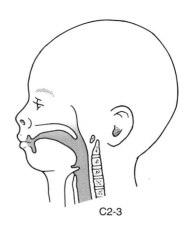

Figure 17-1 In early childhood the larynx is located in a more cephalad position, and descends during growth. (Redrawn with permission from Nichols DG: *Golden Hour*, 2nd edn, Mosby, Philadelphia, 1996.)

C4-5

C2-3

Overall, the most important difference between young children and adults is merely the smaller size. Small nasal passages are more likely to become obstructed with blood or secretions, and tracheal edema is more likely to increase airway resistance in smaller diameter airways since the resistance to flow through a tube is related to the fifth power of the radius of the tube (since this flow is largely turbulent). Of interest, the upper airway of a normal infant is smaller in both inspiration and expiration at 6 weeks of age compared to the neonatal period. This relative narrowing may be caused by postnatal growth of adenoid tissue, or thickening of the mucous membrane lining in response to infection or second-hand smoke exposure.

Dental Development

The 20 primary teeth are identified by a lettering system (Fig. 17-2). They begin to erupt during the first year of life, and are shed at between 6 and 12 years of age. The preoperative physical exam of children in this age group should include a search for loose teeth, which may be dislodged during airway management and accidentally lost within the respiratory tract. Loose or chipped teeth should be documented on the anesthetic record. Significantly loose teeth should be removed by the anesthesiologist (or dentist if one is present) prior to airway instrumentation. This is easily accomplished by grasping the tooth with gauze and rocking the tooth back and

Figure 17-2 The 20 primary teeth are identified by a lettering system, A through T, which begins with the right upper molar and ends at the right lower molar. The picture is viewed as if the patient is facing the examiner with mouth open. (Redrawn with permission from the American Dental Association website.)

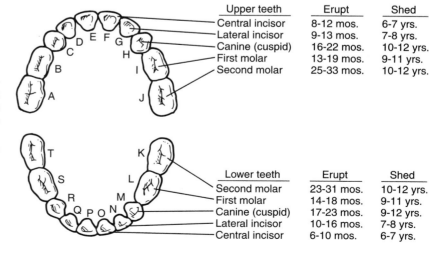

Upper teeth	Erupt	Shed
Central incisor	8-12 mos.	6-7 yrs.
Lateral incisor	9-13 mos.	7-8 yrs.
Canine (cuspid)	16-22 mos.	10-12 yrs.
First molar	13-19 mos.	9-11 yrs.
Second molar	25-33 mos.	10-12 yrs.

Lower teeth	Erupt	Shed
Second molar	23-31 mos.	10-12 yrs.
First molar	14-18 mos.	9-11 yrs.
Canine (cuspid)	17-23 mos.	9-12 yrs.
Lateral incisor	10-16 mos.	7-8 yrs.
Central incisor	6-10 mos.	6-7 yrs.

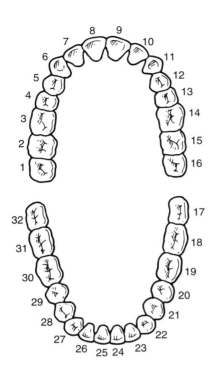

1. 3rd Molar (wisdom tooth)
2. 2nd Molar (12-yr molar)
3. 1st Molar (6-yr molar)
4. 2nd Bicuspid (2nd premolar)
5. 1st Bicuspid (1st premolar)
6. Cuspid (canine/eye tooth)
7. Lateral incisor
8. Central incisor
9. Central incisor
10. Lateral incisor
11. Cuspid (canine/eye tooth)
12. 1st Bicuspid (1st premolar)
13. 2nd Bicuspid (2nd premolar)
14. 1st Molar (6-yr molar)
15. 2nd Molar (12-yr molar)
16. 3rd Molar (wisdom tooth)
17. 3rd Molar (wisdom tooth)
18. 2nd Molar (12-yr molar)
19. 1st Molar (6-yr molar)
20. 2nd Bicuspid (2nd premolar)
21. 1st Bicuspid (1st premolar)
22. Cuspid (canine/eye tooth)
23. Lateral incisor
24. Central incisor
25. Central incisor
26. Lateral incisor
27. Cuspid (canine/eye tooth)
28. 1st Bicuspid (1st premolar)
29. 2nd Bicuspid (2nd premolar)
30. 1st Molar (6-yr molar)
31. 2nd Molar (12-yr molar)
32. 3rd Molar (wisdom tooth)

Figure 17-3   The 32 permanent teeth are identified by a numbering system which begins with the right upper 3rd molar ("wisdom tooth") and ends with the right lower 3rd molar. The picture is viewed as if the patient is facing the examiner with mouth open. **1** = 3rd molar; **2** = 2nd (12-year) molar; **3** = 1st (6-year) molar; **4** = 2nd bicuspid (2nd premolar); **5** = 1st bicuspid (1st premolar); **6** = cuspid ("canine" or "eye tooth"); **7** = lateral incisor; **8** = central incisor; **9–16** = identical sequence in reverse; **17–32** = mirror image of the top row. (Redrawn with permission from the American Dental Association website.)

forth while simultaneously pulling. Minor bleeding in the tooth socket will abate with gentle pressure applied for several minutes.

The 32 permanent teeth begin to appear at the same time as the primary teeth are shed and are identified by a numbering system (Fig. 17-3). Orthodontic hardware can be placed at any time after the eruption of the permanent teeth. If feasible, rubber bands should be removed prior to anesthetic management. During the preoperative physical exam, permanent orthodontic devices should be examined for loose or damaged pieces, and this should be clearly documented on the anesthetic record. If a permanent orthodontic device is in danger of being dislodged during airway management, dental or orthodontic consultation is required before proceeding with the general anesthetic.

Pediatric Airway Assessment

In adults, there are several validated physical characteristics that are associated with the inability to perform mask ventilation or tracheal intubation. No such physical characteristics exist for the pediatric population. Unless syndromic facial anomalies exist (e.g., midface hypoplasia, micrognathia), it is extremely rare that tracheal intubation cannot be accomplished in the prepubertal child. On the other hand, mask ventilation may be difficult for a variety of reasons, including the distorted facial anatomy of the neonate, the relatively large tongue of the child with trisomy 21, and the presence of hypertrophied tonsil and adenoid tissue in toddlers.

PEDIATRIC AIRWAY MANAGEMENT TECHNIQUES

Mask Ventilation

In children aged 4 years and above, mask ventilation is usually uncomplicated and easy to perform. Younger patients may present a challenge to mask ventilation because of the relatively smaller face, larger tongue, and ease with which the anesthesiologist's fingers may compress the soft tissues of the neck and impinge on the upper airway. In the newborns, unintentional jaw pressure from neck flexion, submental pressure, or mandibular pressure during facemask application is associated with upper-airway obstruction. Furthermore, many infants have some degree of laryngomalacia, which renders the supraglottic structures prone to collapse during inspiration.

The most effective mask ventilation technique for infants and young children is for the anesthesiologist to hold the mask over the mouth and nose with the thumb and forefinger, while the middle finger is placed on the bony portion of the mandible (Fig. 17-4). With this

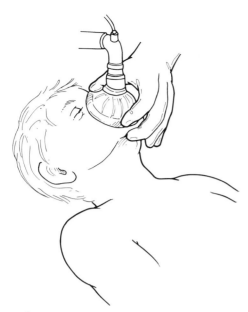

Figure 17-4 The most effective mask ventilation technique for infants and young children is for the anesthesiologist to hold the mask over the mouth and nose with the thumb and forefinger, while the middle finger is placed on the bony portion of the mandible.

technique, the chin can be lifted to provide head extension without compressing the soft tissues of the neck. The upper part of the mask should rest on the bridge of the nose. The most common error of inexperienced practitioners is to hold the mask too low over the nose and compress the nasal passages.

Manual Airway Opening Maneuvers

If mask ventilation becomes difficult owing to upper-airway obstruction, there are a series of manual maneuvers that may improve airflow prior to airway instrumentation. These include chin lift, jaw thrust, and application of continuous positive airway pressure (CPAP). Chin lift will extend the head at the atlantooccipital joint, thus stretching and straightening the airway to decrease the severity of soft tissue obstruction. Jaw thrust will displace the genioglossus in an anterior direction and alleviate obstruction at the levels of the soft palate and epiglottis (via ligaments that connect the genioglossus with supraglottic structures). CPAP distends the soft tissues of the pharynx and larynx, thus counteracting the effects of laryngomalacia and the decrease in pharyngeal dilator tone that is normally seen with loss of consciousness. The use of CPAP, however, often causes unintentional inflation of the stomach. To avoid gastric distention, peak inspiratory pressures should not exceed 15 cmH$_2$O, when possible.

Oral Airway Insertion

When manual techniques have failed to improve upper-airway patency, insertion of an oral airway will establish airflow in almost all cases of children with normal airway anatomy. This is primarily because the oral airway device bypasses the obstruction, which is usually caused by enlarged tonsils and/or adenoids.

The most commonly used airway device in pediatric anesthesia is the Guedel airway, which contains a central lumen for the passage of air flow and for suctioning the posterior pharynx. The insertion technique is similar to that for adults. It can be inserted with the aid of a tongue depressor, or initially inserted with the distal tip oriented cephalad, and then turned 180 degrees when the tip has reached the posterior aspect of the palate.

Oral airways are sized depending on the total length of the device (50–80 mm for most children) or based on an arbitrary scale designated by the manufacturer. The appropriate size is determined by placing the airway adjacent to the child's face to approximate its position in the oral cavity (Fig. 17-5). When appropriately placed, its distal end should snugly curve around the back of the tongue, without the proximal end protruding out of the mouth. Too small an oral airway will push the posterior portion of the tongue against the posterior pharyngeal wall, and too large an oral airway may itself cause upper-airway obstruction at the laryngeal inlet by compressing or distorting the epiglottis (Fig. 17-6). Complications of

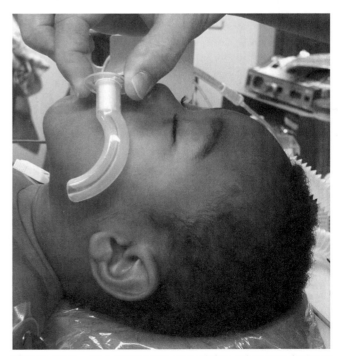

Figure 17-5 The appropriate size of the oral airway device is chosen by placing it adjacent to the face to approximate its position in the oral cavity.

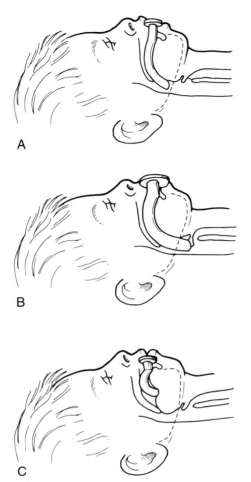

Figure 17-6   **A,** The distal end of the oral airway device should snugly curve around the back of the tongue, without the proximal end protruding out of the mouth. **B,** Too large an oral airway may itself cause upper-airway obstruction at the laryngeal inlet by compressing or distorting the epiglottis. **C,** Too small an oral airway will cause obstruction by pushing the posterior portion of the tongue against the posterior pharyngeal wall. (Redrawn with permission from Coté CJ, Todres ID, Goudsouzian NG, Ryan JF: *A Practice of Anesthesia for Infants and Children*, 3rd edn, WB Saunders, Philadelphia, 2001.)

oral airway use in children are similar to those in adults. If the airway is used to prevent the child from biting on the endotracheal tube during emergence, lip or tooth damage is possible, and a loose tooth is likely to become dislodged and lost in the oral cavity. Therfore, a soft-bite block is recommended for this situation.

Nasal Airway Insertion

A nasal airway may be used as a means to relieve upper-airway obstruction as well as to provide a useful conduit for delivering oxygen and anesthetic gases during surgical procedures in the oral cavity. Nasal airways are available in sizes 12- to 36-French (outer diameter).

A "custom" nasal airway can be fashioned by cutting off the appropriate length of an endotracheal tube.

Prior to insertion, the nasal cavities should be inspected to assure the absence of significant septal deviation, or other causes of narrowing (e.g., polyp) that will obstruct passage of the nasal airway. To avoid trauma and bleeding of the delicate nasal mucosa, the nasal airway should be lubricated and inserted in a posterocaudad direction along the floor of the nasal cavity. A topical vasoconstrictor, such as 0.05% oxymetazoline, can be sprayed on the nasal mucosa prior to nasal airway insertion. The proper diameter is determined by approximating the circular diameter of the nasal opening. The proper length of the nasal airway is estimated by measuring the distance from the nares to the tragus of the ear. When appropriately placed, its distal tip should lie at the level of the angle of the mandible, between the posterior aspect of the tongue and above the tip of the epiglottis. Some red rubber nasal airways are supplied with a movable ring at the proximal end, with which to adjust the proper length at the tip of the nasal opening.

The most common complication from nasal airway insertion is trauma to the nasal or pharyngeal mucosa that results in minor bleeding. Adenoidal tissue may be disrupted and may bleed into the oropharynx. Occasionally, a friable vessel is encountered in the nasal mucosa and bleeding is brisk. A lesser known, though not rare, complication is the insertion of the nasal airway device into a false passage beneath the posterior wall mucosa of the nasal and oral pharynx. This is not usually accompanied by bleeding, so it may be caused by a patent Thornwaldt bursa. Nasal airways should not be inserted in children with a coagulopathy, neutropenia, or suspicion of a traumatic basilar skull fracture.

Laryngeal Mask Airway

The laryngeal mask airway (LMA) is used in pediatric anesthesia as a routine airflow conduit during general anesthesia and as a component of the difficult airway algorithm (see Chapter 18). A variety of sizes are available for pediatric patients (Table 17-1). When the LMA

Table 17-1 LMA Sizes for Children		
LMA Size	Approximate Weight (kg)	Cuff Volume (mL)
1	<5	2–5
1.5	5–10	3–8
2	10–20	5–10
2.5	20–30	10–15
3	30–50	15–20
4	50–70	25–30

was first introduced it was considered to be useful only during situations that were amenable to facemask anesthesia; however, as practitioners have become more comfortable with its use, the LMA has become a substitute for an endotracheal tube in certain cases, such as tonsillectomy or strabismus repair. An LMA that is specially designed with a wire-reinforced shaft is available for use during tonsillectomy or other procedures that would otherwise require an oral RAE endotracheal tube (see below). When compared with an endotracheal tube, the LMA is associated with less laryngeal stimulation and a decreased incidence of airway complications in children with upper respiratory tract infections. In most normal children, positive-pressure ventilation is easily accomplished via an LMA, but peak inspiratory pressure should not exceed 20 cmH$_2$O to prevent gastric insufflation. Because of its inability to seal off the trachea adequately, the LMA is not indicated for use in children at risk for pulmonary aspiration of gastric contents.

The relatively cephalad location of the pediatric larynx does not lend itself to ideal LMA placement. Thus, the smaller the patient, the more difficult it is to achieve ideal LMA positioning in the larynx. Fiberoptic and magnetic resonance imaging (MRI) studies on LMA placement in children have shown a high incidence of malpositioning with the epiglottis situated within the aperture of the LMA, despite seemingly adequate ventilation. In children the LMA is likely to become displaced with patient movement or twisting from its proximal end, and is more likely to result in the deterioration of ventilation after placement when compared with adults.

A variety of methods of LMA placement in children are possible. Besides the direct method of pushing the flattened LMA cuff posterior by applying pressure against the hard palate, the LMA can be inserted with the cuff partially or fully inflated, or inserted with the aperture facing posterior and then turned 180 degrees once in the larynx. There are no advantages to one particular insertion method. A water-based lubricant smeared on the posterior surface of the LMA may decrease the resistance to insertion. Nevertheless, in many children insertion is difficult and is associated with pharyngeal bleeding. Postoperative sore throat is observed after LMA use, though it is not as common as seen after endotracheal intubation.

During emergence from general anesthesia, the LMA can be removed at any time. Removal with the cuff inflated will facilitate removal of blood or secretions that have collected above the cuff. If one chooses to wait until the child is strong and awake before removing the LMA, a bite block should be inserted between the patient's teeth to prevent compression of the lumen of the LMA, which can result in negative-pressure pulmonary edema (see below). Removal of the LMA during the excitement phase of emergence is associated with a

lower incidence of airway complications when compared with removal of an endotracheal tube. Nevertheless, airway complications during emergence are least when the LMA is removed prior to the child regaining airway reflexes and full consciousness. Rapid removal of the LMA may cause displacement of loose teeth.

Endotracheal Intubation

Techniques of endotracheal intubation differ between children and adults. This section will review differences in laryngoscopy, choice of the appropriate type and diameter of the endotracheal tube, confirming proper tracheal placement of the tube, and determining the correct endotracheal tube length.

Laryngoscopy

In most children, laryngoscopy is technically easier than in adults. An unexpectedly difficult view of the glottis is unusual. However, in neonates and small infants, laryngoscopy is often challenging because of the smaller and more cephalad location of the larynx, and the narrower view through the oropharynx. The optimal position for laryngoscopy is attained differently than for adults. The relatively large occiput provides flexion of the head, while the shoulders lie flat on the table. The anesthesiologist's line of sight should be nearly directly over the child's airway, and the laryngoscope blade is inserted almost perpendicular to the OR table to obtain the easiest view of the glottis. This is in contrast to adults, in whom the best glottic view is usually obtained with the laryngoscope blade almost parallel to the OR table.

A variety of pediatric-sized laryngoscope blades are available (Table 17-2). A straight blade is most often used to obtain the best glottic view. In infants and small children, the straight blade is usually inserted into the vallecula to tilt the epiglottis anteriorly to view the glottic opening. The infant's small size and anteriorly placed larynx afford the anesthesiologist the opportunity to use the fifth finger of the nondominant hand to push the larynx in a posterior direction to improve the glottic view (Fig. 17-7).

Endotracheal Tubes

A variety of formulas have been developed by which to determine the most appropriate sized endotracheal tube for children, based on age, weight, or height. All of these formulas have reasonable reliability. The most popular to use with uncuffed oral endotracheal tubes is *Cole's formula*:

$$\text{Internal tube diameter (mm)} = \left[\frac{16 + \text{age (years)}}{4} \right]$$

Another moderately reliable method is to approximate the diameter of the trachea with the diameter of

Table 17-2   Laryngoscope Blade Types and Sizes

Age	Blade Type and Size		
	Miller	Wis–Hippel	Macintosh
Premature neonate	0	–	–
Term neonate	0-1	–	–
1-12 months	1	–	–
1-2 years	1	1.5	2
2-6 years	2	–	2
6-12 years	2	–	3

Modified with permission from Cote CJ, Todres ID, Goudsouzian NG, Ryan JF: *A Practice of Anesthesia for Infants and Children*, 3rd edn, WB Saunders, Philadelphia, 2001.

Table 17-3   Approximate Endotracheal Tube Sizes for Children

Age	Size (mm) and Cuff Type
0-3 months	3.0-3.5 uncuffed
3-10 months	3.5-4.0 uncuffed
10-12 months	4.0 cuffed or uncuffed
2 years	4.5 cuffed or uncuffed
3 years[a]	4.5-5.0 cuffed

[a] For children 4 years of age and older, use Cole's formula. If the value falls in between tube sizes, round down and use a cuffed tube.

the child's fifth finger. Once one gains enough experience with pediatric patients, formulas are abandoned in favor of a "mental" chart (Table 17-3). When using a cuffed endotracheal tube (see below) the choice of its size is less important because the cuff can compensate for the selection of too small a tube.

A RAE (Ring–Adair–Elwyn) endotracheal tube is preformed for oral or nasal use (Fig. 17-8). The proximal end of the oral RAE tube curves onto the chin and is used for oral or ophthalmologic procedures when the surgeon is situated behind the head of the patient. The proximal end of the nasal RAE tube is preformed to rest on the forehead during procedures in the oral cavity or neck. Because a RAE tube is preformed, its length cannot be adjusted once it is properly placed.

Cuffed versus Uncuffed Tubes

Pediatric anesthesiologists have traditionally preferred to use only uncuffed endotracheal tubes in children up to the prepubertal age group. This practice is based on the notion that the unyielding cricoid ring is functionally the narrowest portion of the upper airway, so a cuff is not necessary to seal off the upper portion of the trachea to provide adequate ventilation and prevent pulmonary aspiration. At some uncertain age between 6 and 10 years, the larynx changes shape from conical to cylindrical, and the glottis becomes the narrowest portion; a cuff is then needed to seal off the trachea since the portion of the endotracheal tube that passes the cricoid ring is no longer snug. These hypotheses are

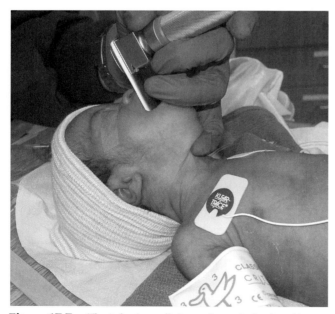

Figure 17-7   The infant's small size and anteriorly placed larynx afford the anesthesiologist the opportunity to use the fifth finger of the free hand to push the larynx in a posterior direction to improve the glottic view.

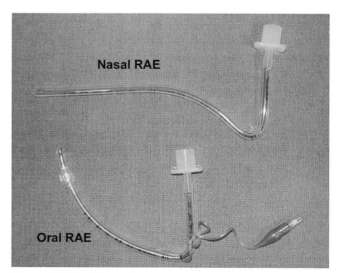

Figure 17-8   The oral RAE tube is preformed for easy attachment to the chin when the surgeon is positioned behind the patient. The nasal RAE tube is preformed to sit on the forehead for procedures in the oral cavity or neck.

based on data obtained from pediatric cadaver specimens, and the clinical observation is that an endotracheal tube will often pass easily through the vocal cords, only to meet resistance at the level of the cricoid ring. Furthermore, an uncuffed endotracheal tube will have a relatively smaller external diameter compared with a cuffed endotracheal tube of the same internal diameter. Therefore, a relatively larger sized internal diameter tube can be inserted comfortably. This will provide relatively less resistance to airflow, and will facilitate suctioning of secretions.

In recent years, a growing number of pediatric anesthesiologists have begun using cuffed endotracheal tubes in smaller children. This trend is a result of the gradual recognition that cuffed tubes are not associated with an increased incidence of airway complications. Furthermore, since spontaneous ventilation in intubated children is not usually performed, the increased resistance of the slightly smaller internal diameter tube will not increase work of breathing. Use of a cuffed endotracheal tube will prevent the need to change the tube if it is incorrectly sized, thus sparing the child from an extra laryngoscopic attempt. The very act of changing endotracheal tubes while the child is anesthetized increases the concentration of inhaled vapors in the OR environment. Avoidance of a leak around the endotracheal tube will also increase the precision of the values and the waveform pattern of the capnographic tracing.

Additional advantages to using a cuffed tube include the ability to ventilate using higher inflation pressures if necessary, and the theoretically decreased risk of pulmonary aspiration.

Confirming Tracheal Location

Once the endotracheal tube has been inserted, it must immediately be determined to be in the trachea and not in the esophagus. Methods for confirming tracheal placement are similar to those for adults and include the characteristic rise of the chest wall and absence of gastric inflation, the presence of breath sounds in the left axilla and absence of breath sounds over the epigastrium, and the characteristic capnographic tracing. These are all confirmed simultaneously in the first several seconds following endotracheal intubation. When the endotracheal tube is placed properly in the trachea, mist should be observed in the proximal end of the tube during exhalation. In small infants, breath sounds are easily transmitted across the epigastrium and chest wall, so auscultation may be less reliable for confirming tracheal placement.

Confirming Tube Dimensions
Tube Diameter
Following insertion of an uncuffed endotracheal tube, the anesthesiologist should determine whether or not it is the appropriate size for the child's trachea. Although standard formulas or guidelines are often used, it is not infrequent that the chosen size is too small or too large. If it is too small, ventilation may be inadequate, and anesthetic vapors will pollute the OR environment. If the endotracheal tube is too large, there may be undue pressure on the tracheal mucosa, resulting in inflammation, injury, and edema, which manifests clinically as postintubation croup. Therefore, it is common practice to determine the fit of the endotracheal tube by performing a "leak test" shortly after the tracheal position is confirmed. This test is performed by auscultating over the mouth or anterior neck while the pop-off valve on the anesthesia machine is progressively closed. The rising airway pressure will reach a point at which air will begin to escape around the wall of the tube, and this can be heard as a characteristic squeak. In children, the pressure at which tracheal damage begins is unknown. However, a leak pressure between 15 and 25 cmH_2O will ensure adequacy of ventilation while minimizing injury to the tracheal wall. When the pressure is above 40 cmH_2O, consideration should be given to changing the endotracheal tube to a smaller size; however, for relatively short surgical procedures, it is unknown whether this tight fit is associated with tracheal injury. Unfortunately, the leak test has been shown to be unreliable and inconsistent between pediatric anesthesiologists on the same child. Furthermore, there are several factors that change the leak, including neck position and degree of neuromuscular blockade.

A modified Cole's formula can be used to estimate the most appropriate size of cuffed endotracheal tube. As long as the cuff is able to be advanced through the vocal cords without much resistance, it is then adjusted to provide a leak between 15 and 25 cmH_2O.

Tube Length
There are several fairly reliable methods for determining the proper length of insertion of the endotracheal tube in children. Four of these are described below.

First, during direct laryngoscopy and insertion of the endotracheal tube through the glottis, the length is noted at which the endotracheal tube has been inserted 2–3 cm past the vocal cords. Some endotracheal tube manufacturers place black line markings at the distal end of the tube that are designed to rest at the level of the vocal cords.

Second, for most children with normal airway anatomy, the proper length in centimeters at which to secure the endotracheal tube at the teeth (or gums for infants) is three times the internal diameter of the tube used (in millimeters), assuming that the proper size of endotracheal tube has been placed.

The two methods noted above will accurately place the endotracheal tube between the vocal cords and the carina in the majority of children with normal tracheal anatomy. However, there are many children in whom the

Article to Know

Khine H, Corddry DH, Kettrick RG et al: Comparison of cuffed and uncuffed endotracheal tubes in young children during general anesthesia. Anesthesiology 86:627–631, 1997.

Henry Khine and his colleagues at the duPont Hospital for Children questioned the traditional wisdom of using uncuffed endotracheal tubes in children. They designed this prospective unblinded study to assess the difference in complications in 488 children from birth to 8 years of age who were randomly selected to receive either a cuffed or an uncuffed endotracheal tube.

- Uncuffed tubes were chosen based on Cole's formula: internal diameter (mm) equal to (16 + age in years)/4.
- Cuffed tubes were chosen based on a modified formula: internal diameter (mm) equal to (16 + age in years)/3.

The authors used an upward rounding approach when the calculated tube size was between sizes, and placed a smaller tube if resistance to passage of the tube into the trachea was encountered. Uncuffed tubes were replaced with the next largest size if a leak around the tube occurred at an inflation pressure <10 cmH_2O.

The authors demonstrated that cuffed tubes were not associated with an increased incidence of complications, such as postintubation croup. On the contrary, the use of a cuffed tube was associated with a greater likelihood that the endotracheal tube fit properly after the first insertion, and a greater likelihood of successfully using 2 L/min total gas flows (Table 17-4). When an uncuffed endotracheal tube was used, the ambient nitrous oxide concentration exceeded 25 parts per million (NIOSH-recommended upper limit of safety) in 37% of cases but did not exceed this limit in any of the cases when a cuffed endotracheal tube was used.

Table 17-4

	Cuffed Tube	Uncuffed Tube	*P*-value
Total patients	251	237	
Patients needing tube changes	3 (1.2%)	54 (23%)	<0.001
Patients needing >2 L/min fresh gas flow	3 (1.2%)	26 (11%)	<0.001

Reproduced with permission from Khine HH et al: *Anesthesiology* 86:627–631, 1997.

The authors concluded that the use of a cuffed tube was advantageous for children because of the avoidance of repeated laryngoscopy, ability to use low total gas flows, theoretical reduction of the risk of aspiration, and the ability to reduce the concentration of anesthetics in the operating room environment. The publication of this study was largely responsible for a change in practice in the pediatric anesthesia community that favored use of cuffed endotracheal tubes in small children. At The Children's Hospital of Philadelphia, we have been routinely using cuffed endotracheal tubes for most children aged over 12 months, without an apparent increase in perioperative airway complications.

trachea is abnormally short, and the use of these methods may place the endotracheal tube in a main bronchus. Therefore, a third, more precise, method of localizing the distal end of the endotracheal tube is warranted. Once it is confirmed that the endotracheal tube is correctly inserted in the trachea, and maximal oxygenation is assured, an assistant manually ventilates the child while the anesthesiologist slowly advances the endotracheal tube and simultaneously listens to breath sounds in the left axilla. At the moment when breath sounds are lost, it can be assumed that the endotracheal tube has passed the carina and has entered the right main bronchus. In rare cases the endotracheal tube will advance into the left main bronchus. If breath sounds are not lost in the left axilla within a reasonable amount of advancing distance, it should be withdrawn and the process should be repeated. If the endotracheal tube still does not appear to enter the right main bronchus, the child's head can be turned to the left, as this maneuver will help guide the tube into the contralateral bronchus. The length of the endotracheal tube at the carina is noted, and it is then pulled back several centimeters so that the optimal location is midway between the vocal cords and the carina. In normal full-term newborns the distance between the vocal cords and the carina is usually 4–5 cm.

Finally, when using a cuffed endotracheal tube, palpation of the cuff in the suprasternal notch usually confirms an adequate position between the glottis and carina.

Effect of Neck Movement on Tube Position

It is very common for head and neck position to change during pediatric surgical procedures. A number of studies have determined the effect of different neck movements on the position of the endotracheal tube in the trachea in children. These studies consistently demonstrate that: (1) neck flexion causes the tip of the endotracheal tube to move toward the carina; (2) neck extension causes the tip to move away from the carina; and (3) lateral rotation causes the tip to move away from the carina, although to a lesser extent than occurs during neck extension. These findings are similar with both orotracheal and nasotracheal tube placement.

Nasotracheal Intubation

Nasotracheal intubation is primarily used for procedures in the oral cavity, and can be safely performed in children of all ages. The tube size chosen is the same as for oral endotracheal tubes. There are various methods that facilitate ease of nasotracheal intubation and decrease the incidence of tissue damage and bleeding. These include softening the nasal tube by soaking it for several minutes in warmed saline, preinsertion of a lubricated soft red rubber catheter through the nasal passage, and administration of a topical vasoconstrictor agent such as cocaine 4% or oxymetazoline 0.05%. The nasal endotracheal tube should be well lubricated, and inserted through the most patent nasal canal.

The technique for insertion of a nasotracheal tube in children is similar to adults and is partially described in the previous section on insertion of nasal airways. In supine, paralyzed children, a Magill forceps is almost always required to direct the tip of the endotracheal tube into the glottic opening. Since nasal endotracheal intubation may cause transient bacteremia, endocarditis prophylaxis is indicated in susceptible children.

RAPID SEQUENCE INDUCTION

The key components of a rapid sequence induction (RSI) of general anesthesia include preoxygenation, apneic oxygenation after administration of a hypnotic agent and muscle relaxant, and application of cricoid pressure to prevent passive regurgitation of gastric contents into the pharynx. Each of these components will be reviewed as they pertain to their usefulness in pediatric patients.

Preoxygenation

Preoxygenation, with the goal of removing nitrogen from the lungs, is performed prior to RSI to lengthen the duration of apnea prior to laryngoscopy. In adults, preoxygenation is easily attained by breathing 100% oxygen for several minutes or asking the patient to take several vital capacity breaths. These maneuvers are not always possible in young uncooperative children who may struggle with facemask application. On the other hand, the relatively smaller ratio of functional residual capacity (FRC) to tidal volume will facilitate a more rapid denitrogenation in children compared with adults. Nevertheless, the optimal length of time for denitrogenation of the pediatric lung has not been determined, although longer preoxygenation times are associated with longer times to desaturation during apnea in children over 2 years of age. Most pediatric anesthesiologists will administer 100% oxygen for at least 1 minute prior to rapid sequence induction, or longer until the oxygen saturation reaches 100% by pulse oximetry.

Apneic Oxygenation

Apneic oxygenation is the process by which the lungs continue to take up oxygen in the absence of spontaneous or controlled breathing movements. It occurs by bulk flow of oxygen from an oxygen source (i.e., anesthesia breathing circuit) through a patent upper airway, trachea, and lower respiratory system. Oxygen will continue to flow into the lungs as it is taken up by the blood passing through the pulmonary vascular bed.

Apneic oxygenation occurs during the phase of rapid sequence induction that follows preoxygenation and administration of a hypnotic agent plus a neuromuscular blocker. This period is required for the neuromuscular blocker to take effect prior to performing laryngoscopy. In healthy, nonobese children, oxyhemoglobin desaturation during apnea may not occur for several minutes. In infants and small children, oxyhemoglobin desaturation during apnea will occur rapidly, despite seemingly adequate preoxygenation and denitrogenation. During apneic oxygenation, a neonate may become hypoxemic within several seconds! This phenomenon is commonly attributed to the infant's relatively lower FRC while anesthetized, combined with a relatively larger oxygen consumption. It is for this reason that, during RSI in infants and small children, positive-pressure ventilation is usually required prior to endotracheal intubation. When this is performed while cricoid pressure continues, it is termed a "modified" rapid sequence induction.

Cricoid Pressure

Cricoid pressure reliably occludes the esophagus in infants and children, even in the presence of a nasogastric tube. In addition, it prevents the entry of gas into the esophagus during mask ventilation. However, in very small infants, cricoid pressure may compress the trachea and prevent adequate air entry into the lungs. The performance of cricoid pressure has not been shown to be associated with a decreased risk of pulmonary aspiration in susceptible patients, but it remains the standard of care for rapid sequence induction in many centers.

Article To Know

Salem MR, Wong AY, Fizzotti GF: Efficacy of cricoid pressure in preventing aspiration of gastric contents in paediatric patients. Br J Anaesth 44:401–404, 1972.

Although published over three decades ago, this article on the efficacy of cricoid pressure in infants is still applicable to current pediatric anesthesia practice. Dr Salem and his colleagues studied the efficacy of cricoid pressure protection against passive regurgitation in a series of three novel experiments. In the first, the authors artificially increased the intragastric pressure to 100 cmH$_2$O in eight infant cadavers, during which cricoid pressure was applied while simultaneously visualizing the pharynx for the presence of colored saline or radiographic contrast material. In the second experiment, the same methodology was used following passage of a nasogastric tube with an outer diameter of 3.1 mm. In the third experiment, three different sizes of nasogastric tubes were inserted into six anesthetized children aged 1–12 years, after being filled with contrast material and then clamped at the proximal end. Lateral neck radiographs were then taken before and after cricoid pressure.

In the first two experiments, firm cricoid pressure prevented passive regurgitation of pressurized saline from the stomach, with or without the presence of the nasogastric tube. The authors concluded that since intragastric pressures in paralyzed infants should not exceed 50 cmH$_2$O, cricoid pressure is an effective method to prevent passive regurgitation. In the last experiment, cricoid pressure did not occlude a nasogastric tube filled with contrast. Thus, it is preferable to retain a nasogastric tube during rapid sequence induction in infants, since it will not interfere with cricoid pressure, and a sudden rise in intragastric pressure can be negated by opening the proximal end of the tube to allow egress of gastric contents.

COMPLICATIONS OF PEDIATRIC AIRWAY MANAGEMENT

Laryngospasm

Laryngospasm describes a powerful self-protective response of the glottic and supraglottic laryngeal adductor muscles that results in partial or complete airway obstruction during attempts at inspiration. Laryngospasm may result from stimulation of a surprising number of anatomic sites, including the nasal mucosa, soft palate, pharynx, epiglottis, larynx, tracheobronchial tree, lung tissue, diaphragm, and abdominal viscera. The vast majority of episodes of laryngospasm in anesthetized children are caused by secretions or blood in contact with the laryngeal mucosa in or around the glottic opening, or by the laryngeal stimulation that occurs during tracheal extubation in a child who has not fully regained consciousness. Risk factors that increase the likelihood of laryngospasm include an active or recent upper respiratory infection and chronic exposure to second-hand tobacco smoke.

Laryngospasm manifests as partial or complete upper-airway obstruction that is not easily relieved by manual airway maneuvers or placement of an oral airway. The distinction between partial and complete upper-airway obstruction is important because the treatment of laryngospasm differs between the two conditions. In partial upper-airway obstruction, which is diagnosed by the presence of high-pitched inspiratory stridor, a small amount of air entry is possible with the administration of positive-pressure ventilation. This will, in many cases, prevent or treat hypoxemia, and allow the passage of anesthetic gases to deepen the level of unconsciousness, thereby alleviating the laryngospasm. Partial laryngospasm can also be alleviated to some extent by applying a jaw thrust maneuver, which is believed to stretch the laryngeal structures in an anterior direction and widen the partially obstructed airway. Some anesthesiologists firmly believe that laryngospasm can be effectively treated within several breaths by applying firm pressure to the anatomical notch posterior to the ear lobe and anterior to the mastoid process. However, this treatment modality has not been scientifically substantiated. In the absence of hypoxemia, partial upper-airway obstruction that does not respond to these conservative measures should be treated by intravenous administration of a nondepolarizing neuromuscular blocker or propofol 1–2 mg/kg. In the presence of hypoxemia, immediate endotracheal intubation or administration of intravenous succinylcholine 0.25–2 mg/kg is indicated. If intravenous access has not been established, intramuscular succinylcholine 4 mg/kg should be administered.

Laryngospasm that causes complete upper-airway obstruction usually results in the rapid development of hypoxemia and is not amenable to application of positive airway pressure. It has been suggested that administration of positive-pressure ventilation during complete upper-airway obstruction will prevent the alleviation of the laryngospasm by forcibly adducting the glottic structures, and may exacerbate gastric distention. Therefore, the trachea should be intubated or succinylcholine should be given without hesitation. Hypoxemia is a potent stimulus for the alleviation of laryngospasm, but it should never be relied upon in lieu of pharmacologic therapy because hypoxemia is associated with the development of negative-pressure pulmonary edema (see below) and/or cardiac arrest.

Pulmonary Aspiration

Pulmonary aspiration of gastric contents is usually diagnosed when a child demonstrates unexplained hypoxemia and respiratory symptoms along with: (1) the direct observation of gastric contents in the pharynx or larynx; or (2) characteristic findings on chest radiography. It is a rare perioperative complication in children, with an estimated incidence ≤0.1% in retrospective studies. Most cases of perioperative pulmonary aspiration in children occur at the time of intubation and, when clinically significant, will cause symptoms within 2 hours. Risk factors for its occurrence include emergency surgery for bowel obstruction or ileus, and lack of sufficient paralysis at the time of laryngoscopy.

In two large retrospective series, the majority of children with directly observed pulmonary aspiration of gastric contents were asymptomatic. Symptomatic children developed cough, wheeze, or unexplained hypoxemia with radiologic changes, and some required postoperative mechanical ventilation, but all eventually recovered.

There are no data to indicate the proper preparative pharmacologic regimen for children suspected of being at risk for pulmonary aspiration. A variety of agents theoretically decrease this risk. Metoclopramide is a prokinetic agent, but most studies in children do not show convincing efficacy for its ability to decrease gastric volume or increase gastric pH at the time of induction of general anesthesia. In addition, metoclopramide should not be administered to children with bowel obstruction or ileus. H_2 antagonists, such as ranitidine and cimetidine, reduce gastric volume and increase gastric pH in children; however, for optimal efficacy, these agents should be administered at least 2 hours prior to surgery. The use of these agents by pediatric anesthesiologists is extremely variable in emergency situations. It is important to keep in mind that the minimal gastric volume or maximal gastric pH that predispose to pulmonary aspiration, or result in clinically important pneumonitis once aspirated into the lung, are unknown.

Treatment of the child with suspected pulmonary aspiration is similar to that for an adult patient, and includes supplemental oxygen and mechanical ventilation as needed for hypoxemia, respiratory distress, or ventilatory failure. Children with mild symptoms such as cough or wheeze should be hospitalized and monitored appropriately. Asymptomatic children who do not require supplemental oxygen after a witnessed intraoperative aspiration may receive routine postoperative care including discharge home, if appropriate. Chest radiography is indicated only in the presence of respiratory distress or unexplained persistent hypoxemia.

Negative-pressure (Postobstructive) Pulmonary Edema

Acute pulmonary edema may develop after brief episodes of severe upper-airway obstruction in children of all ages, and is known as negative-pressure (or postobstructive) pulmonary edema. It most often occurs shortly after alleviation of severe laryngospasm, but it can also be observed after upper-airway obstruction of any cause. Since many cases of negative-pressure pulmonary edema are caused by the child biting on the endotracheal tube or LMA during emergence, a bite block should be inserted prior to emergence.

The exact mechanism of the development of pulmonary edema after upper-airway obstruction is unknown; however, the concomitant development of transient hypoxia appears to be an important contributing factor. Most authors speculate that the substantial negative intrathoracic pressure that results when a child attempts to breath against an obstruction results in a dramatic increase in venous return to the right side of the heart. Hypoxemia that accompanies the obstruction leads to massive sympathetic discharge that promotes systemic vasoconstriction. These two aforementioned processes result in the rapid transudation of fluid and lymph into the alveoli.

The clinical manifestations of negative-pressure pulmonary edema include the rapid development of rales, the appearance of a frothy pink fluid in the endotracheal tube, and a variable degree of hypoxemia. Treatment includes administration of supplemental oxygen, CPAP or PEEP (if mechanically ventilated), and furosemide. An echocardiogram may be indicated to rule out a cardiogenic cause. In healthy children symptoms usually resolve within 12–24 hours.

ADDITIONAL ARTICLES TO KNOW

Borland LM, Sereika SM, Woelfel SK et al: Pulmonary aspiration in pediatric patients during general anesthesia: incidence and outcome. *J Clin Anesth* 10:95–102, 1998.

Dubreuil M, Laffon M, Plaud B, Penon C, Ecoffey C: Complications and fiberoptic assessment of size 1 laryngeal mask airway. *Anesth Analg* 76:527–529, 1993.

Eckenhoff JE: Some anatomic considerations of the infant larynx influencing endotracheal anesthesia. *Anesthesiology* 12:401–410, 1951.

Finholt DA, Henry DB, Raphaely RC: Factors affecting leak around tracheal tubes in children. *Can Anaesth Soc J* 32:326–329, 1985.

Goudsouzian NG, Denman W, Cleveland R, Shorten G: Radiologic localization of the laryngeal mask airway in children. *Anesthesiology* 77:1085-1089, 1992.

Litman RS, Keon TP: Postintubation croup in children. *Anesthesiology* 75:1122-1123, 1991.

Litman RS, Weissend EE, Shibata D, Westesson PL: Developmental changes of laryngeal dimensions in unparalyzed, sedated children. *Anesthesiology* 98:41-45, 2003.

Mason DG, Bingham RM: Laryngeal mask airway in children. *Anaesthesia* 45:760-763, 1990.

Moynihan RJ, Brock-Utne JG, Archer JH, Feld LH, Kreitzman TR: Effect of cricoid pressure on preventing gastric insufflation in infants and children. *Anesthesiology* 78:652-656, 1993.

O'Neill B, Templeton JJ, Caramico L, Schreiner MS: The laryngeal mask airway in pediatric patients: factors affecting ease of use during insertion and emergence. *Anesth Analg* 78:659-662, 1994.

Rotschild A, Chitayat D, Puterman ML et al: Optimal positioning of endotracheal tubes for ventilation of preterm infants. *Am J Dis Child* 145:1007-1012, 1991.

Schwartz RE, Stayer SA, Pasquariello CA: Tracheal tube leak test: is there inter-observer agreement? *Can J Anaesth* 40:1049-1052, 1993.

Videira RLR, Neto PPR, Gomide Do Amaral RV, Freeman JA: Preoxygenation in children: for how long? *Acta Anaesthesiol Scand* 36:109-111, 1992.

Wailoo MP, Emery JL: Normal growth and development of the trachea. *Thorax* 37:584-587, 1982.

Warner MA, Warner ME, Warner DO, Warner LO, Warner EJ: Perioperative pulmonary aspiration in infants and children. *Anesthesiology* 90:66-71, 1999.

Watcha MF, Garner FT, White PF, Lusk R: Laryngeal mask airway vs face mask and Guedel airway during pediatric myringotomy. *Arch Otolaryngol Head Neck Surg* 120:877-880, 1994.

Westhorpe RN: The position of the larynx in children and its relationship to the ease of intubation. *Anaesth Intensive Care* 15:384-388, 1987.

CHAPTER 18

The Difficult Pediatric Airway

RONALD S. LITMAN

Anesthetic management of the difficult pediatric airway is the same as that for adults, with two important exceptions:
1. Awake intubations are rarely feasible.
2. The smaller airway anatomy of the child requires use of smaller intubating equipment that may not be readily available or easy to use.

The broad topic of the difficult airway can be divided into two major aspects: difficult intubation and difficult ventilation. Each of these can be further divided into anticipated or unanticipated. Difficult ventilation can be further subdivided into causes above and below the glottis. Only those entities that cause airway obstruction above the glottis are considered in this chapter. Those that occur below the glottis (foreign bodies, vascular rings, etc.) are considered in separate chapters.

The most important aspect of anesthetic management of the difficult airway is having a clear vision of the plan, as well as the multiple steps of the back-up plans. It is not enough to have only one or even two back-up plans, but rather three or four, and an exact plan for the worse possible situation – the development of life-threatening hypoxemia. Every anesthesiologist must know precisely the method he or she will use to alleviate it and save the child's life. This usually entails a cricothyrotomy or tracheostomy, which are more technically difficult in small children than in adults.

Proper preparation is essential and will depend on the cause of the expected difficulty. A full explanation of the nature of the anesthetic and the risks should be explained to the child's family. An indwelling intravenous catheter is preferred, except when the anesthesiologist feels that provoking or painfully stimulating the child may worsen the upper airway obstruction, as may occur with acute epiglottitis. Pharmacologic preparation consists of an antisialagogue (0.02 mg/kg atropine or 0.01 mg/kg glycopyrrolate) given at least 10–15 minutes prior to the induction of anesthesia. One of the most important aspects of all difficult airway management is the continuous presence of another experienced anesthesiologist or surgeon with airway expertise.

The difficult airway is an important cause of cardiac arrest during anesthesia in children. In the pediatric Perioperative Cardiac Arrest (POCA) Registry, respiratory complications accounted for 30 of the 55 reported cardiac arrests and many of these cases were associated with difficult ventilation or intubation (Table 18-1).

ANTICIPATED DIFFICULT INTUBATION

Unlike adults, normal-appearing children rarely present with an unexpected difficult intubation. Therefore, in this chapter, only the anticipated difficult intubation will be reviewed.

Table 18-1   Respiratory Causes of Cardiac Arrest from the POCA[a] Registry

Mechanism	Number of Cardiac Arrests
Laryngospasm	9
Airway obstruction	8[b]
Difficult intubation	4[c]
Inadequate oxygenation	3
Inadvertent extubation	2
Unclear etiology, presumed respiratory	2
Inadequate ventilation	1
Bronchospasm	1
Total	30

[a]Perioperative Cardiac Arrest.

[b]Two children had macroglossia, one had severe laryngeal papillomatosis, and one had micrognathia. Two of these four died.

[c]All children who arrested because of difficult intubation were 4 months of age or younger: two had congenital heart disease, one had trisomy 18, and one had Pierre–Robin sequence. One of these patients died.

Reproduced with permission from Morray JP, Geiduschek JM, Ramamoorthy C et al: Anesthesia-related cardiac arrest in children: initial findings of the Pediatric Perioperative Cardiac Arrest Registry. *Anesthesiology* 93:6, 2000.

Table 18-2   Examples of Congenital Airway Syndromes

Syndrome	Clinical Characteristics
Beckwith–Wiedemann	Macroglossia, organomegaly, omphalocele, hypoglycemia
Down (trisomy 21)	Macroglossia
Pierre–Robin sequence	Micrognathia, cleft palate, glossoptosis
Treacher–Collins	Hypoplasia of the maxilla and mandible, variable eye and ear deformities
Hemifacial microsomia (e.g., Goldenhar's)	Unilateral or bilateral mandibular hypoplasia, variable microphthalmia, microtia, macrostomia
Apert	Craniosynostosis, syndactyly
Freeman-Sheldon ("whistling face")	Microstomia, facial anomalies, hand anomalies
Mucopolysaccharidoses	Redundant facial and pharyngeal soft tissue
Klippel-Feil	Cervical vertebral fusion
Crouzon	Craniosynostosis
Stickler	Mandibular hypoplasia, myopia, retinal detachment, joint stiffness
Pfeiffer	Craniosynostosis, polydactyly

Preanesthetic Preparation

The most reliable predictor of a difficult intubation is the patient's history. Parents of children who were previously difficult to intubate are frequently concerned with this particular aspect of anesthetic management. Parents of children with congenital airway syndromes will often belong to a support group and will learn about the specific anesthetic problems encountered by children similar to their own. Perhaps the most important predictor of a difficult intubation is a previous anesthetic record. If one is available, it should be reviewed before administration of any subsequent anesthetic.

Physical examination should focus on anatomic anomalies that involve the head, face, or neck, especially if the child carries the diagnosis of a congenital airway syndrome (Table 18-2). Most importantly, the anesthesiologist should evaluate the size and mobility of the mandible. The most likely factor that predicts difficulty with intubation in pediatric patients is a small, malformed, or immobile mandible. Scoring systems that predict the likelihood of a difficult intubation do not exist for children. The Mallampati classification for prediction of the difficult intubation is not useful, except perhaps for larger adolescents.

The technical approach to securing tracheal intubation should be well thought out prior to the time of surgery (Fig. 18-1). All necessary airway equipment should be present in the OR, including the equipment necessary for the second, third, and even fourth options should initial attempts fail. In pediatrics, different sized laryngoscope blades and endotracheal tubes should be within easy reach.

In children with a known difficult intubation, it is preferable to secure venous access while the child is still awake. However, if the child is not amenable, or inspection of the limbs does not show promising possibilities, and if one

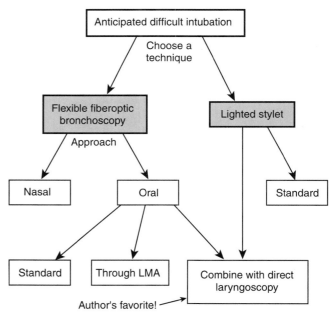

Figure 18-1 Algorithm for the child with an anticipated difficult intubation.

believes the child will not be difficult to ventilate, then general anesthesia may be induced without prior IV access. An antisialagogue should be administered prior to induction, either intravenously (if available) or via the oral route.

An anticipated difficult intubation can be loosely defined as that which the anesthesiologist feels would be too difficult to justify attempts at direct glottic visualization with standard techniques. In other words, the very nature of the anticipated difficult intubation implies that specialized indirect methods are required for tracheal intubation, and direct laryngoscopy should not be attempted first. Although tempting, with each direct laryngoscopy attempt, the severity of airway edema and bleeding will increase and will ultimately decrease the chance of eventual success with more specialized methods.

Techniques

When faced with a potentially difficult intubation, most pediatric anesthesiologists will choose one of two techniques: the lighted stylet, or the flexible fiberoptic bronchoscope. This choice is largely dependent on the experience and personal preference of the anesthesiologist, and may be influenced by the patient's airway anatomy. There is certainly a role in pediatrics for the use of intubating stylets, but if the airway is prospectively identified as difficult, direct methods should not be initially used. Intubating stylets are most effective when direct laryngoscopy reveals at least a portion of the epiglottis, and are used primarily when the difficult intubation was unanticipated.

Lighted Stylet

The lighted stylet (also known as a lightwand) is useful when the child has an anatomically normal larynx that is difficult to visualize with direct methods. This may occur with micrognathia, temporomandibular joint disease (or any condition that limits mandibular mobility), cervical spine instability, or facial trauma. Recent innovative solutions to the size limitations have been overcome, so the lighted stylet can now be used with endotracheal tubes as small as 2.5 mm internal diameter. It is particularly suited to children with limited neck and mandible mobility, but it will not be useful in cases of fixed upper or lower airway obstructive pathology, or the presence of a foreign body. *If the lightwand is used as the first choice for a difficult intubation, the number of attempts should be limited so as not to incur edema or bleeding, should fiberoptic bronchoscopy then be required.*

The use of a lighted stylet for endotracheal intubation in children is not different from adults. The endotracheal tube that contains the lightwand is fashioned in the shape of a hockey stick with a distal bend. The anesthesiologist places a thumb inside the lower teeth and pulls the mandible anteriorly, while the lightwand is introduced

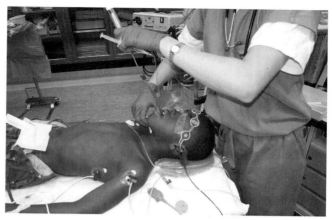

Figure 18-2   Technique for lightwand placement. The mandible is pulled anteriorly as the lightwand is introduced behind the tongue.

into the mouth and immediately posterior to the back of the tongue (Fig. 18-2). It is at this exact point that so many inexperienced practitioners have difficulty because the lightwand is advanced too far too quickly. The first important maneuver is to orient the lightwand anteriorly as soon as it is positioned at the back of the tongue. In children it is easy to advance it into the esophagus sooner than expected. The second important maneuver is to manipulate or twist the lightwand into the midline position by observing the transillumination on the anterior neck. Two common reasons for not seeing a light on the anterior surface of the neck are because it has already passed into the esophagus and because it is not in the midline. Once the bright light is seen in the midline, the lighted stylet is advanced further until the light is seen to form a cone into the trachea. Usually, while advancing the lightwand, one will feel a transient obstruction as the lightwand passes the epiglottis. At this point the lightwand may veer off the midline – it should then be reoriented so that the cone of light projects down into the trachea. The lightwand is then held steady while the endotracheal tube is slid into the trachea. The lightwand itself does not need to be reoriented into the laryngeal inlet prior to passing the endotracheal tube. As long as the cone of light is seen to be directed down into the trachea, the endotracheal tube can be advanced correctly. If the cone of light disappears with caudal advancement, it has most likely entered the esophagus. This can be remedied in subsequent attempts by orienting the lightwand more anteriorly in a higher (more cephalad) position behind the tongue.

An important difference in technique between adults and children stems from the fact that the neck tissues of children are thinner than adults', so the transillumination characteristics will differ. In particular, the light will appear brighter on the skin surface than it does in adults, and may cause some confusion as to its proper placement in the larynx. For this reason it is preferable in smaller children to use a lightwand with an adjustable light source. At The Children's Hospital of Philadelphia, we use a home-grown lightwand for small infants and neonates. It consists of a 20-gauge fiberoptic illuminating lightpipe (Storz Ophthalmics Inc., St Louis, MO) attached to any standard fiberoptic light source (Fig. 18-3).

In children with an immobile mandible, it may be difficult to maneuver the lightwand into an optimal position. In these cases, a particularly useful technique is to combine direct laryngoscopy with a lightwand. Although limited by mandibular immobility, the blade of the laryngoscope may provide greater maneuverability of the lightwand for greater chance of successful tracheal intubation.

Fiberoptic Bronchoscopy

Flexible fiberoptic bronchoscopy is probably the most popular definitive method for difficult tracheal intubation in children. In recent years anesthesiologists have become more adept at manipulating the ultrathin bronchoscope, which may be used inside a 2.5-mm or 3.0-mm internal diameter endotracheal tube (depending on the manufacturer). In addition, the optical aspects of the equipment have improved to allow better screen resolution. An important aspect of its use is that the technique must be practiced on normal children prior to encountering the difficult airway, when its use becomes essential.

There are several reasons why bronchoscopy is different or more difficult in children compared to adults. First, because of the inherently smaller size of children, ultrathin bronchoscopes are required. These ultrathin bronchoscopes may not be manufactured with suction ports. Therefore, secretions or blood are more likely to obscure the view in smaller children. For this reason, it is important to use an antisialagogue prior to beginning the procedure, and then briefly and gently suction the oropharynx prior to the bronchoscopic attempt.

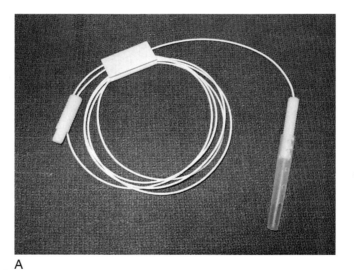

A

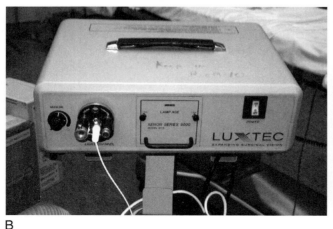

B

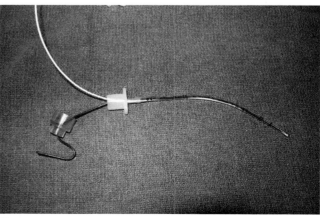

C

Figure 18-3   A, A thin fiberoptic bundle is used as a lightwand. B, The fiberoptic bundle can be attached to any commercially available light source with adjustable light intensity. C, The fiberoptic bundle is inserted alongside a thin pliable stylet into an endotracheal tube.

Table 18-3 Pediatric-sized Laryngeal Mask Airways and Compatible Endotracheal Tubes[a]

LMA Size	Maximum Lubricated *Uncuffed* Standard ETT Inner Diameter (mm)	Maximum Lubricated *Cuffed* Standard ETT Inner Diameter (mm)	Maximum FOB Size[b]
1	3.5	3.0	2.7
1½	4.0	4.0	3.0
2	5.0	4.5	3.5
2½	6.0[c]	5.0	4.0
3	–	6.0	5.0
4	–	6.0	5.0

[a]Based on experiments performed by the author.
[b]As per LMA North America. FOB, fiberoptic bronchoscope.
[c]Largest available uncuffed endotracheal tube available at The Children's Hospital of Philadelphia.

Some ultrathin bronchoscopes do contain a suction port, but it is too narrow to allow effective suctioning of secretions. Furthermore, oxygen insufflation should not be performed via this port in small children because of the possibility of generating dangerously high intrabronchial pressures and development of a tension pneumothorax.

Second, apneic ventilation is usually ineffective in small children because of their limited time to oxyhemoglobin desaturation. This is caused by the markedly reduced functional residual capacity (FRC) in anesthetized small children and their relatively high oxygen consumption. Ventilation can be accomplished during bronchoscopy by the use of a special anesthesia mask that incorporates a conduit for passage of the bronchoscope.

Third, in smaller children, flexible bronchoscopy performed through a laryngeal mask airway (LMA) is more difficult than in adults because LMA placement in children is associated with a higher incidence of malpositioning, which leads to an obscured view of the glottic opening. When possible, fiberoptic bronchoscopy should be initially attempted without an LMA. For those times when an LMA is required for proper visualization of the glottic opening, we keep a reference on hand (taped to the top of the difficult airway cart) of the sizes of endotracheal tubes and fiberoptic scopes that will fit through pediatric LMAs (Table 18-3).

Finally, the unique anatomical variance of infants and children may influence successful fiberoptic bronchoscopy. If a nasal route is chosen, enlarged adenoidal and tonsillar tissue may obstruct the view and is likely to bleed upon contact. The relatively stiff epiglottis of infancy may render glottic visualization more difficult than in adults. This may be overcome by having an assistant provide chin lift with head extension and jaw thrust during the bronchoscopic attempt. The relatively more anterior location of the infant glottis may require more extensive anteflexion of the bronchoscope for adequate visualization of the glottic opening.

There will always be the rare child in whom one of these conventional techniques doesn't work, and the anesthesiologist then must choose an alternative method for securing tracheal intubation. This choice then depends on the urgency and importance of tracheal intubation, and whether or not the surgical procedure is urgent or elective. If the procedure is elective, the anesthesiologist may choose to cancel the case and awaken the child with the eventual plan of trying again on a different day with different personnel. More often, however, the procedure is performed as planned with an alternative means of airway support, such as an LMA, or the trachea is eventually intubated by another method. There are many procedures for which an LMA is not ideal but will suffice instead of an endotracheal tube. These are too numerous to list, and are largely dependent upon the comfort level of the anesthesiologist and surgeon. If either the anesthesiologist or surgeon feels that tracheal intubation is necessary to proceed with the procedure, other alternatives exist for securing tracheal intubation (Box 18-1). These are mainly used by specialists in pediatric anesthesia, and details of these techniques are beyond the scope of this discussion.

Box 18-1 Nontraditional Methods of Pediatric Tracheal Intubation

Digital intubation
Direct laryngoscopy with intubating stylet (gum bougie)
Bullard scope
Anterior commissure scope (used primarily by otolaryngologists)
Combitube in adolescents
Retrograde wire technique (standard or through LMA)
Surgical tracheostomy

The most drastic measures are use of a retrograde wire and surgical tracheostomy. The inherently smaller size of children renders these techniques more difficult to perform, and undesirable side-effects such as bleeding into the airway are more likely. These techniques are used when fiberoptic bronchoscopy has failed because of excessive blood or secretions in the airway, in children with markedly abnormal upper airway anatomy, or when a mass is obscuring the upper airway. A tracheostomy is also helpful when it is known that the child will undergo multiple procedures within the foreseeable future.

Etiologies of Difficult Intubation

Pierre–Robin Sequence

The Pierre-Robin sequence (Fig. 18-4) consists of micrognathia, glossoptosis, and cleft palate. These infants may have an obstructed upper airway from the small anatomic space afforded by their small mandible. The condition is most severe at birth and tends to improve with age. If airway obstruction is severe and life-threatening at birth, tracheostomy is indicated, and is followed by a more definitive mandibular advancement procedure. Concomitant congenital anomalies may lead to other necessary surgical interventions such as cleft palate repair or placement of tympanostomy tubes. Tracheal intubation in these infants may be extremely difficult or impossible. Fortunately, mask ventilation in these infants is often easily accomplished, especially when aided by placement of an oral airway. LMA placement is often essential for establishing ventilation or to provide a guide for tracheal intubation. In many cases, the LMA is used as a temporizing measure to ventilate and oxygenate the infant between attempts at tracheal intubation with either a flexible fiberoptic bronchoscope or a lighted stylet.

Treacher–Collins Syndrome

Treacher-Collins syndrome (Fig. 18-5) consists of hypoplasia of the maxilla and mandible, and variable eye and ear deformities. It results from failure of the first branchial arch to develop between the 3rd and 5th weeks of gestation. These children are notoriously difficult, or impossible, to intubate and may also be difficult to ventilate. Like other severe airway anomalies, the LMA is indispensable for airway management.

Hemifacial Microsomia

The most important anomaly in hemifacial microsomia that renders these children difficult to intubate is mandibular hypoplasia (Fig. 18-6). Additional variable clinical features include microphthalmia, microtia, and macrostomia, which result from a malformation of the first and second pharyngeal arches. These infants are usually easy to mask-ventilate, and may often be easily intubated by direct laryngoscopy. Difficult intubation is likely when the unilateral mandibular hypoplasia is severe, or bilateral (10–33%). As with the aforementioned congenital facial anomalies, the LMA is an effective method for ventilating and facilitating intubation in this patient population.

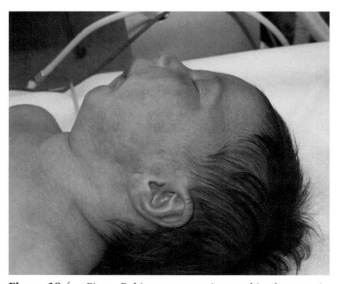

Figure 18-4   Pierre–Robin sequence: micrognathia, glossoptosis, and cleft palate.

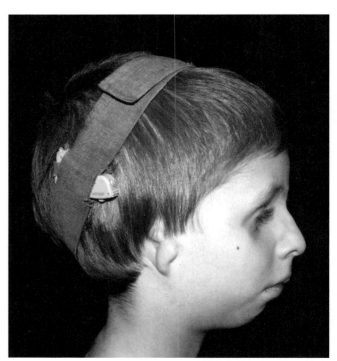

Figure 18-5   Treacher–Collins syndrome: hypoplasia of maxilla and mandible, and variable eye and ear deformities.

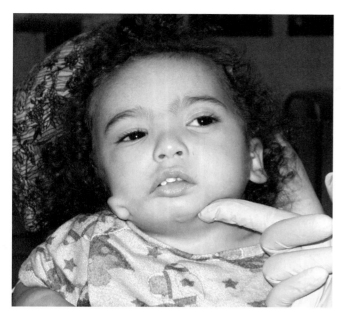

Figure 18-6 Hemifacial microsomia: unilateral mandibular hypoplasia.

ANTICIPATED DIFFICULT VENTILATION FROM UPPER AIRWAY OBSTRUCTION

The expected difficult ventilation is one of the most angst-provoking situations in pediatric anesthesia. There is good reason for this: small children with transient or mild upper airway obstruction may rapidly become hypoxemic. How does one know when a child will be difficult to ventilate? The history and physical exam, and possibly some radiological studies, will almost always indicate the answer to this question. One of the most reliable indicators is previous difficulty with ventilation during a recent anesthetic, assuming there were no clinical changes since that time. Conversely, if the child was easy to ventilate during a recent anesthetic, then one can be reasonably confident that the child will still be easy to ventilate. For these reasons, it is imperative to obtain the previous anesthetic record or directly talk to the anesthesiologist who was present. If there were no previous anesthetics, other aspects of the history can indicate ease of ventilation. Was the child previously sedated for a radiological procedure? If so, were there any ventilation difficulties? How does the child sleep at night? Are there obstructive episodes? Are they related to the position of the child?

On physical exam, signs of clinically important upper airway obstruction include the presence of neck and chest wall retractions, and inspiratory stridor. Intrathoracic airway obstruction is characterized by expiratory stridor or wheezing. The oxyhemoglobin saturation is another indicator of airway patency. A value below 94% on room air is indicative of important upper airway obstruction in the absence of additional lung disease.

If radiological studies have been performed, they should be examined by the anesthesiologist to help determine the possibility of difficulty with ventilation. Important examples include:

1. Lateral neck radiograph for the "thumb sign" of epiglottitis
2. Neck radiograph or computed tomography (CT) for evaluation of the severity of a retropharyngeal abscess
3. Neck CT for evaluation of masses encroaching on the upper airway that are not visible externally (e.g., lymphangioma)

Articles To Know

Markakis DA, Sayson SC, Schreiner MS: Insertion of the laryngeal mask airway in awake infants with the Robin sequence. Anesth Analg 75:822-824, 1992.

Ebata T, Nishiki S, Masuda A, Amaha K: Anaesthesia for Treacher-Collins syndrome using a laryngeal mask airway. Can J Anaesth 38:1043-1045, 1991.

Prospective studies on difficult airway management techniques are scarce. The vast majority of the useful literature on management of difficult airways, especially in the pediatric population, is case reports or case series of successful techniques. Two publications stand out as having influence over the way we practice.

The first article is a report on a series of three infants with Pierre-Robin sequence who were successfully managed by initially placing an LMA while they were awake. Once manual positive-pressure ventilation was confirmed, neuromuscular blockade was administered, and tracheal intubation was accomplished using lighted stylets.

The second publication reported two children with Treacher-Collins syndrome who were successfully managed with laryngeal masks when tracheal intubation had failed.

Reports such as these established the usefulness of the LMA in managing children who were known to be potentially difficult to ventilate. Thus began the era of declining awake intubations in children, and the confidence that children with certain congenital airway syndromes could be adequately managed once anesthetized. Since the publication of these reports, a vast amount of clinical experience in children with congenital airway syndromes has confirmed that use of the LMA in anesthetized children with presumed difficult airways is associated with successful outcomes.

4. Neck and chest CT for evaluation of the extent to which an anterior mediastinal mass impinges on the trachea (a 50% reduction of the tracheal diameter may indicate critical tracheal compression and the inability to ventilate adequately following induction of general anesthesia)

5. Thoracic magnetic resonance imaging (MRI) for diagnosis of a vascular ring, to evaluate the severity of tracheal compression

6. Chest radiograph of a child who has aspirated a foreign body (this may not indicate ease of ventilation but will indicate additional problems that may impact on anesthetic management, such as extent of pneumonitis or degree of unilateral hyperinflation).

When approaching the child who may be difficult to ventilate, the first and most important decision is whether or not to proceed with tracheal intubation with the child awake with mild sedation or fully anesthetized (Fig. 18-7). Awake intubations are rarely performed in children because of their inability to cooperate despite administration of sedative agents. However, if one seriously believes that there exists the real possibility of hypoxemia despite LMA placement, then an awake technique should be performed. Fortunately, this situation is rare in pediatric patients for the very reason that there exist few situations where one feels that LMA insertion would be unsuccessful. *Whether or not an LMA is inserted, the most important principle of airway management is to maintain spontaneous ventilation until it is proven that positive pressure ventilation can be accomplished.*

If an awake intubation is planned, it is helpful to anesthetize the child's upper airway passages with local anesthesia. This is usually performed after the child is sedated. A local anesthetic solution can be administered by nebulizer, but this is variably effective because of the

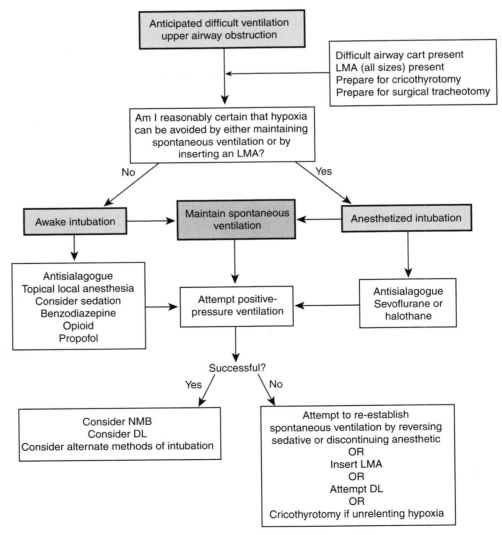

Figure 18-7   Algorithm for the child with anticipated difficult ventilation.

uncooperative nature of children. Most anesthesiologists prefer to sedate children using a combination of a benzodiazepine and opioid because the effects can be rapidly reversed. Others prefer small titrations of ketamine (0.25-mg/kg doses) because of its tendency to preserve upper airway patency at concentrations that reliably impair consciousness. Propofol, when used judiciously, can also be used effectively when one suspects a reasonable chance of being able to successfully ventilate using positive pressure. Inhalational general anesthetic agents may also be used. Sevoflurane will provide rapid loss of consciousness but greater possibility of apnea than halothane. A classic and time-honored technique is to maintain spontaneous ventilation while slowly deepening the level of anesthesia. While maintaining spontaneous ventilation, direct laryngoscopy is performed slowly while progressively applying topical local anesthetic to more distal portions of the pharynx and larynx. If direct laryngoscopy is unsuccessful, specialized techniques such as those discussed in the prior section are then used. If central or obstructive apnea occurs during this procedure, the anesthesiologist must be prepared to either rapidly attempt endotracheal intubation or insert a laryngeal mask to prevent development of hypoxemia.

Etiologies of Difficult Ventilation

Congenital Airway Syndromes

Congenital airway syndromes probably represent the most common reason for an anesthesiologist to suspect difficulty with ventilation. These are discussed in the preceding section.

Trauma

Facial or head trauma is common in children and may cause difficulty with ventilation or intubation. Fiberoptic bronchoscopy may be difficult owing to blood or foreign bodies obscuring the airway. Spontaneous ventilation should be maintained until it is proven that positive-pressure ventilation is possible. The presumed full stomach and possibility of pulmonary aspiration of gastric contents is placed secondary to airway concerns. Unless proven otherwise, cervical spine injuries should be strongly suspected in all cases of head or facial trauma in children.

Masses

Benign tumors that interfere with the upper airway occur commonly in children and include lymphangioma (cystic hygroma) and teratoma. These can be dangerous because of unsuspected airway involvement that may not be apparent from the child's external appearance. Therefore, radiographic studies of the head and neck should be reviewed by the anesthesiologist prior to the time of surgery to obtain information about the likelihood of subsequent airway obstruction with induction of general anesthesia.

Infections

Three important infections occur in children that potentially cause life-threatening airway obstruction: retropharyngeal abscess, laryngotracheobronchitis (croup), and epiglottitis. Each has unique clinical characteristics (Table 18-4).

A retropharyngeal abscess is a bacterial infection that occurs behind the oral pharynx anterior to the

Table 18-4 Comparison of Infectious Causes of Upper Airway Obstruction

	Laryngotracheobronchitis	Epiglottitis	Retropharyngeal Abscess
Organism	Viral: parainfluenza most common	Bacterial: *Hemophilus* influenza type b in children; mixed organisms in adults	Bacterial: usually *Streptococcus* or *Staphylococcus*
Age	6 months to 3 years	2–5 years	2–8 years
Pathology	Inflammation that affects subglottic tracheal mucosa and entire tracheobronchial tree; supraglottic area spared	Supraglottitis: severe swelling of epiglottis, arytenoids, and surrounding tissue	Lymphatic drainage or contiguous spread of pharyngeal or oral infections
Prominent clinical features	Viral prodrome (upper respiratory tract infection), low-grade fever, barking cough, variable degree of inspiratory stridor, hoarseness, rarely progresses to fatigue and respiratory failure	High fever, toxic appearing, seated position and leaning forward preferred, drooling, throat pain, difficulty swallowing, stridor	Sore throat, fever, neck stiffness, difficulty swallowing, neck swelling, tonsillitis, pharyngitis, cervical lymphadenopathy
Radiologic study	Anteroposterior neck radiograph: "steeple" sign indicating tracheal mucosal edema	Lateral neck radiograph: "thumb" sign of swollen epiglottis, prevertebral thickening, hypopharyngeal enlargement on lateral view	Lateral neck radiograph: widening of the retropharyngeal soft tissues; also identified on CT scan
Treatment	Cool mist, steroids, nebulized 2.25% racemic epinephrine	Tracheal intubation until resolved (usually 2–4 days), antibiotics	Tracheal intubation, incision and drainage, antibiotics

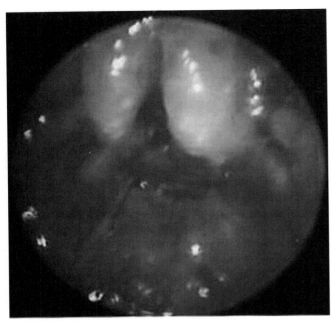

Figure 18-8 Swelling of the epiglottis is seen in a case of acute epiglottitis.

prevertebral fascia. It is characterized by sore throat, fever, neck stiffness, and odynophagia. It is diagnosed by characteristic findings on a lateral cervical spine radiograph or CT scan of the neck. If severe, treatment consists of incision and drainage under general anesthesia with precautions for possible difficult ventilation.

Laryngotracheobronchitis (croup) is a viral-mediated inflammation of the lower portion of the upper airway. It causes edema of the trachea below the glottic level, and is rarely life-threatening. Treatment consists of cool mist, steroids, and nebulized racemic epinephrine in severe cases. Tracheal intubation is rare except in cases of hypoxemia that do not respond promptly to nebulized epinephrine and oxygen therapy.

Epiglottitis is a bacterial infection that actually involves all the supraglottic structures (Fig. 18-8). Since the advent of the vaccination against *Hemophilus* influenza type b, the organism that causes childhood epiglottitis, it is only occasionally seen in children, such as immigrants and those with incomplete immunizations. Nevertheless, when it occurs, it can cause life-threatening upper airway obstruction. The treatment consists of immediate

---

Box 18-2 Epiglottitis Protocol[a]

1. Every attempt should be made to keep the child calm. A parent should be allowed to comfort the child up to and including the induction of general anesthesia. No attempt should be made to place the child supine. If the diagnosis of epiglottitis is seriously entertained, radiographs should not be performed.
2. The following departments should be immediately consulted:
    a. Anesthesiology
    b. Otolaryngology
    c. Surgical suite: If OR space is not immediately available, the child should be taken to the ICU or recovery room; the child should not be transported until appropriate notifications and preparations are complete.
3. Prepare the child for transport:
    a. Have a gurney available to travel with the patient, but do not lay the child supine.
    b. The child can remain in the parent's arms.
    c. A full O₂ tank should accompany the patient and provide supplemental blow-by oxygen.
    d. Have an Ambu-bag with appropriately sized face mask.
    e. Have an intubating laryngoscope with appropriately sized and smaller sized endotracheal tubes.
    f. Have portable suction.
    g. Be ready with atropine 0.02 mg/kg (minimum 0.2 mg, maximum 1.0 mg) and succinylcholine (2 mg/kg).
    h. Transport the child and the parents only when physician experienced in emergency airway management is in attendance. The anesthesiologist attending is always in charge.
4. During the vulnerable period before intubation, handling of the child should be kept to a minimum – no oral examinations and no unnecessary needle sticks. The intravenous catheter is inserted by the best qualified person.
5. When ready for intubation, the anesthesiologist performs an inhalation induction with a volatile agent, with the otolaryngologist present in the room for possible emergency tracheotomy.
6. After the endotracheal tube is appropriately inserted and ventilation is assured, less urgent procedures such as changing to a nasotracheal tube, blood work, and administration of intravenous antibiotics may be performed. Routine paperwork should be dealt with only after the child is safe.
7. Following tracheal intubation, the child is transported to the ICU with adequate sedation and possibly paralysis. Restraints may be required to prevent life-threatening self-extubation.
8. If intensive care monitoring and support are not available, the child should be transported with a physician skilled in emergency airway management to an appropriate facility.

[a]Adapted from Parsons DS, Smith RB, Mair EA, Dlabal LJ: Unique case presentations of acute epiglottic swelling and a protocol for acute airway compromise. *Laryngoscope* 106:1287–1291, 1996.

induction of general anesthesia followed by endotracheal intubation or surgical tracheostomy, followed by a course of antibiotics. Management of epiglottitis begins when the child presents with stridor in the emergency department. Every hospital should have an epiglottitis protocol that consists of immediate consultation with the otolaryngology and anesthesiology services once epiglottitis is suspected in any child (Box 18-2).

Tracheal intubation for epiglottitis should be performed in the OR under deep inhalational anesthesia that maintains spontaneous ventilation until it is proven that positive-pressure ventilation is possible. If feasible, nasotracheal intubation should be performed since the child will be intubated for several days, but this depends largely on the preferences of the pediatric intensive care unit. Although direct laryngoscopy may appear to be easy, difficulty may arise because of severe swelling of all the supraglottic structures with obliteration of the glottic opening. Maintenance of spontaneous ventilation may help the anesthesiologist identify the tiny glottic opening by observing bubbles at the site. If the child is apneic an assistant can push on the child's chest, which may also produce bubbles at the glottic opening. Needless to say, age-appropriate and smaller endotracheal tubes should be on hand with stylets in each. For obvious reasons, an LMA would not be helpful in this situation. If life-threatening hypoxemia occurs prior to tracheal intubation, an immediate surgical tracheostomy or cricothyrotomy is indicated.

Postoperatively, there are several methods used to determine when the child's trachea can be safely extubated. Some physicians will wait until a leak is heard, which indicates a decrease in the amount of glottic swelling. Others may directly inspect the glottis by direct laryngoscopy or flexible bronchoscopy to assess residual glottic swelling. The child should also be afebrile, an indication that the acute bacterial infection is adequately treated.

UNANTICIPATED DIFFICULT VENTILATION

There are several common causes of unanticipated obstruction to ventilation (though some opine that all anesthesiologists should continuously anticipate these complications). They include simple passive airway collapse, obstruction caused by enlarged tonsils or adenoids, and partial or complete laryngospasm. Unanticipated airway obstruction is alarming, especially in small infants because of the rapidity with which hypoxemia develops.

Whatever the cause, the sequence of correctional maneuvers is similar in all cases. The anesthesiologist should first seek to optimally reposition the head and neck while simultaneously checking for appropriate facemask placement. A common error in facemask placement in small children is to place the mask too low on the face such that a portion of the nose is obstructed. Chin lift with or without jaw thrust may also alleviate obstruction at this point. Continuous positive airway pressure (CPAP) can be applied to the upper airway by closing the pop-off valve. Rapid ventilations are delivered at a high inspiratory pressure until the child's chest is seen to rise, and adequate ventilation is confirmed by capnography and rise in oxyhemoglobin saturation. This technique will effectively relieve upper airway obstruction in many cases caused by passive collapse of the pharynx or adenotonsillar hypertrophy, but will not alleviate complete laryngospasm. The next action to take is to place an oral airway. In cases of airway obstruction caused by enlarged tonsils or adenoids, this will almost always be curative unless there is additional cause for the obstruction.

These are the basic maneuvers that should alleviate upper airway obstruction in nearly all cases prior to the development of life-threatening hypoxemia. If these fail, and the oxyhemoglobin saturation is still decreasing, the anesthesiologist is faced with a dire situation and must take immediate action. One of three possible actions is appropriate at this point (or any time earlier in this time sequence):

1. Immediately insert an LMA. Insertion of an LMA will establish adequate ventilation except when the obstruction is caused by laryngospasm or if the LMA is malpositioned, which occurs more often in children than adults. One would have to be very confident that the obstruction is not being caused by laryngospasm if placing an LMA during a severe hypoxic episode. Appropriately sized LMAs should be immediately available in every anesthetizing location.

2. Immediate tracheal intubation can be performed when one is confident of his or her intubating skills and doubts exist as to the cause of the obstruction. This option is commonly considered in neonates. If laryngospasm is occurring, it is usually possible to introduce a styletted endotracheal tube into the glottic opening.

3. Administer succinylcholine. Since laryngospasm is a common cause of unrelenting upper airway obstruction in children, succinylcholine should be administered if conventional methods fail to reverse hypoxemia. It should be administered intravenously if possible, but can also be given via the intramuscular route as well, with relief of laryngospasm within a minute. *One should never withhold succinylcholine during hypoxemia for fear of provoking bradycardia.* If the child developed bradycardia as a result of the hypoxemia, the heart rate will increase with the establishment of normoxemia and will not be made worse because of administration of succinylcholine. If laryngospasm occurs but is not associated with hypoxemia, other options for relief include a bolus of propofol (1-2 mg/kg) or remifentanil (1 µg/kg), or

administration of a nondepolarizing neuromuscular blocker. These would also be viable options if there were absolute contraindications to succinylcholine (e.g., myopathy, malignant hyperthermia (MH)-susceptibility).

Desperate Measures

In the rare instance that none of the above measures is successful, and the child is becoming dangerously hypoxic, desperate last-chance measures must be performed immediately. These include the following:

Reposition the Patient

If an anterior mediastinal mass is suspected and conventional measures (e.g., rigid bronchoscope) have failed to reestablish ventilation and normoxemia, the child should be repositioned to the lateral or prone position. This maneuver may alleviate obstruction of the lower trachea or great vessels surrounding the heart.

Cricothyrotomy

There are several techniques available for creating a surgical airway. A tracheotomy is preferred but may not be rapid enough even if appropriate personnel are available. The most feasible action at this point is usually percutaneous placement of a cricothyrotomy, an opening in the cricothyroid membrane located between the cricoid and thyroid cartilages. Though several commercially made kits are available, the most efficient method is to place a 14- or 16-gauge angiocatheter through the cricothyroid membrane. Once this is properly placed into the child's trachea, one has several options with which to provide oxygenation. *Every anesthesiologist should have a plan for oxygenation through a cricothyrotomy for every case, every day.* One method is to attach a 3.0 endotracheal tube adaptor to the hub of the angiocatheter, which can then be connected to the anesthesia breathing circuit. Another method is to attach the barrel of a 10-mL syringe to the angiocatheter and place a cuffed endotracheal tube within the barrel. Many other successful methods of oxygenation have been described.

It does not matter which method is used, as long as the anesthesiologist has a definite prospective plan should cricothyrotomy be performed. Known complications from this technique in children include pneumothorax, pneumomediastinum, bleeding into the airway, and misplacement of the angiocatheter through the trachea or into a false lumen within the tracheal wall.

Tracheotomy

If a qualified surgeon is present, and it is feasible that a tracheotomy can be rapidly secured, this option may be preferable over cricothyrotomy. However, it cannot be overstated how difficult this technique is in small children. Therefore, this should be regarded as a true last resort in the event that cricothyrotomy is unsuccessful.

ADDITIONAL ARTICLES TO KNOW

American Society of Anesthesiologists Task Force on Management of the Difficult Airway: Practice guidelines for management of the difficult airway. *Anesthesiology* 78:597-602, 1993.

Auden SM: Flexible fiberoptic laryngoscopy in the pediatric patient. *Anesthesiol Clin N Am* 16:763-793, 1998.

Auden SM: Additional techniques for managing the difficult pediatric airway. *Anesth Analg* 90:878-880, 2000.

Davis L, Cook-Sather SD, Schreiner MS: Lighted stylet tracheal intubation: a review. *Anesth Analg* 90:745-756, 2000.

Ebata T, Nishiki S, Masuda A et al: Anaesthesia for Treacher-Collins syndrome using a laryngeal mask airway. *Can J Anaesth* 38:1043-1045, 1991.

Gregory GA: Classification and assessment of the difficult pediatric airway. *Anesthesiol Clin N Am* 16:729-741, 1998.

Iannoli ED, Litman RS: Tension pneumothorax during flexible fiberoptic bronchoscopy in a newborn. *Anesth Analg* 94:512-513, 2002.

Kleeman PP, Jantzen JP, Bonfils P: The ultra-thin bronchoscope in management of the difficult paediatric airway. *Can J Anaesth* 34:606-608, 1987.

Markakis DA, Sayson SC, Schreiner MS: Insertion of the laryngeal mask airway in awake infants with the Robin sequence. *Anesth Analg* 75:822-824, 1992.

CHAPTER 19

Management of General Anesthesia

RONALD S. LITMAN

This chapter details the differences between children and adults in induction and maintenance of, and emergence from, general anesthesia. Principles of use of general anesthetic agents in children are reviewed. These include inhalational and intravenous general anesthetic agents, opioids, and neuromuscular blockers and their antagonists.

INHALATION ANESTHETICS

In the United States, where "ouch-less" hospital environments are a priority, most children requiring surgery receive oral premedication with an anxiolytic agent such as midazolam, followed by an inhalational anesthetic via facemask. Sevoflurane is the induction agent of choice, although many institutions still use halothane. Once the child has lost consciousness, an intravenous catheter is inserted, and an opioid and/or neuromuscular blocker may be administered prior to endotracheal intubation. In this section, the anesthetic agents used for induction of general anesthesia in children will be reviewed.

Sevoflurane

Sevoflurane is an ether type of volatile anesthetic agent that was first described in the 1970s. It was probably not brought to market at that time because its relatively high rate of biotransformation (3–5%) led to concerns about hepatic toxicity. Many believed that the relatively high rate of biotransformation of halothane (20%) was the primary cause of its association with hepatitis. In subsequent years, the cause of "halothane hepatitis" was shown to be unrelated to the metabolism of the agent, and sevoflurane was reintroduced, first in Japan, and later in the United States. In most pediatric centers in the USA, sevoflurane has replaced halothane for inhalational induction of general anesthesia in children because of its less pungent aroma, its lower blood-gas solubility coefficient (0.63) that speeds loss of consciousness, and, perhaps most importantly, its enhanced cardiovascular safety profile.

The minimum alveolar concentration (MAC) of sevoflurane is 3.2% in neonates and infants up to 6 months of age. In school-aged children MAC is 2.5%; the concentration that prevents 95% of children from moving in response to a surgical stimulus (ED_{95}) is 2.9%.

When 60% nitrous oxide is added to sevoflurane, the MAC is lowered to 2.0%. This contribution of N₂O to sevoflurane MAC is relatively less than for halothane.

Induction of general anesthesia with sevoflurane is accomplished by initially setting the vaporizer to the maximal 8% setting. Whether or not this is combined with nitrous oxide, most children will lose consciousness within 5–10 breaths. Sevoflurane depresses ventilation by a dose-dependent reduction in tidal volume. Some studies in children suggest that sevoflurane is a more potent respiratory depressant and causes relatively more upper-airway obstruction than equipotent doses of halothane. Clinically, sevoflurane appears to cause more central apnea than halothane during induction of anesthesia.

During inhalation of sevoflurane, most children develop tachycardia. Twenty percent of children undergoing induction of anesthesia with sevoflurane will develop a nodal rhythm, and infants under 6 months of age will demonstrate lengthening of the QT interval that continues into the postoperative period. These changes, however, do not result in adverse clinical manifestations. Sevoflurane may cause a dose-dependent decrease in heart rate and blood pressure, but to a much lesser extent than halothane, which significantly decreases cardiac output during its administration.

Agitation is commonly observed during the early stages of sevoflurane induction, soon after loss of consciousness. It consists of muscular rigidity and generalized tonic–clonic or myoclonic movements, and may represent a relatively greater propensity for sevoflurane to cause central nervous system (CNS) stimulation than other inhalational agents. Case reports exist that demonstrate exacerbation of electrical seizure activity in children with and without preexisting epilepsy during sevoflurane induction. This effect is accentuated with hyperventilation. These CNS stimulatory effects do not appear to be associated with postoperative sequelae.

Fluoride Toxicity

Sevoflurane is metabolized to inorganic fluoride ion and hexafluoroisopropanol (Fig. 19-1). Plasma concentrations of fluoride >50 μmol/L are associated with nephrotoxicity after administration of methoxyflurane, an obsolete inhalational anesthetic. Although prolonged use of sevoflurane at high concentrations produces fluoride levels in excess of 50 μmol/L, clinical nephrotoxicity with sevoflurane has not been reported. This is most likely secondary to the absence of intrarenal metabolism of sevoflurane, as occurs with methoxyflurane. However, subtle urinary markers of occult renal damage have been demonstrated with prolonged use of sevoflurane. Therefore, prolonged use of sevoflurane is probably contraindicated in children with limited renal reserve.

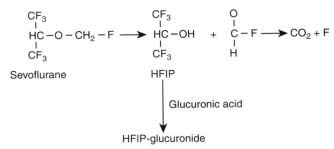

Figure 19-1 Sevoflurane is metabolized to inorganic fluoride ion and hexafluoroisopropanol (HFIP).

Compound A Toxicity

Degradation of sevoflurane by carbon dioxide absorbents produces a variety of compounds (labeled A through E), of which two are produced in significant amounts: compounds A and B. Although compound A is nephrotoxic in rats, the concentration attained in the anesthesia breathing circuit in humans does not cause adverse clinical effects. Factors that increase the level of compound A within the breathing circuit include increased absorbent temperature, decreased absorbent water content, and low flows through the absorbent. Although evidence for compound A toxicity in humans is lacking, sevoflurane should probably not be used with total flows less than 2 L/min, to decrease the accumulation of compound A inside the breathing circuit.

Halothane

Despite halothane's long history of safe use in children, it has been largely replaced by sevoflurane because halothane is associated with slower times to loss of consciousness (blood-gas coefficient 2.3) and a greater chance of clinically significant cardiovascular depression, especially in neonates and small infants. The MAC of halothane is 0.55% in the preterm neonate, 0.87% in the full-term neonate, 1.2% in the 6-month infant, and 0.95% in the older child.

Induction of general anesthesia with halothane is usually accomplished by increasing the concentration on the vaporizer by 0.5% every two to three breaths. After placement of an intravenous catheter and institution of controlled ventilation, the concentration must be decreased to avoid bradycardia and myocardial depression. Cardiac arrests have occurred in situations where the anesthesiologist unintentionally left the halothane vaporizer at its maximal setting of 5% while continuing to increase minute ventilation with positive pressure. Bradycardia and myocardial depression can be attenuated by oral or intravenous premedication with atropine. As an alkane, halothane sensitizes the heart to catecholamines; ventricular arrhythmias are common, especially during periods of hypercapnia or stress-induced catecholamine release.

Desflurane

The most important clinical characteristics of desflurane are its low blood-gas solubility coefficient (0.42), which imparts the fastest onset and offset of all the available inhalational anesthetics, and its extremely low metabolism (0.02%). The MAC of desflurane is 9.2% for neonates, 9.4% for infants 1–6 months old, 9.9% for infants 6–12 months old, 8.7% for patients aged 1–3 years, and 8% for those aged 5–12 years.

Desflurane is extremely pungent and causes substantial airway irritation. Initial clinical pediatric trials demonstrated that the majority of children receiving desflurane for induction of general anesthesia developed respiratory complications consisting of breath-holding, laryngospasm, coughing, increased secretions, and hypoxemia. Therefore, desflurane is contraindicated for induction of general anesthesia in children, but it can be used for maintenance of general anesthesia, even when using a laryngeal mask airway (LMA) or facemask. In most procedures of indeterminate length, children will regain consciousness within several minutes of discontinuation of desflurane.

Nitrous Oxide

Although its clinical advantages are unproven, N_2O is commonly used as an adjunct to inhalational induction of general anesthesia in children because of its ability to reduce the MAC of sevoflurane and halothane, and to speed the onset of unconsciousness via the second-gas effect. It is commonly discontinued when the intravenous catheter is inserted, in preparation for airway management, which is performed after a period of breathing 100% oxygen to increase the margin of safety during the apneic phase.

Nitrous oxide may cause vomiting during induction of anesthesia, and it has been associated with myoclonic movements and even generalized seizures in some case reports. Because N_2O decreases the activity of two vitamin B_{12} enzymes, methionine synthetase and thymidylate synthetase, its use has been implicated in the exacerbation of vitamin B_{12} deficiency with development of neurological symptoms in susceptible patients. Therefore, N_2O should be avoided in children with vitamin B_{12} deficiency.

Alternate Induction Techniques

The majority of children receiving a mask induction of general anesthesia begin by breathing N_2O, up to 70%, and sevoflurane 8% or halothane, incrementally up to 5%. Older children and adolescents who are cooperative may receive a *single-breath induction technique*, which will considerably speed the loss of consciousness. This is performed by priming the anesthesia circuit and ventilation bag with N_2O and the inhalational agent prior to the patient entering the operating room. The distal end of the breathing circuit that is normally connected to the anesthesia facemask is sealed off to prevent the leakage of anesthetic gases into the OR environment. When the child enters the OR, he or she is asked to first blow all the air out of their lungs (it is helpful to practice this technique with the child prior to entering the OR). At the very end of the child's exhalation, the facemask, which is now connected to the open anesthesia circuit, is placed over the child's mouth and nose, and the child is instructed to take "the biggest breath of their life." This technique will invariably result in loss of consciousness soon after the vital capacity breath.

When a child is sleeping prior to entering the OR, one may perform a *steal induction technique*. Exceptional care is taken to avoid awakening the child while he or she is transported into the OR. Once in the OR, the child is not touched or moved to the OR table and no monitors are applied. The anesthesia breathing circuit is primed with N_2O and sevoflurane or halothane, and the mask is moved progressively closer to the child's face without touching it. One must be careful not to move too close to the child's face too quickly, for the child will awaken if he or she smells the pungent anesthetic gas. Once consciousness is lost, the child is moved to the OR table and monitors are applied. Proponents of this technique favor the atraumatic nature of this type of induction, and the child's lack of knowledge of the OR environment. Opponents of this technique fear that a child could suffer psychological harm if he or she awakens from a painful procedure without realizing that it had begun.

Inhalational Agents for Maintenance of General Anesthesia

The majority of pediatric general anesthetics are maintained with an inhalational agent. There are no clear advantages or disadvantages to any agent, except perhaps the lower cost of the older agents, isoflurane and halothane. Sevoflurane and isoflurane are almost identical in their times to awakening and discharge home. Agitation is more commonly seen in the immediate postoperative period with sevoflurane than with other agents. Various theories exist to explain this phenomenon, including more rapid awakening and faster onset of perceived pain, but agitation also occurs following nonpainful procedures such as magnetic resonance imaging (MRI). Postoperative agitation is distressing to the postanesthesia care unit (PACU) staff as well as parents, but it is easily abolished with small intravenous doses of an opioid, midazolam, or clonidine. Desflurane, the least soluble agent, has the advantage of the shortest time to awakening once it is discontinued, but is not associated with improved postoperative outcomes.

INTRAVENOUS ANESTHETICS

In most pediatric centers in the United States, intravenous induction of general anesthesia is reserved for children with previously established intravenous access, children with susceptibility to malignant hyperthermia, and children at risk of pulmonary aspiration of gastric contents who require a rapid sequence induction (RSI) technique. It is rarely used electively, unless the child prefers this method to inhaling gases from a facemask. For children in this latter category, pain can be minimized by using a butterfly needle to access one of the large veins in the antecubital fossa, and an intravenous catheter can then be inserted into a more accessible location (e.g., dorsum of the hand) after the child has lost consciousness. If time permits, one may apply a topical anesthetic cream to several potential intravenous sites.

The most commonly used intravenous induction agents in children are thiopental and propofol, although methohexital, ketamine, and etomidate can also be used.

Barbiturates

Thiopental

Thiopental is the most common barbiturate used for intravenous induction of general anesthesia in children. In doses of 5–7 mg/kg, it provides loss of consciousness within several seconds after administration, without hemodynamic compromise in euvolemic children. Although not studied specifically in children, thiopental administration in the presence of hypovolemia may result in life-threatening hypotension secondary to venous and arterial vasodilatation.

The dose of thiopental used for induction of anesthesia in neonates is less than for older children. This may be due in part to a more immature blood–brain barrier in neonates, and greater bioavailability of the drug, and/or a reduced protein binding in the plasma of neonates. In adults, it is not as effective as equipotent doses of propofol in blunting the airway response to tracheal intubation, and this is probably true for children as well.

Methohexital

Methohexital is shorter-acting than thiopental, but it often causes myoclonic movements immediately after administration and can exacerbate seizures in susceptible children. It is often painful at the site of administration and is associated with postoperative nausea and vomiting. For these reasons, it is used much less often

than thiopental in pediatric anesthesia. The dose for induction of general anesthesia is 1–3 mg/kg.

Nonbarbiturates

Propofol

Propofol is the most common nonbarbiturate agent used for induction of general anesthesia in children. It causes immediate loss of consciousness following administration of 3–6 mg/kg. Children require larger induction doses than adults because of an apparently larger volume of distribution. Maintenance doses are also larger in children because of greater elimination clearance. Propofol is particularly well suited for use in asthmatics, as it blunts airway responses within its clinical dosing range. It has replaced ketamine as the intravenous induction agent of choice for children with asthma.

Propofol usually causes central apnea when administered as a bolus for induction of general anesthesia. If given in titrated doses, apnea can be avoided. However, the apneic dose of propofol is usually less than the dose required to prevent movement in response to a surgical stimulus. Administration of propofol may cause cardiovascular depression in hypovolemic children or those with a preexisting cardiomyopathy.

A particularly difficult problem with propofol is its propensity to cause severe pain in the limb in which it is administered. In general, injection into smaller veins (e.g., dorsum of the hand) produces more pain than injection into larger veins (e.g., antecubital). A variety of studies have attempted to determine the most reliable way to prevent this pain. Methods include concomitant or prior administration of lidocaine or an opioid but are not effective in all children. The most reliable method for preventing propofol-induced pain is to administer a small volume of 1% lidocaine while holding pressure proximal to the vein (i.e., a modified Bier block technique) as the vein distends. Pressure is held for 5–10 seconds to assure that the wall of the vein is anesthetized, after which the propofol is administered. This method effectively blunts the pain in over 90% of children.

Because of propofol's relatively low context-sensitive half-time (see Chapter 2), lack of "hangover," and lack of propensity to cause nausea and vomiting, it is ideally suited to be the major component of a total intravenous anesthesia (TIVA) technique. During unpainful medical procedures that require immobility (e.g., computed tomography (CT), MRI, and radiotherapy) it can be used in moderate infusion doses (150–250 μg/kg/min) that preserve spontaneous ventilation. For painful procedures (e.g., bone marrow biopsy, lumbar puncture, burn dressing changes) and surgical procedures that require a TIVA technique (e.g., rigid bronchoscopy, malignant hyperthermia-susceptible patient), much greater doses of propofol are required to ensure immobility. These larger doses are inevitably associated with central or obstructive apnea, requiring ventilatory assistance. Alternatively, propofol can be combined with an opioid, which will decrease the total required propofol dose, but ventilatory assistance is still often required.

Ketamine

Ketamine is an N-methyl-D-aspartate (NMDA) receptor antagonist that provides excellent dissociative anesthesia in children. It can be used as a sedative or as an induction agent for general anesthesia. At clinically useful doses (1–2 mg/kg), ketamine usually preserves spontaneous ventilation, upper-airway patency, and normal cardiovascular function, while providing analgesia and amnesia during painful procedures. Ketamine stimulates the sympathetic nervous system, which may cause undesirable increases in blood pressure, intracranial pressure, and intraocular pressure. In addition, ketamine is associated with psychomimetic side-effects (e.g., hallucinations, nightmares), increased airway secretions, postoperative nausea and vomiting, and delayed awakening. For these reasons, it has largely been replaced by propofol for almost all clinical uses except brief sedation for painful procedures, and intramuscularly as a sedative for uncooperative developmentally delayed adolescents. Concomitant administration of midazolam may attenuate the psychomimetic side-effects.

Etomidate

Etomidate is mainly used in adults with cardiovascular disease and limited cardiovascular reserve. It may be useful in the traumatized child who is hypovolemic, or in a child with a cardiomyopathy and decreased cardiovascular function. The dose range (0.2–0.3 mg/kg) and side-effects (e.g., pain on injection, myoclonus, vomiting) appear to be similar to those in adults.

ADJUNCTIVE ANESTHETIC AGENTS IN PEDIATRIC ANESTHESIA

Adjunctive anesthetic agents in pediatric anesthesia include opioids and neuromuscular blockers. Their use in pediatric anesthesia will be reviewed in the following sections. More complete details on opioid use in pediatric patients for postoperative analgesia can be found in Chapter 24.

Opioids

Opioids are administered to pediatric surgical patients as a component of a balanced anesthesia technique, to contribute to postoperative analgesia, and to attenuate or prevent postoperative emergence delirium or agitation. The choice of opioid depends on the nature and length of the surgical procedure, and the expected duration of postoperative pain. For example, intranasal or intramuscular fentanyl (2 µg/kg) is often administered to children undergoing myringotomy and tubes because of the lack of an intravenous catheter and the short expected duration of postoperative pain. Intravenous fentanyl is often administered for neurosurgical procedures because of the intense analgesia required intraoperatively, and less analgesic requirements postoperatively. Intravenous morphine is administered for most urologic and abdominal procedures because of the requirement for a relatively longer duration of postoperative analgesia.

Opioids are commonly included as a component of a total intravenous anesthesia (TIVA) technique for painful surgical procedures. Fentanyl or one of its congeners (e.g., alfentanil, sufentanil, and remifentanil) are ideally suited for use in TIVA because of their relatively low context-sensitive half-time. Remifentanil possesses the most favorable profile, as its termination of action is directly related to its metabolism by tissue and plasma esterases. Its effects will usually dissipate within 5–10 minutes of discontinuing the infusion, regardless of the duration of the infusion.

Remifentanil bolus and infusion doses are higher in infants and young children than in adults, reflecting the larger volume of distribution and increased elimination clearance, respectively. Typically, a bolus dose of 1–2 µg/kg will be administered over several minutes, followed by an infusion dose of 0.5 µg/kg/min. This infusion dose is then titrated to achieve the desired analgesic and hemodynamic effects. There is evidence that the use of intraoperative remifentanil in former premature infants may be associated with a decreased incidence of postoperative apnea when compared to halothane for maintenance of general anesthesia. However, it has not been compared with the newer agents, sevoflurane and desflurane, which are described in an earlier section.

Well-established side-effects of opioid use in children include sedation, ventilatory depression, upper-airway obstruction in susceptible children, pruritus, and an increased incidence of postoperative nausea and vomiting. Historically, there has been concern among pediatric anesthesiologists about the increased toxicity profile of opioids when used in newborn infants. This caution relates to the possibility that opioids (especially the less lipid-soluble drug morphine) is allowed greater access through the blood–brain barrier in neonates, and may result in proportionately greater levels in the brain. Furthermore, neonates have been shown to possess increased pharmacodynamic sensitivity, decreased clearance, and a relatively greater depression of CO_2 response curves to opioids when compared with adults. These maturational changes appear to be most pronounced for morphine in comparison with fentanyl and its analogues. However, opioids, like all types of medications administered to neonates, possess substantial interindividual variation in their pharmacokinetic and pharmaco-dynamic properties, so they must be titrated to effect while carefully observing cardiopulmonary side-effects.

Neuromuscular Blockers

Neuromuscular blockers are commonly administered to pediatric patients during induction of anesthesia to facilitate endotracheal intubation and may be continued intraoperatively to enhance optimal surgical conditions and positive-pressure ventilation. Overall, there are probably fewer airway complications in children receiving neuromuscular blockers, even in experienced hands.

There are a number of developmental physiologic differences that affect the pharmacology of neuromuscular blockers. During early childhood, an increase in muscular volume leads to an increase in the number of neuro-muscular receptors; conduction velocity and myelination increase during development; and the rate of acetylcholine release progressively increases. Taken together, these developmental differences are manifested clinically as a greater pharmacodynamic sensitivity of neuromuscular blockers in infants and young children (i.e., neuromuscular blockers are more potent in younger children). In fact, during tetanic stimulation unanesthetized newborns demonstrate significant fade at 50 Hz. This fade in unparalyzed infants suggests that the supply of acetylcholine can be easily exhausted.

The difference in potency among age groups is illustrated as a comparison of the ED_{95} for the neuromuscular blocking agents (Table 19-1). In practice, three (or more) times the ED_{95} is usually administered to assure rapid paralysis and account for pharmacokinetic and pharmacodynamic differences between individual patients. Nondepolarizing neuromuscular blockers tend to be more potent in infants than children, and less potent in children than adults. Clinically, this manifests as a greater duration of action in infants and adults when compared with children.

Since all neuromuscular blockers are water-soluble, and younger children are known to be composed of a relatively greater volume of body water, the volume of distribution for these drugs is larger in younger children (see Chapter 2). Clinically, this translates into a higher bolus dose required to achieve a given plasma level (Table 19-2). However, since neonates and small infants demonstrate enhanced sensitivity to neuromuscular blockers, a lower plasma concentration is required, so the bolus dose is the same as for adults. Neonates and small infants will also demonstrate a prolonged duration of action because of the larger volume of distribution and the decreased liver function in the newborn period. Because of this latter characteristic, the aminosteroidal relaxants, which rely on liver metabolism for their termination of effect, become long-acting agents, often exceeding 60 minutes or more.

Succinylcholine

Succinylcholine, the only depolarizing neuromuscular blocker in use today, remains the fastest acting with the shortest duration of action of any available agent. Despite its many drawbacks to use in children, it retains its place as the agent of choice for rapid sequence induction and as a potential treatment for life-threatening upper-airway obstruction.

Like all other neuromuscular blockers, succinylcholine is water-soluble. Therefore, the intravenous bolus dose required in infants and young children (2 mg/kg) is larger than for older children and adults (1 mg/kg). An intramuscular dose of 4 mg/kg will provide a maximum

Table 19-1 Age-related Differences in Potency of Neuromuscular Blockers

	ED_{95}[a] (mg/kg)		
	Infants	**Children**	**Adults**
Atracurium	0.24	0.33	0.21
Cis-atracurium	<0.06[b]	0.06	0.045
Mivacurium	0.13	0.14	0.08
Pancuronium	0.065	0.095	0.07
Rocuronium	0.25	0.40	0.35
Vecuronium	0.045	0.08	0.04
Succinylcholine	0.61	0.35	0.29

[a] ED_{95} is the dose that produces an average block of 95% in neuromuscular function of the ulnar nerve – adductor pollicis.
[b] Dose–response for cis-atracurium in infants has not been adequately studied.
Reproduced with permission from Brandom BW, Fine GF: Neuromuscular blocking drugs in pediatric anesthesia. *Anesthesiol Clin N Am* 20:45–58, 2002.

Table 19-2 Intubation Doses of Neuromuscular Blockers in Children

Drug	Dose (mg/kg)	Multiple of ED_{95}[a]	Minutes to Intubation	Minutes to T_{25}[b]
Mivacurium	0.3	2–3	1.5	5–15
Rocuronium	0.6	2	1.0	10–30
Cis-atracurium	0.2	5	1.5	45–75
Atracurium	0.5	2	3.0	20–45
Vecuronium	0.1	1–2	2.0	20–60
Pancuronium	0.1	1–2	2.5	45–60
Succinylcholine	2.0	6?	<1.0	3–5

[a] ED_{95} is the dose that produces an average block of 95% in neuromuscular function of the ulnar nerve – adductor pollicis.
[b] T_{25} is the time from injection of blocker to recovery of 25% of baseline neuromuscular transmission or 3 to 4 responses to a train-of-four stimulus.
Reproduced with permission from Brandom BW, Fine GF: Neuromuscular blocking drugs in pediatric anesthesia. *Anesthesiol Clin N Am* 20:45–58, 2002.

Box 19-1	Possible Side-effects and Complications of Succinylcholine

Depolarization-related complications:
  Muscle fasciculation/postoperative myalgia
  Increased intracranial pressure
  Increased intragastric pressure
  Increased intraocular pressure
Prolonged blockade in patients with pseudocholinesterase deficiency
Bradycardia and junctional arrhythmias
Anaphylaxis and anaphylactoid reactions
Rhabdomyolysis leading to myoglobinuria
Hyperkalemia – may be life-threatening
Masseter muscle rigidity/malignant hyperthermia (MH)

onset of blockade in 3–4 minutes and will last for approximately 20 minutes. Its elimination clearance is more rapid in children, so its duration of effect is less than for adults. The major pharmacological differences for succinylcholine that exist between children and adults are not apparent in its beneficial effects, but rather in its adverse effects (Box 19-1).

Bradycardia

Succinylcholine commonly causes vagal-mediated bradycardia, junctional rhythms, or sinus arrest in children. These are commonly seen after the first dose, whereas in adults arrhythmias are usually seen after subsequent doses. For this reason, it is standard practice to administer an anticholinergic agent prior to succinylcholine in pediatric patients. Intravenous atropine (0.02 mg/kg) and glycopyrrolate (0.01 mg/kg) are equally effective in attenuating succinylcholine-induced bradycardia.

Fasciculations

Children under the age of 8 years rarely develop fasciculations or postoperative muscle pain following administration of succinylcholine. This has been attributed to the low overall muscle mass in young children. However, rhabdomyolysis and myoglobinuria can occur after succinylcholine administration despite the absence of fasciculations.

Hyperkalemia

Succinylcholine-induced paralysis results in muscle contraction by simulating the action of acetylcholine. This normally results in potassium release from the intracellular space and a transient and clinically insignificant increase in the plasma potassium level. Patients with obvious or occult muscle atrophy, or disorders associated with up-regulation of extrajunctional acetylcholine receptors (e.g., burns), will demonstrate an exaggerated potassium release after succinylcholine administration. The hyperkalemia that develops can lead to arrhythmias, cardiac arrest, and death.

In the early 1990s the anesthesiology community was alerted to a number of cases of succinylcholine-induced life-threatening hyperkalemia that occurred in young boys with undiagnosed Duchenne muscular dystrophy. As a result, the US Food and Drug Administration (FDA) recommended that succinylcholine no longer be used for routine, elective neuromuscular blockade. When using succinylcholine in an emergency situation, all anesthesiologists should be aware of this possible complication. Hyperkalemia is manifested as tall, peaked T waves on the electrocardiogram, which may develop into a wide complex tachycardia, ventricular fibrillation, and asystole. In the event this occurs, succinylcholine-induced hyperkalemia should be presumed until proven otherwise. The immediate treatment consists of intravenous calcium chloride at a dose of 5–10 mg/kg.

Succinylcholine-induced hyperkalemia can occur in any patient with muscle atrophy, especially when it is due to a progressive myopathy (e.g., Duchenne muscular dystrophy) or following an acute muscle injury or burn. However, normal potassium release after succinylcholine administration is observed in children with cerebral palsy or meningomyelocele.

Malignant Hyperthermia

Succinylcholine is widely considered a triggering agent for malignant hyperthermia (MH). Malignant hyperthermia may manifest clinically as excessive rigidity well after fasciculations are expected to abate. In a previous era when succinylcholine was routinely used for pediatric cases, the incidence of MH was estimated to be 1 in 15,000. Many of these reported cases were likely to be rhabdomyolysis-induced hyperkalemia rather than MH per se. Nevertheless, the possibility of triggering MH is another reason that succinylcholine is no longer used in children on an elective basis.

Masseter Muscle Rigidity

Varying degrees of masseter muscle rigidity (MMR) are observed in children following succinylcholine administration. This response ranges from a mild difficulty with mouth opening to the complete inability to open the mouth ("jaws of steel"). The incidence of this response in children exceeds 1% in some studies. This phenomenon may represent a normal response to succinylcholine, especially if underdosed, or when severe, a harbinger of MH. Up to 50% of patients with a history of severe MMR test positive for malignant hyperthermia susceptibility on halothane/caffeine contracture testing.

If MMR occurs, all volatile anesthetics should be discontinued, and a nontriggering technique with TIVA should be administered. Some experts recommend awakening the patient if the procedure is not emergent and proceeding with the surgery only after a definitive evaluation of MH susceptibility. At the very least, creatine kinase levels should be obtained, along with electrolytes and a blood gas analysis. The patient should be observed

Article To Know

Larach MG, Rosenberg H, Gronert GA, Allen GC: Hyperkalemic cardiac arrest during anesthesia in infants and children with occult myopathies. Clin Pediatr 36:9–16, 1997.

This publication constitutes an analysis of reports received by the Malignant Hyperthermia Association of the United States (MHAUS) and the North American Malignant Hyperthermia Registry from 1990 to 1993, of 25 children with a cardiac arrest within 24 hours of receiving an anesthetic. Cases were examined for causes such as inadequate ventilation, inadequate oxygenation, anesthetic overdose, hypovolemia, and hyperkalemia. Patients were diagnosed as having a myopathy after a pathologic examination of skeletal muscle was performed. Diagnosis of Duchenne muscular dystrophy was made if dystrophin was not detected by immunologic techniques.

Twenty of the cardiac arrests (80%) occurred in the operating room, and the remainder occurred in the recovery room, catheterization laboratory, or intensive care unit. Twenty of the children were previously healthy and were undergoing elective surgical procedures. Two children had an underlying disorder (septicemia and postcardiac surgery). A family history of myopathy was obtained in two children. No history of MH was elicited in any child.

Failure to ventilate or oxygenate was not implicated as a primary cause in any case of cardiac arrest. In addition, anesthetic overdose or hypovolemia was not judged to be present in any case. The presenting cardiac symptoms included wide complex bradycardia, ventricular tachycardia with hypotension, ventricular fibrillation, and asystole.

A potassium level during the cardiac arrest was measured in 18 of 25 patients. Thirteen of these demonstrated hyperkalemia. Mean peak serum K^+ measured 7.4 ± 2.8 mmol/L (median 7.5, range 3.5–14.8). Eight of the 13 patients with hyperkalemia had received succinylcholine and potent inhalational anesthetics, while one patient had received succinylcholine alone, and four had received potent inhalational anesthetics without succinylcholine.

Cardiopulmonary resuscitation was performed for a median time of 42 minutes. In addition to standard pediatric advanced life-support measures, the following medications were given: calcium ($n = 11$), glucose and insulin (6), sodium bicarbonate (20), dantrolene (13), and mannitol (5). Pacemakers were used in two patients, peritoneal dialysis in one patient, and cardiopulmonary bypass was used in two patients. Fourteen patients, including a child with almost certain MH, survived with eventual return of baseline neurological function. One patient survived without meaningful neurological function.

Autopsy was performed on nine of the ten children who died. Four of these nine had a previously undiagnosed myopathy, and an additional three had an unsuspected cardiomyopathy or cardiac hypertrophy. Of the 13 patients with hyperkalemia, eight were eventually shown to have an occult myopathy.

Cases such as these emphasize the importance of preoperative screening for occult myopathies that may manifest subclinically as mild muscle weakness or failure to attain age-appropriate physical milestones. Clinical features of Duchenne muscular dystrophy include calf muscle hypertrophy, toe walking, and a waddling gait. Any suspicion of muscle weakness should warrant a preoperative creatine kinase level; if elevated it may indicate an occult myopathy.

This report highlighted the potential danger in administering succinylcholine to children who were not old enough to manifest clinical symptoms of their myopathy. Duchenne and Becker types of muscular dystrophy may not present until the child is 4 years of age or more. Because of this report, the Anesthetic and Life Support Drugs Advisory Committee of the Food and Drug Administration held hearings and eventually asked the manufacturer to place a black box warning in the package insert of succinylcholine that reads:

"it is recommended that the use of succinylcholine in children should be reserved for emergency intubation or instances where immediate securing of the airway is necessary, e.g., laryngospasm, difficult airway, full stomach, or for intramuscular use when a suitable vein is inaccessible."

This warning ultimately led to the precipitous decline of elective use of succinylcholine in children.

---

closely for signs and symptoms suggestive of an acute MH crisis (see Chapter 21). Dantrolene is not indicated in the absence of signs of MH.

Nondepolarizing Neuromuscular Blockers

The nondepolarizing neuromuscular blockers are divided into two major categories based on structure and mode of elimination.

- The benzylisoquinoliniums, atracurium and cis-atracurium, rely on metabolism by Hofmann degradation and ester hydrolysis by nonspecific plasma esterases for their termination of action, while mivacurium is metabolized by plasma (pseudo) cholinesterase.
- The aminosteroids (vecuronium, rocuronium, and pancuronium) are metabolized in the liver to inactive products that are eliminated by the kidney.

A major advantage of the aminosteroids is their efficacy after intramuscular administration. Rapacuronium, an ultra-short-acting aminosteroid neuromuscular blocker, was recently removed from the market because of concerns that it contributed to life-threatening bronchospasm.

Atracurium

Atracurium is an intermediate-acting (30–40 minutes) neuromuscular blocker that is usually reversible within 20 minutes after administration. Because its metabolism does not rely on hepatic function, its duration of action is predictable, even in neonates. In a dose of 0.5 mg/kg, atracurium produces reliable intubating conditions within 90 seconds after administration. Large doses of atracurium will occasionally result in histamine release that is manifested as a macular rash. Histamine-induced bronchospasm and hypotension are uncommon after atracurium administration in pediatric patients.

Cis-atracurium

Cis-atracurium is a *cis* isomer of atracurium, and possesses a similar clinical and pharmacokinetic profile as atracurium except for its increased potency and its lack of histamine release. Because of the increased potency, its onset to maximum block is slower than that of atracurium. A dose of 0.15–0.2 mg/kg will provide reliable intubating conditions within 2 minutes. Clinical studies in children indicate that administration of cis-atracurium is associated with a longer and less predictable duration of action than atracurium.

Mivacurium

Mivacurium is the shortest-acting neuromuscular blocker in its class (15–20 minutes), primarily due to its metabolism by pseudocholinesterase. Mivacurium was originally marketed as a replacement for succinylcholine, but initial clinical experience demonstrated a lack of satisfactory intubating conditions within 1 minute at the recommended dose (0.15 mg/kg). Therefore, most pediatric anesthesiologists have modified the dose upward to 0.25–0.3 mg/kg, which provides reliable intubating conditions within 1 minute, but is consistently accompanied by a histamine rash and occasional hypotension. These side-effects can be attenuated by increasing the duration over which the drug is administered. Because of its lack of accumulation, mivacurium is particularly suited for multiple repeated dosing or as a continuous infusion. The neuromuscular blockade of mivacurium is usually reversible within 10 minutes following administration of a bolus dose or discontinuation of a continuous infusion. This time to reversibility is relatively shorter than for adults. A disadvantage to the use of mivacurium is the possibility of prolonged duration of action in patients with qualitative or quantitative pseudocholinesterase deficiency.

Vecuronium

Vecuronium is an intermediate-acting neuromuscular blocker (40–75 minutes) that is usually reversible by 20 minutes following its administration. Following a dose of 0.1 mg/kg, reliable intubation conditions are usually achieved within 2 minutes. School-aged children require relatively more vecuronium to achieve a desired effect and recover faster than infants, older children, and adults. Because the termination of vecuronium depends on liver metabolism, the duration of action can be prolonged in neonates and small infants. When given in combination with thiopental, vecuronium can cause crystallization in the intravenous tubing and catheter that can be quite difficult to alleviate. Therefore, when using this combination of drugs the thiopental should be flushed through the tubing prior to injecting the vecuronium. Vecuronium administration is associated with bradycardia when given in combination with fentanyl or one of its analogues. However, vecuronium is not associated with histamine release or bronchospasm.

Vecuronium has been used for rapid sequence induction in children. At a dose of 0.4 mg/kg (four times a typical intubating dose) reliable intubation conditions can be achieved within 1 minute, but at the expense of a prolonged duration of action: reversibility may not be possible for more than 90 minutes. This large dose can be decreased with the concomitant use of an opioid.

Rocuronium

Rocuronium is an intermediate-acting relaxant that possesses a clinical profile similar to vecuronium and atracurium. Its main advantage is its ability to be given in relatively higher doses (1.2–1.6 mg/kg) to achieve reliable intubating conditions within 1 minute. These higher doses are not associated with the prolonged duration of action seen with vecuronium – reversibility is usually possible within 45 minutes. Therefore, rocuronium has become the neuromuscular blocker of choice for rapid sequence induction in children when succinylcholine is contraindicated. Some pediatric anesthesiologists use rocuronium for all RSIs as an alternative to succinylcholine.

Rocuronium can be administered intramuscularly – 1.0 mg/kg for infants and 1.8 mg/kg for children – to provide reliable intubating conditions within 3 minutes in most patients, at the expense of a prolonged duration of action that may exceed an hour. When administering this drug by the intramuscular route, a deltoid injection provides more reliable plasma levels than a quadriceps injection. The bioavailability of rocuronium after intramuscular administration is greater than 80%, and less than 5% of the drug remains in muscle 30 minutes after injection.

Pancuronium

Pancuronium is classified as a long-acting neuromuscular blocker because its duration of effect following an intubating dose is greater than 60 minutes. It is usually reversible by 40 minutes after administration.

Administration of pancuronium commonly causes tachycardia due to a combination of vagal blockade and catecholamine release, so it is ideally suited to counteract the bradycardia that results from administration of fentanyl or its analogues.

EMERGENCE FROM GENERAL ANESTHESIA

This section reviews the principles of emergence from general anesthesia in pediatric patients, with specific emphasis on criteria for tracheal extubation. Emergence is the process by which the patient awakens from general anesthesia and is prepared to recover from the withdrawal of ventilatory and circulatory support.

Until the latter portion of the twentieth century, halothane was routinely used for maintenance of general anesthesia. Because of its delayed excretion and prolonged duration of action, the anesthesiologist was required to predict with reasonable accuracy the time of completion of the surgical procedure. Simultaneously, the brain's concentration of halothane could be regulated with the intention of having the child awaken at or shortly after completion of the surgical procedure. In recent years, however, the majority of pediatric general anesthetics (in the USA) are maintained using isoflurane, sevoflurane, or desflurane. Because of the short duration of action of these agents, titration down toward the completion of surgery requires less skill, especially when using desflurane, which has the shortest duration of action, similar to that of nitrous oxide.

Tracheal Extubation

There are three major criteria for tracheal extubation in children:
- Sufficient muscular strength to ensure upper-airway patency after removal of the endotracheal tube
- The presence of a regular breathing pattern
- A sufficiently high level of consciousness that ensures the presence of airway protective mechanisms.

The first two criteria may appear at any time during emergence, depending on the timing of the administration of reversal agents or discontinuation of the anesthetic agents. The third criterion is usually the last to appear. Each of these criteria will be discussed with particular regard to pediatric patients.

Regular Breathing Pattern

Once all general anesthetic agents have been discontinued, and neuromuscular blockers reversed (if applicable), children will begin to breathe on their own. The first spontaneous breaths may be regular, but as the child begins to regain consciousness, the breaths will become more irregular with alternating periods of breath-holding, and possibly coughing from the stimulus of the endotracheal tube. This phase is temporary and not indicative of wakefulness. During this phase of breath-holding and coughing small infants will often demonstrate profound decreases in oxygen saturation. These episodes can be extremely frightening to the entire operating room staff. During this phase, it is important that the anesthesiologist remains calm and leaves no doubts that he or she is in control of the situation, as the OR staff's emotions are often based on the anesthesiologist's reactions to critical situations. During this phase of breath-holding, coughing, and oxygen desaturation, the child's lungs should be manually ventilated at a fast rate (>30) and with a high enough inflation pressure to cause observable chest wall rise. Air entry is confirmed by listening with a precordial stethoscope, and by watching the capnograph. If the capnograph indicates air exchange, one can be reasonably confident that the oxygen saturation will soon begin to rise. Conversely, if air exchange does not appear on the capnograph, then the anesthesiologist knows he or she must alter the manual ventilation technique, which may often include using unusually high inspiratory pressures. It is only when the child begins to breathe regularly and maintain a normal oxygen saturation that the anesthesiologist can then begin to consider the following two criteria before removing the endotracheal tube.

Sufficient Muscular Strength

Muscular strength at the completion of surgery will depend on the timing of the discontinuation of the anesthetic agent and, if a neuromuscular blocker was administered, the time since the previous dose, as well as administration of an anticholinesterase agent to reverse the neuromuscular blockade (Table 19-3). Administration of anticholinesterase reversal agents should be considered after use of all nondepolarizing neuromuscular blockers, with the possible exception of mivacurium, if more than 15–20 minutes have passed since the most recent dose. Although most studies demonstrate a faster recovery from neuromuscular blockade in children when compared to adults, the acceleration of that

Table 19-3 Antagonism of Neuromuscular Blockade

	Dose (mg/kg)
Anticholinesterase agents	
Neostigmine	0.05–0.07
Edrophonium	0.5–1.0
Anticholinergic agents	
Atropine	0.02 (minimum dose 0.16 mg)
Glycopyrrolate	0.01

recovery by administration of reversal agents is probably not age-dependent. However, as in adults, adequate reversal of a nondepolarizing neuromuscular blocker will not occur until a train-of-four (TOF) monitoring response is detected, with the possible exception of a deep mivacurium blockade. Also similar to adults, neostigmine appears to be a better antagonist of intense neuromuscular blockade than an equipotent dose of edrophonium. Much of what is known about antagonism of neuromuscular blockade is based on studies performed during maintenance of general anesthesia with halothane. Similar studies during sevoflurane or desflurane inhalation have not been performed.

An anticholinergic agent is routinely administered in combination with an anticholinesterase agent to prevent vagotonic bradycardia. Because of similarities in time to onset and duration of action, most anesthesiologists will choose to administer glycopyrrolate with neostigmine, and atropine with edrophonium; however, advantages of using these specific combinations have not been demonstrated experimentally or in clinical practice. Some studies indicate that use of a cholinergic-based reversal agent is associated with a greater incidence of postoperative nausea and vomiting. In contrast to glycopyrrolate, atropine crosses the blood–brain barrier and may possess a central antiemetic effect, thus lowering the incidence of postoperative nausea and vomiting when neostigmine is used.

In the absence of intense neuromuscular blockade, most children will rapidly achieve sufficient strength within several minutes after administration of a reversal agent. In adults, adequate strength is demonstrated by sustained head lift for 5 seconds or a vigorous hand squeeze on command. These criteria cannot be used in small children because of their inability to follow commands. Instead in the author's institution we use the "hip flexion" sign (Fig. 19-2), which indicates that the child has achieved sufficient strength to maintain airway patency independently after removal of the endotracheal tube. In addition, a negative inspiratory force less than $-25\,cmH_2O$ and a vital capacity $>15\,mL/kg$ are indicative of the strength required to sustain a patent upper airway following withdrawal of the endotracheal tube. Recovery of strength based on TOF indices is not routinely required in otherwise healthy children.

Return of Consciousness

The return of consciousness usually occurs last during emergence from general anesthesia. It is not until the child is awake that one can be assured of a regular breathing pattern and a normal airway protective response. In adults, it is relatively easy to detect wakefulness by the response to commands such as "open your eyes." The infant is obviously unable to respond in this manner. The anesthesiologist then must use other criteria such as spontaneous eye-opening, scrunching of the

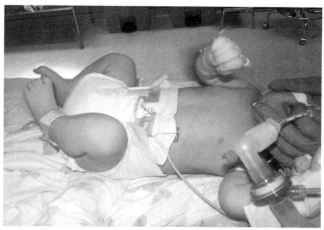

Figure 19-2   The "hip flexion" sign indicates that the child has achieved sufficient strength to maintain airway patency independently after removal of the endotracheal tube.

eyebrows, or crying. One must not confuse involuntary reflexes such as reaching for the endotracheal tube as an indication of wakefulness. In general, harm is not done by leaving the endotracheal tube in too long, only by taking it out too soon. Most experienced pediatric anesthesiologists have observed children who appear to be conscious and strong just immediately prior to tracheal extubation, who then become apneic after the endotracheal tube is removed because of lack of a noxious stimulus. Removal of an endotracheal tube prior to the child regaining full consciousness may also cause laryngospasm via stimulation of laryngeal afferent nerves.

Many pediatric anesthesiologists administer an inspiratory hold, or sigh, up to $30\,cmH_2O$ immediately prior to, and as part of, the last breath before tracheal extubation. The intent of this maneuver is to reverse any existing atelectasis that occurred during the general anesthetic, and restore the function residual capacity (FRC). However, controlled studies on the efficacy of this maneuver have not been performed.

It is not unusual, even in seemingly awake children, for breath-holding to develop immediately after tracheal extubation. This may be caused by the laryngeal stimulation that occurs from the movement of the endotracheal tube. During this phase, provided the patient does not develop hypoxemia, this author prefers to avoid positive-pressure ventilation while maintaining upper-airway patency by chin lift and jaw thrust. In the vast majority of cases, the child will resume spontaneous ventilation within 1 minute and will not develop hypoxemia. In the remainder of children who develop hypoxemia, positive-pressure ventilation is indicated, and laryngospasm should be immediately treated with a small dose of succinylcholine (0.2–0.3 mg/kg).

"Deep" Extubation

Extubation of most children occurs after they have regained consciousness, as outlined above. However, a situation occasionally arises in which it may be detrimental for the child to regain consciousness and airway reflexes with the endotracheal tube still in the trachea. This includes procedures in brittle asthmatics, and certain types of surgical procedures (e.g., ophthalmologic) where coughing may interrupt delicate suture placement. In these cases, it is feasible to remove the endotracheal tube from the trachea prior to the child regaining consciousness and before the child develops the ability to cough. This is commonly referred to as a "deep" extubation. Contraindications to deep extubation in children include suspicion of a greater than normal amount of gastric contents, difficulty with mask ventilation at the beginning of the anesthetic, or difficulty with endotracheal intubation.

A deep extubation can be performed by carrying out a series of progressive steps:

1. Establish a pattern of regular spontaneous ventilation. This can be accomplished by gradually lowering the concentration of inhaled agent and assuring adequate strength by reversing the neuromuscular blockade. During this time the stomach should be emptied with an orogastric tube. None of the inhalational anesthetics have any particular advantage during deep extubation. Desflurane has not been studied and should probably be avoided because of its pungency and tendency to increase airway irritability.

2. Once the child has established a spontaneous, regular breathing pattern, the concentration of the inhaled agent is gradually increased to approximately 2–3 MAC, within the limits of normal vital signs and continuation of spontaneous respiratory effort.

3. The oropharynx is suctioned and the endotracheal tube is removed. Some anesthesiologists prefer to further blunt laryngeal reflexes by administering lidocaine 1.5 mg/kg several minutes prior to extubation. In addition, if excess secretions are present, one may consider the administration of glycopyrrolate prior to extubation.

4. Mask ventilation is then resumed and the inhalational agent is discontinued.

A major disadvantage of performing a deep extubation is that the patient will progress through the lighter stages of anesthesia with an unprotected airway. During this phase, secretions or blood may come in contact with laryngeal structures and precipitate laryngospasm. Therefore, deep extubations should be performed only if the anesthesiologist has the ability to remain with the patient until full consciousness is regained, or if the PACU nursing staff possesses the training and experience to accommodate the emerging child.

ADDITIONAL ARTICLES TO KNOW

Agnor RC, Sikich N, Lerman J: Single-breath vital capacity rapid inhalation induction in children. 8% sevoflurane versus 5% halothane. *Anesthesiology* 89:379–384, 1998.

Barash PG, Glanz S, Katz JD, Taunt K, Talner NS: Ventricular function in children during halothane anesthesia: an echocardiographic evaluation. *Anesthesiology* 49:79–85, 1978.

Baum VC, Yemen TA, Baum LD: Immediate 8% sevoflurane induction in children: a comparison with incremental sevoflurane and incremental halothane. *Anesth Analg* 85:313–316, 1997.

Brandom BW, Fine GF: Neuromuscular blocking drugs in pediatric anesthesia. *Anesthesiol Clin N Am* 20:45–58, 2002.

Brown K, Aun C, Stocks J et al: A comparison of the respiratory effects of sevoflurane and halothane in infants and young children. *Anesthesiology* 89:86–92, 1998.

Cartabuke RS, Davidson PJ, Warner LO: Is premedication with oral glycopyrrolate as effective as oral atropine in attenuating cardiovascular depression in infants receiving halothane for induction of anesthesia? *Anesth Analg* 73:271–274, 1991.

Constant I, Dubois MC, Piat V et al: Changes in electroencephalogram and autonomic cardiovascular activity during induction of anesthesia with sevoflurane compared with halothane in children. *Anesthesiology* 91:1604–1615, 1999.

Davis PJ, Galinkin J, McGowan FX et al: A randomized multicenter study of remifentanil compared with halothane in neonates and infants undergoing pyloromyotomy: I. Emergence and recovery profiles. *Anesth Analg* 93:1380–1386, 2001.

Delphin E, Jackson D, Rothstein P: Use of succinylcholine during elective pediatric anesthesia should be reevaluated. *Anesth Analg* 66:1190–1192, 1987.

Felmet K, Robins B, Tilford D, Hayflick SJ: Acute neurologic decompensation in an infant with cobalamin deficiency exposed to nitrous oxide. *J Pediatr* 137:427–428, 2000.

Friesen RH, Lichtor JL: Cardiovascular depression during halothane anesthesia in infants: a study of three induction techniques. *Anesth Analg* 61:42–45, 1982.

Friesen RH, Wurl JL, Friesen RM: Duration of preoperative fast correlates with arterial blood pressure response to halothane in infants. *Anesth Analg* 95:1572–1576, 2002.

Frink EJ, Green WB, Brown EA et al: Compound A concentrations during sevoflurane anesthesia in children. *Anesthesiology* 84:566–571, 1996.

Galinkin JL, Davis PJ, McGowan FX et al: A randomized multicenter study of remifentanil compared with halothane in neonates and infants undergoing pyloromyotomy: II. Perioperative breathing patterns in neonates and infants with pyloric stenosis. *Anesth Analg* 93:1387–1392, 2001.

Gregory GA, Eger EI, Munson ES: The relationship between age and halothane requirement in man. *Anesthesiology* 30:488–491, 1969.

Gronert GA: Cardiac arrest after succinylcholine: mortality greater with rhabdomyolysis than receptor upregulation. *Anesthesiology* 94:523-529, 2001.

Holzman RS, van der Velde ME, Kaus SJ et al: Sevoflurane depresses myocardial contractility less than halothane during induction of anesthesia in children. *Anesthesiology* 85:1260-1267, 1996.

Kawana S, Wachi J, Nakayama M, Namiki A: Comparison of haemodynamic changes induced by sevoflurane and halothane in paediatric patients. *Can J Anaesth* 42:603-607, 1995.

Kharasch ED, Hankins DC, Thummel KE: Human kidney methoxyflurane and sevoflurane metabolism. *Anesthesiology* 82:689-699, 1995.

Lerman J, Robinson S, Willis M, Gregory GA: Anesthetic requirements for halothane in young children 0-1 month and 1-6 months of age. *Anesthesiology* 59:421-424, 1983.

Lerman J, Sikich N, Kleinman S, Yentis S: The pharmacology of sevoflurane in infants and children. *Anesthesiology* 80:814-824, 1994.

Levine MF, Sarner J, Lerman J et al: Plasma inorganic fluoride concentrations after sevoflurane anesthesia in children. *Anesthesiology* 84:348-353, 1996.

Loeckinger A, Kleinsasser A, Maier S et al: Sustained prolongation of the QTc interval after anesthesia with sevoflurane in infants during the first 6 months of life. *Anesthesiology* 98:639-642, 2003.

Mason LJ, Betts EK: Leg lift and maximum inspiratory force: clinical signs of neuromuscular blockade reversal in neonates and infants. *Anesthesiology* 52:441-442, 1980.

McNeely JK, Buczulinski B, Rosner DR: Severe neurological impairment in an infant after nitrous oxide anesthesia. *Anesthesiology* 93:1549-1550, 2000.

Miller BR, Friesen RH: Oral atropine premedication in infants attenuates cardiovascular depression during halothane anesthesia. *Anesth Analg* 67:180-185, 1988.

Morray JP, Geiduschek JM, Ramamoorthy C et al: Anesthesia-related cardiac arrest in children: initial findings of the Pediatric Perioperative Cardiac Arrest (POCA) Registry. *Anesthesiology* 93:6-14, 2000.

Palmisano BW, Setlock MA, Brown MP, Siker D, Tripuraneni R: Dose-response for atropine and heart rate in infants and children anesthetized with halothane and nitrous oxide. *Anesth Analg* 75:238-242, 1991.

Pounder DR, Blackstock D, Steward DJ: Tracheal extubation in children: halothane versus isoflurane, anesthetized versus awake. *Anesthesiology* 74:653-655, 1991.

Ross AK, Davis PJ, Dear GL et al: Pharmacokinetics of remifentanil in anesthetized pediatric patients undergoing elective surgery or diagnostic procedures. *Anesth Analg* 93:1393-1401, 2001.

Sarner JB, Levine M, Davis PJ et al: Clinical characteristics of sevoflurane in children: a comparison with halothane. *Anesthesiology* 82:38-46, 1995.

Watcha MF, Safavi FZ, McCulloch DA, Tan TS, White PF: Effect of antagonism of mivacurium-induced neuromuscular block on postoperative emesis in children. *Anesth Analg* 80:713-717, 1995.

Zwass MS, Fisher DM, Welborn LG et al: Induction and maintenance characteristics of anesthesia with desflurane and nitrous oxide in infants and children. *Anesthesiology* 76:373-378, 1992.

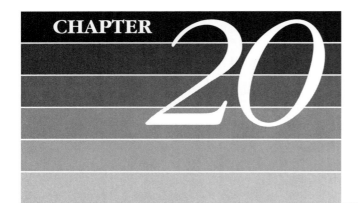

Pediatric Regional Anesthesia

JOSEPH D. TOBIAS

RONALD S. LITMAN

This chapter reviews applications and techniques of the most commonly used regional anesthesia techniques in children. Because young children lack the ability to communicate their analgesic needs and are unable to use a patient-controlled analgesia device, regional anesthesia techniques are preferred for relief of postoperative pain. These techniques can also be used instead of general anesthesia when preexisting anatomic or physiologic alterations increase the risk of general anesthesia. In addition, a benefit of regional anesthesia to an injured extremity is the sympathetic blockade and vasodilatation that increase its distal blood flow.

In contrast to adults, the vast majority of regional anesthesia blocks are performed in children who are anesthetized. The reasons for this are obvious: normal conscious children will not cooperate sufficiently for adequate placement of a regional block. The main disadvantage of this approach is the theoretical injury of a nerve that would have otherwise been detected in a conscious patient by an immediate reaction of extreme pain or a motor response. However, the worldwide experience of regional blocks in thousands of children has shown the occurrence of nerve damage to be exceedingly rare. This knowledge tips the balance in favor of the benefits of regional anesthesia in the anesthetized and immobile child. Another possible disadvantage of performing a regional technique during general anesthesia is the unreliability of the exact location of block placement. Peripheral nerve blocks in anesthetized children are often performed with the assistance of a nerve stimulator and, fortunately, complications as a result of inaccurate block placement are also rare.

CENTRAL REGIONAL TECHNIQUES

Spinal Anesthesia

There are limited applications of spinal anesthesia in children. In adolescents, spinal anesthesia may be offered as an alternative to general anesthesia for low abdominal and lower-extremity procedures. In infants, spinal anesthesia is used when the conduct of general anesthesia with endotracheal intubation is best avoided owing to anatomic or physiologic considerations. The most common use of spinal anesthesia in the pediatric population is for the preterm infant at risk for postoperative apnea following general anesthesia (see also Chapter 22). Spinal anesthesia is easiest to perform in infants weighing less than 3 kg, and is most practical when the duration of the surgical procedure is less than 90 minutes.

Preoperative considerations prior to spinal anesthesia in premature infants include adherence to normal fasting guidelines and assurance of a stable hemoglobin level within normal limits for age. There should be no ongoing acute medical problems. Preoperative application of a topical anesthetic cream over the lumbar spine will decrease pain from the spinal injection. Intravenous access should be obtained prior to performance of the block. Although cardiorespiratory effects are uncommon after spinal block in infants, total spinal blockade can occur. Intravenous access will then facilitate rapid treatment of cardiorespiratory depression. Furthermore, given the relative overactivity of the parasympathetic versus the sympathetic nervous system in neonates, bradycardia may occur during the spinal block and require treatment with atropine. Some pediatric anesthesiologists, however, prefer to perform the spinal block first, and then insert the intravenous catheter on the numb lower extremity.

Different local anesthetics and dosing regimens have been suggested for spinal anesthesia in neonates. The type of local anesthetic is determined by the desired duration of action. Surgical anesthesia will last 30–60 minutes with lidocaine and 60–90 minutes with tetracaine or bupivacaine. Therefore, either tetracaine or bupivacaine is used for most procedures. Most reports in the literature use 1% tetracaine or 0.5–0.75% bupivacaine at doses of 0.4–1 mg/kg. The higher end of the dosing range provides greater reliability and longer duration of surgical anesthesia. A larger dose is required than for adults because of the relatively larger ratio of cerebrospinal fluid (CSF) to bodyweight in neonates (4–6 mL/kg) compared with adults (2 mL/kg) and the resulting dilutional effect. An epinephrine wash should be added to the solution to increase the duration of the anesthetic. It is prepared by withdrawing epinephrine (1 mg/mL) into a tuberculin syringe and then squirting it out, thus leaving a small amount in the syringe. The local anesthetic is then drawn up into the tuberculin syringe, with the same volume of 10% dextrose to create a 1:1 hyperbaric solution.

Spinal anesthesia is difficult to perform in infants. It takes practice and patience. It can be performed in either the sitting or lateral position, and is largely determined by the personal preference of the anesthesiologist. Lumbar puncture is performed at the L3–L4 or L4–L5 interspace because the spinal cord in the small infant ends at a more caudad level (L3) than in older children (L1). The appropriate interspace is found at the intersection of the midline (spinous process) and a line connecting the top of the iliac crest. A 1.5-inch, 22-gauge spinal needle is most often used and inserted approximately 1 cm until a light "pop" is felt as the needle penetrates the dura and subarachnoid membrane. When the stylet is removed, free flow of CSF is obtained, and the syringe is firmly attached to the hub of the inserted spinal needle (a common cause of a failed spinal block is leakage of the local anesthetic solution during injection). Once the syringe is secured to the hub of the spinal needle, CSF is aspirated and the local anesthetic solution is injected over 5–10 seconds. CSF is again aspirated at the end of the injection and then reinjected. This final aspiration and injection clears the small amount of local anesthetic solution remaining in the hub of the needle.

Once the block has been performed, the infant is rapidly and carefully placed supine on the operating room table (Fig. 20-1). Tape is then placed across the legs to prevent them from being lifted up (for placement of the electrocautery pad), which may result in a total spinal block. When the electrocautery pad is placed on the infant's back, the entire infant should be lifted parallel to the table. The blood pressure cuff and pulse oximeter should be placed on a numb lower extremity to minimize stimulation of the conscious infant. Once the spinal block is completed, the anesthesiologist will know within several minutes if the block is successful when the infant's legs become limp. Conversely, if the infant's legs do not become limp within several minutes, the block was probably not successful. When this occurs we do not re-attempt the spinal. Rather, we proceed with general anesthesia for the case.

With a successful spinal block, the anesthesiologist is left with a conscious neonate who must be kept calm during the surgical procedure. Most infants will sleep during the procedure or rest quietly if offered a pacifier dipped in glucose water (Fig. 20-2). What is the course of action when the infant is inconsolable during the surgical procedure? Firstly, the anesthesiologist and surgeon should determine whether the surgical area is properly

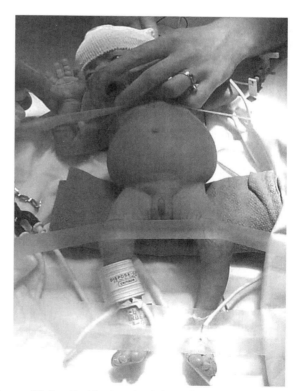

Figure 20-1 Positioning the infant after performing a spinal anesthetic. Tape is placed across the arms and legs to prevent movement and interference with the surgery. The blood pressure cuff and pulse oximeter probe are placed on the anesthetized lower extremities to limit intraoperative stimulation.

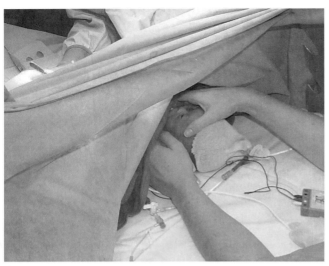

Figure 20-2   The conscious infant must be kept calm when using spinal anesthesia, especially during a hernia repair when crying will push the hernia sac into the wound and increase the difficulty of the surgical repair. This photo shows the anesthesiologist dripping steady amounts of glucose water onto the pacifier to keep the infant from crying during the procedure.

anesthetized. In some cases of a patchy block, the surgeon can administer local anesthesia into the wound with satisfactory results. However, if doubt remains, induction of general anesthesia is the most prudent action. If the infant is merely agitated without pain, and does not become consoled with small sugar-water feedings, the anesthesiologist's options for pharmacologic sedation are limited because the addition of sedative agents of any class will greatly increase the risk of intraoperative and postoperative apnea. One exception to this is the addition of modest concentrations (<50%) of N_2O. However, N_2O does not reliably sedate all infants. If additional sedation is required to complete the surgical procedure, it may be prudent to administer general anesthesia with endotracheal intubation or laryngeal mask airway (LMA) placement.

Complications from spinal anesthesia are not infrequent. Intra- and postoperative apnea, bradycardia, and hypoxemia may occur, necessitating immediate ventilatory assistance and possible atropine administration. A high spinal anesthesia will cause respiratory and neurological depression with rapid onset of hypoxemia. Therefore, the anesthesiologist must maintain vigilance during and after the administration of the spinal anesthetic. Hypotension from a spinal anesthetic-induced sympathetic block does not usually occur in children under the age of 8 years. This may be due to the relatively immature sympathetic nervous system in children compared with adults, or because of the relatively smaller intravascular volume in the lower extremities of children such that lower-extremity vasodilation does not reduce preload to an appreciable extent.

Epidural Anesthesia

Epidural anesthesia can be administered in a variety of ways in children. This decision will depend on the nature and duration of the surgical procedure. For ambulatory patients, a single dose of epidural anesthesia is administered, usually via the caudal canal. For hospitalized patients, whose pain is expected to be prolonged for more than a day, insertion of an epidural catheter will provide continuous postoperative analgesia. The epidural injection or catheter insertion should be ideally located at the level of the surgical incision. In infants, a thoracic epidural can be placed by threading an epidural catheter cephalad via the caudal canal (see below).

In children, epidural anesthesia is administered after the induction of general anesthesia. A commercially available adult epidural tray with a 17-gauge, 3.5-inch needle can be used even in small infants. However, several pediatric epidural kits are commercially available that contain 18- or 20-gauge Touhy or Weiss epidural needles. The Arrow Thera-Cath, contains a radiopaque epidural catheter, which is easily confirmed by routine x-ray examination without injecting contrast material.

Article To Know

Abajian JC, Mellish RWP, Browne AF et al: Spinal anesthesia for surgery in the high-risk infant. Anesth Analg 63:359–362, 1984.

Chris Abajian and his colleagues at the University of Vermont reported their series of spinal anesthetics in prematurely born infants undergoing hernia repair. Although spinal anesthesia for infants had been described many years before, this report served to reawaken the pediatric anesthesia community to the use of spinal anesthesia in infants at risk for postoperative apnea. In this series, spinal anesthesia was attempted in 78 infants for 81 procedures. Eight were unsuccessful after two attempts. The spinal solution consisted of hyperbaric 1% tetracaine in an approximate average dose of 0.25 mg/kg, less than most pediatric anesthesiologists use today. Fourteen infants required intraoperative supplementation with local anesthesia into the surgical field, or intravenous opioids when there was evidence of a patchy block. This report was the impetus for the accelerated use of spinal anesthesia in infants at risk for postoperative apnea following general anesthesia.

The choice of epidural analgesic medications includes a local anesthetic, an opioid, clonidine, or any combination of these. Almost all children will receive a local anesthetic and clonidine may be added in children over 1 year of age. Opioids will usually be used in hospitalized children over 1 year of age who are expected to have severe pain. More specific dosing regimens are discussed in subsequent sections of this chapter and in Chapter 26.

Side-effects and complications from epidural analgesia are the same for children as for adults. Common side-effects include motor blockade of the lower extremities and urinary retention. Relatively common complications include unintentional intravascular injection, and failure of the technique to work adequately. Local anesthesia toxicity from accidental intravascular injection is rare and manifests as seizures in an unanesthetized child or cardiac collapse in an anesthetized child. Additional rare complications include epidural hematoma, epidural abscess formation, intraneural trauma causing a residual neurologic deficit, and unintentional dural puncture with spinal blockade. Postdural puncture headache is rarely seen in children under 8 years of age.

Caudal Epidural Anesthesia

The most popular regional anesthesia technique in pediatric patients is the caudal epidural block, which is relatively easy to perform once the proper landmarks have been identified. It can be performed prior to surgery to be used in combination with general anesthesia, performed after surgery to be used for postoperative analgesia, or used instead of general anesthesia for low abdominal and lower-extremity procedures. A caudal epidural block is performed by placing the patient in the prone or lateral position. The important landmarks are the coccyx and the sacral hiatus located between the two sacral cornua (Fig. 20-3). A 22-gauge short-bevel needle is inserted 1–2 mm caudad from a point midway between the two

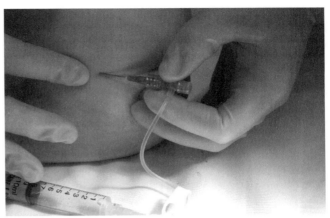

Figure 20-4   When performing a caudal block, the anesthesiologist stands on the opposite side of the OR table. The landmarks are identified with the index finger of the nondominant hand, which is then placed directly over the sacrococcygeal ligament. With the dominant hand, a skin nick is made with an 18-gauge needle and the epidural needle is then placed through this opening into the subcutaneous space. The index finger of the nondominant hand feels the tip of the epidural needle and guides it into the ligament. This finger is then kept in place over the back while local anesthetic solution is injected using a T-piece connector. Lack of subcutaneous swelling confirms proper placement of the needle into the epidural space.

cornua (Fig. 20-4). The needle is inserted at a 30–45 degree angle to the skin and advanced through the sacrococcygeal membrane. As the needle is advanced through the membrane and into the epidural space, a characteristic "pop" or loss of resistance is usually felt. Once the epidural space is entered, care is taken to avoid advancing the needle too far, as the dural sac may extend down as far as the S3 or S4 level in small infants (as opposed to S2 in adults), and an unintentional dural puncture may occur. Since ossification of the sacrum is not complete until adulthood, the epidural needle can be accidentally inserted into the sacrum without much resistance. Many pediatric anesthesiologists feel that a stylet should be used inside the epidural needle. Although many centers use unstyletted needles, they entail the theoretical risk of advancing a plug of dermal or subdermal tissue into the epidural space with the potential for the formation of a dermoid tumor. Some anesthesiologists prefer to make a small nick at the skin with an 18-gauge needle to serve as an entrance way for the block needle and to prevent tissue coring.

Prior to administration of the local anesthetic solution into the epidural space, the anesthesiologist should attempt to rule out unintentional placement of the catheter or needle into the intravascular or intrathecal space. Initially, the epidural catheter or needle is gently aspirated to detect blood or CSF. However, this test is not completely reliable owing to the high compliance of the epidural veins and intrathecal space in children, which collapses easily with even slight negative pressure.

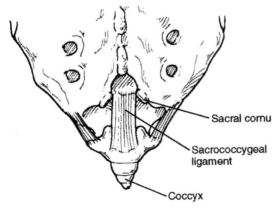

Figure 20-3   Anatomy of the sacrum and coccyx with identification of the sacrococcygeal membrane situated between the sacral cornua.

Although its efficacy is controversial in children, a test dose should then be administered to help detect intravascular placement of the epidural block. In children, the dose of epinephrine that consistently results in hemodynamic changes is 0.5 µg/kg. This translates into a test dose of 0.1 mL/kg of a local anesthetic solution that contains epinephrine, 1:200,000 (5 µg/mL). Sixty seconds is allowed to elapse to assess for intravascular or intraosseous injection. The latter may be particularly relevant in young children as the bones of the sacrum are not completely ossified and thus it is possible to unintentionally place the needle into the sacrum. Although the efficacy of the test dose has been questioned, especially if administered during the use of inhalational anesthetic agents, its reliability can be increased by observing the change in T-wave amplitude, the heart rate, and the blood pressure response. An increase in T-wave amplitude greater than 25% of baseline or increase in heart rate greater than 10 beats/min are indicative of an intravascular injection of epinephrine. Systolic blood pressure has been described to rise by 15 mmHg but is less reliable than heart rate or T-wave changes. Changes in any of these parameters indicate an unintentional vascular injection and the need to reposition the needle. If no response to the test dose is noted, the remainder of the calculated dose is administered over several minutes while the vital signs are continually monitored for evidence of intravascular injection.

A caudal epidural block can be achieved using any local anesthetic agent. The concentration and volume of the solution are usually determined by the height and density of the blockade required. The volume of local anesthetic determines the height of the block, which depends on the level of the surgical incision. Volumes of 1.2–1.5 mL/kg provide analgesia and anesthesia to the T4–T6 dermatome. Doses of 1 mL/kg will provide postoperative analgesia for inguinal procedures, while 0.5–0.75 mL/kg is sufficient for lower-extremity procedures. Dye studies have demonstrated cephalad spread of a caudally injected solution to range between T10 and L1. However, sensory testing demonstrates an anesthetic level that extends five segments higher. Regardless of the volume used, the concentration is adjusted to ensure that no more than 2.5 mg/kg of bupivacaine, ropivacaine, or levobupivacaine is used. With bupivacaine, the majority of experience is with the 0.25% solutions. However, effective postoperative analgesia can be achieved using a 0.125% solution, thereby limiting the total dose and decreasing the severity of motor block.

Caudal ropivacaine provides a faster onset of analgesia and less motor blockade than bupivacaine. A 0.2% solution of ropivacaine has been demonstrated to provide the best efficacy with the least amount of motor blockade. Although peak plasma concentrations of both bupivacaine and ropivacaine will be achieved 20–40 minutes after epidural administration, ropivacaine is

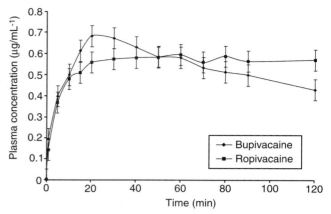

Figure 20-5   Mean (SD) venous plasma total ropivacaine and bupivacaine concentrations after caudal epidural administration of 2 mg/kg of ropivacaine 0.2% or bupivacaine 0.2% in children. Plasma concentrations of both agents peak at between 20 and 40 minutes following caudal administration. However, peak plasma concentrations of ropivacaine are less than equivalent doses of bupivacaine. (Reproduced with permission from Karmakar MK, Aun CS, Wong EL et al: Ropivacaine undergoes slower systemic absorption from the caudal epidural space in children than bupivacaine. *Anesth Analg* 94:259–265, 2002.)

absorbed into the systemic circulation more slowly than equivalent doses of bupivacaine (Fig. 20-5). Ropivacaine is less cardiotoxic than bupivacaine at equipotent plasma concentrations and it is being increasingly used by pediatric anesthesiologists for regional blockade.

Epinephrine can be added to the local anesthetic solution. Its vasoconstrictive properties will slightly prolong the duration of action of the sensory block and limit potentially rapid systemic absorption via epidural blood vessels. The addition of clonidine 1–2 µg/kg will enhance the quality and duration of postoperative analgesia when combined with epidural local anesthetics, and it is now routinely included in the epidural anesthetic solution in many pediatric centers. Epidural administration of the preservative-free S-isomer of ketamine also enhances the quality and duration of analgesia, but it is not currently used in many centers.

A caudal block is most often used in combination with general anesthesia, or to provide postoperative analgesia, but it may be also used as the sole anesthetic for the procedure in much the same manner as with spinal anesthesia as described above (Table 20-1). Various dosing regimens have been suggested when using a caudal epidural block for complete surgical anesthesia, with volumes ranging from 1 to 1.5 mL/kg and concentrations of bupivacaine from 0.25 to 0.375%. The higher volumes are required to provide a block to the T2 dermatome while the higher concentrations are needed to provide more reliable surgical anesthesia. Caution must be observed because the combination of high volume and high concentration can result in local anesthetic toxicity.

Table 20-1	Spinal versus Caudal Epidural Block for the Conscious Infant	
	Advantages	**Disadvantages**
Spinal anesthesia	Lower total dose of local anesthetic (1 mg/kg vs 3–4 mg/kg)	Limited duration of action (60–90 minutes)
	Definite end-point (aspiration of CSF)	Technically difficult in small infants
	Rapid onset	Potential for high block with change in position
	Dense sensory and motor block	
Caudal epidural	High rate of success	High dose of local anesthetic agents required
	Longer duration if catheter inserted	Slow onset of action
	Minimal change in level with change in position	Incomplete motor block

Because of the relatively long plasma elimination times of bupivacaine and levobupivacaine, toxicity may occur when repeated doses are administered for relatively long surgical procedures. To avoid this, some pediatric anesthesiologists use 2-chloroprocaine for continuous caudal anesthesia. Chloroprocaine is rapidly metabolized by plasma esterases (half-life <60 seconds). Therefore, there is a low risk of toxicity with its prolonged use. An initial bolus dose of 1.5–2.0 mL/kg of 3% 2-chloroprocaine is followed by a continuous infusion at 1.5–2.0 mL/kg/h. In one study, serum levels of 2-chloroprocaine were well below the toxic level (zero in the majority of patients) after 2–3 hours of continuous infusion. Additional advantages of 3% 2-chloroprocaine include a rapid onset of action and dense motor blockade.

Thoracic Epidural Analgesia via the Caudal Canal

Segmental anesthesia may be achieved with relatively smaller doses of local anesthetic when the epidural catheter tip is placed in the close vicinity of the spinal segment of the surgical incision. In anesthetized infants, direct thoracic epidural placement would entail the risk of spinal cord trauma. Therefore, when thoracic-level anesthesia is desired, a catheter can be advanced through the epidural space via the caudal canal to the desired level, based on an approximate measurement just prior to the procedure. Minor resistance may be encountered, but the catheter should advance relatively easily. If it does not, it is not positioned correctly. Even when it advances easily, there is a high incidence of malpositioning due to coiling of the catheter within the epidural space. This problem can be minimized by utilizing a styletted catheter, at the expense of a higher incidence of unintentional intravascular and subarachnoid penetration. Once the catheter is thought to be positioned correctly, we inject a small amount of nonionic radiographic contrast (Iohexol–Omnipaque-180) while simultaneously obtaining a radiograph of the chest and abdomen to identify the tip of the level of the catheter and to confirm appropriate placement in the epidural space (Fig. 20-6).

Direct Lumbar or Thoracic Epidural Analgesia

Direct lumbar or thoracic epidural catheter placement in children differs from that in adults. The first major difference is that the distance from the skin to the epidural space is less in children. A rough estimate for the lumbar level is 1 mm of distance for each kilogram of weight between the ages of 6 months and 10 years. The second major difference is that children have a much softer ligamentum flavum than adults. Thus, it is more difficult to identify with certainty during epidural needle placement. An important consequence of these two differences is that unintentional dural punctures are more likely in children than adults. Therefore, the epidural space is approached with caution. The loss-of-resistance technique should be started no greater than

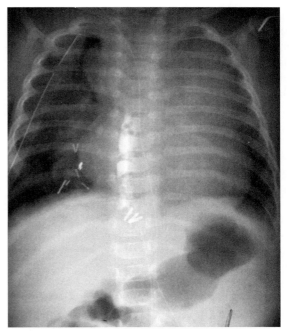

Figure 20-6 Radiograph demonstrating localization of the tip of a thoracic epidural catheter that has been threaded up from the caudal canal. Note the exit of metrizamide dye from the tip of the catheter and the characteristic pattern of the spread of dye into the epidural space.

2 cm beneath the skin, and the needle should be advanced extremely slowly until the epidural space is identified. A small skin nick is made at the site before placing the epidural needle so that the pressure required to advance the epidural needle through the skin does not cause the needle to advance too far and puncture the dura. The loss-of-resistance technique with normal saline is used to identify passage of the needle into the epidural space. Recent evidence suggests that saline is preferred to air because of the possibility of a patchy block if air is injected along a nerve root, and the possibility of a venous air embolus if the needle is situated within an epidural vein. Once the space is identified, an epidural catheter is threaded so that 2-4 cm remain in the epidural space. The catheter is then hung below the level of the heart to look for the outflow of CSF or blood through the catheter. Gentle aspiration for blood or CSF is then performed before local anesthetics are administered. A test dose is given through the catheter using the same diagnostic criteria as described above in the section on caudal block. The initial bolus dose of local anesthesia depends on the level of catheter placement. When the catheter is placed as an adjunct to general anesthesia, 0.25% bupivacaine or 0.2% ropivacaine is used. Suggested starting guidelines for dosing include an initial bolus dose of 0.3 mL/kg (maximum 12 mL) for thoracic epidural placement and 0.5 mL/kg (maximum 15 mL) for lumbar placement.

Complications of epidural catheter placement and analgesia include dural puncture, infection, epidural hematoma, and abscess formation. This technique is contraindicated in children with a coagulopathy (platelet count <100,000/mm^3 or prothrombin time (PT) or partial thromboplastin time (PTT) >1.5 times control) or qualitative bleeding dysfunction (e.g., hemophilia or von Willebrand's disease). Symptoms of epidural hematoma formation include neurologic deficits and back pain.

Neuraxial Opioids

A single administration of a local anesthetic alone may provide up to 12 hours of postoperative analgesia, but in many cases a more prolonged duration of analgesia is required without placing an indwelling catheter. Furthermore, the transient motor blockade that results from administration of local anesthetics is undesirable in some patients. These are indications for administration of opioids into the spinal or epidural space. Unlike local anesthetics, opioids affect sensory neurons without affecting motor or sympathetic function. When used in combination with local anesthetics, there is a synergistic effect with an increase in the duration of the regional anesthetic and an improvement in the quality of analgesia while allowing the use of more dilute solutions of local anesthetics. Thus, inclusion of opioids may lessen the potential for local anesthetic toxicity and side-effects, such as motor blockade.

Intrathecal morphine (5-10 μg/kg per dose) is used to provide prolonged (12-24 hours) postoperative analgesia. Because of its hydrophilic nature, morphine tends to stay within the CSF and travel cephalad to the brain. As a result, caudal or lumbar administration may be used to provide analgesia for thoracic or even craniofacial procedures. It is best administered before the beginning of the surgical procedure since the onset of action is 20-60 minutes. Fentanyl is usually not administered intrathecally because of its short duration of action.

Opioids can also be administered into the epidural space. Since fentanyl is lipophilic, it is rapidly absorbed into the systemic circulation and is no more advantageous than intravenous administration. Therefore, morphine is most commonly administered epidurally. Dose ranging studies in children have demonstrated that 0.03-0.05 mg/kg of epidural morphine provides the best balance between sufficient analgesia and lack of significant respiratory depression.

The most important adverse effect associated with neuraxial opioids is respiratory depression. This is particularly true for morphine since significant concentrations persist in the CSF for up to 24 hours after administration. Delayed respiratory depression is associated with administration of rescue doses of parenteral morphine within 24 hours of the initial epidural morphine dose. When it becomes necessary to use parenteral opioids in children who have received neuraxial opioids, a mixed agonist-antagonist, such as butorphanol or nalbuphine, may have less effect on respiratory function than a pure agonist, such as morphine.

Additional side-effects related to neuraxial opioids include pruritus, nausea, vomiting, and urinary retention. Pruritus tends to be more common with intrathecal morphine, again related to central spread within the CSF. Although the patient may be pain-free, there may be significant distress from the pruritus, requiring treatment with diphenhydramine or a low-dose naloxone infusion. The latter can be used to treat pruritus without diminishing the quality of analgesia. The combination of morphine 30-50 μg/kg and butorphanol 20-30 μg/kg may decrease the incidence of adverse effects when compared to morphine alone.

All patients who receive neuraxial opioids require postoperative respiratory monitoring and are not candidates for home discharge on the day of surgery. In the past, children who had received neuraxial opioids were sent to the pediatric intensive care unit, but with proper training of the nursing staff on regular hospital wards, these children should not require ICU admission. Monitoring should include pulse oximetry when the child is asleep with an evaluation of respiratory rate every 2 hours and sedation scores every 6 hours. With these parameters, changes in respiratory status and increased sedation can be detected early with appropriate intervention.

Monitoring should be continued for 24 hours after neuraxial morphine because of the possibility of delayed respiratory depression.

PERIPHERAL NERVE BLOCKS

Use of peripheral nerve blocks in pediatric anesthesia is an effective way to decrease the side-effects and complications associated with central blocks. When performing a peripheral block in an anesthetized child, a nerve stimulator should be used. This requires avoidance or reversal of neuromuscular blocking agents. The negative electrode attaches to the insulated needle, the positive electrode attaches to the patient using a standard ECG pad, and the nerve stimulator is set to the low-output setting (0.5–1 mA). The needle is then advanced until a motor response is noted in the desired muscle group of the extremity to be anesthetized. The voltage is turned down to 0.2–0.4 mA and a continuing motor response confirms that the needle is in close proximity to the nerve to be anesthetized prior to injecting the local anesthetic. The use of a nerve stimulator, however, theoretically increases the risk of intraneural placement of the tip of the needle. Therefore, when first injecting local anesthetic, a small syringe should initially be used, and any unexplained resistance should warrant adjustment of the needle position.

Regional Anesthesia of the Upper Extremity

Axillary Approach to the Brachial Plexus

The most commonly used method for brachial plexus anesthesia in children is the axillary block. The patient's arm is abducted 90 degrees from the body and the elbow is flexed so that the hand is over the head or behind it. The block is performed using a transarterial, one-injection, or two-injection technique. For the transarterial approach, the artery is fixed against the humerus and a 22- or 25-gauge needle is inserted 1–2 cm away from the axilla, at a 60- to 90-degree angle to the skin, directed toward the arterial pulsation. Constant aspiration is maintained on the plunger of the syringe as it is advanced into the artery. The needle is advanced through the artery until blood is no longer aspirated. One-half of the local anesthetic solution is injected posterior to the artery. The needle is then withdrawn back through the artery until there is no longer blood return and the other half of the local anesthetic is administered in front of the artery. The advantage of this technique is successful blockade of the posterior cord of the brachial plexus which gives rise to the radial nerve. The axillary technique is also a better choice for providing anesthesia of the ulnar nerve, a branch of the inferior trunk of the brachial plexus, which

may be missed with the interscalene approach. However, with the axillary approach, the musculocutaneous nerve is usually missed. A separate musculocutaneous block can be performed through the same needle insertion site as the axillary block, by injecting part of the local anesthetic solution into the body of the coracobrachialis muscle.

An axillary block can also be performed without puncturing the axillary artery. In the one-injection technique, the needle is advanced at an angle of 60–90 degrees to the skin and directed toward the axillary sheath, which is felt manually. As the fascia is pierced, a loss of resistance is felt or an appropriate twitch noted in a distal muscle group if the nerve stimulator is used, and the entire volume of local anesthetic is injected. If a two-injection technique is used, half of the local anesthetic solution is injected and a second needle is positioned more distally and the remainder of the local anesthetic solution injected. If a tourniquet is required for the surgical procedure, a ring of local anesthetic solution can be injected around the proximal medial aspect of the upper part of the arm to anesthetize the intercostobrachial branch of T2.

The total dose of local anesthetic administered into the axillary sheath should equal 1 mL/kg of 0.25% bupivacaine, 0.25% levobupivacaine, or 0.2% ropivacaine up to a maximum of 30 mL, or 0.5 mL/kg of 0.5% bupivacaine, 0.5% levobupivacaine, or 0.3% ropivacaine up to a maximum of 15 mL.

A continuous axillary infusion is accomplished by placing a catheter into the axillary sheath using a catheter-through-a-needle technique or an over-a-wire technique. Several manufacturers make insulated Tuohy needles for use with a nerve stimulator. These kits also have catheters that can be placed through the Tuohy needle. Alternatively, the Seldinger technique can be performed using a single-lumen, 3-French, 5- or 8-cm central line catheter. The 0.018-inch wire included in the kit will pass through a 22-gauge needle and a 0.021-inch wire will pass through a 20-gauge needle. A continuous infusion provides analgesia or sympathetic blockade as adjunctive treatment for distal extremity vascular compromise (e.g., reattachment of severed digits).

Interscalene Approach to the Brachial Plexus

The interscalene approach to the brachial plexus provides anesthesia of the entire upper extremity including the shoulder but is used less frequently in children because of a perceived higher incidence of complications such as pneumothorax. The point of needle insertion is the transection of a horizontal line drawn from the cricoid cartilage to the posterior border of the sternocleidomastoid (SCM) muscle. The interscalene approach anesthetizes the trunks of the brachial plexus as they pass between the anterior and middle scalene muscles. As the trunks of the brachial plexus are organized in a superior to inferior direction, the lower dermatomes of the brachial plexus (C8–T1) are less effectively blocked than with an axillary approach. Therefore, there may be less effective analgesia over the distribution of the ulnar nerve. However, the interscalene approach effectively blocks the musculocutaneous nerve.

A novel approach to the brachial plexus of children was described based on cadaveric evaluation of the anatomy of the neck, and termed a "parascalene" block. It was developed with the goal of finding a needle pathway into the neck that would not injure delicate structures in an anesthetized child. The child is placed supine with a towel roll placed under the shoulders and the head turned away from the side of the block. The landmarks are (1) the midpoint of the upper border of the clavicle, and (2) Chassaignac's tubercle (the transverse process of C6). The latter is identified either by palpation (which can be quite painful in the awake state) or by extending a line from the cricoid ring to the posterior border of the SCM. A line is drawn from Chassaignac's tubercle to the midpoint of the clavicle (Fig. 20-7A). The point of needle insertion is the junction of the upper two-thirds and lower one-third of this line (Fig. 20-7B). An insulated needle is inserted at a 90-degree angle to the skin and advanced until a motor response is noted in the distal upper extremity. The distance from the skin usually ranges from 7 to 30 mm depending on the patient's size. If no response is obtained, the needle is withdrawn and directed more laterally. In the initial reported series ($n = 60$), the brachial plexus was identified on the first or second attempt in 100% of patients and resulted in complete surgical anesthesia in 97%. Local anesthetic solutions used for this block include 0.25% or 0.5% bupivacaine up to 2 mg/kg, 0.2% or 0.3% ropivacaine up to 3 mg/kg, and 1% or 2% lidocaine up to 5 mg/kg. Complications include recurrent laryngeal nerve block, accidental vein puncture, and Horner's syndrome.

Regional Anesthesia of the Lower Extremity

Femoral Nerve, Lateral Femoral Cutaneous Nerve, 3-in-1 Block

The anterior portions of the proximal lower limb and knee are innervated by the femoral, obturator, and lateral femoral cutaneous nerves. The femoral nerve can be anesthetized inferior to the inguinal ligament. While the technique allows direct access to the femoral nerve as it passes under the inguinal ligament, the lateral femoral cutaneous and the obturator nerves are not in the immediate vicinity. As the obturator nerve is a deep structure, isolated blockade is not generally attempted. When obturator nerve anesthesia is required, a fascia iliaca block (see below) is used. Blockade of the lateral femoral cutaneous nerve can be accomplished separately and is frequently combined with a femoral nerve block to anesthetize the lateral aspect of the thigh.

To provide anesthesia to all three nerves, a 3-in-1 block is used. This technique utilizes the fascial sheath that surrounds the femoral nerve as a conduit for local anesthetic to travel proximally to the lumbar plexus and anesthetize the lateral femoral cutaneous and obturator nerves.

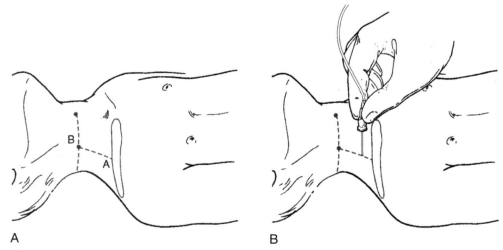

A   B

Figure 20-7 Modification of the interscalene approach to the brachial plexus, also known as the parascalene approach. **A,** The landmarks include the midpoint of the upper border of the clavicle, and Chassaignac's tubercle (the transverse process of C6). The latter is identified either by palpation or by extending a line from the cricoid to the posterior border of the SCM muscle. A line is drawn from Chassaignac's tubercle down to the midpoint of the clavicle. **B,** The point of needle insertion, at an angle of 90 degrees to the skin, is the junction of the upper two-thirds and lower one-third of this line.

A larger volume of local anesthetic than is used for isolated femoral nerve blockade is administered while holding pressure distal to the site of injection. Aside from these two modifications, the technique is the same as an isolated femoral nerve block. The needle is inserted lateral to the femoral artery, 1–2 cm below the inguinal ligament, and advanced at a 45-degree angle in a cephalad direction. As the fascia lata and fascia iliaca are penetrated, a double loss of resistance will be felt. Contraction of the quadriceps muscle can be elicited using an insulated needle with a nerve stimulator. Dosing regimens include 1 mL/kg of 0.25% bupivacaine or 0.5 mL/kg of 0.5% bupivacaine, to a maximum of 40 mL or 2 mg/kg, whichever is less. Ropivacaine can also be used up to 40 mL or 3 mg/kg, whichever is less.

Fascia Iliaca Block

The fascia iliaca block is a modification of the femoral nerve block. At a point that marks the junction of the outer and middle third of a line connecting the symphysis pubis and the anterior superior iliac crest, a perpendicular line is dropped to a point 1–2 cm below the inguinal ligament (Fig. 20-8). This point is at least 2–3 cm lateral to the femoral artery. Injection of local anesthetic solution will spread medially to the femoral nerve and superiorly to anesthetize the obturator and lateral femoral cutaneous nerves. Since the technique is performed several centimeters from the femoral nerve, a nerve stimulator is not used, and unintentional damage to the femoral nerve is minimized.

Penile Block

A penile block provides anesthesia and analgesia for procedures involving the distal penis, such as circumcision, or hypospadias repair. The distal end of the penis is innervated by the dorsal penile nerves, which branch off the pudendal nerve (S2–S4) at the base of the penis and run along the dorsal side, deep to Buck's fascia (Fig. 20-9). These nerves can be anesthetized by injecting 1–2 mL of local anesthetic solution below the deep fascia at the base of the penis at the 2- and 10-o'clock positions. This is commonly referred to as a dorsal penile nerve block (DPNB). Complications of DPNB include subcutaneous hematoma at the site of injection (fairly common), and, rarely, arterial injection.

Alternatively, a penile block can be accomplished with one injection into the subpubic space, which contains the pudendal nerve as it exits from beneath the pubic bone (Fig. 20-10A). The base of the penis is gently stretched downward with one hand while the block needle is advanced along the caudal edge of the pubic bone in the midline (Fig. 20-10B). Initially, a "give" is felt as the needle pierces the superficial fascial layer. The needle is further advanced until another less distinct give is felt as the needle pierces Scarpa's fascia and enters the subpubic space. After gentle aspiration to rule out an intravascular injection, 3 mL of 0.5% bupivacaine is injected. Occasionally a small subcutaneous hematoma will develop but no other complications from this block have been reported.

Local infiltration of the penis is distinguished from a specific nerve block and is traditionally referred to as a ring block (Fig. 20-11). Between 2 and 3 mL of local anesthetic solution are injected below the deep fascial level at the base of the penis in a circumferential fashion. Practitioners who prefer the ring block over the DPNB cite the inconsistent anatomical location of the dorsal penile nerves.

The most common local anesthetics used for injection or infiltration are lidocaine (1% or 2%) and bupivacaine (0.25% or 0.5%). These solutions should not contain

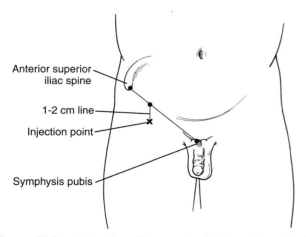

Figure 20-8 Point of needle entry for the fascia iliaca block. A perpendicular line is drawn inferiorly from the junction of the outer (lateral) and middle third of the line connecting the tubercle of the symphysis pubis and the anterior superior iliac crest. The needle is inserted at a point 1–2 cm below the inguinal ligament.

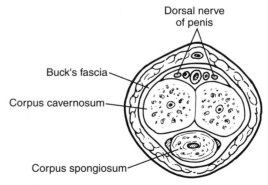

Figure 20-9 Cross-section at the base of the penis. The dorsal penile nerves that originate from the pudendal nerve are usually located at the 2- and 10-o'clock positions and provide sensory innervation to the distal penis. (Redrawn with permission from Litman RS: Anesthesia and analgesia for newborn circumcision. *Obstet Gyne Survey* 56:114–117, 2001.)

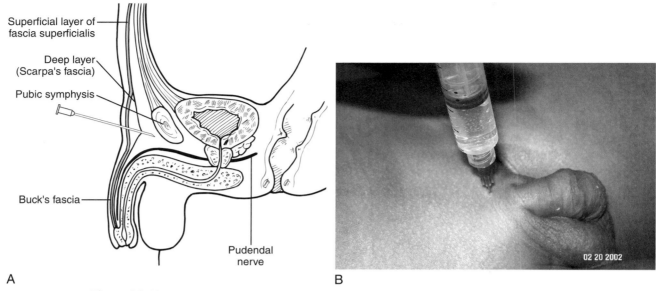

A

B

Figure 20-10   **A**, Drawing of anesthesia of the pudendal nerve by placement of a subpubic space block. **B**, Demonstration of placement of the subpubic space block. (Drawing reproduced with permission from Litman RS: Anesthesia and analgesia for newborn circumcision. *Obstet Gyne Survey* 56:114–117, 2001.)

epinephrine because of the risk of end-arterial vasoconstriction.

Ilioinguinal/Iliohypogastric (Hernia) Block

The ilioinguinal and iliohypogastric nerves originate from the lower thoracic and upper lumbar plexus and travel caudally along the lateral portion of the abdomen between the transversus abdominis and the internal oblique muscles. These nerves provide innervation to the superficial tissues overlying the inguinal ligament and proximal scrotum (Fig. 20-12A), and thus provide analgesia and anesthesia for inguinal procedures. A single injection of local anesthetic is administered 1 cm medial to the anterior superior iliac spine (Fig. 20-12B). The needle is

advanced at a 90-degree angle to the skin and advanced slowly until the deep muscular layer is felt. If the muscular layer is not felt, the needle is advanced until it contacts the ilium and is then withdrawn 1 mm. The local anesthesia solution is injected with the goal of saturating the nerves within the muscle layers. This is accomplished by injecting half the amount of local anesthesia solution while slowly withdrawing the needle. Without removing the needle entirely, the remaining half of the anesthetic solution is injected in a fan-like manner in a medial and caudad direction. For this block, we typically use 1 mL/kg of 0.25% bupivacaine or 0.2% ropivacaine with or without epinephrine.

PHARMACOLOGY OF LOCAL ANESTHETICS IN CHILDREN

There are several clinically relevant differences in local anesthetic pharmacology between children and adults. Local anesthetic metabolism is affected by age, especially in the premature infant and neonate where the hepatic microsomal enzyme system is not fully developed. Protein binding of local anesthetics is decreased owing to the low quantities of albumin and α_1-acid glycoprotein made in the liver during early infancy. This will result in an increased plasma free fraction of the drug, and an increased risk of local anesthetic toxicity. The time it takes for the drug to be absorbed is also a consideration since a rapid rise of the serum concentration is more likely to result in toxicity.

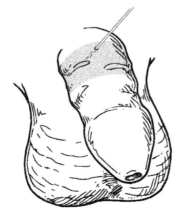

Figure 20-11   Ring block of the penis. (Redrawn with permission from Litman RS: Anesthesia and analgesia for newborn circumcision. *Obstet Gyne Survey* 56:114–117, 2001.)

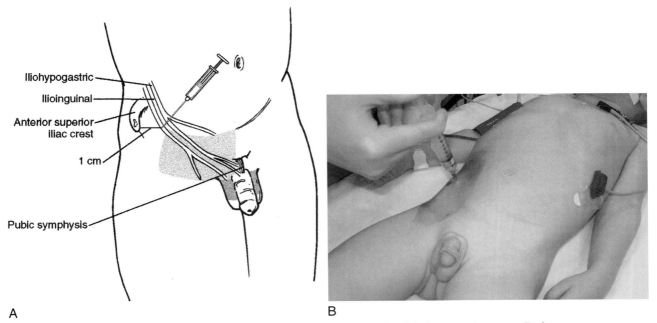

Figure 20-12 **A**, Drawing of innervation of the ilioinguinal and iliohypogastric nerves. (Redrawn with permission from Yaster M, Maxwell LG: Pediatric regional anesthesia. *Anesthesiology* 70:324–338, 1989.) **B**, Administration of an ilioinguinal/iliohypogastric block.

Cardiac output and local blood flow of infants are relatively greater than in adults. Therefore, systemic absorption of local anesthetics is relatively faster in children, as are peak plasma concentrations. Addition of a vasoconstrictor, such as epinephrine, can retard the absorption rate and lower the peak serum concentration by 10–20%.

Anatomical differences between children and adults can affect local anesthetic pharmacology. The fat within the epidural space is sparse and loose in infants. Furthermore, the perineurovascular sheaths that are located around nerve roots and bundles are more loosely attached to underlying structures in children than in adults. It is for these reasons that injected local anesthetics appear to spread more in children, and cover a greater area of innervation. In addition, the endoneurium is relatively loose in young children and allows rapid exposure of the local anesthetic to the nerve. Thus, onset of anesthesia is relatively more rapid than in adults.

With the use of any local anesthetic, regardless of the concentration of the solution, the anesthesiologist must calculate the total milligram dose on a per-kilogram basis to avoid toxic blood levels by administering less than recommended maximum doses (Table 20-2). This is especially important in neonates and small infants. For example, if bupivacaine is used for a caudal anesthetic in a 3-kg baby, the *maximum* dose that should be used is 2.5 mg/kg × 3 kg = 7.5 mg. A 0.25% solution of bupivacaine has 2.5 mg/mL, so a *maximum* of 3.0 mL of the solution should be used. Even with extreme caution and

careful calculation of doses, local anesthetic toxicity can occur.

In summary, the interest in and applications of regional anesthesia in children continue to increase. These techniques may be used to provide an alternative to general anesthesia, an adjunct to general anesthesia, or postoperative analgesia. Any regional anesthetic technique used in the adult population can theoretically be used in the pediatric-aged patient. Given the potential for toxicity, careful calculation of local anesthetic doses (initial bolus dose and continuous infusion) is mandatory.

Table 20-2	Maximum Recommended Doses of Local Anesthetics[a,b]
Local Anesthetic	**Maximum Recommended Dose (mg/kg)**
2-Chloroprocaine	20
Tetracaine	1.5
Lidocaine	7
Mepivacaine	7
Bupivacaine	2.5
Ropivacaine	3.5[c]

[a] Doses should be reduced by at least 30% in infants <3 months of age.
[b] These maximum doses apply to anesthetized children. Doses are reduced in conscious children.
[c] Definitive data are lacking for the maximum dose of ropivacaine.

Article To Know

Giaufre E, Dalens B, Gombert A: Epidemiology and morbidity of regional anesthesia in children: a one-year prospective survey of the French-language society of pediatric anesthesiologists. Anesth Analg 83:904–912, 1996.

This prospective study describes the complications of over 24,000 regional anesthesia techniques in a 1-year period in France. Of approximately 15,000 central blocks (mostly caudal epidurals) performed, there were 23 complications in 22 patients (Table 20-3). Dural puncture, the most common complication, caused total spinal anesthesia in four patients who received intrathecal administration of local anesthetic. Postdural puncture headache occurred in two patients. Intravascular injections were the next most common complication and resulted in immediate seizures in two children and transient cardiac arrhythmias in two children. Two developed delayed cardiac arrhythmias related to systemic absorption of local anesthetic. There were no complications in approximately 9,000 peripheral nerve blocks. The authors suggested that this extremely low incidence of complications after peripheral blocks should encourage more anesthesiologists to use them more often in place of a central block.

Table 20-3

Complications	Spinals (*n*=506)	Caudals (*n*=15,013)	Lumbar Epidurals (*n*=2,396)	Sacral Epidurals (*n*=293)	Thoracic Epidurals (*n*=135)	Peripheral Nerve Blocks and Local Anesthesia (*n*=9,396)	Totals (*n*=24,409)
Dural penetration	0	4	2	2	0	0	8
Uncomplicated	0	0	1	1	0		2
Postdural headaches	0	0	1	1	0		2
Spinal anesthesia	0	4	0	0	0		4
Intravascular injection	1	2	3	0	0	0	6
No clinical effects	1	0	1	0	0		2
Convulsions	0	1	1	0	0		2
Cardiac arrhythmia	0	1	1	0	0		2
Technical problem	0	2	1	0	0	0	3
Delayed installation	0	1	0	0	0		1
Rectal penetration	0	1	0	0	0		1
Catheter knotting	0	0	1	0	0		1
Overdose with cardia arrhythmia	0	1	1	0	0	0	2
Transient paresthesia	0	0	2	0	0	0	2
Postmorphine apnea	0	1	0	0	0	0	1
Skin lesion	0	1	0	0	0	0	1
Morbidity rate (per 1,000)	1 (2.0)	11 (0.7)	9 (3.7)	2 (6.8)	0 (0.0)	0 (0.0)	23 (0.9)

Reproduced with permission from Giaufre et al: *Anesth Analg* 83:904–912, 1996.

Despite the limited use of some of these techniques when compared with the adult population, the reports in the literature demonstrate that these techniques are effective. Ongoing clinical investigations with these techniques are needed to determine optimal dosing regimens and the most effective drug combinations, and to refine these techniques in smaller patients.

ADDITIONAL ARTICLES TO KNOW

Dalens B, Vanneuville G, Tanguy A: A new parascalene approach to the brachial plexus in children: comparison with the supraclavicular approach. *Anesth Analg* 66:1264–1271, 1987.

Dalens B, Vanneuville G, Tanguy A: Comparison of the fascia iliaca compartment block with the 3-in-1 block in children. *Anesth Analg* 69:705–713, 1989.

Doyle E, Morton NS, McNicol LR: Plasma bupivacaine levels after fascia iliaca compartment block with and without adrenaline. *Paediatr Anaesth* 7:121–124, 1997.

Fisher WJ, Bingham RM, Hall R: Axillary brachial plexus block for perioperative analgesia in 250 children. *Paediatr Anaesth* 9:435–438, 1999.

Kinder Ross A, Eck JB, Tobias JD: Pediatric regional anesthesia: beyond the caudal. *Anesth Analg* 91:16–26, 2000.

Nichols DG, Yaster M, Lynn AM et al: Disposition and respiratory effects of intrathecal morphine in children. *Anesthesiology* 79:733–738, 1993.

Paut O, Sallabery M, Schreiber-Deturmeny E et al: Continuous fascia iliaca compartment block in children: a prospective evaluation of plasma bupivacaine concentrations, pain scores, and side effects. *Anesth Analg* 92:1159–1163, 2001.

Tobias JD: Spinal anesthesia in infants and children. *Paediatr Anaesth* 10:5–16, 2000.

Tobias JD: Brachial plexus anaesthesia in children. *Paediatr Anaesth* 11:265–275, 2001.

Tobias JD: Caudal epidural block: a review of test dosing and recognition of systemic injection in children. *Anesth Analg* 93:1156–1161, 2001.

Tobias JD: Regional anaesthesia of the lower extremity in infants and children. *Paediatr Anaesth* 13:152–163, 2003.

Tobias JD, Mencio GA: Popliteal fossa block for postoperative analgesia after foot surgery in infants and children. *J Pediatr Ortho* 19:511–514, 1999.

Tobias JD, Ramsmussen GE, Holcomb GW et al: Continuous caudal anaesthesia with chloroprocaine as an adjunct to general anaesthesia in neonates. *Can J Anaesth* 43:69–72, 1996.

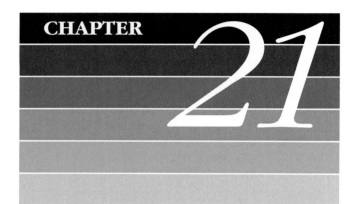

CHAPTER 21

Malignant Hyperthermia

MARY C. THEROUX

Pathophysiology
Children at Risk for Malignant Hyperthermia
Clinical Features and Diagnosis
Treatment of Malignant Hyperthermia
Anesthesia for an MH-susceptible Patient
Malignant Hyperthermia Variants
    Aborted or Subclinical Malignant Hyperthermia
    Masseter Spasm
    Nonanesthetic Malignant Hyperthermia
Malignant Hyperthermia Testing
    Caffeine–Halothane Contracture Test
    Malignant Hyperthermia Association of the United States (MHAUS)
    and the North American Malignant Hyperthermia Registry

In 1960, Denborough and Lovell first described the condition now known as malignant hyperthermia (MH), a potentially fatal disorder of skeletal muscle that manifests as a hypermetabolic crisis in susceptible individuals, and is largely inherited as an autosomal dominant trait. Because MH is considered a dominantly inherited disorder, all first-degree members of a family in which MH has occurred must also be considered MH-susceptible and managed accordingly, unless proven otherwise. It should be noted that those who have had previous anesthetics without problem cannot be certain they are not at risk, because deaths have occurred even though patients have undergone multiple prior uneventful surgeries.

Malignant hyperthermia follows exposure to an inhalational anesthetic or a depolarizing muscle relaxant (e.g., succinylcholine). *There are no other triggering agents*. The incidence might be higher in children (1 in 15,000) than in adults (1 in 50,000). However, these estimates are taken from old data, when succinylcholine was routinely used, and in an era of less sophisticated MH susceptibility testing. Therefore, the true incidence in both adults and children is unknown.

PATHOPHYSIOLOGY

Susceptibility to malignant hyperthermia is conferred by a genetically altered receptor that controls calcium homeostasis within the muscle cell. Over forty such distinct mutations have been found, the most common in genes that code for the ryanodine and dihydropyridine receptors. However, these known mutations account for less than 50% of families.

Gronert described malignant hyperthermia as "a subclinical primary myopathy with secondary systemic pathophysiology; the systemic consequences are marked because MH affects the muscles, which comprise 40% of one's body mass." Normally, muscle cell depolarization leads to the release of calcium from the sarcoplasmic reticulum of the myocyte. When the released calcium combines with troponin, cross-bridges are formed between actin and myosin filaments, leading to muscle contraction. When the depolarization is complete, reuptake of calcium into the sarcoplasmic reticulum causes muscle cell relaxation. The cellular defect associated with malignant hyperthermia renders an individual incapable of this calcium reuptake when he or she is exposed to an anesthetic triggering agent. Calcium then accumulates within the myocyte causing muscular rigidity and a cascade of hypermetabolic reactions that result from unregulated glycolysis and aerobic metabolism. This latter phenomenon results in massive heat production, generation of excess CO_2, and oxygen depletion. Eventual cell death and rhabdomyolysis causes metabolic acidosis, hyperkalemia, and release of myoglobin. Renal damage occurs when large amounts of filtered myoglobin precipitate within the renal tubules and cause obstruction of urine formation and subsequent renal tissue damage.

CHILDREN AT RISK FOR MALIGNANT HYPERTHERMIA

MH-susceptible children are best identified from the preanesthetic history. A previous episode of MH in the patient or a first-degree relative is the most reliable predictor. If this is the case, the anesthesiologist should inquire if a diagnostic muscle biopsy with a caffeine–halothane contracture test was performed (see below). If the biopsy was positive for susceptibility to malignant hyperthermia, the patient is considered MH-susceptible. Unfortunately, most patients and their family members have not undergone biopsy testing. Most often the preanesthetic history reveals a nonspecific episode of anesthetic-related fever or severe illness in a relative, for which the parents have no further information. The record of the anesthetic in question should be reviewed but is usually not available. The anesthesiologist must then decide whether the patient is indeed at risk for malignant hyperthermia, and the type of anesthetic technique to perform. When unsure, many anesthesiologists will conduct an anesthetic devoid of triggering agents. Others may provide this technique only when compelling evidence exists that the patient is MH-susceptible. Many children with a gene defect causing MH-susceptibility will not develop an episode after exposure to a triggering agent. Approximately 50% of MH-susceptible children will have received a triggering agent without developing the acute clinical disease.

Muscle diseases are possibly associated with susceptibility to malignant hyperthermia, but central core myopathy (CCM) is the only entity that possesses a definite genetic link to MH (see also Chapter 5). Other congenital myopathies, such as Duchenne's muscular dystrophy, or myotonic dystrophy have been loosely associated with malignant hyperthermia susceptibility without definitive evidence. However, intracellular calcium abnormalities may exist in these conditions. Exposure to a triggering agent may induce a clinical scenario very similar to the clinical manifestations of malignant hyperthermia. Therefore, many pediatric anesthesiologists will avoid triggering agents in children with a congenital myopathy.

The vast majority of malignant hyperthermia episodes occur in otherwise healthy patients who were not previously known to be at risk for this condition. Resting plasma levels of creatine kinase are elevated in about 70% of MH-susceptible individuals. Yet, this preoperative test is not routinely performed in healthy children.

CLINICAL FEATURES AND DIAGNOSIS

There are no specific clinical signs that positively identify the onset of MH. Common presenting signs are those that are consistent with the onset of a hypermetabolic state (Table 21-1). These include tachycardia, hypertension, and an increase in the production of carbon dioxide, which is manifested as an increase in end-tidal CO_2. Hyperthermia will usually occur but may not be an early sign. Muscle rigidity, despite use of a neuromuscular blocker, is a strongly specific indicator of malignant hyperthermia when other signs are also present, and is almost considered pathognomonic for the disease. Additional findings may include skin mottling, and a brownish discoloration of the urine if myoglobinuria is present. Malignant hyperthermia should be strongly suspected when there is an unanticipated significant increase (two or three times normal) of end-tidal CO_2 that responds only to a very large increase in minute ventilation. This increase may be sudden or may develop gradually over one or two hours. Between patients, there are large variations in the intervals between exposure to a triggering agent and development of symptoms, and the time for the progression of these initial findings into a fulminant life-threatening crisis. The reasons for this are unknown. Presentation of malignant hyperthermia in the postoperative period has been reported, but it is extremely rare beyond the immediate anesthetic period.

A very common scenario, especially in children, is an increase in end-tidal CO_2 that merely represents hypoventilation, and responds to normalization of minute ventilation. This is commonly observed during conditions of bronchospasm, accumulation of endotracheal tube secretions, and bronchial intubation, among many others.

If malignant hyperthermia is suspected, dantrolene should be administered only after confirmation of a mixed metabolic and respiratory acidosis by arterial blood gas analysis without any other explanation. It is also appropriate to begin dantrolene therapy if blood gas analysis cannot be obtained within a reasonable period of time, and the suspicion of MH is high based on clinical signs. Electrolytes and plasma creatine kinase should also be obtained. Unexpected hyperkalemia further

Table 21-1	Clinical Findings Associated with MH
Clinical Signs	**Laboratory Findings**
Hypercarbia	Increased $PaCO_2$
Tachycardia	Decreased pH
Markedly increased minute ventilation	Decreased PaO_2
	Hyperkalemia
Muscle rigidity	Increased CK
Skin mottling	Myoglobin in blood or urine
Hyperthermia	Abnormal coagulation tests
Cola-colored urine	Increased plasma lactate level
DIC	

DIC, disseminated intravascular coagulation.

strengthens the diagnosis. Hyperkalemia may develop rapidly during an acute malignant hyperthermia crisis, and may cause ventricular arrhythmias or asystole. Immediate treatment of hyperkalemia consists of calcium, bicarbonate, and insulin-glucose. Kayexalate delivered by nasogastric tube is also indicated for longer term control. Life-threatening complications of ongoing hypermetabolism and rhabdomyolysis include disseminated intravascular coagulation (DIC), renal failure, congestive heart failure, bowel ischemia, and compartment syndrome of the limbs secondary to profound muscle swelling. DIC is the most frequent cause of death from MH.

There are a number of entities that may present in the perioperative setting that also manifest signs and symptoms of hypermetabolism. These include hyperthyroidism, pheochromocytoma, sepsis, cocaine intoxication, and most commonly, iatrogenic overheating. However, these conditions are not associated with a mixed metabolic and respiratory acidosis. Neuroleptic malignant syndrome, which is rare in children, occurs in patients receiving antipsychotic medications. Although many features of this condition are similar to that of malignant hyperthermia, there is no known association.

TREATMENT OF MALIGNANT HYPERTHERMIA (Box 21-1)

Dantrolene sodium (Dantrium) was first introduced in 1979 as an injectable antidote for acute malignant hyperthermia. It acts by decreasing the release of calcium from the sarcoplasmic reticulum. There is no interaction between neuromuscular blocking agents and dantrolene – they have two different sites of action. Dantrolene is very safe when administered at recommended dosages. Side-effects include nausea, malaise, light-headedness, muscle weakness, and irritation and venous thrombosis at the site of administration due to the high pH of the drug. Limb muscle weakness usually occurs. Respiratory muscle weakness may occur when large doses are used or when administered to debilitated patients.

ANESTHESIA FOR AN MH-SUSCEPTIBLE PATIENT

MH-susceptible patients are commonly anesthetized without problems. A series of preventative steps will ensure that these patients are not accidentally exposed to triggering agents:

Clean Anesthesia Machine

The anesthesia machine should be flushed with oxygen at a flow rate of 10 L/min for 10 minutes. Maintenance procedures for vaporizers should include documentation that the vaporizers do not leak. The time interval required to eliminate anesthetic vapor after the vaporizers are turned off should be known. The vaporizers may be removed to decrease the likelihood of unintentional use. Alternatively, the anesthesiologist can attach large pieces of tape or labels across the vaporizers as a reminder. The CO_2 absorber should be replaced with a fresh absorber.

Nontriggering Technique

A nontriggering technique requires initial placement of an intravenous catheter. This can be facilitated using premedication with oral midazolam, preoperative placement of topical anesthetic over several possible sites, and N_2O inhalation during placement. Any hypnotic agent can be used for induction of general anesthesia followed by maintenance of anesthesia with a continuous infusion of propofol (150–250 µg/kg/min) and opioid supplementation. Core temperature and minute ventilation should be monitored closely in all MH-susceptible patients. Prophylactic dantrolene is not indicated when triggering agents are not administered.

Postoperative Care

Postoperatively, 4 hours of observation is recommended by most experts. However, this time frame is flexible since there are no reported cases of malignant hyperthermia developing in a susceptible patient with a nontriggering technique. Therefore, assuming there are no signs or symptoms of malignant hyperthermia, routine day surgery discharge criteria can apply. Parents should bring their child back to the hospital if fever or brown urine develops.

MALIGNANT HYPERTHERMIA VARIANTS

Aborted or Subclinical Malignant Hyperthermia

Occasionally a patient may develop nonspecific early signs of malignant hyperthermia after a brief exposure to an inhalational anesthetic, with or without succinylcholine. There are no concerns when this occurs until the patient develops postoperative muscle pains or myoglobinuria. Many experts believe this may represent a subclinical or aborted episode of malignant hyperthermia that abated upon discontinuation of the volatile anesthetic. Children with these findings should be observed in the hospital for any signs or symptoms of malignant hyperthermia. Appropriate blood work includes CK and potassium levels. Increased minute ventilation that is out of proportion to the clinical scenario should warrant blood gas testing to determine the presence of a metabolic acidosis. Dantrolene should be administered if there is evidence of ongoing rhabdomyolysis.

Masseter Spasm

The inability to open a child's mouth after administration of a triggering agent is called masseter muscle spasm

Box 21-1 Treatment of Malignant Hyperthermia

Initial Steps

- Call for help.
- Bring the MH cart and dantrolene into OR.
- Notify the surgeon that you suspect MH – finish procedure as rapidly as possible.
- Discontinue volatile agents and succinylcholine.
- Hyperventilate with 100% oxygen at flows of >10 L/min to ensure removal of excess CO_2.
- If surgery must continue, begin nontriggering anesthetic technique to ensure continuing loss of consciousness. Continuous infusion of propofol (100–200 µg/kg/min) is appropriate in combination with an opioid.
- Obtain the core (e.g., esophageal, rectal) temperature.
- Dissolve the 20 mg of dantrolene in each vial with 60 mL of sterile preservative-free water. One vial of dantrolene contains 3 g of mannitol.
- The first dose of dantrolene should be 2.5 mg/kg rapidly. Repeat until end-tidal CO_2 begins to decline (doses in excess of 10 mg/kg may be necessary in some cases). If a dramatic response does not occur within minutes after dantrolene administration, consider alternative diagnoses.
- Ensure adequate intravenous access (consider central line placement).
- Ensure arterial line placement.
- Ensure urinary bladder catheter placement.
- Call MHAUS hotline consultant for management assistance (in the United States: 1-800-MH-HYPER).
- Plan for ICU admission or transfer to fully equipped tertiary care medical center.

Begin Cooling Measures to Achieve Core Temperature Less than 38°C

- Lower temperature in the OR.
- Discontinue all warming measures.
- Place ice packs around the patient.
- Institute iced saline lavage via a nasogastric tube.
- Irrigate the surgical wound with iced saline.

Laboratory Studies

- Serial blood gases
- Electrolytes
- Coagulation studies
- Complete blood count
- Creatine kinase
- Myoglobin
- Lactate
- Urinalysis (if heme positive, confirm probable myoglobinuria by absence of red cells on microscopic examination)
- Urine myoglobin

Treatment of Complications

- Metabolic acidosis: sodium bicarbonate 1–2 mEq/kg. Titrate to achieve normalization of pH.
- Hyperkalemia: hyperventilation, calcium chloride 10 mg/kg or calcium gluconate 10–50 mg/kg; glucose/insulin: 0.15 units of regular insulin/kg and 1 mL/kg of 50% glucose.
- Ventricular arrhythmias: usually respond to treatment of acidosis and hyperkalemia; use standard ACLS protocols except calcium-channel blockers, which may exacerbate hyperkalemia and cause cardiac arrest in the presence of dantrolene.
- Refractory cardiac arrest or pulseless ventricular fibrillation/tachycardia secondary to hyperkalemia: cardiopulmonary bypass as last resort.
- Rhabdomyolysis: Diuresis with furosemide (mannitol already in dantrolene) and bicarbonate to alkalinize urine and prevent precipitation of myoglobin in the kidney.

Continued Management

- Continue IV dantrolene 1 mg/kg every 6 hours for 36 hours or longer if symptoms persist.
- Continue serial laboratory testing every 6 hours.
- Continue to aggressively treat ongoing hyperthermia, acidosis, hyperkalemia, and myoglobinuria. Check blood glucose every 1–2 hours if insulin is being administered.
- Ensure continuous urine output is greater than 2 mL/kg/h.
- Observe for recrudescence of acute malignant hyperthermia signs and symptoms.
- Patient and family should be extensively counseled about the implications of malignant hyperthermia, and should be referred to MHAUS. The anesthesiologist should provide the patient and family with an official letter that provides details of the event.

or rigidity (MMR). It occurs in approximately 1% of children who receive succinylcholine and may be more common in children with strabismus (see Chapter 32). It is not associated with an inability to provide bag/mask positive-pressure ventilation. Although an initial effect of succinylcholine is an increase in masseter muscle tension greater than baseline, this phenomenon, when striking, is called MMR and is thought to be a harbinger of malignant hyperthermia or a clinical clue that the patient is susceptible to malignant hyperthermia. When children with a history of MMR are referred for muscle biopsy testing, up to 50% will test positive for malignant hyperthermia susceptibility. Therefore, when definitive masseter muscle spasm is observed, all triggering agents should be discontinued and, unless it is urgent, the surgical procedure should not be performed. The child should be carefully observed for early signs or symptoms of hypermetabolism, which are then promptly evaluated. Blood levels of creatine kinase and potassium should be obtained immediately. If signs of malignant hyperthermia begin to develop, or if the urine shows a brownish discoloration, a blood gas should be obtained. If a metabolic acidosis is present, the child should be treated for an acute episode of malignant hyperthermia. A rise in CK within 24 hours up to 20,000 U/L or more in a healthy child with MMR indicates probable MH susceptibility.

Nonanesthetic Malignant Hyperthermia

Patients who develop rhabdomyolysis after strenuous exercise, or as a result of heat stroke, have many clinical aspects that are consistent with malignant hyperthermia. In fact, dantrolene may prove useful for treating the initial symptoms. Some anesthesiologists suggest that these episodes occur in individuals with a subclinical muscle abnormality, who should be considered to be susceptible to MH. However, there is currently no evidence that supports this association. An elevated preoperative CK level will raise suspicion that the patient may indeed have a subclinical myopathy. Further neurological evaluation is then necessary, and the patient should undergo a non-triggering anesthetic if surgery is urgent.

MALIGNANT HYPERTHERMIA TESTING

There is no simple diagnostic test available for screening the general population for susceptibility to malignant hyperthermia. The most accurate test involves a biopsy of skeletal muscle from the thigh. It is usually reserved for those with a family history of MH or when a patient has had a previous suspicious reaction to anesthesia. At the time of this writing, the test is available at six medical centers in the United States and three in Canada; a list of those centers is available from MHAUS.

The patient must undergo the test at the biopsy testing center – muscle biopsy samples cannot be sent out for testing.

Caffeine–Halothane Contracture Test

The most reliable existing test for malignant hyperthermia susceptibility is the caffeine–halothane contracture test. A fresh muscle sample from the vastus lateralis is attached to sensitive strain gauges. Each strip is exposed to various concentrations of halothane and caffeine. A contracture of >0.2 g at a concentration of <2 mm caffeine or <2% halothane is considered positive for malignant hyperthermia susceptibility. Based on this test, a patient can be placed into one of three possible categories:

1. Malignant hyperthermia-susceptible: contracture occurs with both halothane and caffeine
2. Malignant hyperthermia-equivocal: contracture occurs with caffeine or halothane but not both
3. Malignant hyperthermia-negative: contracture does not occur with either agent.

The sensitivity (true negative rate) of MH testing is approximately 97%. Specificity (true positive rate) is lower: up to 15% of patients with positive contracture tests may have a false positive test.

Should all patients with suspected MH undergo a muscle biopsy (Box 21-2)? Ideally, yes, because then the

---

Box 21-2   Indications for Muscle Biopsy Testing for MH

Definite Indications

Suspicious clinical history for MH
Family history of MH
Severe masseter muscle rigidity

Possible Indications

Unexplained rhabdomyolysis during or after surgery (may present as sudden cardiac arrest due to hyperkalemia)
Moderate to mild masseter muscle rigidity with evidence of rhabdomyolysis
Exercise-induced rhabdomyolysis

Probably Not Indicated

Sudden, unexpected cardiac arrest during anesthesia or early postoperative period not associated with rhabdomyolysis
Age less than 5 years or weight less than 40 pounds
Neuroleptic malignant syndrome

Reproduced with permission from Rosenberg H, Antognini JF, Muldoon S: Testing for malignant hyperthermia. *Anesthesiology* 96:232-237, 2002.

Case

A 3-year-old 15-kg boy is being anesthetized for emergency appendectomy. His medical history is unremarkable except for symptoms of an upper respiratory tract infection (URI). His symptoms include fever of 38.4°C axillary, cough for three days and runny nose for one week. He receives propofol and rocuronium for induction of general anesthesia. During direct laryngoscopy, the patient moves and is given 40 mg succinylcholine and additional propofol to facilitate endotracheal intubation. Maintenance of general anesthesia consists of isoflurane in oxygen with fentanyl supplementation. Shortly after tracheal intubation, bronchospasm is detected and the $P_{ET}CO_2$ climbs into the high 60s. The esophageal temperature is 38.1°C, and is increasing steadily.

What would you do at this point?

The basic "ABCs" always come first. Manually ventilate the chest while an assistant auscultates over the lung fields. A right main-stem endobronchial intubation is probably the most frequent cause of these symptoms. Manual ventilation will provide an estimate of the patient's lung compliance. Suctioning the endotracheal tube may clear secretions (from the URI) and will increase overall compliance and alleviate wheezing.

The patient's heart rate rises to the 180s, and the $P_{ET}CO_2$ continues to rise, now in the 80s. The temperature has risen to 40.2°C.

There are common causes for this combination of signs in a child with acute appendicitis. The fever may be caused by the underlying illness, the tachycardia may be caused by light anesthesia and fever, and the rise in end-tidal CO_2 is likely caused by hypoventilation from a cause as yet to be determined. However, the astute anesthesiologist should begin to consider the possibility of acute MH. An arterial blood gas with electrolytes is indicated at this time. The bladder should be catheterized. A urine analysis should be immediately performed to detect evidence of myoglobinuria. If the urine is dipstick positive for blood, it must be sent to the microscopy laboratory to detect red blood cells. If none are found, myoglobinuria is strongly suspected.

The results of the arterial blood gas reveal a mixed respiratory and metabolic acidosis: pH = 7.09, K = 6.9 mEq/L. What will you do now?

MH is now strongly suspected. Since early diagnosis and treatment is crucial for successfully treating MH and minimizing morbidity and mortality, additional help should be called for, and the MH cart should be brought into the operating room. All triggering agents should be discontinued, and the patient should be hyperventilated with 100% oxygen in an attempt to bring the end-tidal CO_2 to a normal level. The hyperkalemia should be immediately treated with intravenous calcium chloride 10 mg/kg, and sodium bicarbonate 1 mEq/kg. Glucose and insulin mixture (1 mL/kg) should be prepared and administered. Dantrolene 2.5 mg/kg, should be administered as rapidly as possible. One person should place the diluent, sterile water (60 mL), into the dantrolene bottles; another person shakes it and administers it. Simultaneously, place cold saline bags around the axillae, groin regions, and head. Recheck the patient's respiratory status to monitor how the bronchospasm has evolved. Repeat the arterial blood gas and electrolytes. Additional blood work at this time would include a serum CK, lactate, and myoglobin, complete blood count, and coagulation studies. The surgeon should complete the appendectomy as rapidly as possible and postoperative ICU admission is arranged.

The patient's pH level is now 7.19 and K is 5.9 mEq/L. The urine is cola-colored.

Repeat dantrolene 2.5 mg/kg and sodium bicarbonate 1 mEq/kg. Administer enough intravenous fluids (normal saline or lactated Ringers) to produce a urine output of 2–4 mL/kg/h. Additional doses of dantrolene should be continued until the respiratory acidosis, metabolic acidosis, and hyperkalemia have all resolved. Dantrolene 1 mg/kg should be administered every 6 hours for the next 36 hours unless an acute recrudescence of MH occurs, in which a larger dose is given until symptoms once again abate. The patient should be observed in the ICU until the urine is free of myoglobin. The patient's family should be counseled about MH and referred to the nearest muscle biopsy testing center for further evaluation and diagnosis.

patient and first-degree relatives would know for sure that he or she is either not susceptible (high sensitivity) or probably susceptible (lower specificity). However, not all patients or their families are able to travel to one of the relatively few centers where the biopsy is offered. In addition, many patients' insurance plans will not cover muscle biopsy testing. Furthermore, a muscle biopsy is an invasive, expensive procedure that, for children, requires general anesthesia. In lieu of definitive testing, the patient and first-degree relatives can be considered MH-susceptible and receive nontriggering agents during future anesthetics.

Article To Know

Pollock AN, Langton EE, Couchman K, Stowell KM, Waddington M: Suspected malignant hyperthermia reactions in New Zealand. Anaesth Intens Care 30:453–461, 2002.

This article reviews the clinical features of 123 suspected cases of MH from the New Zealand MH database and correlates these features using a clinical grading scale (Tables 21-2A and B) to the results of contracture testing.

Table 21-2A

Process	Indicator	Score
Rigidity	Generalized muscle rigidity/masseter spasm	15
Muscle breakdown	$K^+ > 6\,mmol/L$	3–15
	Myoglobinuria	
	Elevated CPK	
Respiratory acidosis	Inappropriately elevated minute ventilation	10–15
	Hypercarbia	
Temperature rise	Inappropriate >38.8°C	10–15
	Rapid rise	
Cardiac events	Inappropriate sinus tachycardia	3
	Ventricular tachycardia	
	Ventricular fibrillation	
Other indicators	Response to dantrolene	5–10
	Metabolic acidosis	

Table 21-2B

Score	MH Rank	Likelihood of MH
0	1	Almost none
3–9	2	Unlikely
10–19	3	Somewhat less than likely
20–34	4	Somewhat greater than likely
35–49	5	Very likely
≥50	6	Almost certain

Patients were placed into one of the three groups described in the section on MH susceptibility testing. Of the 123 cases, 93 underwent contracture testing. Of these, 53 were MH-susceptible, 12 were MH-equivocal, and 28 were MH-negative. The correlation of contracture testing with the clinical grading criteria is described in Table 21-3.

Table 21-3

Score	MH Likelihood Ranking	MH-susceptible ($n = 53$)	MH-equivocal ($n = 12$)	MH-negative ($n = 28$)
0	1	–	–	5
3–9	2	4	11	3
10–19	3	11	6	12
20–34	4	15	2	5
45–49	5	17	1	2
≥50	6	6	–	1

Reproduced with permission from Pollock AN et al: *Anaesth Intens Care* 30:453–461, 2002.

The MH-susceptible group included 20 untested individuals who had a clinically fulminant MH reaction and 11 of whom had subsequently died. Of the surviving nine patients, four had declined contracture testing, and the other five were unable to be tested. All five had an immediate relative who had positive contracture testing.

The following are other important results from this analysis:

- An inappropriately high $P_{ET}CO_2$ was the first sign in 70% of MH-susceptible patients.
- Fifteen patients in the MH-susceptible group presented with succinylcholine-induced masseter spasm. Masseter spasm was the only abnormal sign in two of these patients while the others had developed clinical features of MH.

- Tachycardia was present in 95% of MH-susceptible patients. Ventricular ectopy was the earliest presenting sign in three patients, and appeared at another time in the clinical course in 15 of the 53 MH-susceptible patients.
- Increased temperatures ranged from 37.1°C to 43°C in the MH-susceptible group. There were two discernible subgroups: a fulminant group in which the temperature increase closely followed the increase in $P_{ET}CO_2$ (this occurred in 28 of 53 MH-susceptible patients); and a less reactive group that had a slower increase in temperature.
- Low Spo_2 was the earliest sign in only one patient. But Spo_2 monitoring was not available during the entire time that data were collected for this article. Spo_2 was abnormal at some point during the anesthetic (even though it was not the earliest sign) in 10 out of 26 MH-susceptible patients.
- Twenty-seven MH-susceptible patients (50%) had acid–base testing. Eleven of these demonstrated a significant base deficit (>8 mmol/L).
- Generalized body rigidity was present in 16 of 53 MH-susceptible patients. In all but two, this rigidity was associated with succinylcholine administration.
- Creatinine kinase peaked after 24 hours in the MH-susceptible patients; the highest measurement was 165,300 IU. No patient in the MH-equivocal or MH-negative group had a CK higher than 15,000 IU.
- Succinylcholine alone was the triggering agent in one patient in the MH-susceptible group. Twelve patients received a volatile anesthetic only. Thirty-seven patients received both succinylcholine and a volatile anesthetic.
- Eleven patients died, all prior to 1981. These patients were all in the MH-susceptible group.
- Active cooling was employed in 44% of MH-susceptible patients. Dantrolene was given to 24% of MH-susceptible patients, 0% of MH-equivocal patients, and 16% of MH-negative patients. An initial dose of 1.5–2 mg/kg was used; the maximum dose was 17 mg/kg over a 36-hour period.

Malignant Hyperthermia Association of the United States (MHAUS) and the North American Malignant Hyperthermia Registry

In 1981, MHAUS was formed to educate the medical and lay communities about MH and serve as a resource for affected families. In 1987, the North American MH Registry was established to collect and analyze information about clinical episodes of malignant hyperthermia and the results of laboratory tests. These two organizations merged in 1995. A wide variety of educational information for health professionals and the lay public is available at the MHAUS website (www.mhaus.org).

ADDITIONAL ARTICLES TO KNOW

Allen GC, Larach MG, Kunselman AR: The sensitivity and specificity of the caffeine–halothane contracture test: a report from the North American Malignant Hyperthermia Registry. North American Malignant Hyperthermia Registry of MHAUS. *Anesthesiology* 88:579–588, 1998.

Brownell AK: Malignant hyperthermia: relationship to other diseases. *Br J Anaesth* 60:303–308, 1988.

Green Larach M, Rosenberg H, Larach DR, Broennle AM: Prediction of malignant hyperthermia susceptibility by clinical signs. *Anesthesiology* 66:547–550, 1987.

Gronert GA, Mott J, Lee J: Aetiology of malignant hyperthermia. *Br J Anaesth* 60:253–267, 1988.

Gronert GA, Fowler W, Cardinet G et al: Absence of malignant hyperthermia contractures in Becker–Duchenne dystrophy at age 2. *Muscle Nerve* 15:52–56, 1992.

Hopkins PM: Malignant hyperthermia: advances in clinical management and diagnosis. *Br J Anaesth* 85:118–128, 2000.

Ording H, Ranklev E, Fletcher R: Investigation of malignant hyperthermia in Denmark and Sweden. *Br J Anaesth* 56:1183–1190, 1984.

Rosenberg H, Fletcher JE: Masseter muscle rigidity and malignant hyperthermia susceptibility. *Anesth Analg* 65:161–164, 1986.

Rubin AS, Zablocki A: Hyperkalemia, verapamil, and dantrolene. *Anesthesiology* 66:246–249, 1987.

Schwartz L, Rockoff MA, Koka BV: Masseter spasm with anesthesia: incidence and implications. *Anesthesiology* 61:772–775, 1984.

Theroux MC, Rose JB, Iyengar S, Katz MS: Succinylcholine pretreatment using gallamine or mivacurium during rapid sequence induction in children: a randomized, controlled study. *J Clin Anesth* 13: 287–292, 2001.

Van der Spek AF, Fang WB, Ashton-Miller JA et al: The effects of succinylcholine on mouth opening. *Anesthesiology* 67:459–465, 1987.

Van der Spek AF, Fang WB, Ashton-Miller JA et al: Increased masticatory muscle stiffness during limb muscle flaccidity associated with succinylcholine administration. *Anesthesiology* 69:11–16, 1988.

POSTOPERATIVE
CONSIDERATIONS

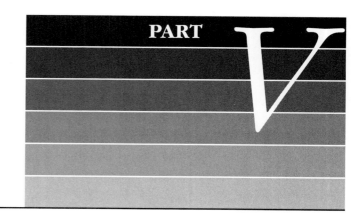

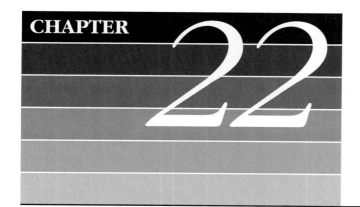

CHAPTER 22

Postoperative Considerations

RONALD S. LITMAN

This chapter discusses routine care and monitoring of pediatric patients in the immediate postoperative period, including discharge criteria standards and management of common postoperative complications. They include nausea and vomiting, emergence delirium, and postintubation croup. Acute postoperative pain management is discussed in Chapter 26 and postoperative fever is covered in Chapter 15.

When an unconscious or partially conscious child arrives in the postanesthesia care unit (PACU), monitoring of vital signs is no different from that used intraoperatively until the child has completely regained consciousness. All children should be monitored with pulse oximetry since the most important postoperative complication is obstructive apnea, which rapidly leads to hypoxemia. Continuous monitoring of heart and respiratory rates will provide early warning of cardiopulmonary complications, such as bradycardia in the small infant who becomes apneic, and opioid-induced respiratory depression. An initial temperature should be obtained when the child arrives at the PACU and monitored at regular intervals until discharge. Electrocardiography and intermittent blood pressure measurement should be determined by the child's clinical condition. Supplemental oxygen administration should be guided by pulse oximetry. In most centers, children are discharged from the phase 1 acute PACU to the phase 2 recovery area (day surgery unit) after regaining consciousness and maintaining stability of vital signs without oxygen supplementation.

DISCHARGE CRITERIA

There are various criteria that one can use to quantify progression of consciousness to allow pediatric patients to be discharged to the phase 2 recovery area and then either to the hospital ward or to home. In 1975, David Steward published a pediatric modification of the standard Aldrete recovery score, with which to monitor the progress of recovery in children (Table 22-1). This score takes into account consciousness and airway patency, with a total score of 9 used to establish appropriate readiness for discharge in most centers. However, this score does not correlate with oxyhemoglobin values in the recovery period, and its relationship to other outcome variables has not been established.

Table 22-1	Steward Postanesthetic Recovery Score	
Patient Sign	**Criterion**	**Score**
Consciousness	Awake	2
	Responds to stimuli	1
	Does not respond to stimuli	0
Airway	Actively crying or coughs on command	2
	Maintains airway patency	1
	Requires assistance to maintain airway patency	0
Movement	Moves limbs purposefully	2
	Moves limbs randomly	1
	Not moving	0

Reproduced with permission from Steward DJ: Simplified scoring system for the post-operative recovery room. *Can Anaesth Soc J* 22:111–113, 1975.

At The Children's Hospital of Philadelphia, more general discharge criteria include adequate hydration, adequate pain control, and minimal nausea and vomiting. Oral intake of fluids is allowed but not encouraged nor required for discharge home. Urinary voiding is also not required for discharge home unless specified by the surgeon based on the performed procedure. Protracted nausea and vomiting is the most common reason for unanticipated hospital admission because of the risk of dehydration and the inability of the child to ingest oral analgesics if continued pain is anticipated. Children with three or more episodes of emesis require evaluation by an attending anesthesiologist who, along with the attending surgeon, will make a determination whether to hospitalize the child overnight for continued intravenous hydration and analgesic therapy. Children with limited home resources may also be hospitalized.

POSTOPERATIVE COMPLICATIONS

Nausea and Vomiting

Postoperative nausea and vomiting (PONV) is probably the most common postoperative complication following general anesthesia in children, and is the most common reason for unanticipated hospital admission. Although PONV is not usually life-threatening, it causes profound discomfort to the child and his or her family. Less common sequelae include electrolyte disturbances, dehydration, and interference with proper surgical healing. Surgical risk factors for PONV include ENT, ophthalmologic, and orthopedic surgery. Anesthetic risk factors include use of inhalational anesthetics and opioids. Patient-related factors include previous PONV and age >3 years. The incidence of PONV can be decreased by use of propofol instead of inhalational agents for general anesthesia, avoidance of opioids by using nonsteroidal anti-inflammatory drugs (NSAIDs) and regional anesthesia, limiting postoperative fluid ingestion, and prophylactic administration of antiemetics. Combination therapy with different classes of antiemetics more successfully prevents and treats PONV than one type of antiemetic alone. The evacuation of stomach contents prior to emergence from general anesthesia does not reduce the incidence of PONV in adults and has not been studied in pediatric patients.

Serotonin Antagonists

Serotonin (hydroxytryptamine) sub-type 3 (5-HT$_3$) antagonists are the first-line treatment of PONV in most pediatric centers because, of all available antiemetic agents, they demonstrate the highest benefit-to-risk ratio. They significantly reduce the incidence and severity of subsequent vomiting in the first 24 hours after surgery.

At the time of this writing, three are licensed in the US: ondansetron, granisetron, and dolasetron (Table 22-2). Ondansetron is the oldest and most widely studied. Although formal comparisons between these agents have not been performed in the pediatric population, they are probably equally efficacious (50–80% percent success in most studies), with slight differences in their side-effect profiles (gleaned from oncological studies). At The Children's Hospital of Philadelphia, nearly all children over the age of 3 years who are anesthetized receive intraoperative administration of ondansetron (average dose 0.05 mg/kg) as a prophylactic measure against PONV. Clinical experience shows that children who vomit despite prophylaxis with ondansetron will not often respond favorably to additional doses in the postoperative period. The optimal dose response has not been determined in this setting.

Dexamethasone

Dexamethasone is a steroid with mineralocorticoid properties that was initially demonstrated to prevent emesis from chemotherapeutic agents and subsequently used for prevention and treatment of PONV. When used in combination with a serotonin antagonist, it significantly lowers the incidence and severity of PONV even further than if a serotonin antagonist was used alone. Dose ranging studies have provided inconsistent results. Most pediatric anesthesiologists use a dose of 0.5–1.0 mg/kg with maximum doses that range from 10 to 20 mg. At these doses, complications or side-effects from dexamethasone are rarely observed and may include hyperactivity and insomnia. At the time of this writing, its efficacy as a treatment for established PONV has not been established.

Table 22-2	**Serotonin Antagonists**	
Agent	Recommended Dose[a]	Side-effects
Ondansetron	0.05 mg/kg	Headache, dizziness, possible increase in LFTs (dose adjustment necessary for liver failure patients)
Granisetron	0.04 mg/kg	Headache, constipation, diarrhea
Dolasetron	0.5 mg/kg[b]	Transient asymptomatic ECG changes in adults, including QT interval prolongation.

[a] Maximum doses have not been established for all agents.
[b] Dose–response studies have not been performed.
LFT, liver function test.

Article To Know

Schreiner MS, Nicolson SC, Martin T, Whitney L: Should children drink before discharge from day surgery? Anesthesiology 76:528–533, 1992.

With this publication, Mark Schreiner and his colleagues at The Children's Hospital of Philadelphia made a major contribution to the practice of postoperative management in children. Before its publication, many centers required children to tolerate ingestion of clear liquids prior to discharge home. These authors set out to determine whether mandatory drinking affected outcome variables such as subsequent vomiting, duration of stay in the postoperative recovery area, and readmission to the hospital.

Nearly one thousand children between the ages of 1 month and 18 years, who underwent outpatient surgery, were randomized to either standard "mandatory drinking" prior to discharge home, or "elective drinking," where oral ingestion of fluids was allowed but not required for home discharge. If a child in this latter group expressed the desire to drink, they were encouraged to drink smaller quantities. Stepwise multiple linear regression analysis was used to determine the effect of drinking on the outcome variables. "Mandatory drinkers" stayed longer in the day-surgery unit and had a higher incidence of emesis prior to discharge home. No patients in either group required hospitalization for protracted vomiting or readmission to the hospital for dehydration. Because of the results of this study, many centers altered their practice and no longer require children to tolerate oral fluids prior to discharge home.

Droperidol

Prior to the advent of the serotonin antagonists, droperidol was considered the most efficacious antiemetic for prevention and treatment of PONV in children. In doses up to 0.075 mg/kg, it effectively prevents PONV in children undergoing high-risk surgical procedures, such as strabismus repair. In comparison studies, droperidol is less effective than serotonin antagonists in preventing or treating emesis, but clinical experience has shown that it is probably more effective for treatment of nausea. Droperidol is a dopamine antagonist, and thus, its side-effect profile includes sedation and extrapyramidal signs. More importantly, in 2001, the FDA mandated that manufacturers of droperidol place a "black-box" warning in the package insert regarding the potential for development of dysrhythmias, including prolongation of the QT interval and torsades de pointes. Most pediatric centers in the US have abandoned its use, mainly for medicolegal reasons.

Metoclopramide

Metoclopramide is a dopamine antagonist that facilitates gastric emptying and may also act as a peripheral or central antiemetic. It is often administered to patients awaiting emergency surgery to decrease gastric volume prior to induction of anesthesia. However, because of the exceedingly low incidence of pulmonary aspiration, its use has not been shown to alter the incidence or severity of this clinically important outcome. It efficacy for prevention or treatment of PONV is inconsistent at best. High doses are usually required for better results (e.g., >0.1 mg/kg), but these higher doses are associated with antidopaminergic side-effects (i.e., extrapyramidal signs).

Nonpharmacologic Treatment of PONV

Acupuncture, acupressure, and electrical stimulation at the Nei-Guan (P6) point on the wrist (slightly proximal to the distal skin crease of the wrist on the ulnar side) have been demonstrated to decrease the incidence of PONV in children but has not been widely adopted in most centers.

Stridor

Stridor in the postoperative period is a worrisome sign of impending airway obstruction and respiratory failure, and must be evaluated immediately. Its management will largely depend on the cause, which is determined by the surgical procedure that was performed, the clinical exam, and the oxyhemoglobin saturation (Spo_2). When stridor is associated with surgery of the upper airway or neck, immediate surgical consultation is warranted. If stridor is associated with a worsening Spo_2 despite oxygen therapy, endotracheal intubation is indicated as an initial management step, and evaluation of the etiology follows. These children may be difficult to ventilate after administration of sedation or induction of general anesthesia. Management principles of an obstructed airway are described in Chapter 18.

Stridor that manifests as a barky or croupy cough, and is not associated with airway surgery, is most likely due to subglottic edema caused by endotracheal tube irritation. This entity is commonly referred to as "postintubation croup." It occurs within 1 hour of tracheal extubation and is associated with tachypnea and use of accessory respiratory muscles and chest wall retractions. The exact location of the edema is unknown but it is presumed to be located at the level of the inflexible cricoid ring. The incidence of postintubation croup is approximately 0.1%. Its occurrence appears to be associated with tight-fitting endotracheal tubes (see Chapter 17), airway surgery (e.g., rigid bronchoscopy), manipulations of the head or neck during surgery, presence of a concurrent upper respiratory tract infection, and a previous bout of infectious croup. As long as the child's Spo_2 is normal with minimal concentrations of supplemental oxygen, no treatment is necessary, although some anesthesiologists may choose to administer dexamethasone, if it has not already been given for prevention of PONV. Ambulatory patients should be observed and can be discharged home when the stridor has abated, and there is no evidence of oxyhemoglobin desaturation (e.g., below 96%) without oxygen supplementation.

If significant airway obstruction is present (Spo_2 less than 96% despite oxygen therapy), treatment with inhaled racemic epinephrine is indicated to provide topical vasoconstriction and help shrink edematous tracheal tissue. Racemic epinephrine is supplied as a 2.25% solution. The dose is 0.05 mL/kg (maximum dose 0.5 mL) diluted in 3 mL of normal saline. It is administered as a nebulized solution every hour if needed, based on clinical symptoms and sympathomimetic side-effects. Administration of racemic epinephrine usually constitutes mandatory overnight or prolonged hospital observation because of its limited duration of effects and possible recurrence of airway obstruction. A persistent Spo_2 less than 90% despite oxygen supplementation is evidence of severe upper airway obstruction, and warrants immediate endotracheal intubation with a smaller sized endotracheal tube than used previously.

Emergence Delirium

Emergence delirium describes a condition of uncontrollable anxiety and agitation upon emergence from general anesthesia. Clinical manifestations include unremitting crying, tachycardia, pupillary dilatation, disinterest in drinking, and the inability to be consoled by the presence of parents. It is a common, benign condition that most likely represents an extension of the state of general anesthesia that most anesthesiologists refer to as "stage 2." It is extremely disconcerting to the parents, PACU staff and adjacent children. External stimuli should be reduced (e.g., lights out) and the child should be swaddled in a warm blanket and encouraged to fall asleep. A low dose of morphine (0.05 mg/kg) will provide sedation and facilitate the onset of sleep. Typically children will awaken approximately one hour later in a more normal state of grogginess. "Stormy inductions" and maintenance of general anesthesia with sevoflurane or desflurane increase the incidence of emergence delirium and the intraoperative administration of fentanyl or morphine decreases its occurrence.

The most important aspect of emergence delirium is the prompt differentiation from more serious events that manifest with the same clinical findings. These include hypoxemia, hypovolemia, hypoglycemia, pain, and severe anxiety that is easily treated by having the child's parents present.

ADDITIONAL ARTICLES TO KNOW

Abramowitz MD, Oh TH, Epstein BS, Ruttimann UE, Friendly DS: Antiemetic effect of droperidol following outpatient strabismus surgery in children. *Anesthesiology* 59:579-583, 1983.

Cravero J, Surgenor S, Whalen K: Emergence agitation in paediatric patients after sevoflurane anaesthesia and no surgery: a comparison with halothane. *Paediatr Anaesth* 10:419-424, 2000.

Litman RS, Keon TP: Postintubation croup in children. *Anesthesiology* 75:1122-1123, 1991.

Litman RS, Wu CL, Catanzaro FA: Ondansetron decreases emesis after tonsillectomy in children. *Anesth Analg* 78:478-481, 1994.

Martin TM, Nicolson SC, Bargas MS: Propofol anesthesia reduces emesis and airway obstruction in pediatric outpatients. *Anesth Analg* 76:144-148, 1993.

Pappas ALS, Sukhani R, Hotaling AJ et al: The effect of preoperative dexamethasone on the immediate and delayed postoperative morbidity in children undergoing adenotonsillectomy. *Anesth Analg* 87:57-61, 1998.

Soliman IE, Patel RI, Ehrenpreis MB, Hannallah RS: Recovery scores do not correlate with postoperative hypoxemia in children. *Anesth Analg* 67:53-56, 1988.

Steward DJ: Simplified scoring system for the post-operative recovery room. *Can Anaesth Soc J* 22:111-113, 1975.

Tyler DC, Woodham M, Stocks J, Leary A, Lloyd-Thomas A: Oxygen saturation in children in the postoperative period. *Anesth Analg* 80:14-19, 1995.

Ummenhofer W, Frei FJ, Urwyler A, Kern C, Drewe J: Effects of ondansetron in the prevention of postoperative nausea and vomiting in children. *Anesthesiology* 81:804-810, 1994.

Watcha MF, Bras PJ, Cieslak GD, Pennant JH: The dose–response relationship of ondansetron in preventing postoperative emesis in pediatric patients undergoing ambulatory surgery. *Anesthesiology* 82:47-52, 1995.

Weinstein MS, Nicolson SC, Schreiner MS: A single dose of morphine sulfate increases the incidence of vomiting after outpatient inguinal surgery in children. *Anesthesiology* 81:572-577, 1994.

PEDIATRIC PAIN MANAGEMENT

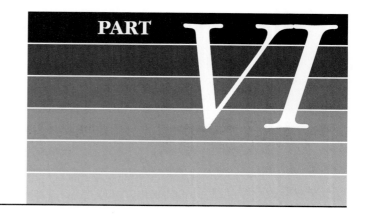

PART

VI

Pediatric Pain Assessment

JOHN B. ROSE

DEIRDRE E. LOGAN

At What Age Are Children Capable of
    Experiencing Pain?
Assessing Pain in Children

Pediatric pain is often not recognized and ineffectively managed. Perhaps this is caused by the inability of children to effectively describe the location and severity of their pain. But healthcare workers unknowingly contribute to the inadequate treatment of pain in children. The basis for this is speculative, and may include a lack of knowledge about pathophysiology of pediatric pain or pharmacology of analgesics in pediatric patients. Other possible explanations include ignorance of appropriate pediatric pain assessment tools and available treatment options, as well as an inability to recognize the large variability in pain experienced by different patients with similar types of pain.

Many healthcare professionals still believe that pain is an inevitable, expected consequence of illness and injury, and that pain is less harmful than the risks associated with the analgesic interventions. Furthermore, many parents believe that their child's pain is unavoidable. Inflexible prescribing practices that use PRN regimens with inappropriately low or infrequent analgesic doses still occur. Fear of side-effects such as nausea, vomiting, and respiratory depression, as well as fear of long-term sequelae (e.g., drug dependence and addiction) also cause inadequate treatment of pain in children. The fact is, however, that a variety of analgesic therapies can be provided safely to children, even prematurely born neonates.

Lack of adequate pain treatment of children is partially caused by the lack of approved labeling of potent analgesics. Pharmaceutical companies have been unwilling to fund necessary studies to obtain pediatric labeling because the market size is limited. This has resulted in a paucity of pharmacokinetic and pharmacodynamic data and a lack of information about adverse effects.

AT WHAT AGE ARE CHILDREN CAPABLE OF EXPERIENCING PAIN?

To experience pain, one must possess the ability to perceive a peripheral noxious stimulus via a functioning nociceptive system, and develop a motor, autonomic, metabolic, psychological, behavioral, or emotional response. Neonates sense noxious stimuli and routinely demonstrate all these responses. In the developing fetus, cutaneous sensation begins in the 7th week of gestation in the perioral region and soon spreads to the face, hands, feet, and trunk. By the 15th week of gestation, cutaneous sensation has spread to the extremities, and by the 20th week, sensory perception is present in all cutaneous and mucosal regions. Substance P appears in fetal nerve tissue by the 10th week and endogenous opioids are detected at 22 weeks. Synapses begin to form between peripheral sensory neurons and dorsal horn neurons by this time. Myelination of nerve tracts in the spinal cord and brainstem begins during the 22nd week of gestation and is complete by the third trimester. Peripheral nerve myelination is not fully completed until after birth. However, one of the major nociceptive neurons is unmyelinated (C-fibers) and the other is thinly myelinated (A-δ fibers). This does not mean that noxious signals are not transmitted, but that they are transmitted more slowly.

Centrally, the cerebral cortex begins to develop at 8 weeks and will contain 10 billion neurons by the 20th week of gestation. Fetal electroencephalographic patterns, though intermittent and unsynchronized, appear by the 22nd week; by the 27th week, signals are synchronized in both hemispheres. By the 30th gestational week, cortical evoked potentials can be detected. At the beginning of the third trimester, all elements of the nociceptive system required to process noxious stimulation are present. The only component of the nociceptive system that is not present at birth is the descending inhibitory pathway, which develops during the first 6 months of antenatal life. Thus, the neonate is not capable of attenuating nociceptive signals. The dorsal horn cells of the neonate that are responsible for transmitting nociceptive signals centrally have wider receptive fields and lower excitatory thresholds than in older subjects. These properties mature quickly in the postnatal period. Excitatory thresholds of dorsal horn neurons are further lowered by repetitive minor injuries such as neonatal surgery and daily heal lancings. Neonates may experience more pain in response to a given noxious stimulus than older children or adults.

Some practitioners erroneously assume that since neonates cannot remember a painful event, it is of no consequence. But the metabolic and behavioral stress response that accompanies neonatal pain is associated with increased morbidity and mortality. This response can be reduced by using regional anesthesia, opioids, or general anesthesia prior to painful procedures.

Though little is known about neonatal consciousness and the perception of pain, there is evidence of complex, integrated cortical responses to nociceptive stimulation. Neonates subjected to noxious events (circumcision, repeated heel lancing, phlebotomy, etc.) demonstrate abnormalities in short-term behavior such as periods of increased crying, and feeding and sleeping abnormalities. Furthermore, painful experiences during early infancy affect future responses to painful events. In some instances physiologic responses are enhanced while behavioral responses are blunted. Opposite changes may occur under different circumstances. For example, infants who were circumcised at birth without anesthesia will demonstrate an exaggerated pain response to immunizations in the first year of life when compared with infants who received adequate anesthesia during newborn circumcision.

To summarize, neonates may not be able to interpret or remember painful events but even premature newborns are capable of perceiving noxious events and mounting a variety of physiological and behavioral responses. These responses may translate into short- and long-term behavioral changes during subsequent painful stimuli. Since these stress responses and adverse outcomes can be reduced by the judicious use of analgesics, pain should be anticipated whenever possible and treated appropriately.

ASSESSING PAIN IN CHILDREN

One of the challenges of pediatric pain management is the assessment and treatment of pain in preverbal children, as well as patients with neurological or cognitive impairment who cannot adequately communicate their experience of pain.

The Joint Commission on Accreditation of Health Care Organizations (JCAHO) has mandated that all patients have a basic right to pain assessment and management. In fact, JCAHO considers pain assessment to be the "5th vital sign." Pain assessment is not performed for the purpose of recording pain scores to fulfill JCAHO requirements. Rather, it is the first step in managing pain and is always used to plan subsequent analgesic therapy.

When children are experiencing pain, they may deny its existence or indicate they are comfortable for a variety of reasons. They may fear that if they report it, additional painful interventions will occur, or they will be separated from their parents, or both. They may believe that their pain is a form of punishment and their acknowledgement of it is equivalent to an admission of guilt. Some children have been taught to mistrust strangers and they will not talk to doctors or nurses but will tell their parents how they are feeling. Lastly, some children believe that doctors and nurses will just intuitively know when they are having pain and will automatically institute proper treatment without being told.

Proper assessment of pain will facilitate its treatment. For example, it is inconceivable that one would know when to begin antihypertensive therapy without measuring blood pressure. Similarly, pain treatment cannot begin without a measure of its severity or the response to treatment. The severity of one's pain is always subjective and difficult to measure, yet it can be measured in everyone. Occasionally the measurement is approximate, indicating that all pain is either absent, possible, probable, or definite. More often, however, we use specific tools to measure pain less ambiguously.

Pain assessment tools exist for children at different ages, stages of development, and under a variety of circumstances. Ideally, these pain assessment tools would be practical and easy to use. Unfortunately, some tools do not fulfill this criteria and further work is required to refine assessment instruments for young preverbal patients and cognitively impaired patients.

Pain assessment is most accurate when the child can describe its location, nature, and severity. With appropriate words and tools, children over 3 years of age can reliably communicate their pain. In children under 3 years, one must rely on a combination of behavioral clues and physiologic signs. Many of these signs are also seen in conditions other than pain. These include parental separation, hunger, fear, and anxiety. Thus, misinterpretation is common. Parents can determine whether their child is in pain by learning specific behaviors in their child that distinguish pain from distress or anxiety.

Perception, expression, and treatment of pain will depend on the child's age and developmental stage. As an example, consider a 3-month-old infant with epidermolysis bullosa (Fig. 23-1). This tragic congenital dermatologic condition is similar to a severe burn that requires

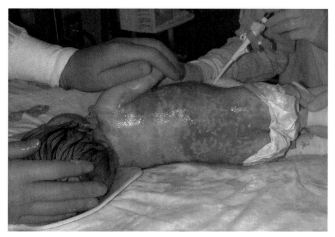

Figure 23-1   A 3-month-old infant with epidermolysis bullosa.

twice-daily dressing changes. The infant has no understanding of her pain and no ability to tell us about it. Therefore pain assessment is based on observation of behavioral and physiologic responses.

Piaget described four developmental stages of childhood. During the initial sensorimotor stage (approximately 0–2 years) children have little or no understanding of pain and no language ability. During this stage, we rely on behaviors (posture, activity, crying, feeding, sleeping, etc.) and physiologic signs (e.g., tachycardia, hypertension, diaphoresis, and oxyhemoglobin saturation) to determine the severity of an infant's pain. Pain scores that are useful during this developmental stage include the

ATTIA, CRIES, and CHEOPS scores (Table 23-1). The CRIES score uses five indicators (*C*rying; *R*equires oxygen; *I*ncreased heart rate and blood pressure; *E*xpression; and *S*leeplessness) which are graded from 0 to 2; this gives a total between 0 and 10 (Table 23-2). A score over 4 indicates that additional analgesics are required.

The second Piaget developmental stage is the preoperational stage (approximately 2–7 years), in which children acquire some language ability and can localize pain, differentiate "a little" and "a lot," and can use simple terms to describe their pain such as "boo-boo," "ouch," "hurt," and "owee." This stage is notable for its egocentrism – children see the pain as a punishment for being bad. Pain assessment tools commonly used during this developmental stage include CHEOPS and FACES (Fig. 23-2). Mature children in this stage may be able to use patient-controlled analgesia.

During Piaget's concrete operations stage (approximately 8–12 years) children think logically and can be taught methods of cognitive and behavioral pain control such as distraction, relaxation, guided imagery, and hypnosis. They can relate details about their pain such as how the pain varies with activity or time of day. FACES, a numeric, or a visual analog scale (VAS) can be used to assess pain in this stage. The numeric tool is a simple verbal 11-point scale (0–10) on which 0 represents no pain and 10 represents the worst pain imaginable. The VAS score consists of a 10-cm line with 0 at the left and 10 at the right. The child indicates the severity of his or her pain by placing a mark on the line. Patient-controlled analgesia is preferred during this developmental stage.

Table 23-1   Pain Assessment Tools for Children

Scale	Type	Population	Comments
ATTIA	Observational (behavioral)	Infants <1 year	10 indicators scored 0, 1, or 2. 0 = no pain, 20 = maximum pain
CRIES	Observational (behavioral and physiological)	Infants <1 year	5 indicators scored 0, 1, or 2. 0 = no pain, 10 = maximum pain
Neonatal Infant Pain Scale (NIPS)	Observational (behavioral and physiological)	Infants <7 months	6 indicators scored 0, 1, or 2. 0 = no pain, 7 = maximum pain
Toddler-Preschooler Postoperative Pain Score (TPPPS)	Observational (behavioral)	Postoperative children 1–5 years	7 indicators scored 0 or 1. 0 = no pain, 7 = maximum pain
Children's Hospital of Eastern Ontario Pain Score (CHEOPS)	Observational (behavioral)	Postoperative children 1–7 yrs	6 indicators rated 4 = no pain, 13 = maximum pain
Objective Pain–discomfort Scale (OPS)	Observational (behavioral)	Postoperative adolescents	6 indicators rated 0, 1, or 2. 0 = no pain, 12 = maximum pain
Oucher	Self report	Children 3–12 years	Photographs of child in 6 states of increasing pain
Faces	Self report	Children 3–12 years	Numerous faces scales exist; see Fig. 23-2 as example
Numeric	Self report	Children >7 years	Simple verbal 11-point scale 0 = no pain, 10 = maximum pain
Visual Analog Scale (VAS)	Self report	Children >7 years	10-cm line, 0 = no pain, 10 = maximum pain

Table 23-2   CRIES Scale for Postoperative Pain

	0	1	2
Crying	No	High-pitched	Inconsolable
Requires $Spo_2 > 95\%$	No	$F_IO_2 < 30\%$	$F_IO_2 < 30\%$
Increased vital signs	Heart rate and blood pressure equal to or less than preoperative values	Less than 20% of preoperative values	Greater than 20% of preoperative values
Expression	None	Grimace	Grimace/grunt
Sleeplessness	No	Awakens frequently	Awake

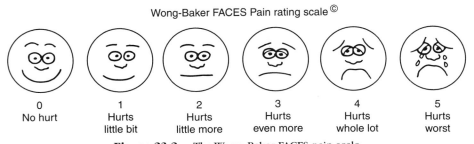

Wong-Baker FACES Pain rating scale ©

0	1	2	3	4	5
No hurt	Hurts little bit	Hurts little more	Hurts even more	Hurts whole lot	Hurts worst

Figure 23-2   The Wong–Baker FACES pain scale.

Case

A 1-month-old 4.2-kg male infant is scheduled to have a right thoracotomy and right lower lobectomy for a congenital cystic adenomatoid malformation of the lung.

Is this infant capable of mounting a stress response and experiencing pain after this surgery?

The nociceptive circuitry required to transmit and perceive noxious stimuli is present at birth. Since descending inhibitory pathways are not fully developed for up to 6 months after birth, this infant may experience more pain after thoracotomy than an older child. Severe pain in neonates can result in short- and long-term alterations in behavioral and physiologic responses to pain. Untreated pain may result in a significant physiologic stress response that may adversely affect recovery.

How can you tell whether this infant is having pain?

The best approach is to a look for a variety of behavioral and physiological clues. These include facial expressions, increased crying, altered sleeping and feeding patterns, inability to suck on a pacifier, increased heart rate and blood pressure, mottled skin, and diaphoresis. Pain in an infant can result in breath-holding, irregular and ineffective respirations, and oxyhemoglobin desaturation. Several validated, age-appropriate pain assessment tools are available to determine this infant's degree of discomfort.

When should you start planning for this patient's postoperative pain management?

Pain management planning should begin during the preanesthetic evaluation. In the author's institution the standard analgesic regimen for a neonate undergoing a thoracotomy includes a continuous infusion of epidural local anesthetics. The parents should be told about the risks and benefits of epidural analgesia versus systemic opioid therapy. In this infant, we would use epidural analgesia by advancing a catheter through the caudal canal to the T6 level. An initial intraoperative bolus dose would consist of 3 mL of 0.2% ropivacaine. Postoperatively we would continue epidural analgesia with a continuous infusion of 0.1% ropivacaine at 1 mL/h.

Article To Know

Lidow MS: Long-term effects of neonatal pain on nociceptive systems. Pain 99:377-383, 2002.

This article reviews the emotional and behavioral responses of neonates during painful procedures, and the resulting changes in neural circuitry responsible for transmission and modulation of nociceptive information. Neonates who experience severe and/or repeated noxious stimuli may suffer long-lasting consequences that will alter their response to painful events in the future. Excessive neonatal exposure to noxious stimuli can result in a decrease in behavioral responses and an increase in physiological responses to subsequent painful stimuli. In other words, a neonate who is subjected to repeated heel lancing, and who then undergoes surgery at a later time, may not demonstrate characteristic pain behaviors such as grimacing and crying but can have more pronounced cardiovascular changes and a greater stress response. Some studies indicate that these changes in behavioral and physiological responses to pain in infants diminish over time and disappear. However, other studies involving extremely low birthweight neonates who spent several weeks to months in neonatal intensive care demonstrate persistent alterations in pain behavior as well as other behavioral disturbances until 16 years of age.

In the final stage of child development, Piaget's formal operations stage, abstract thought is possible. Adolescents can more precisely characterize their pain with adjectives like burning, stinging, throbbing, or stabbing. They can articulate subtle changes in severity of pain with different treatments. Numeric or VAS scores are appropriate for this age group. Patient-controlled analgesia is preferred in this age group. A variety of nonpharmacologic techniques can be used as adjuncts to control pain. These include imagery, hypnosis, distraction, relaxation, and biofeedback.

ADDITIONAL ARTICLES TO KNOW

Anand KJS, Hickey PR: Pain and its effects in the human neonate and fetus. *N Engl J Med* 317:1321-1329, 1987.

Anand KJS, Hickey PR: Halothane–morphine compared with high-dose sufentanil for anesthesia and postoperative analgesia in neonatal cardiac surgery. *N Engl J Med* 326:1-9, 1992.

Anand KJS, Maze M: Fetuses, fentanyl, and the stress response: signals from the beginnings of pain? *Anesthesiology* 95:823-825, 2001.

Anand KJS, Sippell WG, Aynsley-Green A: Randomised trial of fentanyl anaesthesia in preterm babies undergoing surgery: effects on the stress response. *Lancet* i (8524):62-66, 1987.

Anand KJS, Hansen DD, Hickey PR: Hormonal–metabolic stress responses in neonates undergoing cardiac surgery. *Anesthesiology* 73:661-670, 1990.

Beyer JE, McGrath PJ, Berde CB: Discordance between self-report and behavioral pain measures in children aged 3-7 years after surgery. *J Pain Sympt Manag* 5(6):350-356, 1990.

Breau LM, Finley GA, McGrath PJ, Camfield CS: Validation of the non-communicating children's pain checklist: postoperative version. *Anesthesiology* 96:528-535, 2002.

Kain ZN, Cicchetti DV, McClain BC: Measurement of pain in children: state of the art considerations. *Anesthesiology* 96: 523-526, 2002.

Sturla Franck L, Miaskowski C: Measurement of neonatal responses to painful stimuli: a research review. *J Pain Sympt Manag* 14(6):343-378, 1997.

Tyler DC, Tu A, Douthit J, Chapman CR: Toward validation of pain measurement tools for children: a pilot study. *Pain* 52:301-309, 1993.

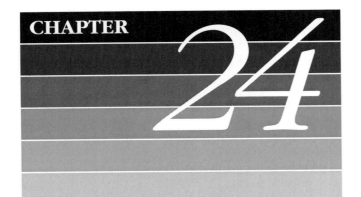

Pediatric Analgesia Pharmacology

JOHN B. ROSE

Pharmacokinetic Considerations
Analgesic Agents
    Antipyretic, Analgesic, and Nonsteroidal
      Anti-inflammatory Drugs (NSAIDs)
    Tramadol
    Ketamine
    Opioids
      Morphine
      Fentanyl
      Hydromorphone (Dilaudid)
      Meperidine (Demerol)
      Methadone
      Codeine
      Oxycodone
      Nalbuphine
      Naloxone

An important reason why pediatric pain is insufficiently treated is a lack of knowledge about the pharmacology of analgesic medications in this age group. This is partly due to the fluctuating pharmacokinetic and pharmacodynamic properties of analgesics during development. Although many analgesic medications have undergone thorough pharmacologic investigation in adults, similar studies have not always been performed in children.

PHARMACOKINETIC CONSIDERATIONS

Developmental changes in the composition of body compartments, plasma protein binding capacity, hepatic-enzyme systems, renal function, as well as changes in metabolic rate, oxygen consumption, and respiratory function may all significantly impact on analgesic drug distribution, metabolism, clearance, and action in pediatric patients. Reduced protein binding in neonates compared with older children and adults is the result of decreased quantities of albumin and α_1-acid glycoprotein,

the presence of a qualitatively different albumin that binds proteins less effectively, higher free fatty acid and bilirubin concentrations, and a lower plasma pH. Opioids and local anesthetics are heavily bound to α_1-acid glycoprotein in older children and adults, but neonates may have increased unbound concentrations of these drugs leading to increased analgesic effects as well as an increased potential for respiratory and central nervous system depression, and cardiovascular toxicity. Several conditions (e.g., burns, inflammatory bowel disease, malignancy, infection, and trauma) are associated with increased α_1-acid glycoprotein levels, and are associated with an increased bound fraction and decreased free fraction of drug in the blood. Thus, the administration of the usual dose of an analgesic may result in subtherapeutic effects in this patient population.

Body composition affects pharmacokinetics. Total body water content is approximately 85% of bodyweight in the premature neonate, compared to 75% in a full-term infant and 60% in an adult. This results in an increased volume of distribution for water-soluble drugs. It also results in an increased duration of action and therefore the need to increase the dosing interval for some drugs. Muscle mass and fat content are likewise reduced in preterm neonates (15% and 3% of bodyweight, respectively) compared to full-term infants (20% and 12%, respectively) and adults (50% and 18%, respectively). Smaller fat and muscle stores in neonates result in higher plasma concentrations of drugs since there is less uptake of drugs in these pharmacodynamically inactive sites. This, coupled with the fact that a greater proportion of cardiac output goes to the neonatal brain, means that there is a more rapid delivery of drugs to active sites. Furthermore, some have suggested that the blood–brain barrier is immature at birth and facilitates entry of drugs into brain tissue. Thus the brain concentration of many drugs may be higher in neonates than in older children and adults.

Most analgesics are lipophilic substances whose effects are diminished, and eventually ended, by a series of chemical reactions that transform them into water-soluble, inactive, substances that are able to be excreted. This transformation process, which is referred to as drug metabolism, often involves two phases and occurs primarily in the liver. Phase I reactions include oxidation, reduction, hydroxylation, and hydrolysis. Phase II reactions include conjugation processes such as glucuronidation, glycosylation, sulfation, methylation, and acetylation. The most important phase I enzyme family is the cytochrome P-450 system. This mixed oxidase system is dependent upon nicotinamide adenine dinucleotide phosphate (NADPH) and oxygen and is responsible for both oxidation and reduction reactions. Acetaminophen, nonsteroidal anti-inflammatory agents (NSAIDs), tramadol, and opioids are all metabolized in part by cytochrome P-450. At birth, hepatic enzyme systems responsible for oxidative metabolism (especially cytochrome P-450) and conjugation (including glucuronosyl transferases) are severely deficient. Hepatic enzymes responsible for drug metabolism, though present in limited quantities at birth, develop rapidly and approach adult levels over the first few months of life. Because of the relatively large liver size in children aged 2–6 years, metabolic capacity actually exceeds that of the adult and then declines to adult levels by puberty. Thus, children aged 2–6 years may require increased doses, shorter dosing intervals, and higher infusion rates of analgesics than younger or older patients in order to achieve comparable degrees of analgesia. In addition to age, several pathophysiologic conditions – including hypoxemia, hypotension, and increased intraabdominal pressure – can also affect drug metabolism by decreasing hepatic or renal blood flow and function. An example of this is the neonate who has undergone repair of omphalocele or gastroschisis and has increased intraabdominal pressure. Another important metabolic pathway consists of tissue and blood esterases which are responsible for remifentanil metabolism.

Water-soluble metabolites and, to a lesser extent, parent compounds are excreted primarily by the kidney in the urine but also by the liver in bile. In patients with a reduced glomerular filtration rate such as newborns, parent drug or active metabolite accumulation can lead to increased toxicity. For example, morphine undergoes phase II hepatic metabolism to yield morphine-6-glucuronide which is an active metabolite approximately 100 times more potent than morphine. Fortunately, this metabolite is less soluble in lipids and it does not penetrate the blood–brain barrier and brain tissue as readily as does morphine. Nevertheless, in patients with renal failure, this and other metabolites accumulate and may result in increased toxicity, including somnolence, coma, and/or respiratory depression. Likewise, normeperidine

may accumulate in patients with renal insufficiency receiving meperidine and result in seizures.

The immaturity of various respiratory functions and the high metabolic demands of the neonate have important implications for opioid therapy. Neonates and infants are more prone to develop atelectasis and respiratory failure when medical conditions or surgical procedures increase their work of breathing and/or metabolic demands since they have more compliant chest walls, poor control of lingual and pharyngeal muscles, smaller caliber airways, more compliant or collapsible laryngeal and tracheal cartilage, a decreased percentage of type 1 (fatigue resistant) diaphragm muscles, and a functional residual capacity that approaches the alveolar closing volume. Neonates have diminished ventilatory responses to carbon dioxide and oxygen, and they have an increase in metabolic rate with an oxygen consumption of 8 mL/kg/min. If ventilatory drive is depressed by opioid analgesics, a condition that readily occurs if sedatives or general anesthetics have also been administered, hypoventilation with hypercarbia and acidosis ensues. In this setting, irregular respirations with pauses or apnea can quickly lead to hypoxemia and cardiac arrest.

ANALGESIC AGENTS

Antipyretic, Analgesic, and Nonsteroidal Anti-inflammatory Drugs (NSAIDs)

NSAIDs are useful in the treatment of a large number of mild to moderately painful conditions and can be used effectively in combination with opioids for the treatment of severely painful conditions. In the last decade, these drugs have been extensively studied and found to be efficacious for the treatment of postoperative pain in children, particularly following ambulatory surgery (Table 24-1). Unlike opioid analgesics, antipyretic, analgesic, and NSAIDs do not depress respirations, result in sedation, or lead to dependence with long-term use. They act by inhibiting cyclooxygenase (COX) which is responsible for metabolizing arachidonic acid to form a variety of prostaglandins and thromboxanes. These are hyperalgesic substances thought to work by sensitizing peripheral nerve endings. They are also vasodilators and produce erythema and swelling along with the pain that accompanies inflammation or trauma. When arachidonic acid is released from traumatized cell membranes, it can also be metabolized by a lipoxygenase pathway to leukotrienes. When COX inhibitors are used, excessive leukotriene production is thought to be the mechanism responsible for producing aspirin-induced bronchoconstriction in some individuals.

Two principal COX isoenzymes have been identified. The constitutive form of COX (COX-1) is widely present in many tissues. The production of prostaglandins and

Table 24-1 Antipyretics and NSAIDs

Drug	Preparation	Dose	Interval	Maximum Daily Dose	Comments
Aspirin	*Tabs:* 81 mg, 325 mg *Chewable tab:* 81 mg	PO: 10-15 mg/kg	4-6 h	90 mg/kg/day	Contraindicated in children with viral syndrome, NSAID allergy, or syndrome of asthma, rhinitis, and nasal polyps
Acetaminophen	*Tabs:* 325 mg, 500 mg *Chewable tabs:* 80 mg, 160 mg *Elixir:* 160 mg/5 mL *Drops:* 80 mg/0.8 mL *Suppositories:* 80 mg, 120 mg, 325 mg, 650 mg	PO: 10-15 mg/kg. Rectal (single dose): 35-45 mg/kg Rectal (repeated dose): 20 mg/kg	Oral (children): 4 h Rectal (newborns, infants, children): 6 h Rectal (premature newborns, 28-32 postconceptual weeks): 12 h	Children: lesser of 100 mg/kg/day or 4 g/day. Infants: 75 mg/kg/day Newborns: (>32 post-conceptual weeks) 60 mg/kg/day; (28-32 postconceptual weeks) 40 mg/kg/day	Hepatic failure and necrosis with overdoses.
Ibuprofen	*Tabs:* 200 mg, 400 mg, 600 mg, 800 mg *Chewable tabs:* 50 mg, 100 mg *Elixir:* 100 mg/5 mL *Drops:* 50 mg/1.25 mL	PO: 6-10 mg/kg	4-6 h	Lesser of 40 mg/kg/day or 2.4 g	Prolonged use increases the risk for gastric irritation, ulceration, and hemorrhage; bleeding disorders; altered renal function.
Naproxen	*Tabs:* 220 mg, 250 mg, 375 mg, 500 mg *Elixir:* 25 mg/mL	PO: 5-10 mg/kg	12 h	20 mg/kg/day	Prolonged use increases the risk for gastric irritation, ulceration, and hemorrhage; bleeding disorders; altered renal function.
Ketorolac	*Injects:* 15 mg/mL, 30 mg/mL	IV: 0.5 mg/kg	6 h	Lesser of 2 mg/kg/day or 120 mg	No more than 5 days of therapy due to risk of gastric irritation, ulceration, and hemorrhage; bleeding disorders; altered renal function

IV, intravenously; PO, by mouth; NSAID, nonsteroidal anti-inflammatory drug.

thromboxanes in these tissues is essential for mediating important physiologic functions. These functions include protection of the gastric mucosa, renal blood flow regulation, and platelet aggregation. The inducible COX (COX-2) is found in traumatized or inflamed cells. COX-1 inhibition is responsible for the unwanted side-effects of NSAIDs (gastric ulceration and hemorrhage, disturbances in blood clotting, alterations in renal blood flow and function, and bronchoconstriction) and COX-2 inhibition produces the therapeutic effects. Most drugs in this class are nonselective COX inhibitors and interfere with the normal physiologic functions described above as well as producing anti-inflammatory and analgesic effects. New classes of drugs that are relatively selective COX-2 inhibitors have appeared recently but studies in children have been few. Since acetaminophen is a weak

COX inhibitor and has no peripheral anti-inflammatory effects, its analgesic action, like its antipyretic effect, is believed to be mediated by central COX inhibition.

Acetylsalicylic acid (aspirin) is the oldest known drug in this class but is rarely used in pediatrics now because it is associated with Reye's syndrome. It is still useful in juvenile rheumatoid arthritis and other rheumatologic conditions. It is administered orally at a dose of 10-15 mg/kg every 4 hours. The maximum daily dose is 90 mg/kg.

Acetaminophen is the most popular antipyretic and analgesic used in pediatric patients. It does not inhibit peripheral COX and therefore has none of the unwanted effects of other NSAIDs. A clear dose-response effect of rectally administered acetaminophen up to 60 mg/kg has been demonstrated in pediatric ambulatory surgery patients. It is estimated that 50% of pediatric ambulatory surgery patients who receive rectal acetaminophen 35 mg/kg intraoperatively will not require morphine in the pediatric acute care setting. Effective analgesic plasma concentrations are not known but antipyretic effects are seen with levels of 10–20 μg/mL and can be achieved within 30 minutes after oral doses of 10–15 mg/kg. Absorption following rectal administration is variable, with peak concentrations attained 2–3 hours after administration. Orally administered acetaminophen 10–15 mg/kg can be given every 4 hours. The maximum daily dose of acetaminophen is 100 mg/kg in children, 75 mg/kg in infants, 60 mg/kg in neonates born at 32 weeks' gestation or greater, and 40 mg/kg in preterm neonates born at 28–32 weeks' gestation. When acetaminophen 35–45 mg/kg is administered rectally, subsequent doses should be reduced to 20 mg/kg and the dosing interval lengthened to every 6–8 hours. Acetaminophen is metabolized primarily in the liver through glucuronidation and sulfation. Under normal circumstances only a small fraction is oxidized by the cytochrome P-450 system. However, with acetaminophen overdose, the oxidation pathway is enhanced and results in the production of the hepatotoxic metabolite N-acetyl-*p*-benzocinon-imine, and fulminant hepatic failure and necrosis can occur unless treatment with N-acetylcysteine is started.

Several other NSAIDs are now commonly used for the management of a variety of painful conditions in children. There is little difference in analgesic efficacy between the many drugs that are now available. Choice of an agent depends upon other factors such as the desired dosing interval and the patient's fasting status. Ibuprofen is the most widely used drug in this class and is available in several formulations for pediatric administration. Adverse events are rare when used for a short time. Some studies claim superior analgesia with ibuprofen versus acetaminophen but others have failed to demonstrate a difference. For analgesia, ibuprofen can be given as a single dose of 15 mg/kg orally. However, for repeated doses in children aged 6 months to 12 years, ibuprofen should be given as 10 mg/kg every 6 hours orally (maximum daily dose 40 mg/kg).

Naproxen has a longer half-life than ibuprofen, allowing it to be given every 8–12 hours. Its safety in newborns and infants has not been established. The usual dose is 5–10 mg/kg orally (maximum daily dose 20 mg/kg). In the United States, ketorolac is the only NSAID available as an intravenous as well as oral preparation. It has been used effectively in selected pediatric postoperative patients who are not at risk for bleeding since it, like all the nonselective COX inhibitors, interferes with platelet aggregation. Ketorolac should not be used for more than 5 days because of the risk for gastric ulceration and hemorrhage. The recommended dose of ketorolac is 0.5 mg/kg intravenously every 6 hours (the maximum daily dose being the lesser of 2 mg/kg and 120 mg).

Tramadol

Tramadol is an effective and safe analgesic for postoperative pain in children. It is an atypical opioid structurally related to codeine, whose unique mechanism of action involves both central inhibition of norepinephrine and reuptake of serotonin. Animal studies indicate that naloxone only partially reverses tramadol analgesia, which indicates that nonopioid mechanisms may predominate. Tramadol has one-tenth the affinity for the μ receptor as codeine, and appears to be 10–15 times less potent than morphine in adult clinical trials. Tramadol is also similar in chemical structure to the antidepressant venlafaxine, a unique selective serotonin receptor inhibitor.

Tramadol has a favorable side-effect profile compared to opioid analgesics, making it an attractive alternative for analgesic therapy in children. When used according to dosing guidelines, it does not cause respiratory depression, sedation, or constipation. Analgesic tolerance has not been a problem with long-term tramadol administration, and although psychological dependence occurs, it is rare. However, the incidences of nausea, vomiting, and dizziness are not different from those associated with opioid analgesics. Seizures are a rare complication of tramadol therapy. Exceeding dosing guidelines, prescribing tramadol in patients taking psychoactive medications (tricyclic antidepressants, selective serotonin reuptake inhibitors, monoamine oxidase inhibitors, and neuroleptics, and other drugs known to reduce seizure thresholds), and administering tramadol to patients with a known seizure disorder or head injury, all appear to increase the risk for seizures. Tramadol is available as a 50-mg scored tablet. It is also available in combination with acetaminophen (37.5 mg tramadol/325 mg acetaminophen). The recommended dose of tramadol is 1–2 mg/kg (maximum dose 100 mg) every 6 hours (maximum daily dose the lesser of 8 mg/kg/day or 400 mg/day). It is not yet FDA-approved for use in pediatric patients.

Ketamine

The phencyclidine derivative and dissociative anesthetic, ketamine, is a potent analgesic in subanesthetic doses and has been administered orally, rectally, intramuscularly, and intravenously to provide analgesia for short painful procedures in children. Analgesic effects may be mediated via N-methyl-D-aspartate (NMDA) receptor antagonism as well as σ opioid receptor agonism. However, naloxone administration does not result in antagonism of ketamine analgesia. Ketamine also has an affinity for central muscarinic receptors and anticholinesterase agents may partially reverse its effects.

Administration of ketamine is associated with a unique set of side-effects and potential complications.

Ketamine is known to be a negative inotrope. However, owing to its ability to release endogenous catecholamines, cardiovascular function is well preserved unless the patient is severely hypovolemic. Ketamine is a respiratory depressant and attenuates the ventilatory response to carbon dioxide. Although laryngeal reflexes remain intact, aspiration of gastric contents can occur and has been reported following its use in children for short painful procedures. Ketamine is a bronchial smooth muscle dilator. Salivary and bronchial secretions are increased by ketamine but can be prevented by prior administration of atropine or glycopyrrolate. Central nervous system effects include an increase in cerebral blood flow and oxygen consumption, and thus intracranial pressure may rise dangerously in children with decreased intracranial compliance. Also, ketamine is associated with psychomimetic effects including recurrent hallucinations and nightmares. Prior administration of a benzodiazepine may attenuate or prevent these effects.

Intravenous doses of ketamine as low as 0.25–0.5 mg/kg may produce intense analgesia for 10–15 minutes. However, higher doses (e.g., 1–2 mg/kg) may be needed to produce profound analgesia for short painful procedures such as fracture reduction. The bioavailability of oral ketamine is 20–25%. Oral ketamine 1.25–2.5 mg/kg will often result in adequate analgesia without loss of consciousness. Nevertheless, close observation and monitoring by an individual with expertise in recognizing and managing respiratory depression is required. Furthermore, equipment and medications necessary for emergency airway management should be present whenever ketamine is administered. The author's practice always includes the administration of oral midazolam 0.5 mg/kg and atropine 0.02 mg/kg prior to oral ketamine 1.25 mg/kg for children who require analgesia for a painful procedure.

Opioids

Opioids are useful in the treatment of moderate to severe nociceptive pain and may occasionally be useful in the treatment of neuropathic pain. Other indications for opioids include cough suppression and the treatment of dysentery. Unlike NSAIDs, which act by enzyme inhibition, opioids exert their pharmacologic effects primarily by binding to pre- and post-synaptic cell membranes in the central nervous system via specific opioid receptors, resulting in neuronal inhibition. Neuronal inhibition may occur by at least two mechanisms: the inhibition of excitatory neurotransmitter release from presynaptic terminals and/or hyperpolarization of the neuron. Opioid receptors are linked to regulatory G proteins when bound to an opioid analgesic. By regulating ion channels, G proteins cause hyperpolarization of the neuron, rendering it less excitable.

Several types and subtypes of opioid receptors have been identified. The μ receptor (so named because of its affinity for morphine) is found in the cortex, thalamus, and periaqueductal gray regions of the brain as well as in the substantia gelatinosa of the spinal cord. The μ receptor has been further subtyped to include μ_1 (mediating supraspinal analgesia and dependence) and μ_2 (mediating respiratory depression, intestinal dysmotility, sedation, and bradycardia). Most opioids in clinical use today exert their analgesic effects when administered systemically at supraspinal μ receptors. However, with spinally administered opioids, effects are predominantly mediated by μ receptors in the substantia gelatinosa of the spinal cord.

The κ receptor is found primarily in the substantia gelatinosa of the spinal cord but is also found in the brain. It is associated with spinal analgesia, sedation, miosis, inhibition of antidiuretic hormone, and mild respiratory depression. The δ receptor mediates analgesia and euphoria and has been located in the pontine nucleus, amygdala, and deep cortex. Sigma (σ) receptor activation by some opioids, especially the mixed agonist–antagonist drugs like butorphanol and nalbuphine, is thought to mediate unpleasant psychomimetic effects including dysphoria and hallucinations.

Opioids are classified as strong or weak, or as naturally occurring, semisynthetic, or synthetic. However, it is more useful to consider opioids as agonists, partial agonists, mixed agonist–antagonists, or antagonists. An agonist, upon binding and occupying a receptor, initiates a change in cellular function that produces a pharmacologic effect. Examples include morphine, meperidine, hydromorphone, methadone, oxycodone, codeine, fentanyl, and remifentanil. An antagonist is a drug that by binding to a receptor prevents access of the agonist to the receptor site and therefore antagonizes the pharmacologic effect of the agonist. Examples include naloxone, naltrexone, and nalmefene. A partial agonist such as buprenorphine binds the receptor but in doing so results in less than a maximal response of a pure agonist. The mixed agonist–antagonists nalbuphine and pentazocine may bind to multiple receptor types and exert agonist effects at some while antagonist effects at others.

Side-effects of all opioid analgesics are similar and include nausea, vomiting, sedation, pruritus, urinary retention, respiratory depression, ileus, and constipation. Less common effects include myoclonic movement, dysphoria, hallucinations, and seizures. However, there is great individual variability in the side-effect profiles of specific opioids. Thus if a child on a patient-controlled analgesia pump receiving morphine experiences an intolerable side-effect such as vomiting, it is worthwhile to try a different opioid such as hydromorphone. Often, this is an effective way to alleviate an undesirable side-effect.

The recommended doses of several opioids used routinely at The Children's Hospital of Philadelphia are provided in Table 24-2. There is wide individual variability in analgesic response to opioids, so the doses recommended are intended to guide initial dosing. Careful and repeated assessment of patients receiving analgesics is required in order to determine analgesic efficacy and to look for analgesic complications. Commonly the initial dose selected will need to be modified upward or downward based on clinical circumstances.

Table 24-2   Opioid Dosing Regimens

Opioid	Routes/Age Groups	Dose/Interval
Morphine	*Oral, immediate release*:	
	Infants and children	0.3 mg/kg every 3–4 h
	Oral, sustained release:	
	Infants and children	0.25–0.5 mg/kg every 8–12 h
	IV bolus:	
	Preterm neonate[a]	10–25 µg/kg every 2–4 h
	Full-term neonate[b]	25–50 µg/kg every 3–4 h
	Infants and children[c]	50–100 µg every 3 h
	IV infusion:	
	Preterm neonate[d]	2–5 µg/kg/h
	Full-term neonate[d]	5–10 µg/kg/h
	Infants and children	15–30 µg/kg/h
	Epidural bolus:	
	Infants and children	25–33 µg/kg single dose
	Epidural infusion:	
	Infants and children	4–8 µg/kg/h
Hydromorphone	*Oral*:	
	Infants and children	40–80 µg/kg every 4 h
	IV bolus:	
	Infants and children	10–20 µg/kg every 3–4 h
	IV infusion:	
	Infants and children	3–5 µg/kg/h
	Epidural infusion:	
	Infants and children	1–3 µg/kg/h
Fentanyl	*Oral transmucosal*	10–15 µg/kg (oralet)
	Intranasal	1–2 µg/kg
	Transdermal	25, 50, 75, 100 µg/h (duragesic patches)[e]
	IV bolus	0.5–1 µg/kg every 1–2 h
	IV infusion	0.5 µg/kg/h
	Epidural bolus	0.5–1 µg/kg
	Epidural infusion	0.2–1 µg/kg/h
Meperidine[f]	*IV bolus*:	
	Infants and children	0.8–1 mg/kg every 3–4 h
Methadone	*Oral or IV bolus*:	
	Infants and children	0.1–0.2 mg/kg every 12–36 h
Nalbuphine	*IV bolus*:	
	Preterm neonate	10–25 µg/kg every 2–4 h
	Full-term neonate	25–50 µg/kg every 2–4 h
	Infants and children	50–100 µg/kg every 2–4 h
	IV infusion:	
	Preterm neonate	5–10 µg/kg/h
	Full-term neonate	10–15 µg/kg/h
	Infants and children	20 µg/kg/h
Codeine	*Oral*	0.5–1 mg/kg every 4 h
Oxycodone	*Oral*	0.1–0.15 mg/kg every 4 h

[a] Newborns ≤37 weeks of gestation.
[b] Newborns >37 weeks gestation.
[c] Infants >3 months of age.
[d] Significant risk for respiratory depression in neonates with a natural airway and spontaneous ventilation.
[e] Not for acute pain management but for the opioid-tolerant patient with chronic pain; patches may not be cut into smaller sizes.
[f] Avoid long-term use since a metabolite, normeperidine, may accumulate and cause seizures.
IV, intravenous.

Morphine

Morphine is the prototypical opioid analgesic against which all others are compared. It is administered to children by many routes for the management of many types of pain. Morphine is primarily metabolized in the liver by glucuronidation to form morphine-3-glucuronide (M3G), an inactive metabolite, and morphine-6-glucuronide (M6G), an active metabolite. Both M3G and M6G are excreted by the kidneys. The morphine glucuronidation pathway is present in even premature newborns but the capacity for glucuronidation matures quickly with age. Although morphine's volume of distribution (V_d) remains relatively constant in children of all ages (2.8 ± 2.6 L/kg), clearance (Cl) and termination half-life ($t_{1/2}$) appear to change with age. In a recent metaanalysis of morphine pharmacokinetics, clearance was 2.2 ± 0.7 mL/min/kg in preterm neonates, 8.1 ± 3.2 mL/min/kg in term newborns 0–57 days old, and 23.6 ± 8.5 mL/min/kg for infants and children over 11 days old. The terminal half-life of morphine was reported to be 9.0 ± 3.4 hours in preterm neonates, 6.5 ± 2.8 hours in full-term neonates aged 0–57 days, and 2.0 ± 1.8 hours in infants and children over 11 days old. These values represent pooled estimates from a number of studies. There is tremendous variability among individuals and even in the same individual over time. Although the data from several studies involving preterm neonates up to 1 week of age correlated well and these patients clearly represent a separate group, the exact age at which term newborns transition to the older infants, children, and adults with regard to morphine $t_{1/2}$ and Cl is unknown. Some term newborns achieve adult values for these parameters by 2 weeks of age but many take up to 2 months of age to attain these values.

Studies to determine the effective plasma morphine concentration for analgesia in children have yielded inconsistent results. This is in part due to the fact that pain is a subjective experience and the amount of pain reported by children after similar surgeries is quite variable. Therefore it is important to monitor the degree of analgesia and the types and severity of side-effects produced by any dose of morphine and to adjust the dose accordingly.

Fentanyl

Fentanyl is highly lipophilic enabling it to readily penetrate cell membranes, and is a hundred times more potent than morphine. It has a relatively rapid onset and short offset making it a preferred analgesic for short, painful procedures. Its short duration of effect is due to redistribution of the drug from active sites, not its metabolism. In fact, fentanyl has a relatively long total body elimination half-life: 233 ± 137 minutes in 3- to 12-month-old infants, 244 ± 79 minutes in infants aged over 1 year, and 129 ± 42 minutes in adults. This means that with high doses, repeated doses, or continuous infusions, fentanyl can accumulate in the plasma and its duration of effects such as analgesia and respiratory depression becomes dependent upon its metabolism and excretion. Fentanyl and related compounds are highly bound to α_1-acid glycoprotein in the plasma. Thus, newborns that have reduced α_1-acid glycoprotein have a higher percentage of free unbound fentanyl. Fentanyl undergoes glucuronidation in the liver to form inactive metabolites which are excreted by the kidneys.

In addition to intravenous and epidural administration, fentanyl can be administered by intranasal, transmucosal, and transdermal routes. Intranasal fentanyl has been administered intraoperatively to children undergoing myringotomy and tube insertion to provide postoperative analgesia. Fentanyl is also available in a candy matrix (fentanyl oralet) for transmucosal absorption and is administered as a premedication for children undergoing painful procedures. Transmucosal absorption is approximately 25–33%, bypasses the hepatic first-pass effect, and is therefore more efficient than oral administration. Analgesic effects begin within 20 minutes of transmucosal administration, and last for approximately 2 hours. If somnolence is observed the oralet should be taken away from the child.

Fentanyl can be administered transcutaneously by a patch that consists of a semipermeable membrane and a drug reservoir. The fentanyl patch is applied to the skin with a contact adhesive. The patches come in a variety of strengths to deliver fentanyl at a rate of 25, 50, 75, or 100 μg/h for 3 days. There is a relatively long time to onset, but after the patch is removed a small depot of fentanyl remains in the skin. The fentanyl patch is not appropriate for opioid-naive patients with acute pain since the analgesic effects cannot be achieved rapidly and the dose of fentanyl cannot be safely titrated.

Hydromorphone (Dilaudid)

Hydromorphone is a synthetic derivative of morphine. Many clinicians who are familiar with this drug believe that it produces less nausea, vomiting, pruritus, and sedation than morphine. It is approximately 10 times more lipophilic and 5 times more potent than morphine. It has a longer duration of action (4–6 hours) and elimination half-life (3–4 hours). Hydromorphone has been used by a variety of routes (see Table 24-2) and is often used for patient-controlled analgesia.

Meperidine (Demerol)

Meperidine is a synthetic opioid derived from phenylpiperidine. It is one-tenth as potent as morphine, and has a similar pharmacokinetic profile. It is metabolized in the liver by hydrolysis and N-demethylation, and has an elimination half-life of approximately 3 hours. Meperidine has an active metabolite, normeperidine, which is one-half as potent as an analgesic but twice as potent at causing seizures. Once thought to be less of a respiratory depressant than morphine, in equianalgesic doses, meperidine appears to produce the same amount of respiratory depression. Controversy exists as to whether it has less of an effect on the Sphincter of Oddi and biliary tract pressure than morphine. Some clinicians believe it is the opioid of choice for treating severe pain associated with biliary colic or pancreatitis. Meperidine administration is associated with a 20% reduction in cardiac output and tachycardia. In high doses it may slow the electroencephalogram. It is rarely used repeatedly in pediatrics because a metabolite, normeperidine, may accumulate in this setting and produce tremors or seizures. A catastrophic syndrome of excitation, delirium, hyperpyrexia, and convulsions has been seen in patients who received meperidine concomitantly with monoamine oxidase inhibitors and in patients with hyperthyroidism. It is still used to treat postoperative shivering as well as shivering associated with amphotericin or blood product administration.

Methadone

Methadone is a synthetic opioid that is equipotent or slightly more potent when compared to morphine. It has the longest and most unreliable elimination half-life of any of the opioid drugs in common use, ranging from 13 to 100+ hours. Its analgesic effects as well as respiratory and central nervous system depressant effects can last 12–36 hours and sometimes longer after a single dose. Methadone also has excellent bioavailability, roughly 80%, after oral dosing. Although traditionally used orally to wean opioid-dependent patients, there is interest in administering methadone to patients with acute pain to provide stable, continuous levels of analgesia. With intravenous administration, peak effects can be seen within 10–15 minutes after a single dose. Thus titrating methadone with incremental doses of 0.05 mg/kg IV every 15 minutes is possible. Once satisfactory analgesia is achieved, additional methadone at 0.05–0.1 mg/kg can be administered every 4–12 hours as needed. The drug should be held if somnolence or adequate analgesia is present. In addition to being a μ receptor agonist, methadone is also an NMDA receptor antagonist. This may explain the phenomenon referred to as "incomplete cross-tolerance" which is used to describe the observation that methadone is more potent as a respiratory and central nervous system depressant than predicted by conversion formulas from morphine. Instead of a 1:1 conversion ratio for morphine to methadone, the ratio may actually be closer to 1:0.1. Failure to recognize this can result in severe respiratory depression and death.

Codeine

Codeine is a derivative of morphine and must undergo O-demethylation in the liver by a P-450 oxidase pathway to produce morphine in order to produce effective analgesia.

Approximately 5–10% of administered codeine is converted to morphine in the majority of subjects. However, depending on the ethnic group studied, anywhere from 4% to 10% of the population is devoid of the enzyme required for this conversion, so these individuals do not derive analgesic benefit from the drug. After oral administration, codeine has 60% bioavailability. Analgesic effects are seen within 20 minutes with peak effects at between 1 and 2 hours. Its elimination half-life is 2.5–3 hours. Codeine is usually administered with acetaminophen for conditions that are moderately painful. Because a significant number of people do not experience analgesic benefits from codeine, and because codeine is associated with severe nausea and vomiting in some patients, in the author's institution we prefer to use oxycodone as a first-line oral opioid analgesic in children. Only when a child has been on codeine in the past, and the family requests codeine because it worked well, do we continue to prescribe this drug.

Oxycodone

Oxycodone is a semisynthetic thebaine derivative produced by modifying morphine. It has an equivalent potency to morphine when given intravenously and is 10 times more potent than codeine when administered orally. After oral administration, it has a bioavailability of 60%. Analgesia begins within 20–30 minutes and peaks at between 1 and 2 hours. Oxycodone has an elimination half-time of 2.5–4 hours and duration of effect of 4–5 hours. Oxycodone and its active metabolite oxymorphone may accumulate in patients with renal insufficiency, leading to respiratory depression if the dose and interval are not adjusted. Some investigators believe that oxycodone produces less nausea but otherwise the side-effect profile is similar to that of all potent opioid analgesics. Specifically, oxycodone at equianalgesic doses produces similar degrees of respiratory depression and sedation. A sustained-release form is now available but many families resist this drug because of the negative press it has received related to its abuse.

Nalbuphine

Nalbuphine possesses agonist properties at the κ receptor and antagonist effects at the μ receptor. It is mainly metabolized in the liver and has a plasma half-life of about 5 hours. At intravenous doses up to 200 μg/kg it is roughly equivalent to morphine with respect to analgesia. However, nalbuphine appears to have a ceiling effect, as increasing the dose beyond this point does not result in greater analgesia. Kappa-mediated effects (e.g., sedation, dysphoria, and euphoria) may occur with increasing doses or with repetitive lower doses. Nalbuphine has been used to antagonize μ-mediated effects such as nausea, vomiting, pruritus, urinary retention, and respiratory depression in patients receiving morphine, fentanyl,

Article To Know

Gunter JB, Varughese AM, Harrington JF et al: Recovery and complications after tonsillectomy in children: a comparison of ketorolac and morphine. Anesth Analg 81:1136-1141, 1995.

Adenotonsillectomy is a common procedure in children and recovery can be painful and complicated by nausea, vomiting, dehydration, bleeding, and airway obstruction. This article is important because it addresses this clinical scenario. It is the report of a randomized, double-blind investigation of the effect of ketorolac 1 mg/kg IV or morphine 0.1 mg/kg IV administered in the operating room after tonsillectomy by electrocautery dissection under a standard halothane anesthetic in 96 children aged 1-12 years. All subjects received rectal acetaminophen 15-20 mg/kg on admission to the postanesthesia care unit (PACU). Intravenous morphine 0.05 mg/kg could be administered twice in the PACU as a rescue analgesic at the discretion of the anesthesiologist. This study was discontinued after the first 97 subjects were enrolled because of an increased incidence of major bleeding and a greater number of bleeding episodes during the first 24 hours in patients who received ketorolac ($n = 49$). No differences existed between the two study groups with respect to demographics and surgical management. Two subjects in the ketorolac group required reoperation for hemorrhage (on the day of surgery and 5 days after) compared to one child in the morphine group on postoperative day 6. Ketorolac patients had more bleeding episodes than the morphine subjects (0.22 episodes per subject vs 0.04 episodes per subject) in the first 24 hours after surgery. Among subjects who bled, the ketorolac group had more severe bleeding than the morphine group. One-third of each study group required morphine rescues in the PACU. There were no differences in awakening times, recovery, or discharge readiness times. One patient in the morphine group and three in the ketorolac group required supplemental oxygen to maintain oxyhemoglobin saturation >95% after discharge from the PACU. Emesis occurred with the same frequency in both groups but the median number of emetic episodes was less in the ketorolac vs morphine group (1 [0-3] vs 3 [0-4]). The authors concluded that ketorolac 1 mg/kg at the conclusion of tonsillectomy resulted in less severe postoperative vomiting but did not result in morphine-sparing in the PACU, more rapid recovery and discharge readiness times, or rates of unplanned admission to the hospital. Furthermore, postoperative ketorolac administration was associated with a higher incidence of major bleeding. Based on this and other evidence from studies looking at preoperative ketorolac administration, ketorolac is contraindicated in pediatric patients undergoing adenotonsillectomy.

or hydromorphone. Other primarily μ-mediated effects such as physical dependence are reported much less frequently with chronic nalbuphine administration. Patients receiving μ agonists for long periods may experience withdrawal symptoms if they are transitioned to nalbuphine abruptly. As with pentazocine and butorphanol, nalbuphine may cause less elevation of biliary tract pressure than pure μ agonists and has therefore been used for the treatment of pain associated with biliary tract pathology. Nalbuphine is primarily administered intravenously but has been administered orally. Oral bioavailability is only 20-25%.

Naloxone

Naloxone is a potent μ, δ, and κ antagonist. It is used to antagonize respiratory depression (up to 10 μg/kg IV) and sedation, and in low doses (1-2 μg/kg/h) it is useful in treating intractable pruritus associated with opioid administration. It will also antagonize all other μ effects including analgesia, urinary retention, nausea, and vomiting. A syndrome of hypertension, tachycardia, dyspnea, tachypnea, pulmonary edema, nausea, vomiting, and ventricular fibrillation has been reported in opioid-dependent patients or in patients who are receiving high doses of opioids for severe pain and who receive excessive doses of naloxone rapidly for the treatment of respiratory depression

and coma. It is preferable in these circumstances to provide ventilatory assistance while titrating smaller amounts of naloxone (0.5-1 μg/kg IV) to the desired effect.

Naloxone is rapidly metabolized in the liver and has a plasma elimination half-life of 60 minutes. Therefore, its duration of action is less than that of the μ agonists it is intended to antagonize. Continued close observation is required in all patients who have received naloxone to reverse respiratory depression in order to prevent a catastrophic return of respiratory depression when the effects of naloxone are gone.

ADDITIONAL ARTICLES TO KNOW

Andersson BJ, Holford NH, Wollard GA et al: Perioperative pharmacodynamics of acetaminophen analgesia in children. *Anesthesiology* 90:411-421, 1999.

Berde CB, Sethna NF: Analgesics for the treatment of pain in children. *N Engl J Med* 347:1094-1103, 2002.

Berde CB, Beyer JE, Bournaki MC et al: Comparison of morphine and methadone for prevention of postoperative pain in 3- to 7-year-old children. *J Pediatr* 119:136-141, 1991.

Finkel JC, Rose JB, Schmitz ML et al: An evaluation of the efficacy and tolerability of oral tramadol hydrochloride tablets for the treatment of postsurgical pain in children. *Anesth Analg* 94:1469-1473, 2002.

Kart T, Christrup LL, Rasmussen M: Recommended use of morphine in neonates, infants, and children based on a literature review: 1. Pharmacokinetics. *Paediatr Anaesth* 7:5–11, 1997.

Kart T, Christrup LL, Rasmussen M: Recommended use of morphine in neonates, infants, and children based on a literature review: 2. Clinical use. *Paediatr Anaesth* 7:93–101, 1997.

Kendrick WD, Woods AM, Daly MY et al: Naloxone versus nalbuphine infusion for epidural morphine-induced pruritis. *Anesth Analg* 82:641–647, 1996.

Kokki H, Hendolin H, Maunukseal EL et al: Ibuprofen in the treatment of postoperative pain in small children: a randomized double-blind placebo controlled parallel group. *Acta Anaesth Scand* 38:467–472, 1994.

Korpela R, Korvenoja P, Meretoja OA et al: Morphine-sparing effect of acetaminophen in pediatric day-case surgery. *Anesthesiology* 91:442–447, 1999.

Lynn AM, Opheim KE, Tyler DC: Morphine infusion after pediatric cardiac surgery. *Crit Care Med* 12:863–866, 1984.

Lynn AM, Nespeca MK, Opheim KE, Slattery JT: Respiratory effects of intravenous morphine infusions in neonates, infants, and children after cardiac surgery. *Anesth Analg* 77:695–701, 1993.

Parker RI, Mahan RA, Giugliano D et al: Efficacy and safety of intravenous midazolam and ketamine as sedation for therapeutic and diagnostic procedures in children. *Pediatrics* 99:427–431, 1997.

Singleton MA, Rosen JI, Fisher DM: Plasma concentrations of fentanyl in infants, children, and adults. *Can J Anaesth* 34:152–155, 1987.

Local Anesthetics and Adjuvant Analgesics

JOHN B. ROSE

OVERVIEW

All local anesthetics in use today are synthetic derivatives of cocaine, the first local anesthetic to be discovered, and a plant alkaloid obtained from the leaves of the South American coca plant. Cocaine is a benzoic acid derivative coupled to a tertiary amine compound by an ester linkage. It is a weak base that is poorly soluble in water. Similarly, all local anesthetics contain a lipophilic benzoic acid derivative linked to a hydrophilic tertiary amine by an ester or amide chain and exist in ionized (cationic) and unionized forms (weak base). The lipophilic and hydrophilic components of local anesthetics enable their penetration into both lipid and aqueous membranes. It is this essential property that permits local anesthetics to traverse perineurium and axonal walls and block neural transmission without affecting cellular function or metabolism. Sodium conductance (i.e., depolarization) is prevented when an adequate concentration and volume

of local anesthetic surround the nerve. The external opening of the Na^+ channel is not the site of action of local anesthetics. Rather, the lipophilic, uncharged base form of the local anesthetic penetrates the neuronal cell wall and reaches the axoplasm where it again exists in equilibrium as both a charged ionized salt and an uncharged base. The relative concentration of these forms depends on the tissue pH and the pKa of the compound. Once in the axoplasm, the charged base or cationic form enters the internal opening of the sodium channel and blocks Na^+ conductance. During repolarization, K^+ efflux through K^+ channels is not disrupted by local anesthetics.

Local anesthetic metabolism is determined by the chemical linkage. Those with an ester linkage are metabolized by plasma esterases and those with an amide linkage are metabolized in the liver. Compounds with ester linkages are more likely to cause allergic reactions. The degree of lipid solubility of a local anesthetic determines its potency. This should not be surprising given the fact that the neuronal cell wall is a lipid structure. However, the relationship between lipid solubility and potency is not linear. The onset of action of a local anesthetic is correlated with its specific dissociation constant, or pKa – the pH at which 50% of the drug is present as the uncharged base and 50% as the cationic form. The unionized base is required to penetrate the cell wall. All local anesthetics have a pKa greater than 7.4. The lower the pKa of a local anesthetic, the greater the number of uncharged molecules available to traverse the lipid cell membrane, and the more rapid its onset of action.

The duration of action of a local anesthetic is determined by its protein binding capacity. After traversing lipid membranes, the local anesthetic enters the sodium channel, a protein structure, in order to exert its pharmacologic effect. Therefore, duration of action is directly correlated with degree of protein binding.

Frequency-dependent blockade is another important characteristic of local anesthetics. Most local anesthetics enter the sodium channel only when it is open during depolarization. Thus neurons with high-frequency depolarization (i.e., sensory and pain fibers) are more readily blocked than fibers that have low-frequency depolarization (i.e., motor nerves). The dissociation of sensory and motor blockade is clinically useful. Lidocaine and bupivacaine are dependent on the frequency of depolarization but tetracaine and etidocaine do not depend on it. Hence, etidocaine causes a relatively greater amount of motor block, and is therefore not useful in epidural infusions for postoperative analgesia.

A final property of local anesthetics that deserves mention is tissue penetrance. This characteristic has not been the subject of many investigations and is not quantifiable. Nevertheless, the onset of action of local anesthetics is not solely dependent upon the drug's dissociation constant. Chloroprocaine has a pKa of 9.1 and one would predict that it would have a slow onset time. However, it has a rapid onset time. In order to explain this phenomenon the concept of tissue penetrance was proposed. Chloroprocaine has a high tissue penetrance since it is able to penetrate perineural tissues rapidly.

Toxicity of local anesthetics can be divided into three categories: allergic reactions, neurotoxicity and systemic toxicity. Rare allergic reactions are mainly associated with ester local anesthetics, which are metabolized by plasma esterases to form para-aminobenzoic acid (PABA), the probable allergenic component. PABA is present in sunscreens and it is recommended that ester local anesthetics not be administered to patients with a history of sunscreen allergy. Skin testing is available to diagnose true local anesthetic allergy. The amide local anesthetics are safe in patients with a true allergy to ester anesthetics as cross-reactivity between ester and amide local anesthetics has not been demonstrated.

Every local anesthetic is capable of producing neurotoxicity. However, this complication is rare. True local anesthetic neurotoxicity is usually mild and resolves completely over time. More common is a neuropathy that follows a nerve injury due to needle trauma or a direct intraneural injection of epinephrine-containing local anesthetics in high concentrations. Lidocaine 5% for spinal anesthesia has been a particular concern because of its association with transient neurologic symptoms (TNS). This syndrome is characterized by the appearance of back pain that radiates to the buttocks within 24 hours of the block, the absence of motor and sensory deficits, and resolution within 3–10 days. The lowest effective concentration of local anesthetic should be used when performing any regional block. Preservatives in local anesthetics may also cause neurotoxicity. A 2-chloroprocaine preparation containing 0.2% bisulfite was associated with neurotoxicity following caudal and epidural analgesia. A preservative-free preparation is now available.

Excessive blood levels of a local anesthetic may cause systemic toxicity. Most commonly this occurs from an unintentional intravascular injection. However, delayed toxicity can occur from systemic absorption of excessive doses of local anesthetics used for epidural or peripheral nerve blocks. All local anesthetics appear to have a similar therapeutic index for central nervous system toxicity. In the conscious patient this consists of ringing in the ears, tingling around the lips, other abnormal and disturbing sensory findings, or a change in mental status. Seizures are often preceded by twitching movements. Local anesthetics do not produce irreversible neurological damage by themselves. However, permanent neurological injury may occur as a result of hypoxemia related to airway obstruction during a convulsion. Local anesthetic toxicity is additive. Therefore after one has administered the maximum recommended dose of one local anesthetic, it is neither safe nor advisable to administer a second local anesthetic.

Cardiovascular depression or cardiac arrest is the most severe form of local anesthetic toxicity. The blood level required to produce cardiac changes is higher than that required to produce neurologic toxicity.

There is additional toxicity associated with individual local anesthetics. Prilocaine is metabolized to ortho-toluidine which can produce methemoglobinemia. Prilocaine is a component of the topical anesthetic EMLA (eutectic mixture of local anesthetics). Methemoglobinemia is highly unlikely if one adheres to the dosing recommendations for EMLA. Bupivacaine and etidocaine have a more profound effect on cardiac conduction tissue than lidocaine and are associated with development of reentrant arrhythmias and asystole. These effects may be seen with plasma concentrations only slightly higher than those required to produce seizures. Successful resuscitation is more likely with the rapid restoration of adequate oxygenation and ventilation, use of high-dose epinephrine to treat electromechanical dissociation, and administration of antiarrhythmics other than lidocaine. Cardiopulmonary bypass has been successfully used while waiting for the cardiotoxic effects of bupivacaine to dissipate.

PHARMACOLOGY OF LOCAL ANESTHETICS

Tetracaine

Tetracaine is an ester local anesthetic with a high pKa of 8.5, slow onset, and long duration of action (60–360 minutes). It is among the most potent local anesthetics in clinical use today. It is also among the most toxic. The maximum dose is 1 mg/kg. Tetracaine is most commonly used for spinal anesthesia (usual dose 0.2–0.6 mg/kg) and topical anesthesia of the eye. For spinal anesthesia in children it comes in two forms – a lyophilized crystal that is reconstituted, or a 1% solution that is diluted with distilled water, cerebrospinal fluid, or dextrose to produce hypobaric, isobaric, or a hyperbaric solution, respectively. The duration of action of tetracaine is prolonged by addition of epinephrine. It is also available as an ophthalmic solution as tetracaine hydrochloride 0.5%. The usual dose is 1-2 drops per eye.

2-Chloroprocaine

2-Chloroprocaine is gaining popularity for pediatric epidural analgesia. Because it is rapidly metabolized by plasma esterases, accumulation in the plasma is unlikely, and systemic toxicity is rare. Chloroprocaine has a relatively high pKa of 9 and only about 5% of the drug is present in the unionized form at physiologic pH. Chloroprocaine has a rapid onset of action (5-10 minutes) because of its high tissue penetrance. It has a short duration of action (45 minutes) that can be prolonged (to 70-90 minutes) with addition of epinephrine. It has roughly a quarter of the potency of tetracaine or bupivacaine.

Use of epidural chloroprocaine decreased in the 1980s because of neurotoxicity associated with its 0.2% bisulfite preservative. Currently, chloroprocaine is available without preservatives for epidural use. Even with preservative-free chloroprocaine, a syndrome of back pain after large epidural doses has been described in adults. Epidural anesthesia is achieved by administering up to 1 mL/kg of 2-chloroprocaine (2% or 3%) with epinephrine 1:200,000 (maximal dose of chloroprocaine, 20-30 mg/kg). Continuous epidural analgesia has been used in infants aged under 6 months using 1.5% chloroprocaine at 0.6-0.8 mL/kg/h.

Lidocaine

Lidocaine was the first amide local anesthetic introduced and remains the most popular local anesthetic in use today. Lidocaine has a relatively low pKa of 7.9 and 25% of the drug is nonionized at physiologic pH. It has a rapid onset and an intermediate duration of action (60-90 minutes) that is prolonged by adding epinephrine. It has one-eighth the potency of bupivacaine or tetracaine. The maximum dose of 5 mg/kg can be increased to 7 mg/kg by adding epinephrine. In addition to epidural and peripheral nerve blockade, lidocaine can be administered transcutaneously in the form of a skin patch (Lidoderm). It is also available as an oral formulation (mexiletine) for the treatment of neuropathic pain, and it is the only anesthetic recommended for intravenous regional blockade.

Bupivacaine

Bupivacaine has a relatively low pKa of 8.1 and is 15% unionized. Therefore, its time to onset is relatively slow.

Bupivacaine is highly protein bound and thus has a long duration of action which is not prolonged by adding epinephrine. However, addition of epinephrine will reduce the rate of systemic absorption, and thus lower the peak plasma concentration, which is an important consideration given the potential toxicity of bupivacaine. Bupivacaine is one of the most potent local anesthetics in use today. Its L-enantiomer, levobupivacaine, may have less cardiac toxicity but it has equal anesthetic potency. The maximum dose of both bupivacaine and levobupivacaine is 2.5 mg/kg. Severe cardiovascular depression at plasma levels slightly above those considered necessary to produce signs and symptoms of neurotoxicity has been observed with bupivacaine. Bupivacaine has more depressant effects on the cardiac conduction system than lidocaine, but is no more toxic than lidocaine with regard to its effects on blood pressure and cardiac output. Bupivacaine can reduce conduction time and increase the potential for reentrant rhythms. Its duration is long because it is highly protein-bound and thus takes a long time to "wash out" from the sodium channel. Thus, resuscitation can be prolonged but is not impossible.

Ropivacaine

Ropivacaine is the newest of the amide local anesthetics and was developed because of the cardiotoxicity associated with bupivacaine. It is chemically similar to bupivacaine, having a propyl side-chain whereas bupivacaine has a butyl side-chain. Its pKa is 8.0 and a slightly greater percentage of the drug is present in the unionized form at physiologic pH. Ropivacaine is slightly less protein-bound than bupivacaine, so it is not surprising that it has a faster onset but slightly shorter duration of action (150-300 minutes). Like bupivacaine, the duration of blockade is not prolonged by adding epinephrine.

Ropivacaine is produced only as the L-enantiomer. One feature common to all the amide anesthetics is that their L-form possesses less cardiotoxicity. Ropivacaine appears to possess more sensorimotor discrimination than bupivacaine when administered to produce equivalent analgesia. It is estimated that ropivacaine is about three-quarters as potent as bupivacaine. It is available as 0.2% and 0.5% solutions and is dosed similarly to bupivacaine for epidural and peripheral nerve block with a maximum dose of 2.5-3.0 mg/kg, or 4 mg/kg when epinephrine is added.

Eutectic Mixture of Local Anesthetics

Eutectic mixture of local anesthetics (EMLA), which consists of lidocaine 2.5% and prilocaine 2.5%, is a topical anesthetic. It is used prior to heel lancing, venipuncture, intravenous cannulation, dural puncture, and even neonatal circumcision. It is an invaluable aid for children

Article To Know

Hansen TG, Ilett KF, Reid C et al: Caudal ropivacaine in infants: population pharmacokinetics and plasma concentrations. Anesthesiology 94:579-584, 2001.

Ropivacaine is the newest amino-amide local anesthetic. It is commercially available as the L-enantiomer and has a long duration of action similar to bupivacaine. Like bupivacaine, it produces a frequency-dependent block and therefore produces minimal motor block when used in low concentrations (<0.2%). Most importantly, it possesses less potential for cardiac toxicity when compared to equipotent doses and plasma concentrations of bupivacaine.

This paper describes the pharmacokinetics of caudally administered ropivacaine in two groups of infants under 12 months of age. Group 1 consisted of 15 patients 0-3 months of age, and group 2 consisted of 15 patients 3-12 months of age. During a standardized general anesthetic, all subjects received 0.2% ropivacaine 1 mL/kg (2 mg/kg) in the caudal epidural space. Venous blood was sampled at 0, 15, 30, 45, 60, 120, 150, 240, 360, 540, and 720 minutes after ropivacaine administration. Total and free plasma ropivacaine concentrations were collected to describe pharmacokinetic parameters: volume of distribution, clearance, and absorption and elimination half-times.

The highest total ropivacaine plasma concentrations in groups 1 and 2 were similar. The highest individual total ropivacaine concentration was seen 150 minutes after dosing in a 76-day, 4.7-kg infant. The highest free ropivacaine concentrations were significantly higher in the 0- to 3-month-old patients ($p < 0.0002$). The highest individual free plasma ropivacaine concentration was seen 150 minutes after dosing in a 36-day, 4.2-kg infant. The median fraction of free ropivacaine was significantly greater in group 1 vs group 2 ($p < 0.01$), 10% vs 5%, respectively. The mean absorption and elimination half-lives for both groups together were 0.43 and 5.1 hours, respectively. The clearance of ropivacaine for the combined groups was 310 mL/h/kg. This value is at the lower end of the range of ropivacaine clearance that these authors reported for children with a mean age of 2.1 and 3.3 years (0.35-0.67 L/h/kg). The authors also state that age and percentage of free ropivacaine were significant covariates of clearance. Lower clearance was associated with younger patients and higher free ropivacaine fractions. The authors believe that the capacity to metabolize ropivacaine, though present in the newborn, is reduced. A maturation process occurs that reaches adult levels at 6-12 months of age.

Ropivacaine levels associated with toxicity in children have not been reported but are believed to be greater than levels of bupivacaine known to produce systemic toxicity (2000-10,000 µg/L). However, adults have tolerated total and free plasma ropivacaine concentrations of 1000-3000 µg/L and 10-150 µg/L, respectively, without signs of toxicity. The total and free plasma ropivacaine concentrations in infants after caudal ropivacaine, 2 mg/kg, are similar to those reported in older children and adults and well below the levels of bupivacaine associated with CNS and cardiac toxicity (>2000 µg/L).

who must undergo repeated venipuncture on a regular basis. However, it must be applied 60-90 minutes prior to the procedure as its onset time is slow. The recommended dose of EMLA in neonates is 0.5 g applied 60 minutes prior to the procedure.

PHARMACOLOGY OF ADJUVANT ANALGESICS

Clonidine

Clonidine is an α_2-adrenergic agonist that was developed primarily as a nasal decongestant because of its peripheral vasoconstrictor properties. It was soon recognized to have hypotensive effects and was primarily then used as an antihypertensive agent in adults. More recently, its anxiolytic and antinociceptive effects have been useful in the perioperative setting. For sedation and anxiolysis, clonidine can be administered orally at a dose of 4 µg/kg. It possesses the ability to reduce intraoperative anesthetic requirements, reduce postoperative opioid consumption, and stabilize hemodynamic responses to laryngoscopy and surgery.

Clonidine is used as an analgesic adjuvant in the management of acute and chronic pain in children. It dramatically prolongs the duration of peripheral nerve, epidural, and spinal blocks when combined with a local anesthetic or when given separately as an oral dose. Clonidine alone can produce analgesia when injected in the epidural or intrathecal space, or in the proximity of peripheral nerves. However, because of the large doses required, side-effects of hypotension, bradycardia, and sedation limit its utility as a sole analgesic agent. Clonidine is also used to control withdrawal symptoms in children with opioid or benzodiazepine dependence.

The mechanism by which clonidine exerts its analgesic effects are uncertain. In the superficial laminae of the dorsal horn of the spinal cord and in certain brainstem nuclei, α_2-receptors are abundant. Central sympatholysis is believed to be responsible for its antihypertensive effect. The prevention of norepinephrine release from presynaptic nerve terminals by clonidine is believed to be partially responsible for producing analgesia. However, there is evidence that clonidine increases acetylcholine release from neurons in the dorsal horn of the spinal cord, thus activating spinal acetylcholine receptors.

This may enhance local anesthetic blockade of C and A-δ fibers by augmenting potassium conductance.

Clonidine can be administered by a variety of routes. As an epidural additive, the dose is 1–2 μg/kg which may be followed by an infusion of 0.05–0.33 μg/kg/h. When given orally, it is almost totally absorbed from the GI tract. Once in the systemic circulation, its high lipid solubility allows it to penetrate the spinal cord and brain. Clonidine comes in an injectable form as well as a tablet (0.1, 0.2, and 0.3 mg) and transdermal patch (0.1, 0.2, and 0.3 mg). The patches may be cut in half or quarters to deliver fractional doses, and need to be changed every 7 days. The oral and transdermal dose of clonidine is 4–8 μg/kg/day. The oral dose is usually administered in two divided doses. Clonidine cannot be abruptly discontinued after prolonged administration, because severe hypertension and other symptoms similar to an abstinence syndrome may occur.

Anticonvulsants

Anticonvulsants are useful for managing a variety of neuropathic pain conditions including complex regional pain syndrome, phantom limb pain, and post-herpetic neuralgia. However, few studies in children exist and the use of this class of drugs in children is based on extrapolation from adult literature and from growing anecdotal pediatric experience. Although early adult experience established the efficacy of phenytoin, carbamazepine, and valproic acid as analgesic adjuvants, gabapentin is now the first-line anticonvulsant used for this purpose.

Gabapentin

Gabapentin was developed as a gamma amino benzoic acid (GABA) agonist for relief of muscle spasticity but was later recognized to be more effective as an anticonvulsant. The mechanism of action of gabapentin has not been clearly delineated. It does not appear to interact with receptors or sodium channels, and may enhance extracellular GABA concentrations by altering GABA transport. Gabapentin is not metabolized and is entirely dependent on renal excretion for elimination. It is not protein-bound and has a half-life of 5–9 hours. The most common adverse effects include abdominal pain, dizziness and ataxia, tremor, nystagmus, somnolence, and mood and behavior disturbances. However, gabapentin is generally well tolerated and the side-effects can be largely avoided by slowly increasing the dose of gabapentin on a daily basis until analgesia results or intolerable side-effects appear. In the author's institution we start with 2 mg/kg (maximum dose 100 mg) at bedtime on the first day, 2 mg/kg twice-daily on the second day, and then 2 mg/kg thrice-daily. We continue to increase the daily dose in this fashion by 2 mg/kg/day.

If somnolence is bothersome we administer half the daily dose at bedtime. The maximum daily dose is 50 mg/kg/day.

Carbamazepine

Carbamazepine is an anticonvulsant that is believed to produce analgesia by sodium-channel blockade. Carbamazepine is metabolized by the liver. Therapy is initiated in children aged over 6 years with an oral dose of 10 mg/kg/day divided in 2–4 doses and increased to the usual maintenance dose of 15–30 mg/kg/day. Severe adverse effects including aplastic anemia, agranulocytosis, congestive heart failure, sedation, fatigue, ataxia, slurred speech, and hepatitis have been reported. A complete blood count and liver function studies should be obtained prior to and during therapy.

Valproic Acid

Valproic acid is an adjuvant treatment for neuropathic pain accompanied by a mood disturbance, and prophylactic therapy for migraine headaches. At least three mechanisms of action have been proposed for valproic acid: (1) increased production and release of GABA in central neurons; (2) reduced neuronal excitation initiated by NMDA-type glutamate receptors; and (3) direct membrane stabilizing effects. The usual oral starting dose of 10–15 mg/kg/day may be increased to 60 mg/kg/day in 2–3 divided doses. Anorexia, nausea and vomiting, weight gain or loss, and sedation are common side-effects. The most serious side-effects include hepatotoxicity, hyperammonemia, platelet dysfunction, and pancreatitis.

Tricyclic Antidepressants

The tricyclic antidepressants have proven efficacy in adult patients with chronic neuropathic pain. When added to an analgesic regimen, they improve sleep, mood, and overall daily functioning. Prospective controlled studies of tricyclic antidepressant therapy for chronic pain in children have not been performed. These drugs are believed to produce analgesia by central serotonin and norepinephrine reuptake inhibition, thus augmenting descending inhibitory pathways. This class of drugs causes anticholinergic side-effects: dry mouth, sedation, orthostatic hypotension, constipation, urinary retention, and tachycardia. Sudden death from arrhythmias has been reported in children on tricyclic antidepressants for the treatment of depression. Prior to initiating tricyclic antidepressant therapy, we obtain a thorough history for palpitations, syncope, and cardiac conduction disturbances. An electrocardiograph should be obtained to rule out prolonged Q_T interval. Nortriptyline may produce less daytime somnolence and fewer anticholinergic effects than amitriptyline. However, when insomnia accompanies chronic neuropathic pain we prefer to use amitriptyline. Analgesic therapy with amitriptyline or nortriptyline is initiated at 0.1–0.2 mg/kg at bedtime and increased by 0.1–0.2 mg/kg every 3–4 days to a maximum of 1 mg/kg/day or 50 mg.

Local Anesthetics

The local anesthetic lidocaine and its oral formulation (mexiletine) are referred to as membrane stabilizers because they block sodium channels, prevent membrane depolarization, and block excitatory impulses along neural pathways. They are used to treat neuropathic pain in adults and increasingly have been used in pediatric patients with mixed results. To determine whether the pain syndrome under question responds to lidocaine, we administer an intravenous bolus of 1 mg/kg and follow with an infusion at 1 mg/kg/h initially, with gradual increases to achieve a plasma lidocaine concentration of 2–5 mg/mL. If this test regimen produces adequate analgesia, oral therapy with mexiletine is begun. Adverse side-effects of mexiletine include nausea and vomiting, ataxia, diplopia, and sedation; these frequently limit its use.

ADDITIONAL ARTICLES TO KNOW

Agarwal R, Gutlove DP, Lockhart CH: Seizures occurring in pediatric patients receiving continuous infusion of bupivacaine. *Anesth Analg* 75:284–286, 1992.

Bourlon-Figuet S, Dubousset AM, Benhamou D, Mazoit X: Transient neurological symptoms after epidural analgesia in a five-year-old child. *Anesth Analg* 91:856–857, 2000.

Collins J, Kerner J, Sentivany S et al: Intravenous amitriptyline in pediatrics. *J Pain Symptom Manage* 10:471–475, 1995.

Constant I, Gall O, Gouyet L et al: Addition of clonidine or fentanyl to local anaesthetics prolongs the duration of surgical analgesia after single-shot caudal block in children. *Br J Anaesth* 80:294–298, 1998.

De Negri P, Ivani G, Visconti C et al: The dose–response relationship for clonidine added to a postoperative continuous epidural infusion of ropivacaine in children. *Anesth Analg* 93:71–76, 2001.

Hansen TG, Ilett KF, Lim SI et al: Pharmacokinetics and clinical efficacy of long-term epidural ropivacaine infusion in children. *Br J Anaesth* 85:347–353, 2000.

Kohane DS, Sankar WN, Shubina M et al: Sciatic nerve blockade in infant, adolescent, and adult rats: a comparison of ropivacaine and bupivacaine. *Anesthesiology* 89:1199–1208, 1998.

Maxwell LG, Martin LD, Yaster M: Bupivacaine-induced cardiac toxicity in neonates: successful treatment with intravenous phenytoin. *Anesthesiology* 80:682–686, 1994.

McCloskey JJ, Haun SE, Deshpande JK: Bupivacaine toxicity secondary to continuous caudal epidural infusion in children. *Anesth Analg* 75:287–290, 1992.

Mikawa K, Nishina K, Maekawa N et al: Oral clonidine premedication reduces postoperative pain in children. *Anesth Analg* 82:225–230, 1996.

Taddio A, Goldbach M, Ipp M et al: Effect of neonatal circumcision on pain during vaccination in boys. *Lancet* 345:291–292, 1995.

Taddio A, Stevens B, Craig K et al: Efficacy and safety of lidocaine–prilocaine cream for pain during circumcision. *N Engl J Med* 336:1197–1201, 1997.

Tobias JD, Rasmussen GE, Holcomb GW et al: Continuous caudal anaesthesia with chloroprocaine as an adjunct to general anaesthesia in neonates. *Can J Anaesth* 43:69–72, 1996.

Wheeler DS, Vaux KK, Tam DA: Use of gabapentin in the treatment of childhood reflex sympathetic dystrophy. *Pediatr Neurol* 22:220–221, 2000.

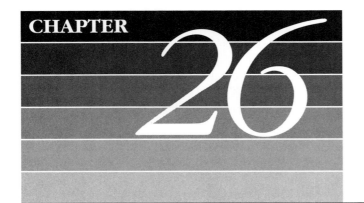

CHAPTER 26

Acute Pain Management in Children

JOHN B. ROSE

Pain is termed "acute" when it results from tissue injury, inflammation, or infection. It is most intense initially and gradually resolves as the injured or inflamed tissue heals over the course of days to weeks. This classic type of nociceptive pain is usually responsive to opioids, nonsteroidal anti-inflammatory drugs (NSAIDs), and regional anesthesia.

Nociception consists of: (1) transduction of an inflammatory, mechanical, or thermal stimulus into a neural impulse; (2) transmission of the neural impulse from the periphery to the central nervous system; (3) modulation of the impulse; and (4) perception of the stimulus. The first three processes are relatively consistent among individuals. The fourth is influenced by behavioral, familial, and cultural factors. Consequently, the perception of pain resulting from similar injuries or conditions is highly variable among individuals.

PATHOPHYSIOLOGY OF ACUTE PAIN

Tissue injury is associated with the release of inflammatory and algesic substances such as histamine, bradykinin, serotonin, substance P, leukotrienes, and potassium and hydrogen ions. Arachidonic acid is released from cell membranes and transformed into many of these substances by cyclooxygenase and lipoxygenase. Substance P, which is produced in the spinal and gasserian ganglia, and stored in somatic and visceral neurons, is released when peripheral cells are injured. By increasing vascular permeability and vasodilatation, it exacerbates the edema and erythema that accompany injury and inflammation. Substance P is also believed to recruit additional nociceptive fibers and lower depolarization thresholds.

Nociceptors, which respond to a wide variety of noxious mechanical and thermal stimuli, transmit signals via A-δ (myelinated) and C (unmyelinated) fibers. Unlike other sensory nerves which fatigue and develop higher thresholds after repeated stimulation, prolonged stimulation of nociceptors lowers excitation thresholds and causes peripheral sensitization. Furthermore, stimuli which are not normally noxious can be carried from the periphery to the central nervous system (CNS) via A-α and A-β fibers where they are transformed into pain signals. Hyperalgesia, an increased response to a noxious stimulus, indicates peripheral sensitization. Allodynia is pain in response to a stimulus which is normally not noxious, and also indicates peripheral sensitization. Repeated noxious stimulation sensed by the CNS causes amplification of pain intensity and duration. This is referred to as "wind-up" or "central sensitization." Many of these changes occur in the dorsal horn of the spinal cord where sensory and nociceptive signals from the periphery converge. These signals are processed and modified through complex and multiple synaptic connections and biochemical influences.

The dorsal horn of the spinal cord is anatomically divided into several laminae; lamina I is the most dorsal or superficial layer. A-δ and C fibers form synapses with second-order neurons mostly in laminae I (substantia gelatinosa), Iii, Iio, and V. Other sensory neurons synapse in laminae Iii, III, IV, and V. Lamina V contains a large number of wide dynamic-range neurons (WDR) that receive input from both nociceptive and non-nociceptive sensory fibers from somatic and visceral structures. Referred visceral pain may result from signal processing activities in these neurons. Following signal selection, processing, and modification in the dorsal horn, the second-order neurons project centrally via tracts in the anterior and anterolateral aspect of the contralateral spinal cord. These spinal pain pathways are called the spinothalamic, spinoreticular, and spinomesencephalic tracts. The lateral spinothalamic tract is the most important pain tract. These three tracts form two other tracts, the neospinothalamic and the paleospinothalamic tract. Pain from the head and neck is similarly projected via the trigeminal nerve to the neo- and paleo-trigeminothalamic tracts. The neospinothalamic tract comprises large myelinated fibers which synapse within the thalamus and then project to the somatosensory cortex, making few synapses along the way. This tract is believed to be responsible for relaying information about the location and severity of the pain so that immediate action can be taken to escape further injury. The paleospinothalamic tract carries nociceptive information to brain structures that are important in the formation of memories and emotions. This tract relays that an injury has occurred, and promotes memory and learning so that similar injuries are avoided in the future.

Peripheral nociceptive signals are attenuated centrally by an inhibitory descending pathway. This pathway arises from the cerebral cortex and synapses with neurons in laminae I, IIo, and V of the dorsal horn at every level of the spinal cord. Serotonin and norepinephrine are the important neurotransmitters in this inhibitory pathway. Tricyclic antidepressants, tramadol, and clonidine may exert their analgesic effects at least in part by activating this descending inhibitory pathway.

This brief anatomical overview demonstrates that viewing pain as the simple transmission of neural impulses from the periphery to the cerebral cortex is inaccurate. Signals can be augmented or attenuated at many different levels. In addition, nociceptive pathways have multiple synapses in the limbic system, frontal cortex, and medial thalamus where pain is influenced by emotions, behavior, past experiences, cultural orientation, and emotional states, among other factors. Successful acute pain management targets all the elements in this complex system of pain signal transduction, transmission, modulation, and perception. Balanced analgesia with a combination of opioid therapy, regional anesthesia and NSAIDs are increasingly administered to pediatric patients with success. A balanced approach results in a reduction in systemic opioid administration and opioid-related side-effects.

Until very recently, moderate to severe pediatric pain was treated with intermittent opioid analgesics administered on a PRN basis by the intramuscular or intravenous route. But these regimens continued to cause pain and suffering for a number of reasons. The doses and dosing intervals were often inadequate and there was no adjustment of these parameters because of a fear of adverse events. Intramuscular injections are painful and frightening; children with needle phobia would rather endure their pain than receive an intramuscular injection.

Also, patients or their families would be required to ask their nurse for analgesic medication. Delays occurred because the nurse would have to respond to the call, check the orders, obtain the medication, and administer the drug. Plasma opioid concentrations fluctuated widely from the time of dosing until the next dose was administered. Peak plasma opioid concentrations were high within an hour of dosing and side-effects such as nausea, vomiting, sedation, and respiratory depression occurred. Some children would refuse analgesic therapy in order to avoid these symptoms. Severe pain also resulted when trough plasma opioid concentrations were very low just prior to the subsequent dose. These techniques did not take into account the large variability in the amount of pain experienced by children with similar conditions, or the wide variability in their responses to analgesics. Children normally have fluctuating analgesic needs. During rest, analgesic requirements are less than when attempting to change position, breathe deeply, or undergo dressing changes, diagnostic tests, therapeutic procedures, or nursing care.

Effective pediatric pain management considers all these variables and includes a proactive plan for managing background and breakthrough pain. In the author's institution we accomplish this goal using four specialized techniques: patient-controlled analgesia, continuous intravenous opioid infusions, continuous epidural analgesia, and patient-controlled epidural analgesia. Less frequently used techniques include nurse- and parent-controlled analgesia and continuous peripheral nerve blockade, and will not be discussed further.

PATIENT-CONTROLLED ANALGESIA

Patient-controlled analgesia (PCA) has been used for pediatric pain management for nearly 20 years. It is the most common analgesic intervention utilized at The Children's Hospital of Philadelphia for managing moderate to severe acute pain in children over 6 years old. It is popular because it is safe, effective, and highly satisfactory in the view of patients and their families, as well as nurses and physicians. Occasionally children under 6 years can effectively use PCA. Usually these youngsters have had repeated or prolonged pain associated with malignancy. PCA is considered safe because if a patient has a high demand for opioid, he or she will eventually become somnolent and stop using the demand button. However, if another individual pushes the button for the patient, there is potential for severe CNS and respiratory depression; thus only the patient is allowed to press the button. PCA is effective because it allows patients to titrate the amount of analgesic they desire based on the amount of pain they are experiencing. Plasma concentrations of opioids are maintained in a narrower range with lower peak levels and higher trough levels than with intermittent injections. This results in less respiratory and central nervous system depression. PCA is well suited to deal with the variable amount of pain between patients with similar conditions, as well as the different levels of pain that an individual patient will experience from external factors.

Computerized PCA infusion pumps are programmed to deliver a specified (demand) dose of opioid when the patient pushes a button. The pump is programmed to administer only one demand dose in a specified period of time (lockout interval) regardless of how many times the patient presses the button. The pump is also programmed to deliver no more than a specified maximum amount of opioid in the course of one hour (1 hour limit). The pump records the patient's history of attempts and actual opioid injections. This facilitates tracking analgesic requirements.

The infusion pumps may be programmed to deliver a continuous (basal) infusion of opioid regardless of whether or not the patient uses the demand button. The adult literature does not support the use of PCA basal infusions because they result in an increased incidence of side-effects without improving analgesia. However, it is the author's experience that many children benefit from a low basal infusion during their early postoperative course as it allows them to sleep without having to awaken and press the PCA button for nighttime pain relief. Teenagers who have had a major procedure such as posterior spinal fusion will benefit from a basal infusion during their first two postoperative days. Even with a basal opioid infusion, some children will have severe pain if they have been resting or sleeping comfortably for a prolonged period without pressing the demand button. In this situation it is almost impossible for the patient to get caught up quickly by pressing the demand button. Therefore, in addition to the PCA orders, an intravenous rescue medication (e.g., morphine 50 μg/kg every 3 hours) is ordered for breakthrough pain. Standing orders for treating complications of opioids normally include naloxone 10 μg/kg IV for respiratory depression and unresponsiveness, ondansetron 50 μg/kg IV every 8 hours for nausea and vomiting, and nalbuphine,

50 μg/kg IV every 4 hours for pruritus and moderate breakthrough pain.

Morphine is usually the first-line analgesic for PCA in children, but this choice will depend on an individual patient's medical and analgesic history. The most common agents used in the author's institution, along with the programmed parameters, are described in Table 26-1.

CONTINUOUS INTRAVENOUS OPIOID INFUSION

Continuous intravenous opioid infusion (CIV) is used in children under 7 years of age or in cognitively impaired or physically disabled children aged over 7 years who are not able to use a PCA device. The advantages of CIV over intermittent opioid administration are the attainment of stable plasma opioid levels without wide plasma opioid fluctuations. There is less reliance on nursing staff for analgesic administration. However, a constant infusion will not cover pain that increases intermittently, so analgesic rescue administration will be required. Delays in receiving these rescue doses can result in severe breakthrough pain. If the goal of the infusion is to eliminate all pain (background and breakthrough), the patient may experience significant respiratory or CNS depression during inactivity or resting, and side-effects will occur more frequently.

The choice of opioid depends on the patient's history and preference. The initial infusion rate depends on the patient's age and history. In general, a healthy opioid-naive child with a severely painful condition receives a continuous infusion at a rate equal to the maximum basal infusion rates listed in the PCA table. If a child is at increased risk for central nervous system or respiratory depression, the rates are reduced by 25–50%.

The most common opioid used for CIV in the author's institution is morphine, with doses adjusted for age (Table 26-2). Morphine infusions are associated with an increased risk of respiratory depression in preterm and full-term neonates, so further reductions in infusion rates are required in this age group. Rescue medications are the same as for children receiving PCA opioids.

Table 26-1 PCA Dosing Guidelines

Drug	Demand Dose (μg/kg)	Lockout Interval (min)	Basal Infusion (μg/kg/h)	1-hour Limit (μg/kg)	PRN IV Rescue Dose (μg/kg)
Morphine	20	8–10	0–20	100	50
Hydromorphone	4	8–10	0–4	20	10
Fentanyl	0.5	6–8	0–0.5	2.5	0.5–1.0
Nalbuphine	20	8–10	0–20	100	50

Table 26-2   Continuous Morphine Infusion Dosing

Age Range	Dose
Newborns (0-2 months)	5-10 μg/kg/h
Infants (3-6 months)	10-15 μg/kg/h
Infants >6 months	15-20 μg/kg/h
Children >1 year	20-30 μg/kg/h

Table 26-4   Adjuvant Medications for Patients Receiving Epidural Analgesia

Symptom	Medication
Nausea or vomiting	Ondansetron 0.1 mg/kg IV every 8 hours
Breakthrough pain, pruritus, nausea, or vomiting	Nalbuphine 50 μg/kg IV every 4 hours
Breakthrough pain	Ketorolac 0.5 mg/kg IV every 6 hours (maximum 20 doses)
Muscle spasm	Diazepam 0.1 mg/kg PO/PR every 6 hours

CONTINUOUS EPIDURAL ANALGESIA

Continuous epidural analgesia (CEA) provides pain relief for surgical procedures below the fourth thoracic dermatome. Patients who receive CEA experience incomparable dermatomal analgesia as a result of blockade of nociceptive impulses arising from the surgical field. The postoperative epidural analgesic solution may contain a single agent or a combination of different classes of analgesics (Table 26-3).

Since epidural analgesia begins in the operating room, good communication is required between the anesthesiologist and postoperative pain management personnel. This communication should include the patient's medical history, the precise surgical procedure planned, the location of both the epidural insertion site and the tip of the epidural catheter, the length of catheter inserted into the epidural space, and the types of epidural analgesia administered intraoperatively.

Administration of CEA requires the presence of a pain management service that can immediately respond to problems. It should be comprised of nurses and physicians who have expertise in CEA and who make daily rounds to evaluate patients and ensure that CEA is running as ordered and that analgesia is adequate. The pain management team should proactively address expected adverse effects such as nausea, vomiting, pruritus, motor block, and epidural site inflammation, as well as less frequent and more severe sequelae such as respiratory and CNS depression (Table 26-4).

Standard orders for patients receiving CEA should include a warning that additional parenteral or enteral opioids are not to be administered while the patient is receiving epidural opioids. This is because of the increased risk for respiratory and CNS depression when systemic and epidural opioids are administered concurrently. Additional orders include the use of a cardiorespiratory monitor, recording of respiratory rate every hour for 24 hours and then every 4 hours, and the recording of pain scores, blood pressure, heart rate, and mental status every 4 hours. A functioning intravenous line must be maintained during CEA, as well as a list of who to call with questions or help. In the author's institution we routinely order a bag, mask, oxygen, and suction immediately available at the bedside. We also order administration of 100% oxygen by face mask and SQ naloxone 10 μg/kg, to be given for a respiratory rate <12 or unresponsiveness.

The most common problem with CEA is ineffectiveness. This usually results when the tip of the epidural catheter is too far from the midpoint of the surgical dermatome. Other reasons include catheter problems (e.g., obstruction,

Table 26-3   CEA Dosing Guidelines

Patient	Bupivacaine or Ropivacaine (mg/mL)	Fentanyl (μg/mL)	MSO$_4$[a] (μg/mL)	Clonidine (μg/mL)	Rate (BUP or ROP mg/kg/h)
Newborn 0-2 months (natural airway, spontaneous ventilation)	1 (0.5-1.0)	N/A	N/A	N/A	0.2 (0.15-0.25)
Newborn 0-2 months (endotracheal tube, mechanical ventilation)	1 (0.5-1.0)	2	N/A	0.6	0.2 (0.15-0.25)
Infant	1 (0.5-1.25)	2 (2-5)	25	0.6	0.25 (0.15-0.3)
Child (lumbar)	1 (0.5-1.25)	5 (2-5)	25-50	0.6-1.2	0.25 (0.2-0.4)
Child (thoracic)	1 (0.5-1.25)	5 (2-5)	NR	Investigational	0.2 (0.2-0.4)

[a]Lumbar epidural analgesia only.
BUP, bupivacaine; ROP, ropivacaine; N/A, not applicable; NR, not recommended.

Case

A 4-week-old, 4.2-kg female infant with biliary atresia is scheduled for a Kasai procedure through a 5-cm transverse right upper-quadrant incision. The anesthesiologist does not anticipate postoperative ventilatory management or ICU admission.

What options exist for managing postoperative pain in this patient?

Three general options exist for managing postoperative pain in this infant: continuous epidural analgesia (CEA), continuous intravenous morphine infusion, and intermittent intravenous morphine administration on either a scheduled or PRN basis. Because of the wide fluctuations in plasma morphine concentrations, and because this baby is expected to experience severe postoperative pain, intermittent opioid administration would be this author's last choice for this infant. A continuous intravenous morphine infusion may result in accumulation of morphine as a result of reduced capacity for liver metabolism and subsequent respiratory depression. Thus, I would not choose a continuous morphine infusion for this infant. CEA with bupivacaine will result in superior postoperative analgesia. Systemic opioid administration can be minimized or eliminated, which is desirable in a 4-week-old infant on a general surgical floor.

The anesthesiologist inserted a caudal epidural catheter and successfully advanced the tip to the T8 level. In the operating room the infant received 0.25% bupivacaine 4 mL at the beginning of the surgical procedure, 2 hours ago. What epidural analgesic solution will you use postoperatively?

Ideally, one should be able to use only a local anesthetic solution and avoid epidural opioid administration in this infant. Since the tip of the epidural catheter is at a good position in the area of the surgical dermatome, local anesthetic alone is likely to produce adequate postoperative analgesia. This author would choose bupivacaine 1 mg/mL at 0.8 mL/h. This rate is roughly equivalent to bupivacaine 0.2 mg/kg/h, slightly less than the maximum recommended dose in this age group. Since the tip of this epidural catheter is near the center of the surgical dermatomes, this should be a sufficient rate. I would avoid addition of clonidine in an infant of this age since it can cause sedation and respiratory depression and should be reserved for use in the intensive care setting.

Approximately 36 hours after the epidural infusion begins, the infant is comfortable and lying very still but appears pale, poorly perfused, and has a heart rate of 84/min with a respiratory rate of 32/min, blood pressure of 84/42 mmHg, and oxyhemoglobin saturation of 97% in room air. What might be happening and what will you do?

Accumulation of bupivacaine can result from immature hepatic metabolic pathways in young infants. For this reason, it is inadvisable to run epidural infusions beyond 48 hours. In addition, plasma protein binding capacity is reduced, thus increasing the amount of unbound plasma bupivacaine. The free fraction of bupivacaine is primarily responsible for producing systemic toxicity. This infant has biliary atresia – both her capacity for hepatic metabolism and her protein binding may be further reduced. She is at increased risk of systemic bupivacaine toxicity in spite of the fact that she was receiving only 0.2 mg/kg/h of epidural bupivacaine, less than the maximum recommended dose in this age group.

Signs of systemic toxicity may be very subtle in the neonate. The early signs of central nervous system toxicity are often absent in this age group. Cardiac toxicity may be the first indication of an elevated plasma bupivacaine level. Therefore it is advisable to discontinue the epidural infusion and continue to closely monitor the infant for signs of further deterioration. Although bupivacaine levels are not immediately available in most hospitals, sending a level would help establish this diagnosis.

kinking, leakage, or breakage), pump failure, inappropriate infusion solution or rate, or accidental displacement of the catheter from its original position. In the event of motor block, the concentration of the local anesthetic solution can be decreased. If opioid-related side-effects occur, the dose of the epidural opioid should initially be reduced by 25–50% before discontinuing its use if the symptoms persist. A rare but serious complication is the development of local anesthetic toxicity as a result of systemic absorption. This is extremely unlikely if one adheres to the concentrations and infusion rates listed in the table. A notable exception to this is a patient with a reduced capacity for local anesthetic metabolism and excretion (e.g., a neonate with biliary atresia who has undergone a Kasai procedure).

PATIENT-CONTROLLED EPIDURAL ANALGESIA

Patient-controlled epidural analgesia (PCEA) combines the benefits of epidural analgesia and patient-controlled analgesia. This technique is usually suitable for children over 7 years of age who are capable of using a

Article To Know

Jylli L, Lundeberg S, Olsson GL: Retrospective evaluation of continuous epidural infusion for postoperative pain in children. Acta Anaesthesiol Scand 46:654-659, 2002.

This article addresses the safety and efficacy of postoperative epidural analgesia in a large series of pediatric patients. The study included all children treated with continuous epidural analgesia for postoperative pain over a 5-year period. Epidural catheters were placed after the induction of anesthesia in all subjects. All catheters were inserted at the L2-L3 (abdominal surgery) or the L4-L5 (lower-extremity surgery) levels. Bupivacaine 1.25 mg/mL was used in all cases. Infusion rates of 0.2-0.3 mg/kg/h were used for children aged 0-3 years, and in older children the maximum rate was 0.5 mg/kg/h. Opioids (morphine 30 µg/kg or fentanyl 0.5-4 µg/kg/h) were not used routinely but were added in 48 cases of children in the intensive care unit. Ward nurses assessed pain every 3 hours using a behavioral scale, FACES scale, or visual analog scale depending on the patient's age. These data were recorded during visits by the Acute Pain Treatment service and used to assess the overall efficacy of epidural analgesia which was rated as good, adequate, or inadequate. The efficacy of epidural analgesia was rated inadequate if supplemental systemic opioids were required. Complications were also assessed during visits by the Acute Pain Treatment service. Complications were rated as related to the drug, epidural technique, caregivers, technical problems, or miscellaneous. Also recorded for each patient was the reason for discontinuing the epidural infusion: no further need – satisfactory analgesia; unsatisfactory analgesia; complications; need to mobilize the patient; or miscellaneous.

Four hundred and seventy-six children received 518 epidural infusions during this 5-year period. Gastrointestinal surgery, lower-extremity orthopedic surgery, and urologic surgery accounted for 220, 185, and 113 procedures, respectively. The median duration of the epidural infusion was 50 hours (range <12 hours to >96 hours). The mean number of visits by the Acute Pain Treatment service was 3.6 visits per patient (range 1-17). During the visits, epidural analgesia was rated as good during 76% of the visits, adequate in 16%, and inadequate in 8%. No complications were reported in 81% of patients. Ninety-five complications were reported in 81 patients, but none was serious or had long-lasting effects. Complications reported by at least 2% of patients included: leakage around catheter ($n = 15$); catheter dislodgement ($n = 13$); and nausea or vomiting ($n = 11$). Epidural catheters were routinely removed on the morning of the third postoperative day. The majority of patients (63%) had satisfactory analgesia and catheters were removed because of lack of further need. However, catheters were removed prematurely owing to unsatisfactory analgesia in 21% of patients. Other common reasons for prematurely discontinuing epidural analgesia included complications ($n = 41$) and the need for the patient to mobilize ($n = 20$). In comparing the 108 patients who had unsatisfactory epidural analgesia with the 325 patients who had satisfactory epidural analgesia, the authors found that there was a higher incidence of unsatisfactory analgesia in older patients, patients with supraumbilical incisions, abdominal surgery, and long duration of surgery.

This study describes a systematic approach for delivering effective postoperative epidural analgesia to pediatric patients. It is a labor-intensive technique requiring at least daily visits of a team with expertise in epidural analgesia. Of interest is the fact that the Acute Pain Treatment service routinely omitted opioids from their epidural infusions and used only bupivacaine 1.25 mg/mL (0.2-0.5 mg/kg/h) with few cases of motor block ($n = 2$) or other complications.

Several weaknesses of this report should be mentioned. This is a retrospective review of pediatric epidural analgesia. Pain scores were recorded but not used to determine efficacy. The lack of need for rescue analgesics was used to determine whether epidural analgesia was adequate. However, the authors do not describe how they determined the need for rescue analgesics. This study did not involve any patients who underwent thoracic surgery or had thoracic epidural analgesia. The finding that patients with supraumbilical incisions were at greater risk for inadequate analgesia is not surprising since epidural catheters were placed at the level L2-L3 for this type of surgery and hydrophilic epidural opioids were not routinely administered.

PCA demand button. The management strategy is similar to CEA with respect to all the same safety precautions, and a similar rule that only the patient may press the button. In the author's institution our standard analgesic solution includes bupivacaine 0.75 mg/mL, and either fentanyl 5 µg/kg (thoracic PCEA) or morphine 50 µg/kg (lumbar PCEA). Ropivacaine 0.75-1.0 mg/mL can also be used when available. Our initial PCEA pump parameters include a demand dose of 0.05-0.1 mL/kg, a lockout interval of 20-30 minutes, basal infusion of 0.1-0.2 mL/kg, and a 1-hour limit of 0.2-0.4 mL/kg (maximum 19.9 mL).

DRUG TRANSITION

The transition from specialized techniques like CIV, PCA, CEA, and PCEA is often challenging. Oral analgesic therapy can begin when the child's pain subsides and oral medications are tolerated. Epidural techniques, particularly those that involve opioids, are discontinued before oral analgesics are started. The same is true for CIV. Patients receiving PCA may be started on oral analgesics and allowed to use demand-only PCA (no basal infusion) for a brief period to make certain that the dose of oral analgesics is sufficient. A co-analgesic agent such as acetaminophen 10-15 mg/kg PO every 4 hours, ibuprofen 10 mg/kg PO every 4 hours, or ketorolac 0.5 mg/kg IV every 6 hours may be helpful for smoothing the transition. Rescue analgesic medications such as morphine 50 μg/kg IV every 3 hours or nalbuphine 50 μg/kg IV every 3 hours should also be ordered. During the transition, close observation of the patient by the pain management service can detect problems early and adjust the medications or doses to ensure the patient's comfort. Oxycodone 0.1-0.15 mg/kg PO every 4 hours with acetaminophen or ibuprofen is the standard oral regimen in the author's institution, but we occasionally use hydromorphone or tramadol.

ADDITIONAL ARTICLES TO KNOW

Berde CB: Convulsions associated with pediatric regional anesthesia. *Anesth Analg* 75:164-166, 1992.

Bray RJ, Woodhams AM, Vallis CJ et al: Morphine consumption and respiratory depression in children receiving postoperative analgesia from continuous morphine infusion or patient controlled analgesia. *Paed Anaesth* 6:129-134, 1996.

Caudle CL, Freid EB, Bailey AG et al: Epidural fentanyl infusion with patient-controlled epidural analgesia for postoperative analgesia in children. *J Pediatr Surg* 28:554-559, 1993.

Collins JJ, Geake J, Grier HE et al: Patient-controlled analgesia for mucositis pain in children: a three-period crossover study comparing morphine and hydromorphone. *J Pediatr* 129:722-728, 1996.

Karl HW, Tyler DC, Krane EJ: Respiratory depression after low-dose caudal morphine. *Can J Anaesth* 43:1065-1067, 1996.

Krane EJ: Delayed respiratory depression in a child after caudal epidural morphine. *Anesth Analg* 67:79-82, 1988.

Krane EJ, Tyler DC, Jacobson LE: The dose-response of caudal morphine in children. *Anesthesiology* 71:48-52, 1989.

Luz G, Innerhofer P, Bachmann B et al: Bupivacaine plasma concentrations during continuous epidural anesthesia in infants and children. *Anesth Analg* 82:231-234, 1996.

Monitto CL, Greenberg RS, Kost-Byerly S et al: The safety and efficacy of parent-/nurse-controlled analgesia in patients less than six years of age. *Anesth Analg* 91:573-579, 2000.

Neely JK, Trentadue NC: Comparison of patient-controlled analgesia with and without nighttime morphine infusion following lower extremity surgery in children. *J Pain Symptom Manage* 13:268-273, 1997.

CHAPTER 27

Chronic Pediatric Pain

JOHN B. ROSE

DEIRDRE E. LOGAN

Pain is considered "chronic" when it is constant and lasts for more than 3 months. It may persist because of ongoing tissue inflammation, as seen in children with inflammatory bowel disease or juvenile rheumatoid arthritis. It may also occur without tissue inflammation when peripheral or central nervous system neurons become abnormally modified – neuropathic pain. Neuropathic pain syndromes are an enigmatic and heterogenous group of disorders that have been recognized by a variety of names for over 100 years and continue to baffle physicians, patients, and their families. This perplexity stems from the lack of known precise pathophysiologic mechanisms responsible for the debilitating symptoms. Authorities believe that neuropathic pain syndromes are caused by abnormalities of the peripheral, central, and autonomic nervous system, coupled with myofascial dysfunction and/or psychological distress.

Neuropathic pain is not as uncommon during childhood as once thought. The most common type of neuropathic pain in children is complex regional pain syndrome type 1 (CRPS-1), which is the focus of this chapter.

COMPLEX REGIONAL PAIN SYNDROME

In 1993, the International Association for the Study of Pain (IASP) recommended that neuropathic pain syndromes should be grouped together and called complex regional pain syndromes (CRPS). CRPS is divided into two different types depending on the initiating injury: CRPS type 1 (formerly called reflex sympathetic dystrophy) follows soft tissue injury, and CRPS type 2 (formerly called causalgia) follows a peripheral nerve injury. CRPS-2 is rare in children and will not be discussed further in this chapter.

The differential diagnosis of a painful condition involving the distal extremity is long (Box 27-1). It is usually possible to eliminate most conditions based on the results of prior diagnostic evaluations, history, and physical examination. Furthermore, the diagnosis of CRPS-1 is excluded by the existence of conditions that would otherwise account for the degree of pain and dysfunction. Unfortunately, there are no tests that can confirm the diagnosis of CRPS-1. The IASP has established diagnostic criteria for CRPS-1 (Box 27-2). However, it remains a diagnosis of exclusion.

Delayed diagnosis of CRPS-1 is common and may exceed a year from the time symptoms begin. Diagnostic delays lead to prolonged pain, suffering, and disability,

---

Box 27-1   Differential Diagnosis of Distal Limb Pain in a Child

Osteomyelitis
Septic arthritis
Cellulitis
Lyme disease and other rheumatologic conditions
Bone fracture or sprain
Neoplasm
Osteoid osteoma
Entrapment neuropathy
Small fiber neuropathy (i.e., diabetic neuropathy)
Deep venous thrombosis
Vascular insufficiency
Lymphedema
Erythromelalgia
Psychiatric etiologies (e.g., somatization or conversion disorders)

Box 27-2   IASP Diagnostic Criteria for CRPS Type 1

Presence of an initiating noxious event, or a cause for immobilization
Continuing pain, allodynia, or hyperalgesia with pain disproportionate to any inciting event
Presence of edema at some time during the illness
Changes in skin blood flow as evidenced by skin color changes or skin temperature differences of at least 1.1°C from the homologous body part
Abnormal sudomotor activity (increased or decreased sweating) in the region of the pain

---

and may result in harmful therapies such as splinting or casting. Immobilization of the effected extremity may exacerbate the condition.

There are several aspects of CRPS-1 in children that may provide clues to the proper diagnosis. As with adults, females are affected more than males by a ratio of 4:1, but unlike adults, the lower extremities are most often affected. A history of trauma, albeit trivial, can be elicited in many children. Frequently the trauma occurs during an organized sporting event. At the time of diagnosis, many of these children are disabled and unable to attend school or participate in normal activities. Some children with lower-extremity CRPS-1 are able to ambulate with crutches but others are bedridden or wheelchair bound.

Children diagnosed with CRPS-1 often manifest psychological symptoms that contribute to their pain and disability. These include fear, anxiety, anger, depression, maladaptive coping skills and behaviors, and sleep disturbances. In three large pediatric reports, psychological disorders were identified in 25–77% of patients.

Clinical Signs and Diagnosis

The clinical presentation of children with CRPS-1 includes a combination of sensory, motor, and autonomic signs and symptoms. However, no single physical finding is pathognomonic.

Sensory changes consist of a continuous, spontaneous pain that affects multiple dermatomes. It is often described as deep, burning, sharp, or stinging.

Motor changes include a decreased range of motion, weakness, tremors, and abnormal postures such as equinovarus deformity of the foot and clenched fist in the hand. Continued immobilization can worsen or perpetuate the disease.

Autonomic changes include skin color changes, temperature alteration, edema, and sudomotor abnormalities.

Commonly, the skin overlying the affected extremity takes on a red, purple, blue, mottled, or ashen gray discoloration. However, skin color varies between patients and within the same patient over time. Edema gives the skin a smooth appearance and is present in every patient at some point in the illness. The affected area may feel cooler or warmer than surrounding unaffected areas and the opposite extremity. Sudomotor abnormalities include hyperhidrosis (abnormal moistness) or hypohidrosis (abnormal dryness). Most children with CRPS-1 experience allodynia (severe pain in response to stimuli not usually associated with pain) and hyperalgesia (severe pain in response to stimuli which usually produces less discomfort).

Physical exam of the affected extremity can range from normal to severely atrophic. Changes related to disuse of the extremity include muscle atrophy, increased hair and nail growth, and hyperkeratosis. Children will tend to guard the involved extremity and may refuse close examination. Frequently, personal hygiene of the involved extremity has been neglected. There may be radiographic evidence of osteopenia.

Therapies

Reported therapies include NSAIDs, tricyclic antidepressants, opioids, anticonvulsants, corticosteroids, sympathetic blocks, physiotherapy, transcutaneous electrical nerve stimulation (TENS), and psychological therapies. While most of these achieve modest success, none has proven effective in prospective, controlled, doubleblinded clinical trials. Yet children with CRPS-1 appear to be more responsive to therapy than adults. Combinations of the above therapies result in resolution of symptoms in 46–69% of children, the average recovery time being 7 weeks (range 1–140 weeks). In one particularly notable study for its lack of medications and sympathetic blocks, a program of intensive physical therapy that included 4 hours of aerobic exercise per day, 1–2 hours of hydrotherapy per day, desensitization therapy, and psychological counseling resulted in complete resolution of symptoms in 92% of children in 14 days (range 1–90 days). In those children followed for at least 2 years, 88% remained symptom-free, 10% had continued pain but were fully functional, and 2% had functional limitations. Of the children who were symptom-free at 2 years, 31% eventually experienced a relapse. The differences in outcomes cited above may reflect differences in patients as the diagnostic criteria were not the same in all reports.

Children with CRPS are best cared for by an experienced multidisciplinary team of individuals that includes a physician, a psychologist, and a physical therapist. The physician confirms the diagnosis, coordinates physical and psychological therapies, and when appropriate starts medications or performs sympathetic blocks to facilitate participation in physical therapy.

Case

A 12-year-old, 48-kg female is referred to your office for evaluation and treatment of right foot and leg pain that began 7 weeks ago when she twisted her right ankle while playing soccer. Radiographs of her foot revealed minimal soft tissue swelling around the lateral aspect of her ankle and no bony injury. Because of severe pain, ecchymosis, and swelling she was placed in a short leg cast for 3 weeks. After the cast was removed, the pain persisted and radiographic evaluation of the area was normal. Although the pain was originally limited to the dorsum of her right foot and the lateral aspect of her ankle, it has now spread to involve her entire right foot and extends above her ankle circumferentially involving the distal 6 inches (15 cm) of her lower leg. The pain prevents her from sleeping and the resulting fatigue prevents her from attending school regularly. She cannot bear weight on her right foot and requires crutches to ambulate. She is also unable to wear a sock or shoe on her right foot. When she sleeps at night she elevates her leg to avoid its contact with the mattress or bed linens. Prior to this injury she was in excellent health, and has no other current systemic findings. She has been taking acetaminophen 650 mg PO every 6 hours, ibuprofen 600 mg PO every 6 hours, and oxycodone 5 mg PO when the pain is severe. None of these medications provides any relief. She is an "A" student in the 7th grade, enjoys sports, and lives at home with her mother, father, older sister and two younger brothers. Physical exam is remarkable for a swollen, mottled right foot that is moist and cool to touch (Fig. 27-1). She has severe pain to light touch circumferentially around her toes, foot, ankle, and lower leg, and she refuses to move her foot or toes.

What is this child's diagnosis and on what basis did you make the diagnosis?

This patient fulfills all the IASP diagnostic criteria for CRPS type 1. Specifically, she has continual nondermatomal pain, hyperalgesia, allodynia, and edema of her foot and lower leg. There are skin temperature and color changes and sudomotor findings. She has a history of a trivial soft tissue injury and immobilization of her extremity. Finally, this patient was seen by three other physicians and underwent numerous investigations prior to her referral. The results of her previous work-up exclude all other conditions that could explain her findings.

What would be your initial management?

This patient was hospitalized for 3 weeks to facilitate treatment strategies. The oxycodone, ibuprofen, and acetaminophen were discontinued, and she was administered amitriptyline 25 mg PO at bedtime to promote sleep. The patient received physical therapy twice a day and she and her family were seen by a pain management psychologist. Therapeutic activities and goals were facilitated with the help of child life and occupational therapists. Physical therapy goals for this patient included normal gait ambulation without assistive devices, full active range of motion and normal strength of her right lower extremity, the ability to wear shoes and socks on both feet continuously for 8 hours daily, and the independent performance of a home exercise program. These goals were achieved with a variety of pool and land activities.

What is her prognosis?

This type of multidisciplinary approach with medical management of her symptoms, psychological evaluation and treatment, and physical therapy can result in the complete resolution of symptoms in the majority of subjects. However, a small number of children develop chronic disability and are never able to regain full function.

Daily physical therapy is the cornerstone of treatment for children with CRPS-1. It should focus on desensitization, full weight-bearing, and functional usage of the extremity. The goal is to return the affected extremity to normal functioning, rather than only pain relief. The therapist should acknowledge the presence of pain during initial treatments but continue nonetheless. It is thought that the pain of CRPS-1 results when the body misinterprets sensory information and responds as though an acute injury is in progress. Physical therapy halts this inappropriate response and reestablishes normal neuronal responses. The central nervous system is bombarded with "normal" sensory information such as the perception of touching or weight-bearing by using the affected body part in functional activities.

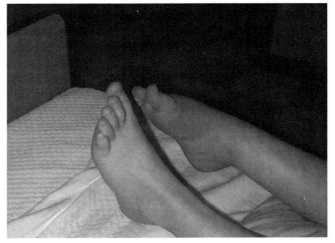

Figure 27-1   Painful, mottled, swollen, warm, moist right foot, ankle, and lower leg.

Additional therapies such as hot and cold packs, TENS, and ultrasound are not usually effective. Immobilization of the affected limb is contraindicated since it may enhance progression of the disease.

Psychological Assessment

The purpose of psychological assessment is to estimate the severity of the child's and the family's pain-related distress and dysfunction. The psychologist will attempt to gain an understanding of their expectations for treatment, their coping styles and skills, recent stressful events and other life changes, and developmental and social histories. The psychologist will help the child and family understand the mechanism of the pain, and will teach coping strategies, relaxation techniques, techniques that maximize function, and cognitive restructuring techniques to address negative thinking. The psychologist will evaluate symptoms of depression and anxiety, and teach the child and family how to increase their sense of self-control over the pain and disability.

Some families may resist psychological involvement because they view it as an indication that the pain is psychosomatic. Therefore, the medical team should present psychological therapy as an integral component of the global pain management program and inform families of the ways in which psychological techniques can be useful in gaining control over the pain. The treatment team should emphasize the mind–body connection so that patients understand that pain is not necessarily a medical or psychological entity, but rather that pain treatment requires medical and psychological approaches.

Clinical Course and Progression

The clinical course and progression of CRPS-1 is highly variable and difficult to predict with reasonable accuracy. Most children will experience a remission of symptoms but many will relapse at the original site or at a new location. A few children never experience a remission. Although some of these children have reduced pain and may return to their premorbid activities, others have a chronic, progressive course with severe pain and disability.

In summary, CRPS-1 is a chronic pain disorder associated with significant morbidity. Its inciting factors and pathophysiology are not fully known. Prompt intervention by an experienced multidisciplinary team can lead to resolution of severe symptoms in most children. However, remissions that are marked by persistent pain and disability are common.

ARTICLES TO KNOW

Lee BH, Scharff L, Sethna NF et al: Physical therapy and cognitive-behavioral treatment for complex regional pain syndromes. *J Pediatr* 141:135–140, 2002.

Murray CS, Cohen A, Perkins T, Davidson JE, Sills JA: Morbidity in reflex sympathetic dystrophy. *Arch Dis Child* 82:231–233, 2000.

Raja SN, Grabow TS: Complex regional pain syndrome I (reflex sympathetic dystrophy). *Anesthesiology* 96:1254–1260, 2002.

Sherry DD, Wallace CA, Kelley C, Kidder M, Sapp L: Short- and long-term outcomes of children with complex regional pain syndrome type 1 treated with exercise therapy. *Clin J Pain* 15:218–233, 1999.

Wilder RT, Berde CB, Wolohan M et al: Reflex sympathetic dystrophy in children: clinical characteristics and follow-up of seventy patients. *J Bone Joint Surg* 74-A:910–919, 1992.

PEDIATRIC SURGICAL PROCEDURES

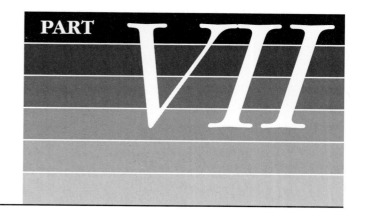

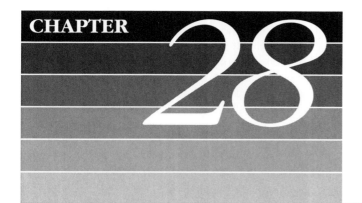

CHAPTER 28

Anesthesia for Pediatric General and Abdominal Surgery

RONALD S. LITMAN

Abdominal surgery in infants and children presents a number of unique anesthetic challenges that are reviewed in this chapter. The first section consists of a discussion of anesthetic concerns for intraabdominal procedures, especially in neonates and small infants. This discussion is general in nature, and the reader should remember that there exists a wide spectrum of patient conditions and surgical techniques for which the anesthetic technique is individualized. The second section reviews unique aspects of a number of common pediatric surgical conditions of the abdomen that are of interest to anesthesiologists. Anesthetic considerations for indwelling vascular access placement (e.g., Hickman or Broviac catheters) are also covered.

GENERAL CONSIDERATIONS

Intraabdominal procedures in children run the gamut from simple hernia repairs in healthy children to complex bowel resections in extremely ill premature infants

(e.g., for necrotizing enterocolitis). Therefore, these general guidelines are intended to be modified for each individual patient, depending on the nature of the surgical procedure and the severity of the illness.

Preoperative assessment should consist of investigation of comorbidities and evaluation of volume resuscitation. Many abdominal diseases will present with vomiting, diarrhea, and sequestration of fluid within the abdominal cavity. Therefore, estimation of volume status is crucial, and preoperative volume resuscitation is often required.

The preoperative physical exam is focused on determination of vital signs, cardiorespiratory stability, and evaluation of the child's upper airway. Signs of dehydration include dry mucous membranes, poor skin turgor, lethargy, weight loss, tachycardia, cold mottled skin, poor peripheral capillary refill, and a sunken fontanel in the young infant. Additional systemic findings include metabolic acidosis, oliguria, and hypotension.

Abdominal distension may be caused by bowel edema, accumulation of fluid or air in the bowel, and pneumoperitoneum if intestinal perforation has occurred. It can cause elevation of the diaphragm, which decreases functional residual capacity, and in the small infant can result in alveolar closure during normal tidal breathing, and lead to hypoxemia and respiratory failure.

Small infants with abdominal processes require a full set of preoperative laboratory studies, including a complete blood count with platelets, electrolytes, and coagulation tests. A type-and-crossmatch should be obtained if there is a possibility of blood loss requiring red cell transfusion. When bowel ischemia is likely, such as with necrotizing enterocolitis, a blood gas analysis is indicated to determine the severity of the underlying metabolic acidosis. Liver and kidney function tests are also appropriate in children with abdominal pathology that is likely to cause dysfunction of these organ systems.

Premedication should be administered when indicated for pain, anxiety, or prophylaxis against pulmonary aspiration of gastric contents. This includes an opioid for pain relief and a benzodiazepine for anxiolysis. Some anesthesiologists may choose to administer a H_2-antagonist to reduce gastric acidity; however, there is no proven benefit to this practice. Metoclopramide, a prokinetic agent, should not be administered if there is the possibility of an intestinal obstruction.

Primary intraoperative anesthetic considerations include management of dehydration, hypovolemia, acidosis, and hypothermia. Standard monitors are usually sufficient but the disease process should determine the need for either direct arterial measurement or central venous access. All measures to ensure normothermia should be used (see Chapter 15). These include core temperature monitoring (esophageal or rectal), warming the operating room (OR), humidification of the breathing circuit, use of an intravenous fluid warming device, and use of a forced warm-air heating blanket underneath and around the child. Overhead radiant heaters can be used for neonates and small infants during placement of monitors and induction of anesthesia. In tiny infants, an esophageal catheter can be advanced too far and into the stomach, where it becomes warm from the OR lights during a laparotomy, thus producing an artifactual elevation in temperature. An indwelling urinary catheter is indicated if the procedure will last more than 3-4 hours, or if large intraoperative fluid fluctuations are anticipated. A urinary collection bag is utilized in small neonates or premature infants.

Insensible losses are often high when a large surface area of bowel is exposed (at least 10 mL/kg/h) and will warrant liberal fluid administration. Hypovolemia can occur rapidly from unanticipated bleeding or third-space losses from bowel exposure or edema. Neonates with large abdominal defects such as gastroschisis often require more than 50 mL/kg of isotonic fluid over the duration of the procedure. Many pediatric anesthesiologists will insert two intravenous catheters. Isotonic crystalloid solutions are appropriate for most volume resuscitations; albumin or other colloid solutions are rarely used. Some pediatric anesthesiologists, however, prefer to administer 5% albumin to extremely premature infants undergoing extensive bowel surgery, to maximize the duration that the solution will remain in the vascular space. The occasional child may require inotropic therapy with dopamine (see Chapter 38) if hypotension persists despite seemingly adequate volume resuscitation, especially when there is an intraabdominal process associated with sepsis.

Virtually all infants and children presenting for urgent abdominal surgery are considered to have a full stomach, and thus at increased risk for pulmonary aspiration of gastric contents during the loss of consciousness that accompanies induction of general anesthesia. Decreased gastric emptying in these patients may be caused by the pathologic abdominal process, or administration of medications with anticholinergic effects, such as opioids. Children undergoing elective abdominal procedures that are minor and not associated with pathologic processes that interfere with normal gastric emptying can be managed with normal fasting guidelines (see Chapter 12).

In children presumed to be at risk for pulmonary aspiration of gastric contents during induction of anesthesia, rapid sequence intubation (RSI) with administration of cricoid pressure is indicated. Succinylcholine 2 mg/kg or high-dose rocuronium (1.2-1.6 mg/kg) are both effective for this purpose. A modified rapid sequence induction is preferred in small infants who will likely develop oxyhemoglobin desaturation during brief periods of apnea, and will therefore require assisted ventilation prior to endotracheal intubation. Awake intubations are rarely, if ever, performed on neonates by pediatric anesthesiologists, except during episodes of severe hemodynamic instability.

Many children will present for abdominal surgery with an indwelling nasogastric tube, which should be suctioned immediately prior to induction of general anesthesia. It can then be removed to facilitate airway management, and replaced following insertion of the endotracheal tube.

Maintenance of general anesthesia during abdominal procedures depends primarily on the severity of the child's illness. For healthy children undergoing procedures that are not expected to require postoperative mechanical ventilation, a balanced technique is chosen, including an inhalational agent and an opioid. In children who are expected to require postoperative mechanical ventilation, an opioid-based technique is preferred, as it has fewer deleterious effects on the cardiovascular system when compared to inhalational agents, and can be continued into the postoperative period to decrease the child's overall stress response and provide ongoing analgesia and sedation. Small infants and neonates tend to remain hemodynamically stable after relatively large amounts of opioids in the absence of hypovolemia. N_2O is avoided during all but superficial abdominal wall procedures (e.g., simple hernia repair). Regional analgesia via the lumbar or caudal epidural route can be considered when the child is hemodynamically stable and does not demonstrate evidence of bacteremia or sepsis.

Neonates who undergo major abdominal surgery will benefit from postoperative mechanical ventilation for several days. This allows liberal titration of opioids and a decreased stress response without the risk of apnea during this phase of large fluid requirements and intravascular fluid shifts secondary to intestinal "third spacing."

ANESTHETIC MANAGEMENT OF INDIVIDUAL PROCEDURES

Choledochal Cyst

A choledochal cyst is an abnormal dilatation of the common bile duct that, when sufficiently large, obstructs the egress of bile from the liver. It is commonly diagnosed in infants within the first year but may occur in older children. The classic triad of symptoms includes pain, jaundice, and a right upper-quadrant abdominal mass. Chronic biliary obstruction may cause secondary liver damage.

The important aspects of anesthetic management for children undergoing choledochal cyst removal consist of attention to liver function abnormalities and provision of postoperative analgesia. High lumbar or low thoracic epidural analgesia is preferred.

Congenital Diaphragmatic Hernia

A congenital diaphragmatic hernia (CDH) is a malformation of the diaphragm that allows the abdominal contents to enter and remain within the thoracic cavity during fetal life (Fig. 28-1). It occurs in approximately 1 of every 2500 live births and is often detected by prenatal ultrasound. The most critical consequence of this anomaly is the prevention of normal prenatal lung growth.

SITES OF CONGENITAL DIAPHRAGMATIC HERNIA

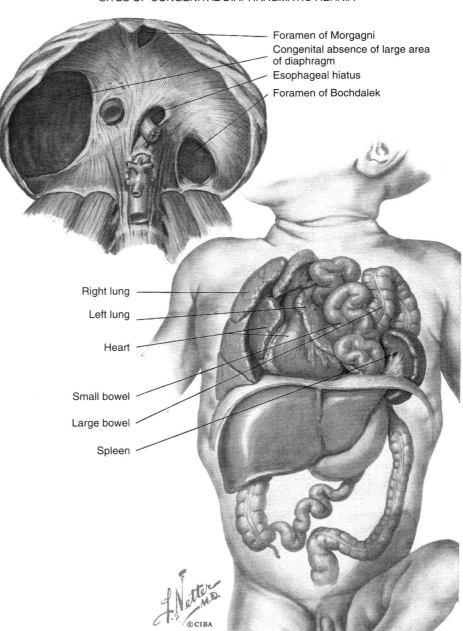

Foramen of Morgagni
Congenital absence of large area of diaphragm
Esophageal hiatus
Foramen of Bochdalek

Right lung
Left lung
Heart
Small bowel
Large bowel
Spleen

Figure 28-1 Sites of congenital diaphragmatic hernia. (Reproduced courtesy of Ciba–Geigy.)

Severe cases cause significant lung hypoplasia that is incompatible with maintenance of normoxemia at birth. Most commonly, CDH occurs on the left side, posteriorly through the foramen of Bochdalek. Right-sided or anterior defects through the foramen of Morgagni occur infrequently, and are not usually associated with severe pulmonary hypoplasia, but rather signs of intestinal obstruction.

Severe defects manifest immediately after birth as respiratory distress. Newborns with CDH will demonstrate chest wall retractions, tachypnea, hypoxemia, absence of breath sounds on the affected side, and the classically appearing scaphoid abdomen that indicates a lack of organs within the abdominal cavity. Diagnosis is confirmed by radiography, which demonstrates bowel in the thoracic cavity and a gasless abdominal cavity. Infants with mild defects and normal lung growth may not be diagnosed until many months after birth, when a chest radiograph is obtained for unrelated reasons.

Pulmonary hypoplasia and hypoxemia trigger a number of deleterious effects in the newborn period, the most critical of which is persistent pulmonary hypertension and failure to transition normally from fetal to adult circulatory function (see Chapter 1). The pressure on the right side of the heart remains high, and right-to-left shunting continues across the ductus arteriosus, which also fails to close secondary to persistent hypoxemia, hypercarbia, and acidosis. Additional right-to-left shunting can occur through a patent foramen ovale or ventricular septal defect, if present. This process sets up a vicious cycle that is difficult to abort in the absence of normoxemia and normal lung function. Concomitant congenital heart disease contributes to the pathologic process and reduces overall survival.

Medical management at birth consists of immediate tracheal intubation and institution of mechanical ventilation. Bag-and-mask positive pressure ventilation should be minimized in an effort to reduce gastric distention since the stomach or small intestine may be contained within the thoracic cavity. A nasogastric tube should be immediately inserted to decompress the upper digestive tract. Until the late 1980s, these infants were rushed to surgery in an attempt to remove the abdominal contents from the thoracic cavity and allow reexpansion of the hypoplastic lung. This practice did not improve survival since the compressed lung is hypoplastic, not atelectatic. Current medical management includes medical stabilization; corrective surgery is performed on a semi-elective basis within the first few weeks of life.

Initial medical management consists of optimization of oxygenation and ventilation, administration of sedatives and neuromuscular blockers, establishment of normothermia, and placement of intravenous and arterial access lines. The goal of ventilatory management is a Pao_2 greater than 60 mmHg and a Pco_2 less than 45 mmHg,

to minimize increases in pulmonary arterial pressures. The inability to reduce the Pco_2 or reduce the alveolar-to-arterial oxygen gradient to less than 500 mmHg despite maximal ventilatory techniques (e.g., using the oscillator or jet ventilator) is associated with a poor outcome and is an indication for institution of extracorporeal membrane oxygenation (ECMO). Pulmonary vasodilator therapy with inhaled nitric oxide is infrequently successful.

Surgical correction of CDH occurs in the operating room after medical stabilization, or in the neonatal intensive care unit (NICU), while the patient remains on ECMO life support. The surgery consists of an abdominal or thoracic reduction of the herniated viscera, and placement of an ipsilateral chest tube. Some surgeons will insert a contralateral chest tube to protect against pneumothorax from aggressive ventilator therapy. Unexplained intraoperative decreases in lung compliance, hypoxemia, or hypotension are suggestive of a contralateral pneumothorax and should warrant chest tube placement. The diaphragmatic defect is closed by primary repair or by using a synthetic patch.

Ventilatory management during CDH repair consists of a balance between avoidance of barotrauma and avoidance of factors that increase PVR, such as hypoxemia, hypercarbia, and acidosis. Simultaneous pulse oximetry at preductal (right upper-extremity) and postductal (lower-extremity) sites allows early detection of right-to-left shunting from development of pulmonary hypertension. Cannulation of the right radial artery will allow continuous blood pressure measurement and measurement of preductal oxygenation.

Additional anesthetic priorities during CDH repair include provision of adequate volume expansion, especially when high ventilatory pressures are required, and reduction of sympathetic tone using a high-dose opioid technique to minimize elevations in PVR. Mechanical ventilation is continued in the postoperative period in all but the most minor defects.

Extrahepatic Biliary Atresia

Extrahepatic biliary atresia describes a congenital malformation of the hepatic ducts between the biliary system of the liver and the duodenum, such that bile cannot be emptied properly from the liver. This disease manifests as direct hyperbilirubinemia within the first several weeks of life. Infants with biliary atresia require a surgical anastomosis between the duodenum and an intrahepatic biliary duct (Kasai procedure). Anesthetic concerns are primarily those of decreased hepatic function and its sequelae, such as clotting factor deficiency, and avoidance of medications that are metabolized in the liver. Postoperative epidural analgesia is preferred in the absence of a coagulopathy. Long-term postoperative complications after the Kasai procedure include recurrent ascending cholangitis and chronic cirrhosis. Therefore, some of these children will ultimately require a liver transplant.

Hirschsprung's Disease

Hirschsprung's disease (congenital aganglionic megacolon) is defined as the absence of parasympathetic ganglion cells in the lower colon. It is the most common cause of large bowel obstruction in the newborn, and presents in the first few days of life as a failure to pass meconium and abdominal distention. On rare occasions these children may become very ill with toxic megacolon, peritonitis, and colonic perforation. Treatment consists of a colostomy at the time of diagnosis, and definitive therapy (pull-through procedure) some time later in the first year of life, although some surgeons may now choose to perform this procedure in the neonatal period. In many centers, laparoscopy is being utilized during a large part of the intraabdominal resection prior to the perineal repair.

During the latter portion of the procedure when the perineum is repaired, the child will be placed at the far end of the OR table in the lithotomy position. The anesthesiologist should anticipate this relocation and adjust the lengths of the monitoring wires, breathing circuit, and IV tubing accordingly.

Imperforate Anus

Imperforate anus (anal atresia) is diagnosed shortly after birth on physical exam, or after an evaluation for failure of the infant to pass meconium in the first days of life. This anomaly ranges in severity from a mild stenosis with a thin obstructive band that is punctured at the bedside, to a more severe atresia that is associated with other anomalies. Anal atresia is a component of the VATER syndrome: Vertebral anomalies, Anal atresia, Tracheo-Esophageal fistula, and Renal/genitourinary malformations. An updated acronym is VACTERL to include Cardiac and Limb anomalies.

Anal atresia is considered an urgent surgical procedure. A colostomy is performed shortly following diagnosis. It is less urgent in female infants with a rectovaginal fistula that allows passage of meconium. The corrective procedure, a posterior sagittal anorectoplasty (Pena procedure), is often performed during the first year of life. Unique anesthetic concerns include the delineation of coexisting anomalies, and assessment of fluid and electrolyte imbalance. The procedure usually begins in the prone position; some surgeons will turn the child and complete the procedure in the supine or lithotomy position.

Indwelling Intravenous Access

One of the most commonly performed surgical procedures in children is the intraoperative placement of an indwelling venous catheter (Broviac, Hickman, Port-a-Cath, etc.) into the central venous system. The catheter is inserted into one of the central veins of the neck or groin, and a portion of it is tunneled underneath the skin for improved stability and to discourage infection at the site of the vein. Children with different types of chronic diseases will require this procedure for long-term parenteral nutrition, administration of antibiotics, or administration of chemotherapy, among many other conditions.

Preoperative evaluation of the patient should consist of complete delineation of comorbidities. A preoperative anxiolytic can be administered orally or intravenously if access has been established. There are no unique considerations for induction and maintenance of general anesthesia. The procedure is performed with the child in the Trendelenburg position, with the head hyperextended and turned to one side. Therefore, airway access is limited, and for this reason all children undergo endotracheal intubation for the procedure.

General anesthesia is also utilized in many children who require removal of their tunneled catheter. The tunneled central catheter can be used to administer intravenous induction agents but should not be removed prior to establishing peripheral venous access. Significant blood loss can occasionally occur from a tear in the vein that contained the tunneled catheter. Endotracheal intubation is not required for this procedure, which often takes less than 10 minutes to perform and in which surgical draping is minimal.

Inguinal Hernia

Inguinal hernia repair is one of the most common surgical procedures in children. A unilateral hernia is usually diagnosed on routine physical exam in healthy school-aged children. Bilateral hernias commonly occur in extremely premature infants and, because of the potential risk of incarceration, will usually be repaired before the child is discharged from the hospital. Therefore, these children will present with all the usual medical problems associated with prematurity (see Chapters 10 and 11).

There are many ways to anesthetize these children. Different factors are taken into consideration, including the health of the child, preference of the surgeon, and the skills of the anesthesiology provider. Older children with uncomplicated unilateral hernias can receive maintenance of general anesthesia by mask or laryngeal mask airway (LMA). When laparoscopic examination of the contralateral side is performed, endotracheal intubation and neuromuscular blockade may be indicated, depending on the preference of the surgeon. Small infants who are at risk for development of postoperative apnea may benefit from spinal anesthesia for inguinal hernia repair (see Chapter 20).

Intussusception

Intussusception is the telescoping of a portion of bowel (usually the distal ileum) into the adjacent more distal portion with subsequent swelling and obstruction. Occasionally, this obstruction may be severe and lead to intestinal ischemia. The cause is largely unknown but is associated with a polyp or enlarged intestinal lymph nodes (Peyer's patches). These children are usually between the ages of 2 months and 5 years, and present with vomiting, bloody (currant jelly) stools, and abdominal distention. Bowel ischemia and sepsis may be present in severe or protracted cases. The diagnosis is confirmed radiographically. In many cases, the intussusception can be reduced using a barium enema. All others must undergo exploratory laparotomy and manual reduction. The primary anesthetic considerations for this procedure consist of fluid resuscitation, maintenance of normothermia, and provision of postoperative analgesia.

Laparoscopic Surgery

A variety of pediatric abdominal procedures are now being performed through the laparoscope. These include appendectomies, pyloromyotomies, hernias, Nissen fundoplications, and bowel resections, to name just a few. In older children, the laparoscopic methods and anesthetic implications are the same as for adults. In younger children and infants, increases in intraabdominal pressure (IAP) may result in cardiopulmonary compromise. In several studies, an IAP less than 12 mmHg appears to be safe in this young patient population. IAP above 12 mmHg has been associated with hypotension, bradycardia, and difficulty with ventilation secondary to a loss of functional residual capacity (FRC) and a decrease in lung compliance. IAP greater than 6 mmHg may cause increased PVR and result in right-to-left shunting in cyanotic children with congenital heart disease.

Malrotation and Midgut Volvulus

Malrotation is defined as an abnormal twisting of the intestine as it migrates back into the fetal abdominal cavity from its embryonic extraabdominal location during the latter part of the first trimester. When this twisting compromises the blood supply of the intestine (superior mesenteric artery), the condition is known as a *volvulus*. Infants who develop volvulus from malrotation usually become symptomatic sometime in the first 2 months of life, although mild cases can remain asymptomatic for many years. Symptoms include bilious vomiting or signs of intestinal perforation and ischemia. These infants can present quite ill with a sepsis-like picture; the condition can be fulminant and even fatal. Severely ill children may require fluid and blood resuscitation, and endotracheal intubation in the preoperative period. Children with malrotation often have additional congenital anomalies that should be investigated prior to surgery.

The treatment of volvulus consists of urgent exploratory laparotomy and surgical reduction (Ladd's procedure). The bowel is untwisted along the mesentery and fixed in an unrotated position. Most children are awakened and extubated in the operating room and require only routine postoperative care. However, depending on the severity of the child's illness, consideration should be given to leaving the child's trachea intubated and institution of mechanical ventilation postoperatively, especially if a "second-look" laparotomy is planned to assess bowel viability.

Meckel Diverticulum

A Meckel diverticulum is a persistence of the omphalomesenteric duct after fetal life that presents as painless rectal bleeding sometime in the first few years of life. Definitive treatment is surgical resection via exploratory laparotomy. Clinically significant anemia is uncommon. The major anesthetic consideration is relief of postoperative pain, for which epidural analgesia is recommended.

Necrotizing Enterocolitis

Necrotizing enterocolitis (NEC) is a multifactorial disorder that affects 6–10% of prematurely born infants weighing under 1500 g. Risk factors include administration of hypertonic enteral feedings, decreased bowel perfusion, and infection with enteric organisms (Fig. 28-2). It is a fulminant disease that initially manifests as abdominal distention and bloody stools, and can progress rapidly to severe intestinal ischemia, sepsis, and shock. Additional signs and symptoms include cardiovascular instability, respiratory failure, temperature instability, metabolic acidosis, thrombocytopenia, and disseminated intravascular coagulation (DIC). Mortality ranges between 10% and 30%. Infants who survive an episode of NEC are more likely to suffer from neurodevelopmental morbidity.

Pathologic findings range from mild mucosal ulceration to bowel perforation and severe peritonitis. Bowel ischemia causes damage to the intestinal mucosa, which allows bowel gas to penetrate the submucosal region and enter the mesenteric veins and portal venous system. Diagnosis is usually made on the basis of an abdominal radiograph that reveals pneumatosis intestinalis (air bubbles within the intestinal wall), or free air within the abdominal cavity or portal venous system.

Mild cases of NEC can be managed conservatively with medical therapy that consists of gastric decompression, antibiotics, and volume resuscitation with isotonic fluids and blood products. Surgical exploration is indicated for infants with radiographic evidence of intestinal perforation

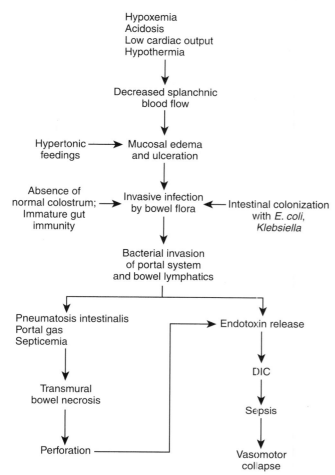

Figure 28-2 Possible factors in etiology and outcome of neonatal necrotizing enterocolitis. (Reproduced with permission from Burrington JD: Necrotizing enterocolitis in newborn infants. *Clin Perinatol* 5:29–44, 1978.)

ischemia and severity of the underlying disease. Lower birthweight infants have poorer outcomes.

Omphalocele and Gastroschisis

Although each represents a distinct anatomical defect, omphalocele and gastroschisis are discussed together because their anesthetic considerations are nearly identical. Each is a congenital defect that allows a portion of the intestinal viscera to remain outside the abdominal cavity, and requires surgical repair as soon as possible after birth.

An omphalocele occurs when the visceral organs fail to migrate from the yolk sac back into the abdomen early in gestation; the defect occurs at the insertion of the umbilicus (Fig. 28-3). Gastroschisis is thought to result from an occlusion of the omphalomesenteric artery during early development. As a result, the abdominal viscera herniate through a rent in the abdominal wall, usually to the right of the umbilicus (Fig. 28-4). Omphalocele is more likely than gastroschisis to be associated with prematurity and additional congenital anomalies. It is a component of the Beckwith–Wiedemann syndrome, which consists of hypertrophy of multiple organs. In this syndrome, enlargement of the tongue may compromise the upper airway, and pancreatic enlargement causes hyperinsulinism, which results in hypoglycemia. Infants with gastroschisis are usually born at full term, and it is usually an isolated defect. The major pathophysiological difference between the two defects is that, in omphalocele, the intestinal contents remain covered with the peritoneal membrane which protects the intestinal mucosa from the irritative effects of amniotic fluid, and there is less

(i.e., free air) or rapidly worsening disease. Inotropic support may be necessary to support cardiovascular function.

Anesthetic considerations include management of acidosis, hypovolemia, anemia, electrolyte imbalance, coagulopathy, and support of cardiovascular function. An arterial line is recommended to monitor blood pressure closely and facilitate frequent collection of blood samples. Central venous cannulation will facilitate volume replacement.

An exploratory laparotomy is performed to examine the bowel in its entirety. Perforations may be repaired or surgically excised. A variable amount of ischemic bowel may be removed. This procedure is associated with large amounts of fluid and possibly blood loss. The anesthesiologist should be prepared to resuscitate the infant with isotonic fluid (normal saline or Lactated Ringers solution) and blood products as needed. Postoperatively these infants remain intubated, sedated, and mechanically ventilated while supportive therapy continues. Recovery and survival are dependent on the extent of bowel

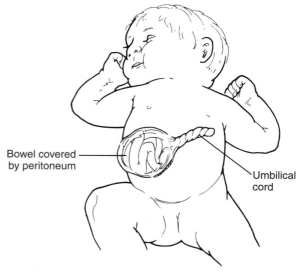

Figure 28-3 An omphalocele occurs when the visceral organs fail to migrate from the yolk sac back into the abdomen early in gestation. The abdominal organs are covered by the peritoneal membrane.

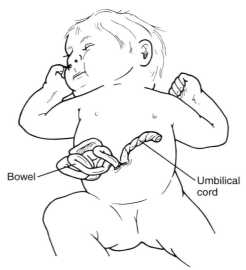

Bowel

Umbilical
cord

Figure 28-4   A gastroschisis is thought to occur as a result of an occlusion of the omphalomesenteric artery. As a result, the abdominal viscera herniate through a rent in the abdominal wall, usually to the right of the umbilicus, and the intestinal contents are not covered by a membrane. Therefore, the infant is at higher risk of fluid and temperature loss and development of sepsis.

evaporative fluid and temperature loss after delivery than with gastroschisis. Because infants with gastroschisis lack this "protective" covering, they are more prone to dehydration, hypothermia, "third-space" fluid accumulation, electrolyte imbalance, acidosis, bleeding, and sepsis.

Whether diagnosed *in utero* or at birth, management begins immediately after delivery. The extruded abdominal contents are covered with warm saline dressings and are encased in a sterile plastic bag to decrease fluid and temperature loss, and discourage infection. A nasogastric tube is placed for gastric decompression, normovolemia is maintained with intravenous hydration, and associated comorbidities are addressed prior to surgical repair.

Considerations for induction of general anesthesia are similar to those for any newborn infant with a presumed increased risk of a "full stomach" secondary to intestinal obstruction. A modified rapid sequence intubation (RSI) is performed after suctioning the nasogastric tube. Some pediatric anesthesiologists will prefer to temporarily remove the nasogastric tube during endotracheal intubation.

Achieving a primary repair is the major surgical priority, for failure to place all the intestinal contents into the abdominal cavity increases postoperative morbidity significantly. However, in many cases where the abdominal cavity is too restrictive, a partial replacement is performed, and the remaining external viscera is encased in a synthetic silo mesh. Complete repair is accomplished as a staged procedure, allowing for the reduction of intestinal swelling over several days.

A number of intraoperative adverse physiologic derangements may occur when the surgeon attempts to place a large volume of abdominal contents into a restrictive abdominal cavity. Cephalad displacement of the diaphragm

Article To Know

Yaster M, Buck JR et al: Hemodynamic effects of primary closure of omphalocele/gastroschisis in human newborns. Anesthesiology 69:84-88, 1988.

Few articles exist in the pediatric anesthesia literature that have contributed important information concerning anesthetic management of complex neonatal procedures. This article represents one of those publications. Myron Yaster and his colleagues at Johns Hopkins were interested in predicting the outcome of primary surgical repair of omphalocele and gastroschisis based on the intraoperative abdominal pressure. They expanded upon their own animal experiments which demonstrated that acute elevations in intraabdominal pressure are associated with reductions in cardiac output and regional blood flow. They designed an observational study to determine whether increased gastric pressure at the time of the primary repair is associated with postoperative organ system failure.

The authors studied 11 newborns undergoing primary closure of an omphalocele or gastroschisis within the first 24 hours of life. Intragastric pressure was continuously measured using a fluid-filled 12-French orogastric tube, and cardiac output indices were measured intraoperatively. Primary repair could not be accomplished in three infants. In the remaining eight infants, four required reoperation within 24 hours (group 1) and four had unremarkable postoperative courses (group 2). Indications for reoperation of the group 1 infants included low or absent urine output, or other evidence of poor cardiac output. Two of these infants were found to have ischemic or necrotic bowel during reoperation. Infants in group 1 who required reoperation had significantly greater increases in intragastric pressure and central venous pressure and decreases in cardiac index during the primary repair than infants who did not require reoperation. In group 1 the intragastric pressures ranged from 6 to 18 mmHg; in group 2 the range was 22-28 mmHg. Furthermore, an increase of central venous pressure (CVP) by 4 mmHg or more predicted reoperation. These results were subsequently confirmed in a prospective management study by the same group, and by a separate study that utilized bladder pressures. The results indicate that intraabdominal pressures greater than 20 mmHg are associated with critical decreases in organ perfusion. Anesthesiologists should use liberal neuromuscular blockade and tailor their ventilatory parameters to remain below this level whenever possible.

can significantly decrease functional residual capacity (FRC) and tidal volume, and lead to hypoxemia. During the repair, the anesthesiologist must frequently use manual ventilation in response to rapid changes in lung compliance and the need for increased inspiratory pressures to maintain adequate tidal volumes. The presence of hypoxemia despite maximal ventilation may preclude completion of a primary repair.

Increased intraabdominal pressure may result in an abdominal compartment syndrome. Venous compression leads to decreased preload and hypotension, and lower-limb venous congestion. Arterial compression causes renal artery compression and oliguria, and decreased perfusion to the lower extremities. Bowel ischemia may also occur. The anesthesiologist must ensure adequate volume and blood replacement, and full neuromuscular blockade must be maintained throughout the procedure. The surgeon is intent on performing a primary repair, but is often limited by respiratory and circulatory compromise, which must be adequately communicated by the anesthesiologist. This procedure provides the anesthesiologist with the opportunity to act in concert with the surgeon as each continually communicates their respective priorities.

All infants, except those with the most trivial repairs, remain intubated and mechanically ventilated in the postoperative period. Abdominal compartment syndrome may continue postoperatively; therefore, paralysis and adequate sedation with an opioid infusion are essential for optimal management.

Pyloric Stenosis

Pyloric stenosis describes an abnormality that occurs within the first several weeks of life, in which a hypertrophied pylorus obstructs the passage of food from the stomach to the small intestine. With an incidence of up to 1 in 300 live births, it represents one of the most common procedures requiring general anesthesia within the first weeks of life. Clinical manifestations include projectile nonbilious vomiting after feeds, and when severe or protracted, dehydration and failure to thrive. The diagnosis is confirmed by characteristic findings on physical exam (palpation of the hypertrophied pylorus), barium swallow, or ultrasound examination. Chronic emesis causes loss of hydrochloric acid from the stomach, which leads to a hypochloremic, hypokalemic metabolic alkalosis.

Once the condition is diagnosed, these children should be hospitalized and given intravenous therapy to correct the dehydration and electrolyte abnormalities. A nasogastric tube is inserted and all feedings are stopped. Rehydration consists of normal saline for reestablishment of normovolemia (some infants may require in excess of 50 mL/kg), and maintenance fluids consisting of D5-1/4NS

with potassium chloride added. Pyloric stenosis is never considered a surgical emergency. Perioperative morbidity and mortality are associated with surgical correction prior to normalization of fluid and electrolyte derangements. Serum potassium should be in the normal range, and serum chloride should be ≥90 mEq/L prior to surgery. The kidney will retain chloride as a result of volume contraction. A urine chloride >20 mEq/L suggests that volume status has been adequately restored.

Prior to induction of general anesthesia, the infant's nasogastric tube should be suctioned and removed, and a large-bore suction catheter (e.g., 14-French) is inserted orally into the stomach and suctioned while tilting the infant in all directions to evacuate any remaining gastric contents. This procedure will completely empty the stomach in nearly all infants. The most common anesthetic induction technique at The Children's Hospital of Philadelphia is a modified rapid-sequence technique that consists of preoxygenation, followed by administration of propofol or thiopental, and a nondepolarizing neuromuscular blocker. Positive-pressure ventilation is provided by mask while an assistant provides cricoid pressure prior to endotracheal intubation. A true rapid-sequence technique using succinylcholine is not often used because oxyhemoglobin desaturation will usually occur prior to intubation, and the incidence of pulmonary aspiration is exceedingly low. "Awake" intubations are no longer performed on children with pyloric stenosis. Maintenance of general anesthesia can consist of any inhalational agent; however, desflurane is preferred because of its ability to be rapidly eliminated. Opioids are not administered, unless a remifentanil infusion is chosen for the duration of the procedure.

Surgical correction consists of a pyloromyotomy, in which the pylorus is partially split lengthwise to loosen the constriction. It is performed as an open procedure or by laparoscopy. Following the myotomy, the surgeon will often request insufflation of the stomach with air via an orogastric tube to test the integrity of the pyloric mucosa. Fluid and blood losses are minimal. Local anesthesia should be administered by the surgeon to the skin and subcutaneous tissues.

Although definitive data are lacking, the clinical experience of many pediatric anesthesiologists has been that these infants take longer than usual to emerge from general anesthesia and will often manifest central apnea in the postoperative period. Some attribute this to the underlying electrolyte imbalance and metabolic alkalosis associated with pyloric stenosis. This author's practice is to minimize these complications by using short-acting anesthetic agents (e.g., propofol for induction, desflurane for maintenance), and discontinue the anesthetic agent at the time of the myotomy. Mivacurium is used for neuromuscular blockade. Use of continuous remifentanil as the primary maintenance agent has been associated with less postoperative apnea compared to halothane.

Case

A 3-week old, 1.4-kg male infant is scheduled for emergency exploratory laparotomy for NEC. The infant was born at 28 weeks' gestation at a weight of 1.2 kg, and was mechanically ventilated during the first week of life. The infant had been doing well until 2 days ago when he developed abdominal distention and bloody stools. An abdominal radiograph revealed pneumatosis intestinalis and air in the portal system. Antibiotics were begun, enteral feeds were immediately stopped, and a nasogastric tube was inserted for continuous gastric decompression. His current vital signs are: temperature 36.4°C, heart rate 168/min, respiratory rate 54/min, and blood pressure 66/28 mmHg. Recent laboratory findings include: WBC 5.4, Hgb 9.3, and platelets 70,000; electrolytes Na 132, K 5.5, Cl 99, CO$_2$ 19; and glucose 77. Arterial blood gas analysis while breathing 1 liter oxygen by nasal cannula revealed pH 7.20, Pco_2 36 mmHg, Po_2 83 mmHg, and base excess −7.8.

What else would you like to know before proceeding with general anesthesia and the exploratory laparotomy?

This small infant with NEC is teetering on the brink of becoming extremely ill, as evidenced by his low core temperature, anemia, thrombocytopenia, hyponatremia, and metabolic acidosis. There is also a high risk of developing central apnea for which institution of mechanical ventilation will be required. Therefore, surgery should not be delayed for very long. My primary preoperative objectives at this point include volume resuscitation and correction of his anemia. Normal saline boluses, 10 mL/kg, should be administered until urine output reaches at least 1 mL/kg/h. Packed red blood cells should be transfused prior to surgery if time permits. The blood bank should be alerted about this child, and should be asked to prepare packed red cells, platelets, and fresh frozen plasma.

What intraoperative monitors are required for this child?

In addition to standard monitors, I would consider direct arterial cannulation to closely follow blood pressure and facilitate frequent intraoperative blood sampling for hemoglobin, electrolytes, and blood gas analysis. Two free-flowing intravenous lines should be inserted prior to the beginning of the procedure for blood and fluid administration, and provision of a continuous glucose and electrolyte solution. The surgeons may place an indwelling central venous catheter to facilitate postoperative fluid administration and parenteral nutrition.

Hypothermia commonly occurs in small infants with a large amount of skin or intestinal surface exposed. Esophageal or rectal temperature monitoring will closely approximate core body temperature. The OR should be warmed and an overhead radiant heater used during induction of anesthesia and placement of monitors and invasive lines. During the procedure, a forced warm air blanket should be placed underneath and around the infant and should cover all nonoperative exposed body parts, including the face and head. Intravenous fluids should be warmed.

How would you induce anesthesia in this infant?

My primary concerns at induction of general anesthesia include avoidance of pulmonary aspiration of retained gastric contents and hemodynamic deterioration secondary to underlying anemia and possible hypovolemia and sepsis. Previous generations of pediatric anesthesiologists would have performed endotracheal intubation prior to induction of general anesthesia; this is no longer performed in most pediatric centers. The most commonly performed induction technique is a modified rapid sequence induction following administration of intravenous atropine and evacuation of the stomach via the nasogastric tube. Small doses of thiopental or propofol can be administered along with fentanyl that is administered in small amounts and titrated to the infant's blood pressure and heart rate. A nondepolarizing neuromuscular blocker is administered at a sufficiently high dose so as to ensure adequate paralysis and intubating conditions within 1 minute (see Chapter 19). Cricoid pressure can be performed during positive-pressure bag–mask ventilation, with or without the presence of the nasogastric tube (see Chapter 17). A 3.0 styletted endotracheal tube is then inserted when adequate muscular relaxation has been obtained.

How will you maintain general anesthesia in this infant?

Maintenance of general anesthesia will consist primarily of an opioid-based technique with a low-dose inhalational agent, and avoidance of N$_2$O. Small doses of fentanyl (e.g., 1–2 µg/kg) will be administered intermittently throughout the procedure and titrated to the infant's vital signs. The oxygen concentration should be continuously adjusted to maintain the preductal oxyhemoglobin saturation between 92% and 95%.

What fluids would you administer for this procedure?

One intravenous line will infuse the infant's maintenance solution that contains glucose, potassium, and possibly calcium. Unless the infant demonstrated preoperative hypoglycemia, I will usually halve the usual maintenance rate in an attempt to avoid hyperglycemia related to the intraoperative stress response. This is unlikely in prematurely born infants because of the lack of glycogen stores, which primarily accumulate during the third trimester. Nevertheless, glucose levels will be monitored at least hourly throughout the procedure and the infusion will be adjusted accordingly.

Case   *Cont'd*

The other intravenous line will be used for administration of crystalloid volume replacement (e.g., normal saline) and blood products. Third-space fluid accumulation and evaporative losses usually result in the administration of at least 20 mL/kg/h during the procedure. Red cells should be transfused to maintain the infant's hemoglobin of at least 10 mg/dL. Additional calcium should be administered along with red cells. Platelets and fresh frozen plasma are indicated for generalized nonsurgical bleeding during the procedure. Sodium bicarbonate is indicated for continuing metabolic acidosis that results in a pH of less than 7.15.

Would you extubate this infant's trachea at the completion of the procedure?

Postoperatively, a substantial amount of third-space fluid accumulation and fluid shifts are expected. Therefore, this infant should remain sedated and mechanically ventilated for at least several days. This will also facilitate analgesic management with a continuous opioid infusion without risking ventilatory depression. Furthermore, depending on the extent of intestinal ischemia, this infant's medical condition may worsen over the first several postoperative days and necessitate administration of inotropic agents. In addition, these infants are often returned to the OR for a "second-look" procedure to evaluate ongoing bowel necrosis.

Is there any role for regional analgesia in this infant?

Regional analgesia, in the form of epidural administration of local anesthetics, is not indicated in this infant because of the possibility of bacteremia or sepsis, and will not be necessary in the intubated patient receiving continuous opioids.

ADDITIONAL ARTICLES TO KNOW

Andropoulos DB, Heard MB, Johnson KL, Clarke JT, Rowe RW: Postanesthetic apnea in full-term infants after pyloromyotomy. *Anesthesiology* 80:216–219, 1994.

Bissonnette B, Sullivan PJ: Pyloric stenosis. *Can J Anaesth* 38:668–676, 1991.

Bozkurt P, Kaya G, Yeker Y, Tunali Y, Altintas F: The cardiorespiratory effects of laparoscopic procedures in infants. *Anaesthesia* 54:831–834, 1999.

Davis PJ, Galinkin J, McGowan FX et al: A randomized multicenter study of remifentanil compared with halothane in neonates and infants undergoing pyloromyotomy: I. Emergence and recovery profiles. *Anesth Analg* 93:1380–1386, 2001.

Galinkin JL, Davis PJ, McGowan FX et al: A randomized multicenter study of remifentanil compared with halothane in neonates and infants undergoing pyloromyotomy: II. Perioperative breathing patterns in neonates and infants with pyloric stenosis. *Anesth Analg* 93:1387–1392, 2001.

Wolf AR, Lawson RA, Dryden CM, Davies FW: Recovery after desflurane anaesthesia in the infant: comparison with isoflurane. *Br J Anaesth* 76:362–364, 1996.

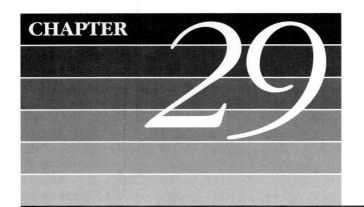

CHAPTER 29

Anesthesia for Pediatric ENT Surgery

RONALD S. LITMAN

DANIEL S. SAMADI

JOSEPH D. TOBIAS

Ear, nose, and throat (ENT) surgery represents a large proportion of pediatric surgeries and remains one of the most challenging because of the frequency of airway obstruction in infants and small children. The anesthesiologist must be familiar with a variety of airway management techniques that are unique for each type of procedure, as well as the different types of airway instruments used by otolaryngologists.

This chapter reviews the anesthetic implications for the most common ENT procedures performed in children.

ENT emergencies that manifest as life-threatening airway obstruction are extensively reviewed in Chapter 18.

EAR SURGERIES

Myringotomy and Tube Placement

Otitis media is a bacterial infection that develops within a transudate in the middle ear in susceptible children. It is usually caused by chronic eustachian tube obstruction from either congenital narrowing or adenoidal hypertrophy. Myringotomy and tube placement consists of the insertion of tiny ventilating tubes through the tympanic membrane to drain fluid from the middle ear and prevent future fluid collections. It is the most common surgical procedure requiring general anesthesia in children, who frequently present with fever and upper respiratory tract infections that will not abate until the ear fluid is drained. The major focus of the preoperative assessment is to ensure that the child does not have any lower airway symptoms that indicate acute reactive airway disease or pneumonia.

The standard anesthesia technique for myringotomy and tube placement consists of an inhalational induction, usually with sevoflurane and N_2O, although halothane is still used in many centers. Once the child has reached a depth of unconsciousness sufficient to prevent response to a painful stimulus, the anesthesiologist turns the child's head to the side while maintaining mask anesthesia, and the tubes are placed by the surgeon using a microscope (Fig. 29-1). Intravenous access is usually not necessary. Each ear tube insertion typically lasts no more than 5 minutes. Many children will manifest upper airway obstruction when the head is turned. This usually abates with application of continuous positive airway pressure (CPAP) or placement of an oral airway. Laryngospasm may occur if the depth of anesthesia is insufficient for the procedure. Central or obstructive

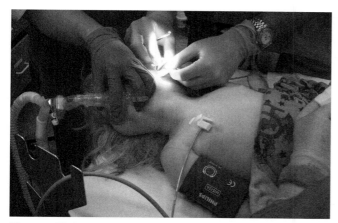

Figure 29-1 Anesthetic management of myringotomy tube placement. While maintaining mask ventilation, the anesthesiologist turns the patient's head to the side to allow the surgeon to perform the myringotomy and insertion of ventilating tubes by visualizing the ear drum with a microscope. Upper airway obstruction is common while the child's head is turned.

apnea may occur and is treated with positive-pressure ventilation.

Postoperative pain is severe in some children immediately after the procedure and can occasionally last a few hours. Thus prophylactic analgesia is indicated. Choices include oral (15 mg/kg) or rectal (40 mg/kg) acetaminophen, ibuprofen 10 mg/kg, codeine 0.5–1 mg/kg, or oxycodone 0.1 mg/kg. Intranasal or intramuscular fentanyl 1–2 µg/kg, administered while the child is anesthetized, provides adequate postoperative analgesia and decreases agitation during emergence from general anesthesia without prolonging discharge times. Similar results are attained using intranasal butorphanol 25 µg/kg. Postoperatively, children with preexisting upper respiratory tract infections may develop hypoxemia and require oxygen therapy.

Tympanomastoidectomy

Indications for a tympanomastoidectomy include chronic otitis media or presence of a cholesteatoma. The surgery is performed through an incision behind the ear to expose the ear canal and tympanic membrane, or through the ear canal. The ear canal is widened and a portion of the mastoid bone is removed. The eardrum is rebuilt and the cholesteatoma is removed if present. These children are usually otherwise healthy, but may have hearing loss. The procedure is performed in the supine position with the child's head turned away from the side of the surgery. The OR table is turned 90–180 degrees away from the anesthesia machine. Therefore, the anesthesiologist must anticipate the requirement of a breathing circuit with sufficient length. During the procedure, the head and neck are completely covered with

drapes, so access to the airway is difficult. There is minimal blood loss or third-space fluid losses. If the surgeon requests facial nerve monitoring, and paralysis is desired for endotracheal intubation, an intermediate-acting neuromuscular blocker should be chosen and used for intubation only. The use of N_2O should be discussed with the surgeon who may request that it be discontinued prior to placement of a tympanic graft. A temporary urinary catheter should be considered for procedures greater than 4 hours duration. Hyperthermia is possible if a warming blanket is used. The main postoperative concern is nausea and vomiting, so antiemetic prophylaxis should be administered. Postoperatively, children may be discharged home if they are well hydrated and do not have severe pain.

Tympanoplasty

A tympanoplasty is repair of a perforated ear drum using a temporalis fascia graft. It may also involve reconstruction of the bones of the middle ear. A postauricular approach is most often used. Virtually all anesthetic implications and techniques are the same as those for tympanomastoidectomy.

NASAL SURGERY

Nasal Cautery

Nasal cautery is performed in children who have chronic nose bleeds secondary to friable blood vessels along the anterior portion of the nasal septum. The children are usually healthy. The procedure consists of brief electrocauterization and typically lasts no more than 10–15 minutes. Some anesthesiologists may choose to provide mask anesthesia while intermittently removing the mask for the surgeon to cauterize the vessels. Laryngeal mask airway (LMA) or endotracheal tube placement are reasonable options, especially if the child is expected to bleed into the back of the pharynx. Postoperative analgesia is minimal and easily treated without opioids.

Nasal Fracture Reduction

Nasal fractures are common in children following facial trauma. Reduction and fixation is rarely a surgical emergency. The children are scheduled for elective closed or open reduction as an outpatient. Closed reduction consists of the manipulation of the nasal bones externally with the assistance of instruments through the nasal openings. Bleeding is typical, though not enough to be clinically important. However, there is a significant amount of blood that enters the nasopharynx. For this reason, most pediatric anesthesiologists will choose LMA placement or endotracheal intubation for airway management, and will thoroughly suction the pharynx prior to removal. Postoperative pain may require opioid analgesia. Since postoperative nausea and vomiting is common, a prophylactic antiemetic is indicated.

Juvenile Angiofibroma Resection

A juvenile angiofibroma is a benign vascular tumor of the posterior nasopharynx that can spread into contiguous structures. Adolescent boys are most often affected and present with chronic nasal obstruction or painless nasal bleeding that is not associated with trauma. Many patients will undergo preoperative embolization to limit intraoperative bleeding, which may be severe. Additional preoperative assessment includes a complete blood count, coagulation studies, and a type-and-crossmatch. Induction and maintenance of anesthesia are routine. Once consciousness is lost, two large-bore intravenous catheters are inserted for volume replacement and possible blood transfusion. An arterial line is often placed, depending on the size of the tumor and extent of the procedure. Airway management consists of a straight or RAE oral endotracheal tube, depending on the surgical approach. A temporary urinary catheter should be placed if the anticipated duration of the surgery is more than 3–4 hours. The surgical approach is dependent on the size and exact location and spread of the tumor. The main intraoperative concern is blood loss. At the end of the procedure the nasal cavity is frequently packed. Depending on the extent of the surgical resection these children may remain intubated at the end of the procedure and mechanically ventilated in the ICU until their vital signs and fluid status have stabilized.

UPPER AIRWAY SURGERY

Tonsillectomy

Tonsillectomy remains a common childhood surgical procedure. There are two indications: recurrent infection (usually in children older than 4 years) and sleep apnea (usually in children under 4 years). When performed for children with sleep apnea, adenoidectomy is usually performed at the same time. Anesthetic implications of children with sleep apnea are discussed in Chapter 4.

Most routine tonsillectomies are performed as outpatient surgery. Certain groups of children with a high risk of postoperative upper airway obstruction should be scheduled for overnight hospital admission. This includes children less than 4 years of age and those with severe sleep apnea. In addition, children with coexisting medical problems (e.g., trisomy 21, obesity, bleeding disorders) should be hospitalized postoperatively.

Some surgeons require preoperative hemoglobin testing and coagulation studies, even though there is little support in the literature for this practice, unless there is

a history of a bleeding disorder in the child or the family. Nonsteroidal anti-inflammatory drugs (NSAIDs) should be discontinued at least 3 days prior to surgery. Aspirin is discontinued 2 weeks prior to surgery. A preoperative oral anxiolytic should be administered at a decreased dose in young children with significant airway obstruction. Oral acetaminophen 15 mg/kg may be added to the premedication to help decrease postoperative pain.

The goals of anesthetic management for tonsillectomy are a motionless patient during the procedure, a rapid and smooth emergence, postoperative pain relief, and control of postoperative nausea and vomiting. Following induction of anesthesia, an oral RAE endotracheal tube is inserted to accommodate the mouth opening device used by the surgeon. There are several types of these devices; each is designed to secure the endotracheal tube against the tongue in the midline, and allow maximal surgical exposure of the pharynx. A growing number of pediatric anesthesiologists routinely use an LMA for airway management during tonsillectomy. Advantages and disadvantages of LMA use during tonsillectomy are listed in Box 29-1. Adjuvant medications include an opioid for pain and a 5-HT$_3$ antagonist to help prevent postoperative nausea and vomiting. Dexamethasone also decreases the incidence of postoperative nausea and vomiting, is associated with improved postoperative fluid intake, and lessens the severity of postoperative pain. Neuromuscular blockers are administered by some anesthesiologists. Maintenance of anesthesia can consist of a combination of an inhalational agent, N$_2$O, or continuous infusion of propofol. Propofol maintenance is associated with less postoperative nausea and vomiting.

Once the anesthesiologist has taped the endotracheal tube or LMA appropriately, the OR table is turned 90 degrees. A rolled-up sheet or similar "shoulder roll" is

---

Box 29-1   LMA for Tonsillectomy

Advantages

Easy to insert
Allows for lighter level of general anesthesia
Smoother emergence without tracheal stimulation
Can be removed at completion of procedure prior to
  patient regaining full consciousness
Decreased incidence of postoperative sore throat

Disadvantages

May retract more cephalad in pharynx and obscure
  surgical view
Appropriate size for child may not fit under surgeon's
  mouth-opening device
May not completely protect against secretions entering
  the glottic opening

placed underneath the shoulders of the patient, and the head is placed in extension. When the surgeon inserts the mouth gag, the child's mouth is maximally opened (Fig. 29-2). During this process the endotracheal tube may be pulled out of the trachea or critically compressed. Therefore, the anesthesiologist should ensure that ventilatory parameters remain the same as before the gag was placed. In addition, because of the surgeon's viewpoint from above the head of the child, he or she may not notice that certain portions of the lips and tongue have become pinched by the gag. The anesthesiologist must carefully observe this process to ensure that injury does not occur.

During tonsillectomy, there are several anesthetic concerns. Blood loss varies and may be significant, but is difficult to measure. However, it is rarely severe enough to warrant transfusion. Fluids should consist of an isotonic solution to replace the preoperative deficit, blood loss, and minimal insensible losses. Some surgeons prefer to infiltrate the tonsillar fossae with a local anesthetic to decrease postoperative pain. Others, however, feel that this practice results in a higher incidence of postoperative bleeding. At the end of the procedure, the surgeon may pass a soft catheter to suction gastric contents. However, blood is rarely recovered, and there is no evidence that this practice influences the incidence of postoperative nausea and vomiting. Once the surgeon has completed the procedure the table is turned back to the anesthesiologist and an oral airway or bite block is inserted into the mouth to prevent the child from biting down and compressing the endotracheal tube during emergence. The nasal passages are gently suctioned for secretions and excess blood. The catheter should go no farther than the anterior nasal cavity to avoid dislodging

a fresh clot from the adenoid bed in the nasopharynx. Similarly, oral suctioning should be gentle and limited to the anterior midline of the oral cavity so that the tonsillar fossae are avoided. Bright red blood that is continually suctioned during emergence should prompt a reexploration before the child is awakened.

There are two schools of thought with regard to the safest and most appropriate method for emergence and tracheal extubation following tonsillectomy: wide-awake versus deep extubation. The major advantage of a wide-awake extubation is the patient's conscious ability to maintain airway patency immediately following the procedure. The main purported disadvantage is an increased tendency for bleeding secondary to coughing and bucking during emergence, which may disrupt clots at the surgical site. The main advantage of a deep extubation is the avoidance of bleeding during emergence, and the facilitation of throughput in a busy surgical suite. Disadvantages include possible respiratory depression and failure to maintain airway patency, and laryngospasm during the semiconscious phase of emergence as a result of secretions or blood in the larynx.

Following an awake tracheal extubation, the child is carefully observed for several minutes to ensure airway patency and the ability to maintain spontaneous ventilation without hypoxemia. The child should be kept in the operating room until he or she demonstrates the ability to maintain a patent airway without jaw thrust or chin lift. Occasionally, an oral airway may be left in place during transport to the postoperative care unit. The classic "tonsil position" with the child lying on one side and with the head lower than the body will facilitate upper airway patency and draining of blood and secretions from the mouth. This may be the case for the relatively unconscious child. In practice, however, this is rarely utilized since the supine position is preferred for airway management during transport.

At The Children's Hospital of Philadelphia, a wide-awake extubation technique is preferred. Coughing during emergence is minimized by administering a moderate dose of intraoperative morphine (0.075–0.15 mg/kg) and low concentrations of inhalational agent. Neuromuscular blockade is usually administered. Box 29-2 describes our standard anesthetic protocol. Using this technique, bleeding during emergence and postoperative laryngospasm are exceedingly rare.

Other centers, however, are equally adamant about the efficacy and safety of the deep extubation technique. This technique requires a relatively greater use of inhalational agent and less opioid, to facilitate adequate airway patency following tracheal extubation. Local anesthetic infiltration is also recommended. If deep extubation is routinely used, the institution must develop a culture within the postoperative recovery site that facilitates expedient treatment of transient airway obstruction and laryngospasm.

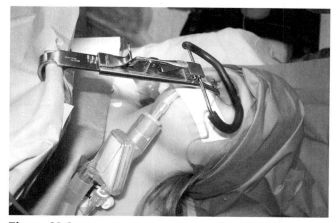

Figure 29-2   Tonsillectomy positioning. The OR table is turned 90 degrees away from the anesthesiologist. The surgeon inserts a mouth-opening gag (a MacGiver device is shown in this photo) that stabilizes the oral RAE endotracheal tube on the chin. During mouth opening, the endotracheal tube can become compressed or kinked, or unintentional trauma to the mouth or lips may occur.

Box 29-2   Anesthesia Protocol for Tonsillectomy at The Children's Hospital of Philadelphia[a]

Premedication

Oral midazolam 0.5 mg/kg; maximum dose 10 mg (for small children with sleep apnea, some anesthesiologists choose to halve this dose)
Oral acetaminophen 10-15 mg/kg

Induction

Sevoflurane, 8% and adjusted downward as child loses consciousness
N_2O, 70% in oxygen – discontinued when intravenous access is established
Vecuronium 0.1 mg/kg
Morphine 0.075-0.125 mg/kg

Maintenance

Desflurane (concentration titrated to hemodynamic variables)
N_2O, 70% in oxygen

Emergence

Reversal of muscle relaxant with neostigmine and atropine or glycopyrrolate
Extubation when awake

Adjuvant Intraoperative Therapy

Ondansetron 50-100 μg/kg
Dexamethasone 0.5 mg/kg; maximum dose 10 mg

Postoperative

Morphine 0.05 mg/kg titrated to pain relief or onset of sleep
Ondansetron 50-100 μg/kg for continued emesis
Oxygen as needed to maintain SpO_2 > 94% prior to discharge from PACU

[a]All medications are administered intravenously, except for premedication.

The most important postoperative concern following tonsillectomy is upper airway obstruction. The precise cause is unknown and may be related to airway edema, residual effects of general anesthesia, or a combination of the two. It occurs more often in children less than 3 years of age, and in children with preexisting sleep apnea. It most often manifests within the first postoperative 30 minutes. Delayed upper airway obstruction is uncommon. Initial treatment consists of optimal placement of the head and neck in a position that is most consistent with airway patency, cool mist in oxygen, and administration of steroids if not already given. If these measures fail to relieve continuing hypoxemia (SpO_2 < 90%), placement of a soft lubricated nasopharyngeal airway is indicated.

Most children with distress secondary to upper airway obstruction will allow placement of this device without much of a struggle. Should this measure be necessary, the child should be admitted to a postoperative hospital unit with close nursing supervision (e.g., PICU). Should the child remain hypoxemic despite placement of a nasopharyngeal airway, tracheal intubation is then indicated, with a trial of extubation at a later time.

The most common postoperative concerns following tonsillectomy are pain relief and postoperative nausea and vomiting. Opioids should be titrated to achieve sufficient analgesia while avoiding respiratory depression and upper airway obstruction. Many children will alternate between crying in pain and falling asleep and becoming hypoxemic. This is a continual challenge for the anesthesiologist and postoperative care staff. Outpatients with moderate pain may be given oxycodone or equivalent analgesic syrup prior to leaving the facility. NSAIDs are not administered to tonsillectomy patients for 2 weeks because of the increased incidence of postoperative bleeding.

Nausea and vomiting occur in up to 75% of children following tonsillectomy. They are likely caused by residual swallowed blood that irritates the lining of the stomach, or other unknown factors related to the site of the surgery or the anesthetic technique (e.g., opioids). Vomiting can result in exacerbation of bleeding from the tonsillectomy site, and dehydration. Treatment includes maintenance of intravenous fluid therapy, antiemetics, and continuous observation for hypovolemia and anemia. Continued presence of blood in the vomitus should initiate examination for a primary bleed. Additional doses of a 5-HT_3 antagonist may be administered, but are generally less effective for treating nausea alone. Droperidol is often effective, especially for nausea. However, at the time of this writing it is no longer used by most centers because of the "black box warning" concerning its association with a prolonged Q_T interval. Metoclopramide is usually ineffective in this setting. Most centers will employ one of a number of other antiemetics for refractory vomiting. Children with ongoing postoperative nausea and vomiting should have their intravenous access maintained to provide continuous hydration. If vomiting is continuous and severe, hospital admission is warranted for continuation of intravenous hydration and antiemetic therapy. The vast majority of children will no longer manifest postoperative nausea and vomiting by the second postoperative day.

Additional postoperative complaints following tonsillectomy include otalgia, fever, uvular swelling, and velopharyngeal insufficiency.

Peritonsillar Abscess Incision and Drainage

A peritonsillar abscess results when bacterial tonsillitis spreads to the tonsillar fossae and soft palate. It produces fever, severe sore throat, dysphagia, and trismus from pterygoid muscle spasm. Patients may be dehydrated from the fever and the inability to drink. Preoperative considerations include administration of antibiotics, intravenous isotonic fluids, and a MRI or CT scan of the neck to estimate the spread of the infection and severity of airway obstruction. Airway evaluation is often difficult due to the presence of trismus. Preoperative sedatives are avoided if airway obstruction is evident.

Induction of anesthesia will depend on the likelihood of a difficult intubation. If the anesthesiologist suspects a potential difficult ventilation or intubation, spontaneous ventilation should be maintained during induction of anesthesia until it is known that positive-pressure ventilation is successful. If a difficult airway is not suspected, a rapid sequence induction and tracheal intubation are indicated. The trismus will abate upon administration of general anesthesia. The anesthesiologist should consider that the abscess may rupture during direct laryngoscopy, and be prepared with a double-suction set-up, various sized styletted, cuffed, oral RAE endotracheal tubes, and an extra working laryngoscope. Visualization of the glottic opening may be difficult secondary to altered pharyngeal anatomy. The intraoperative anesthetic implications are the same as for a tonsillectomy. Tracheal extubation should take place when the child is fully awake to optimize upper airway patency. However, postextubation airway obstruction may occur from residual pharyngeal swelling.

Bleeding Tonsil

Bleeding following tonsillectomy can be severe and life-threatening. Primary bleeding occurs in the first 24 hours and is a direct result of residual operative bleeding. Secondary bleeding occurs 5–14 days postoperatively as a result of scab dislodgement. These cases are usually considered surgical emergencies. It is difficult to estimate the blood actually lost. Most is swallowed, and some children will vomit this swallowed blood but estimates of its volume are inaccurate. Therefore, anesthesiologists should assume hypovolemia and anemia until proven otherwise. The preoperative history should focus on the duration of the vomiting, and presence of any indicators of hypovolemia or anemia, such as dizziness or fainting. Physical exam should focus on detection of hypovolemia or anemia by checking skin turgor, signs of dehydration, and presence of pallor. Preoperatively, IV access is obtained, and blood samples are sent for a CBC and coagulation studies. An additional blood sample should be retained for possible type-and-cross if the hemoglobin level is low. Aggressive fluid hydration with an isotonic solution is geared toward normalization of vital signs and adequate urine output. Children often remain normotensive despite hypovolemia and anemia. Unless the bleeding is active and brisk, normalization of fluid status is the goal prior to surgery. The anesthesiologist should review an available anesthetic record from the original surgery to determine the presence of problems or issues that would influence the subsequent anesthetic technique (e.g., difficult ventilation or intubation). Small doses of intravenous midazolam may be administered shortly before surgery under the direct supervision of the anesthesiologist. Some anesthesiologists may wish to administer intravenous metoclopramide (0.1 mg/kg) to facilitate gastric emptying. The OR should be prepared with a double-suction set-up, several different sized styletted, cuffed, oral RAE endotracheal tubes, and an extra working laryngoscope.

Rapid sequence induction of anesthesia and tracheal intubation is indicated using sodium pentothal or propofol, and succinylcholine or rocuronium. If hypovolemia is suspected, lesser doses of these hypnotic agents should be used to avoid hypotension upon induction of general anesthesia. Alternatively they can be combined with ketamine, or ketamine can be used alone. Occasionally the anesthesiologist will encounter a situation whereby the pharynx is filled with blood, thereby impeding adequate visualization of the laryngeal inlet. Simultaneous hypotension secondary to systemic vasodilation in a child with preexisting hypovolemia may occur. These are tense moments – the ENT surgeon should be present in the OR during induction, and the most qualified anesthesiologist available should be managing the airway. Once the airway is secured by tracheal intubation, the stomach can be suctioned. Intraoperative anesthetic considerations are the same as for a routine tonsillectomy with the exception of more vigilant attention to blood loss and fluid replacement. Tracheal extubation should occur with the child fully awake because of the possibility of residual blood in the stomach. Postoperative concerns are the same as after routine tonsillectomy and include pain and emesis.

Adenoidectomy

Adenoidectomy is primarily indicated in young children with chronic nasal obstruction, chronic sinusitis, and middle ear infections caused by eustachian tube blockage. Upper respiratory illnesses are extremely common, and often do not abate until after the surgery has been performed. Perioperative anesthetic considerations are essentially the same as for tonsillectomy, except for a lesser amount of postoperative pain, and less chance for postoperative upper airway obstruction. Morphine is often limited to 0.05 mg/kg intraoperatively, and then titrated to achieve analgesia in the intensive care unit.

Esophageal Foreign Body

In the course of placing objects in their mouths, toddlers will occasionally swallow these objects, which may become stuck in the esophagus. Most commonly, a coin becomes lodged in the proximal esophagus and must then be removed under general anesthesia with endotracheal intubation. Severe pain or airway obstruction are the only reasons this procedure becomes an emergency. Otherwise, the child should be admitted, made nil-by-mouth (NPO), and intravenous access obtained with administration of maintenance fluids. A radiograph should be obtained just prior to surgery to confirm that the coin has not already passed into the stomach. In the preoperative holding area, intravenous midazolam may be titrated to effect. Induction and maintenance of anesthesia is routine, with the expectation that this procedure will last no more than 5–10 minutes. If the anesthesiologist suspects a residual full stomach, then rapid sequence induction and tracheal intubation are indicated. Cricoid pressure may or may not be applied, depending on the location of the foreign body. The OR table is turned 90 degrees away from the anesthesiologist and the surgeon uses a rigid esophagoscope to remove the object. Postoperative pain is usually mild and does not ordinarily require opioids.

Frenulectomy

A frenulectomy is an elective procedure that entails cutting the frenulum, which is the midline structure below the tongue. It is indicated for ankyloglossia, a condition of restricted tongue movement due to congenital overgrowth of the frenulum. It may be performed by a dissection technique and sutures, or using electrocautery, or both. Children are usually healthy. Airway management varies depending on the preference of the surgeon and anesthesiologist. Spontaneous ventilation via mask anesthesia or nasopharyngeal airway is easily accomplished if the surgeon is amenable. Others will feel more comfortable with placement of an LMA or endotracheal tube, because of the possibility of bleeding into the back of the pharynx. Postoperative pain is mild to moderate and responds to small doses of opioids and/or ketorolac.

Dental and Oral Surgical Procedures

The most common dental procedures requiring general anesthesia in children consist of extractions and restorations of teeth. Children are often scheduled for this procedure with general anesthesia because of a previous failure to cooperate using sedative techniques. Another reason to use general anesthesia is when mild sedation is untenable because of the presence of developmental delay or other behavioral problem. Many children have preexisting comorbidities. These should be completely investigated prior to the day of the procedure. Premedication with an anxiolytic is usually indicated. Uncooperative adolescents with developmental delay

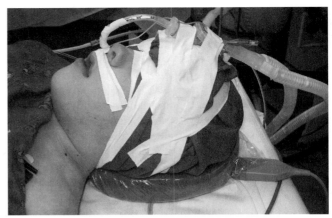

Figure 29-3 During dental and oral surgery procedures, a nasal RAE endotracheal tube is secured to the forehead using a head wrap. Care is taken to ensure that the bend of the tube does not abut against the tip of the nose, and cause compression ischemia.

may refuse oral premedication and require intramuscular administration of ketamine (see Chapter 12).

An inhalational induction of general anesthesia is usually performed. Neuromuscular blockade is optional. After the child loses consciousness, a head wrap is snugly applied to the head to use as a secure attachment for the endotracheal tube (Fig. 29-3). A nasotracheal intubation is performed using a nasal RAE tube, aided by a Magill forceps. The OR table may be turned 90 degrees away from the anesthesiologist. All connections of the breathing circuit must be checked and appropriately tightened prior to beginning the procedure. Fluid requirements are minimal. Hyperthermia is possible during long procedures. Unintentional breathing circuit disconnections or obstructions of the capnograph line are possible hazards. The dentist or oral surgeon will usually infiltrate a moderate amount of local anesthesia. Administration of acetaminophen and/or ketorolac may help alleviate postoperative residual soreness. Small doses of an opioid may also be required.

LARYNGEAL SURGERY

Laryngoscopy and Bronchoscopy

Direct laryngoscopy and flexible or rigid bronchoscopy are used as part of a diagnostic work-up in the evaluation of respiratory compromise (e.g., laryngomalacia, subglottic stenosis), as a therapeutic tool for the treatment of laryngeal lesions (e.g., papilloma, cysts), and for the removal of foreign bodies from the upper or lower airways.

A variety of medical conditions may cause airway abnormalities that require diagnostic or therapeutic intervention. As an example, children born prematurely are especially prone to develop subglottic stenosis, and are frequently evaluated for chronic stridor, or inability to be successfully weaned from mechanical ventilation. The one common theme among children presenting for laryngoscopy and bronchoscopy is an obstructed upper or lower airway that may worsen with the loss of pharyngeal muscle tone that accompanies induction of general anesthesia, or present difficulty with endotracheal intubation.

The preoperative history should consist of a thorough review of previous anesthetics and optimization of comorbid conditions. Physical exam is focused on upper airway anatomy and the severity of existing airway obstruction. In the case of potentially significant airway obstruction, the history and physical exam will determine the anesthetic approach to securing the airway (see Chapter 18). There are no specific requirements for preoperative laboratory testing. Radiographic studies of the head and neck region should be reviewed to assess the potential for airway obstruction during induction of general anesthesia.

Preoperative anxiolysis is tailored to the age and medical condition of the patient. Sedative medications may exacerbate existing airway obstruction and lead to life-threatening hypoxemia. Intravenous atropine or glycopyrrolate is frequently administered to dry airway secretions, to prevent vagal-induced bradycardia, and to attenuate cholinergic-mediated bronchoconstriction during airway manipulation. All appropriate equipment and personnel for dealing with a potentially difficult airway, including surgical equipment for tracheostomy, should be available. Preoperative communication with the surgeon will facilitate a precise understanding of the procedural components and will enable the anesthesiologist to develop a plan for airway management and the subsequent anesthetic technique.

Flexible bronchoscopy allows for dynamic assessment of the upper airway during spontaneous respiration, as well as for an evaluation of the peripheral tracheobronchial tree. It is particularly helpful for the evaluation of laryngomalacia, tracheomalacia, and bronchomalacia. Flexible bronchoscopy is performed soon after the patient loses consciousness so that spontaneous respiration is maintained. It is commonly performed through a device attached to the anesthesia mask to allow concomitant inhalation of oxygen and inhalational anesthetic during the procedure.

A rigid bronchoscope is a stainless steel hollow tube that is used for diagnostic and therapeutic procedures within the airway below the glottis. The distal end is blunt, and the proximal end contains a ventilation side-port that attaches to the standard anesthesia breathing circuit. A thinner telescope with an optical eyepiece is placed coaxially within the rigid bronchoscope and allows for magnified and illuminated visualization of the airway (primarily below the glottis) while retaining the ability to provide adequate ventilation (Fig. 29-4). When the telescope is removed, instruments can be passed through

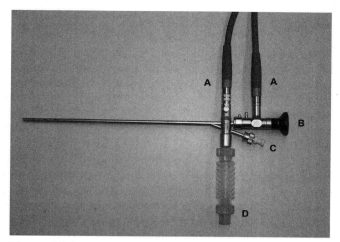

Figure 29-4 Rigid bronchoscope. The distal end of the rigid bronchoscope is blunt, and the proximal end contains a ventilation side-port (D) that attaches to the standard anesthesia breathing circuit. A thinner telescope with an optical eyepiece (B) is placed coaxially through the proximal end and allows for magnified and illuminated visualization of the airway. The rigid bronchoscope as shown contains additional ports for attachment of a light source (A) and a suction port (C).

the bronchoscope to retrieve foreign bodies, resect masses, etc., while maintaining oxygenation and ventilation. The rigid bronchoscope is particularly suited for difficult airway management because of its ability to bypass laryngeal and tracheal lesions that compress the airway and contribute to difficult ventilation or intubation. It may be life-saving in the case of a mediastinal mass that is compressing the bronchial tree below the carina (see Chapter 8).

There are a variety of sizes and lengths of pediatric bronchoscopes that are chosen on the basis of the age and size of the child (Table 29-1). The bronchoscope size is chosen to give the surgeon the best possible view while causing the least amount of trauma to the glottis and subglottic tissues. The time taken to perform

Table 29-1	Size Characteristics of the Rigid Bronchoscope			
Size	Length (cm)	ID (mm)	OD (mm)	Age
2.5	20	3.5	4.2	Premature
3.0	20, 26	4.3	5.0	Premature, newborn
3.5	20, 26, 30	5.0	5.7	Newborn to 6 months
3.7	26, 30	5.7	6.4	6–12 months
4.0	26, 30	6.0	6.7	1–2 years
5.0	30	7.1	7.8	3–4 years
6.0	30, 40	7.5	8.2	5–7 years
6.5	43	8.5	9.2	Adult

ID, inner diameter; OD, outer diameter.
Reproduced with permission from Bluestone D ed: *Pediatric Otolaryngology*, 4th edn, WB Saunders, Philadelphia, 2002.

bronchoscopy should be as short as possible to decrease the risk of obstructive edema secondary to vocal cord and subglottic trauma. In some cases, the surgeon may choose to examine the glottis and the subglottis with the telescope alone to minimize trauma to this region. In this case, simultaneous ventilation is not possible; preoxygenation will increase the duration of apnea before hypoxia intervenes.

Various successful methods have been reported for anesthetizing children for bronchoscopy. Anesthetic induction can be accomplished using inhaled sevoflurane or an intravenous hypnotic agent. Following loss of consciousness, and prior to airway manipulation, intravenous and topical lidocaine can be administered to prevent the occurrence of protective airway reflexes such as gag and laryngospasm. Topical lidocaine within the lower airway may precipitate reflex bronchoconstriction unless preceded by intravenous lidocaine. Small doses of an opioid can be carefully titrated to maintain spontaneous ventilation, which is maintained during flexible bronchoscopy to evaluate dynamic function of the airway. Spontaneous ventilation should always be maintained with a potentially difficult ventilation or intubation. Neuromuscular blockers are administered only after adequate positive-pressure ventilation has proved successful. Flexible bronchoscopy is initially performed with the head of the OR table facing the anesthesiologist, so that mask ventilation can be optimally continued throughout the procedure.

The anesthetic plan for rigid bronchoscopy will be largely determined by the *a priori* choice of spontaneous or positive pressure ventilation during the bronchoscopy. This choice is influenced by the personal preferences of the anesthesiologist and surgeon, who must agree on an acceptable technique prior to administration of anesthesia. There are times, however, when this decision will be made during the case, depending on the surgeon's findings and the patient's clinical condition. With either ventilatory method, these procedures entail a large percentage of time that the child's airway is open (i.e., exposed to the atmosphere when the surgeon removes the optical eyepiece or removes the bronchoscope). For this reason, a total intravenous anesthesia (TIVA) technique is preferred to decrease OR pollution from inhalational agents and provide an uninterrupted source of general anesthesia to the patient.

There are advantages and disadvantages of both spontaneous and controlled ventilation methods during rigid bronchoscopy. If spontaneous ventilation is maintained, continuous ventilation is occurring, despite interruptions in the anesthesia breathing circuit. For some obstructive lesions, negative-pressure breathing may provide better oxygenation and ventilation. Disadvantages of spontaneous ventilation include the requirement to maintain a sufficient depth of anesthesia to obliterate airway reflexes and

prevent patient movement during instrumentation, yet maintain sufficient ventilatory function and hemodynamic stability. Thus, topical anesthesia to the airway is an important component of this technique.

A controlled ventilation technique, which usually consists of administration of a neuromuscular blocker, relies on intermittent positive-pressure breaths between apneic periods when the surgeon instruments the airway, or uses the laser. Its advantages include the ability to provide optimal oxygenation and ventilation during the breathing phase, and assurance of lack of patient movement to airway manipulation. Its obvious disadvantage is that during periods of apnea, even with preoxygenation, there is a limited time before oxyhemoglobin desaturation will occur, and the child will require additional positive-pressure breaths. Another significant disadvantage is the lack of assurance that positive-pressure ventilation will be successful with an obstructive lesion within the airway. In the case of a foreign body lodged within the bronchial tree, a theoretical disadvantage of positive pressure is the unintentional movement of the object further distally. This can worsen airway exchange or create a ball-valve effect with hemodynamic consequences secondary to lung compression of vascular structures. Fortunately, this complication is extremely rare.

Once the child is adequately anesthetized, and just prior to performing rigid bronchoscopy, the OR table is turned 90 degrees away from the anesthesiologist, while mask ventilation is continued from a side position (Fig. 29-5) or by an assistant at the head of the table until the surgeon is optimally prepared to instrument the airway. The goal of the entire process should be a smooth, coordinated, sharing of the child's airway with a combination of optimal oxygenation, ventilation, and surgical exposure.

Suspension Laryngoscopy

Suspension laryngoscopy is used mainly for procedures of the upper airway with the carbon dioxide laser. The child's head is fixed in a constant position that provides an optimal view of the larynx (Fig. 29-6). An endotracheal tube can be held in place by the suspension laryngoscope. If the endotracheal tube remains in place during the laser treatment, it must be wrapped with aluminum tape to decrease the chances of an airway fire. Alternatively, several commercial laser-safe endotracheal tubes are available. Removing the endotracheal tube during the laser treatments will optimize visualization for the surgeon and remove a possible source of an airway fire. Oxygenation and ventilation is then provided by one of two methods: either intermittent endotracheal tube placement between apneic laser treatments, or insufflation of oxygen using a jet ventilator device that is inserted into the side port of the suspension laryngoscope

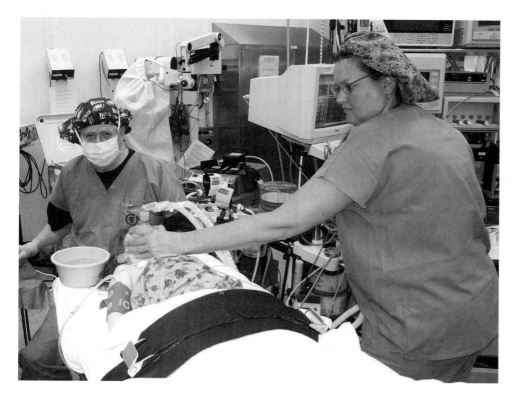

Figure 29-5   Anesthesia for rigid bronchoscopy. Once the child is adequately anesthetized, and just prior to performing rigid bronchoscopy, the OR table is turned 90 degrees away from the anesthesiologist, while mask ventilation is continued by the anesthesiologist from a side position or by an assistant at the head of the table until the surgeon is prepared to instrument the airway.

proximal to the glottis. The jet ventilator device is attached to a standard 50 psi wall outlet and a valve is used to decrease the driving pressure required for adequate chest excursion (usually 10–15 psi) and to avoid barotrauma. The valve is manually opened 15–20 times per minute to provide alveolar ventilation.

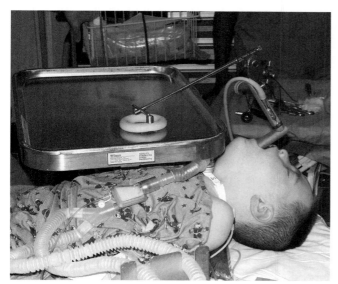

Figure 29-6   Suspension laryngoscopy. The child's head and neck are fixed with the suspension laryngoscope to provide optimal visualization of the larynx.

Alternatively, spontaneous ventilation can be maintained during laryngoscopy by insufflating continuous 100% oxygen through the side-port of the suspension laryngoscope. As with rigid bronchoscopy, a TIVA technique is preferred. Capnography is impossible during jet ventilation or insufflation techniques. If it is essential that $P\text{CO}_2$ be monitored, transcutaneous carbon dioxide monitoring will provide a reasonable estimate.

If suspension laryngoscopy is used in combination with the CO_2 laser, all usual laser precautions should be strictly followed. The child's eyes should be securely covered with wet saline gauze, and all skin surfaces are completely covered with sheets or drapes. If the endotracheal tube remains within the airway during the laser treatment, it must be completely wrapped with aluminum tape or a commercially available laser tube should be used. If a cuffed endotracheal tube is used, the cuff should be filled with water or saline. Some anesthesiologists inject methylene blue into the saline that goes into the cuff to better detect its breakage by the laser. Oxygen concentrations should be as low as possible and N_2O should be avoided to minimize combustibility.

Tracheostomy

The term given to creating a hole in the trachea is a matter of debate, with the names *tracheotomy* and *tracheostomy* used interchangeably. In general, *tracheotomy* is the temporary surgical cutting of the trachea through the anterior neck tissues, whereas *tracheostomy* entails a more permanent opening into the trachea and placement of the tracheostomy tube.

Over the last decade, there has been a decrease in the number of pediatric tracheostomies being performed, largely due to improvements in airway management by pediatric anesthesiologists. However, with an increase in the length of survival of children with complex medical problems, a new population of patients requiring tracheostomy is emerging. Several studies have shown that once a tracheostomy is placed, the duration that it is left in place has increased over time due to the increased number of chronically ventilated children. A recent trend shows that the procedure is being performed in younger children, with a peak incidence in patients aged under 12 months.

The three most common indications for a tracheostomy in children are: (1) prolonged mechanical ventilation (>50%), (2) upper airway obstruction (40%), and (3) pulmonary toilet (10%). Within each category there are congenital, traumatic, metabolic, infectious, and neoplastic conditions that require tracheostomy. Although the underlying medical conditions may be numerous, the most common diagnoses in pediatric tracheostomy patients are bronchopulmonary dysplasia and neurologic disorders.

The decision to perform an elective tracheostomy is complex and depends on several factors, including the child's underlying medical condition, the severity of airway obstruction, and the difficulty and length of intubation. In general, a child who is chronically ventilated is initially managed with an endotracheal tube, with the timing of conversion to a tracheostomy somewhat age-dependent. Neonates may tolerate endotracheal tube intubation for several months with minimal laryngeal injury owing to a more pliable airway. On the other hand, in older children and adolescents the laryngeal cartilage is firmer, requiring a tracheostomy to be performed after 2–3 weeks of tracheal intubation.

In an emergency airway situation, procedures such as direct endotracheal intubation and rigid bronchoscopy should be attempted first. If these are unsuccessful, the next procedure of choice is cricothyrotomy, which reduces the risk of injury to the esophagus and the major neurovascular structures of the neck, compared to tracheostomy. In infants and children, the cricothyroid membrane may be easily identified in experienced hands. Tracheostomy should be reserved as the last resort in an emergency pediatric airway management.

Early tracheostomy tubes were made of stainless steel or silver. These tubes had the advantages of causing minimal tissue reaction and avoiding tracheal collapse. However, their rigidity caused significant discomfort to the patient owing to injury to the tracheal mucosa.

Most manufacturers currently use tubes that have minimal tissue reactivity and conform to the structure of the airway.

The ideal tracheostomy tube should be made of a material that causes minimal tissue reactivity, can be easily cleaned and maintained, and is available in a variety of sizes and lengths. The tube needs to be rigid enough to prevent kinking or collapse, yet soft enough to be comfortable for the patient. Modern tracheostomy tubes have a 15-mm male connector for the attachment of standard respiratory equipment. The ideal tube also contains an inner cannula that may be removed and cleaned.

Tracheostomy tubes for small children do not contain a cuff. In larger children and adolescents, cuffed adult tracheostomy tubes may be used. In selecting the appropriate tracheostomy tube, both the diameter and length should be considered. The external diameter determines the size of the tube that may be inserted, whereas the inner diameter determines the actual airway size. The diameter of the tube should be large enough to allow adequate air exchange, easy suctioning, and clearance of secretions. If the indication for tracheostomy is assisted ventilation, the size of the tube should be adjusted to prevent excessive air leak. Predictors of the appropriate tube size include the child's age and the size of a preexisting endotracheal tube. Too large a tube will compromise the capillary flow in the tracheal wall, which may result in mucosal ulceration and development of fibrous stenosis. Overinflation of a cuffed tracheostomy tube for a prolonged period may produce similar injuries. This complication may be avoided by selecting the proper sized tracheostomy tube (Table 29-2) and adjusting the cuff pressure to less than 20 cmH$_2$O. The choice of the tube size is also influenced by visualizing the size of the tracheal lumen.

The length of the tube is important, especially in neonates and infants. A tube that is too short may result in accidental decannulation or the development of a false passage. If a tube is too long, the tip may abrade the carina or rest in the right main bronchus. Some plastic tubes may be cut to the desired length. Extra-long custom-made tubes may be helpful in unusual situations, such as tracheomalacia or tracheal stenosis, to span the involved area.

Unless airway obstruction is immediately life-threatening, pediatric tracheostomy procedures should be performed in the operating suite. This creates a well-controlled environment for the child and the personnel performing the procedure. The operating suite provides optimal illumination, proper positioning of the child, and expert nursing care. In addition, a full range of laryngoscopes and bronchoscopes are available to control the airway if necessary.

In children with an indwelling endotracheal tube, the choice of induction and maintenance of general anesthesia is unimportant. However, if the tracheostomy is

Table 29-2   Size Comparison of Endotracheal and Plastic Tracheostomy Tubes

Cannula	Approx. French	Inner Diameter (mm)	Outer Diameter (mm)	Overall Length
Endotracheal tube[a]				
2.5		2.5	3.6	12 cm
3.0		3.0	4.3	14 cm
3.5		3.5	4.9	16 cm
4.0		4.0	5.6	18 cm
4.5		4.5	6.2	20 cm
5.0		5.0	6.9	22 cm
5.5		5.5	7.5	25 cm
6.0		6.0	8.2	26 cm
Bivona[b]				
2.5	12	2.5	4.0	30 mm
2.5	12	2.5	4.0	38 mm
3.0	14	3.0	4.7	32 mm
3.0	14	3.0	4.7	39 mm
3.5	16	3.5	5.3	34 mm
3.5	16	3.5	5.3	40 mm
4.0	18	4.0	6.0	36 mm
4.0	18	4.0	6.0	41 mm
4.5	20	4.5	6.7	42 mm
5.0	22	5.0	7.3	44 mm
5.5	24	5.5	8.0	46 mm
Franklin[c]				
3.5		3.5	5.0	44 mm
4.0		4.0	6.0	44 mm
4.5		4.5	6.7	48 mm
5.0		5.0	8.0	51 mm
5.5		5.5	8.5	54 mm
6.0		6.0	9.3	57 mm
Portex				
3.0		3.0	5.0	36 mm
3.5		3.5	5.8	40 mm
4.0		4.0	6.5	44 mm
4.5		4.5	7.1	48 mm
5.0		5.0	7.7	50 mm
5.5		5.5	8.3	52 mm
Shiley[d]				
00 Neonatal		3.1	4.5	30 mm
00 Pediatric		3.1	4.5	39 mm
0 Neonatal		3.4	5.0	32 mm
0 Pediatric		3.4	5.0	40 mm
1 Neonatal		3.7	5.5	34 mm
1 Pediatric		3.7	5.5	41 mm
2 Pediatric		4.1	6.0	42 mm
3 Pediatric		4.8	7.0	44 mm
4 Pediatric		5.5	8.0	46 mm

[a] The endotracheal tubes are marked with the inner diameter, usually with the outer diameter, and with the length.

[b] The Bivona tube is manufactured by the Bivona Corporation of Gary, IN. Both the inner and outer diameters are marked on the tubes.

[c] The Franklin tube is of the Great Ormond Street design, manufactured in England and distributed by Inmed Corporation Norcross, GA. The tubes are stamped with just the inner diameter.

[d] The Shiley tube is manufactured by Shiley Laboratories, Irvine, CA. The tubes are stamped with the size and inner and outer diameters.

Reproduced with permission from Bluestone D ed: *Pediatric Otolaryngology*, 4th edn, WB Saunders, Philadelphia, 2002.

being performed for acute airway obstruction, principles of difficult airway management will apply (Chapter 18). Prior to performing the procedure, the surgeon and anesthesiologist should discuss the method of choice for obtaining and securing the airway. All alternatives should be discussed in the event that the child cannot be intubated successfully. It is preferred to perform the tracheostomy with the child intubated under general anesthesia with paralysis. In certain situations of severe upper airway obstruction, it may be necessary to perform the tracheostomy with mild sedation and infiltration of local anesthesia.

The tracheostomy is performed supine with the child's neck extended using a shoulder roll. The child should be breathing 100% oxygen in anticipation of a temporary interruption of ventilation. If a nasogastric tube is present it should be removed so as not to alter normal neck anatomy. Lidocaine with epinephrine is infiltrated into the subcutaneous tissue one to two fingerbreadths above the sternal notch. A horizontal skin incision is then made at the same site. A vertical midline dissection is performed to expose the tracheal rings. Traction sutures are placed in a paramedian position at the level of the second or third tracheal ring, to rapidly open the airway should accidental decannulation occur before the tract is established. The trachea is incised vertically in the midline to expose the underlying endotracheal tube. While directly observing the endotracheal tube, the anesthesiologist gradually pulls it back to just above the incision as the surgeon inserts the tracheostomy tube. The anesthesia breathing circuit is then connected to the tracheostomy tube; correct placement is confirmed by listening for bilateral breath sounds and observing a normal capnographic tracing. *Prior to these final confirmations, the endotracheal tube should never be completely withdrawn out of the trachea.* Flexible bronchoscopy is then performed to identify the distal position of the tracheostomy tube. Proper adjustment or possible replacement of the tracheostomy tube with a different size is done at this stage. The previously placed endotracheal tube is removed just prior to leaving the operating room or after arrival at the intensive care unit. A postoperative chest radiograph is obtained to further confirm tube position and rule out pneumothorax.

Postoperatively, humidified air by collar or ventilator is provided to prevent excessive dryness and thickening of tracheal secretions. The first tracheostomy tube change is done on the fifth to seventh postoperative day after a well-formed tract has been established. The traction sutures are also removed at this time.

Anesthesiologists should be aware of the various complications related to pediatric tracheostomy. Bleeding can occur from superficial tissues, thyroid vessels, or vascular anomalies such as a high-riding innominate artery, and can obstruct the surgeon's view of the opened trachea. Air entry into the subcutaneous tissues may cause a pneumomediastinum, pneumothorax, subcutaneous emphysema, or any combination of those. Anatomic injury to the neurovascular structures in the neck, including the recurrent laryngeal nerve, can also occur. During placement, the tracheostomy tube can be unintentionally placed into a false lumen adjacent to the trachea, or into the esophagus. For these reasons, the endotracheal tube should never be fully removed before final confirmation that the tracheostomy tube is functional.

LOWER AIRWAY SURGERY

Bronchial Foreign Body

A variety of different types of edible and inedible foreign bodies commonly become lodged in the distal bronchial tree. Toddlers are most affected because of their underdeveloped ability to coordinate swallowing of small food items such as peanuts. Bronchial foreign bodies are likely to cause distal airway obstruction with development of emphysema, atelectasis, and pneumonia. Children may present with a respiratory illness that runs the gamut from tachypnea and fever to respiratory failure and hypoxemia. A bronchial foreign body is suspected when a toddler presents with the sudden onset of respiratory distress that usually begins with a choking episode. The foreign object may or may not be observed. Confirmation of the diagnosis consists of radiological demonstration of the foreign body if it is radiopaque, or unilateral emphysema from a ball-valve effect of the distal obstruction. An aspirated peanut will exacerbate the condition by causing a lipoid pneumonitis.

This procedure is usually considered a surgical emergency. Preoperative assessment should be focused on determining respiratory function, administration of antibiotics, and bronchodilator therapy if bronchospasm is present. An intravenous catheter should be inserted. Intravenous midazolam can be titrated to achieve anxiolysis in the preoperative holding area under direct supervision of the anesthesiologist. An anticholinergic agent should also be administered. A rapid sequence induction and tracheal intubation is indicated if a full stomach is suspected. Induction and maintenance of general anesthesia is the same as described above for rigid bronchoscopy, with a choice between spontaneous or controlled ventilation.

NECK SURGERY

Thyroglossal Duct Cyst

A thyroglossal duct cyst is a small collection of fluid in the soft tissue of the midline of the neck. It is believed to be a remnant of the connection between the tongue and the thyroid gland in fetal life. During childhood it can become infected and enlarged, and requires excision. These children are usually otherwise healthy. Preoperative assessment, and induction and maintenance of general anesthesia, are no different from usual. The anesthesiologist may wish to place a towel wrap around the head with which to secure the endotracheal tube over the forehead. The child is positioned similarly to tracheostomy with the neck extended for a transverse midline incision. The anesthesiologist may be asked to depress the base of the tongue to move the cyst to facilitate surgical identification. Surgical risks include unintentional trauma to vascular or airway structures in the neck. Postoperative concerns include hematoma formation with subsequent airway compression.

Branchial Cleft Cyst

Branchial cleft cysts are found on the side of the neck and develop from a failure of involution of one of the branchial clefts during embryonic development. These children are otherwise healthy; perioperative and postoperative anesthetic implications are essentially the same as for the thyroglossal duct cyst.

Neck Mass Biopsy and Excision

When unclassified neck masses in children do not respond to conventional antibiotic therapy, an excisional biopsy is indicated to rule out malignancy or

(rarely) tuberculosis. The vast majority of these cases are straightforward; the anesthetic implications are described above. However, when a lymphoma is suspected, the anesthesiologist must be aware that there may be an occult anterior mediastinal mass that carries the potential for life-threatening airway obstruction following induction of general anesthesia (see Chapter 8). Preoperative symptoms that are suggestive of an anterior mediastinal mass include coughing or dyspnea in the supine position that is relieved when the child assumes the sitting or prone positions.

Cystic Hygroma

Another name for a cystic hygroma is a lymphangioma. It is a malformation of lymphatic vessels in and around the neck region. They are strongly associated with Turner syndrome, trisomy 21 (Down syndrome), trisomy 18 (Edwards syndrome), and Noonan syndrome, although many otherwise normal children are affected.

Article To Know

Groudine SB, Hollinger I, Jones J, DeBouno BA: New York State guidelines on the topical use of phenylephrine in the operating room. The Phenylephrine Advisory Committee. Anesthesiology 92:859–864, 2000.

The pediatric anesthesia community was shocked with the report of an intraoperative death of an otherwise healthy 4-year-old undergoing routine adenoidectomy. The course of events that led to this tragedy began with the intraoperative topical instillation of phenylephrine into the child's nasopharynx, and subsequent treatment of severe hypertension with a beta-blocker (labetalol). This publication summarizes the findings of a panel that was convened by the New York State Department of Health to investigate this and other similar cases, to determine the mechanism of cause of death, and to recommend guidelines for future use of phenylephrine in the operating room.

Although it is becoming less frequent, some surgeons continue to use phenylephrine (0.25–1%) as a topical vasoconstrictor during upper airway surgery. Total absorbed doses are difficult to calculate. However, there are a number of published reports of systemic absorption of topical phenylephrine that resulted in severe hypertension. The New York State panel that reviewed these cases noted a recurrent pattern associated with poor outcomes: the development of severe, refractory pulmonary edema and cardiac failure following treatment with beta-blockers. Table 29-3, taken from this article, details these cases.

Table 29-3 New York State Phenyleprine Morbidity

Patient #	Age (years)	Phenylephrine (%)	Hypertensive Treatment	Pulmonary edema	Cardiac Arrest
1	3	0.25	None	Yes	No
2	4	0.5	L, AD	Yes	Yes
3	7	0.25	L	No	No
4	9	?[a]	L, AD	Yes	Yes
5	23	1.0[a]	AD, E, Ca	Yes	No
6	26	0.5[a]	L, AD	Yes	Yes
7	36	1.0[a]	AD	Yes	No
8	40	1.0[a]	AD	Yes	No
9	47	0.5[a]	L, AD	Yes	No

[a]Lidocaine with 1:100,000 epinephrine was also injected into the surgical field.

L, labetalol; AD, anesthesia deepened; E, esmolol; Ca, calcium-channel blocker

Article To Know *Cont'd*

Phenylephrine administration causes stimulation of α_1 receptors and increases total peripheral resistance by vasoconstriction. Administration of β-blockers will impair the heart's ability to maintain cardiac output by increasing contractility and heart rate. This cardiac depression, coupled with the shifting of blood into the pulmonary vasculature, results in pulmonary edema as seen in the patients described in the article.

The following are this author's recommendations for use of phenylephrine in children; they are adapted from the Phenylephrine Advisory Committee's guidelines:

1. Phenylephrine should not be used as a topical vasoconstrictor during airway procedures in children. Oxymetazoline, 0.025%, is equally effective and is not associated with adverse effects in children.
2. If phenylephrine is used in children, the initial dose should not exceed 20 µg/kg. During its use, blood pressure and pulse should be closely monitored.
3. Phenylephrine-induced hypertension is transient and benign in otherwise healthy children. It should not be initially treated unless it persists or results in electrocardiographic abnormalities or pulmonary edema. It is reasonable, however, to transiently increase the concentration of inhalational agent while closely monitoring hemodynamic status.
4. Antihypertensive agents that are direct vasodilators or α-receptor antagonists (e.g., nitroprusside, hydralazine) are appropriate treatments. Beta-blockers and calcium-channel blockers should be avoided since their use is associated with worsening of cardiac output and development of pulmonary edema.

Cystic hygromas are often found at birth and tend to enlarge during early childhood. The majority of children present for surgical excision for cosmetic reasons. The occasional child will present for reduction and/or tracheostomy due to respiratory distress from airway compression (Fig. 29-7). Cystic hygromas tend to grow inward and compress the airway. The preoperative assessment should always include MRI examination to delineate its spread and evaluate airway patency. A hemoglobin level and type-and-screen should be obtained preoperatively if an extensive dissection and excision is planned, or if the mass is located near the vascular structures of the neck. Induction and maintenance of general anesthesia is practitioner dependent and will vary with the severity of the mass and the degree of airway obstruction. Principles of management of the difficult airway will apply if upper airway obstruction is suspected. Intraoperative concerns include blood loss, fluid management, and hypothermia if the dissection is extensive, and the possibility of nerve monitoring. A temporary urinary catheter should be placed if the procedure is expected to last more than 3–4 hours.

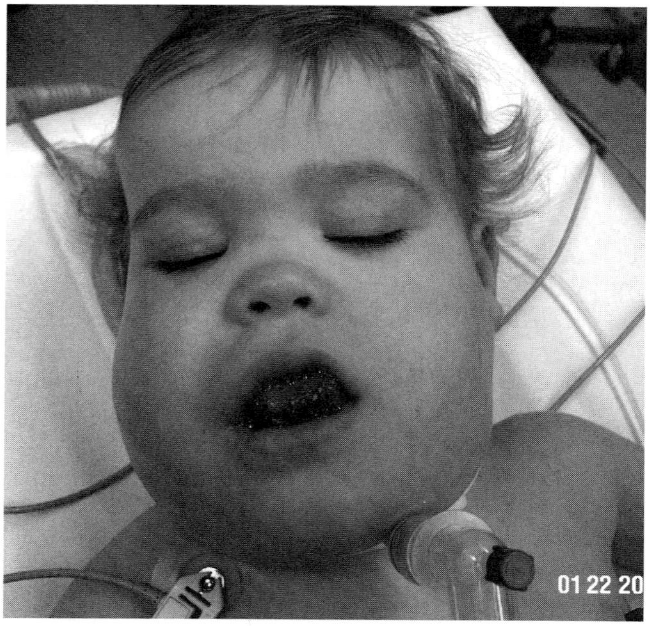

ADDITIONAL ARTICLES TO KNOW

Aouad MT, Siddik SS, Rizk LB et al: The effect of dexamethasone on postoperative vomiting after tonsillectomy. *Anesth Analg* 92:636–640, 2001.

Catlin FI, Grimes WJ: The effect of steroid therapy on recovery from tonsillectomy in children. *Arch Otolaryngol Head Neck Surg* 117:649–652, 1991.

Furst SR, Rodarte A: Prophylactic antiemetic treatment with ondansetron in children undergoing tonsillectomy. *Anesthesiology* 81:799–803, 1994.

Gallagher MJ, Muller BJ: Tension pneumothorax during pediatric bronchoscopy. *Anesthesiology* 55:685–686, 1981.

Goldstein NA, Armfield DR, Kingsley LA et al: Postoperative complications after tonsillectomy and adenoidectomy in children with Down syndrome. *Arch Otolaryngol Head Neck Surg* 124:171–176, 1998.

Hawkins DB, Joseph MM: Avoiding wrapped endotracheal tube in laser laryngeal surgery: experiences with apneic anesthesia and metal laser-flex endotracheal tubes. *Laryngoscope* 100:1283–1287, 1990.

Figure 29-7 Large cystic hygroma. This child required tracheostomy to relieve airway compression from a large cystic hygroma.

Helfaer MA, McColley SA, Pyzik PL et al: Polysomnography after adenotonsillectomy in mild pediatric obstructive sleep apnea. *Crit Care Med* 24:1323-1327, 1996.

Holinger LD, Konior RJ: Surgical management of severe laryngomalacia. *Laryngoscope* 99:136-142, 1989.

Hudgins PA, Siegel J, Jacobs I et al: The normal pediatric larynx on CT and MR. *Am J Neuroradiol* 18:239-245, 1997.

Hunton J, Oswal VH: Anaesthesia for carbon dioxide laser laryngeal surgery in infants. *Anaesthesia* 43:394-396, 1988.

Keon TP: Death on induction of anesthesia for cervical node biopsy. *Anesthesiology* 55:471-472, 1981.

Litman RS, Wu CL, Catanzaro FA: Ondansetron decreases emesis after tonsillectomy in children. *Anesth Analg* 78:478-481, 1994.

Litman RS, Ponnuri J, Trogan I: Anesthesia for tracheal or bronchial foreign body removal in children: an analysis of ninety-four cases. *Anesth Analg* 91:1389-1391, 2000.

Morton S, Rosen C, Larkin E et al: Predictors of sleep-disordered breathing in children with a history of tonsillectomy and/or adenoidectomy. *Sleep* 24:823-829, 2001.

Pappas ALS, Sukhani R, Hotaling AJ et al: The effect of preoperative dexamethasone on the immediate and delayed postoperative morbidity in children undergoing adenotonsillectomy. *Anesth Analg* 87:57-61, 1998.

Pounder DR, Blackstock D, Steward DJ: Tracheal extubation in children: halothane versus isoflurane, anesthetized versus awake. *Anesthesiology* 74:653-655, 1991.

Randall DA, Hoffer ME: Complications of tonsillectomy and adenoidectomy. *Otolaryngol Head Neck Surg* 118:61-68, 1998.

Rowe RW, Betts J, Free E: Perioperative management for laryngotracheal reconstruction. *Anesth Analg* 73:483-486, 1991.

Satyanarayana T, Capan L, Ramanathan S et al: Bronchofiberscopic jet ventilation. *Anesth Analg* 59:350-354, 1980.

Splinter WM, Roberts DJ: Dexamethasone decreases vomiting by children after tonsillectomy. *Anesth Analg* 83:913-916, 1996.

CHAPTER 30

Anesthesia for Pediatric Neurosurgery

RONALD S. LITMAN

Pediatric neurosurgical patients present a unique set of anesthetic challenges that include treatment of increased intracranial pressure (ICP), the use of positions other than supine, and the anesthetic implications of neurophysiologic monitoring. These and other general considerations are addressed in the first part of this chapter, followed by a discussion of anesthetic techniques for common pediatric neurosurgical procedures.

PATHOPHYSIOLOGY AND TREATMENT OF INCREASED ICP

There are structural and functional differences in cranial anatomy between children and adults that influence cerebral physiology and management of increased ICP. Whereas the normal adult ICP measures between 8 and 18 mmHg, normal ICP in small children ranges from 2 to 4 mmHg. The skull of newborns does not completely fuse until the latter part of the first year of life. Consequently, the intracranial space is relatively compliant and the dura is able to expand when brain tissue becomes edematous as a result of trauma or mass lesions. Therefore, neonates and small infants may not exhibit signs and symptoms of

the early stages of pathologic processes that increase brain mass. An important clinical correlate is that, when a small infant or neonate presents with signs or symptoms of increased ICP, there may already be advanced disease. Later in childhood, after fusion of the cranial sutures, children may exhibit less intracranial compliance than adults. This is postulated to be caused by a relatively higher percentage of brain tissue to CSF and blood vessels in children. Thus, children may be at higher risk of dangerous increases in ICP with relatively less edema or tumor mass.

In cases of increased ICP, the general management goal is to achieve an ICP <20 mmHg in all ages. Numerous studies have verified that cerebral perfusion pressure (CPP), the difference between the mean arterial pressure and the ICP, varies directly with age. In other words, younger children require lower CPP. In children younger than 8 years a CPP >40 mmHg is recommended, whereas in older children the CPP should be >60 mmHg. It is unknown whether it is more important to decrease ICP or optimize CPP during conditions of acutely increased ICP. Nevertheless, in pediatric patients, CPP values <40 mmHg are strongly correlated with worse outcomes at any ICP.

Methods to lower ICP are the same in children as in adults. Standard therapies include elevation of the head, avoidance of jugular kinking by keeping the head positioned in the midline, hyperventilation to decrease P_{CO_2}, and administration of diuretics such as mannitol and furosemide. Recent reports of the efficacy of hypertonic saline are encouraging as another possible treatment modality.

Administration of volatile anesthetics will cause generalized cerebral vasodilation. In adults, an acute increase in ICP will render the patient more susceptible to the deleterious effects of volatile anesthetics. This is probably true in the pediatric population as well. Furthermore, neonates and infants appear to maintain the same degree of cerebral vasoconstriction in response to decreased P_{CO_2} as seen in adults. However, there is evidence that in anesthetized infants and children, cerebral vasodilation may occur at lower levels of P_{CO_2} than observed in adults.

There has been a major shift in the way P_{CO_2} is managed during adult neurosurgery, and this has extended into pediatric practice. In general, the P_{CO_2} is no longer maintained below 30 mmHg for fear of vasoconstriction-induced aggravation of cerebral ischemia. Rather, mild hyperventilation (P_{CO_2} in low-to-mid 30s) is most often employed, the major reason being to offset the possible vasodilatory effects of general anesthetics. However, in the face of acutely increased ICP, lowering the P_{CO_2} below the previous level will usually result in cerebral vasoconstriction and, at least temporarily, decrease ICP. This principle may extend to P_{CO_2} levels below 20 mmHg. When managing increased intracranial pressure, F_IO_2 (fractional inspired oxygen concentration) should always be set to 1.0 to maximize oxygen delivery to the brain cells.

PREOPERATIVE ASSESSMENT

Most children presenting for neurosurgery have been hospitalized for evaluation of a recently diagnosed brain mass or malfunctioning shunt. In the course of this hospitalization, it is expected that normal baseline laboratory studies have been performed. Other children with known brain pathology have had their evaluation as an outpatient, and may be admitted to the hospital on the day of the surgery. Required blood tests include a hemoglobin, and in most tumor cases, a type and screen. Electrolytes should be obtained if there is a possibility of hormonal alterations of sodium homeostasis. Many children who present for neurosurgery are being treated with anticonvulsants. Unless the drug regimen is changing, or the child's seizures are uncontrolled, preoperative anticonvulsant levels are not indicated.

The majority of children presenting for neurosurgery will benefit from preoperative anxiolysis. Since most

Article To Know

Chambers IR, Treadwell L, Mendelow AD: Determination of threshold levels of cerebral perfusion pressure and ICP in severe head injury by using receiver–operating characteristic curves: an observational study in 291 patients. J Neurosurg 94:412–416, 2001.

When increased ICP occurs as a result of acute head trauma, there is uncertainty as to whether management should be guided by controlling the increased ICP or optimizing CPP. The authors of this study collected data on 207 adults and 84 children who had sustained severe head trauma (Glasgow Coma Scale score ≤8) and who had continuous measurement of ICP. Receiver/operating characteristic curves were developed based on this data and coupled with outcome variables (severity of disability) to determine the prognostic accuracy of ICP and CPP. The significant findings of this study were: (1) children tolerated lower CPP values than adults: a CPP of 45 mmHg in children and 55 mmHg in adults was associated with good outcomes; (2) an ICP value <35 mmHg was associated with a good outcome (same level for adults) but was not as robust a predictor as the CPP.

Prospective observational studies are often difficult to interpret. Since there is no prospective assignment to a specific targeted group based on ICP or cerebral perfusion pressure, it is impossible to determine cause and effect, only association. For example, it is feasible that the worse injuries that were destined to be associated with worse outcomes were associated with, but not caused by, a higher ICP and a lower CPP. Yet, this type of data is still useful as it provides prognostic indicators that help clinicians develop management strategies based on specific values of ICP and CPP. It infers that, in children with severe head trauma, we should attempt to maintain a CPP of at least 45 mmHg and an ICP <35 mmHg.

Article To Know

Robertson CS: Management of cerebral perfusion pressure after traumatic brain injury. Anesthesiology 95:1513–1517, 2001.

This succinct review of current concepts of head trauma management appeared in the December 2001 issue of *Anesthesiology* in the Clinical Concepts and Commentary section. This article is mandatory reading for all anesthesiologists. Dr Robertson discusses the most recent guidelines for management of acute head trauma that are published by the Brain Trauma Foundation (see additional readings). She then summarizes and compares two innovative approaches to acute head trauma management. The first is the optimization of the cerebral perfusion pressure (Rosner technique). The second emphasizes reduction of capillary hydrostatic pressures to minimize brain edema (Lund technique). Finally, Dr Robertson discusses alternative strategies that stress an etiology and time-based approach. These concepts and recommendations are appropriate for both pediatric and adult patients.

of these children already have indwelling intravenous catheters, intravenous midazolam can be titrated to effect in the preoperative holding area. Oral or rectal midazolam may also be administered in children without IV access. Intravenous fentanyl can also be administered if the child is having ongoing pain. There is a concern in neurosurgical patients that administration of preoperative sedation will lead to hypoventilation and, thus, hypercarbia which contributes to worsening of increased ICP. However, this situation is unusual in children. Those children with acutely increased ICP will present emergently and are often obtunded or too ill to benefit from preoperative anxiolysis.

It is commonly believed that increased ICP slows gastric emptying and renders the patient at risk for aspiration of gastric contents. Yet very few data exist, especially in children, to substantiate this fact. In addition, clinical experience has shown that aspiration is quite rare in this population. Therefore, premedication with H_2-antagonists and metoclopramide is rarely indicated unless the procedure is emergent and the child had a recent meal, or if there are other reasons to suspect that the child has abnormally increased gastric contents.

ANESTHETIC TECHNIQUES

A modified rapid sequence induction of general anesthesia is the preferred technique because of the possibility of increased gastric contents in patients with increased ICP. Any IV induction agent can be used, along with a nondepolarizing neuromuscular blocker, while an assistant provides cricoid pressure during bag-mask positive-pressure ventilation. Succinylcholine is generally avoided because of its propensity to increase ICP. If, however, a reasonable risk of pulmonary aspiration of gastric contents exists, a full rapid sequence induction using succinylcholine or high-dose rocuronium is indicated. Alternatively, if the child does not have an indwelling intravenous catheter, and there is no reasonable risk of pulmonary aspiration of gastric contents, then an inhalational induction can be performed. Cricoid pressure is applied as soon as the child loses consciousness, and IV access is rapidly attained to permit continuation of a modified rapid sequence technique.

Succinylcholine is traditionally avoided in neurosurgery because of its ability to transiently increase ICP. Although the precise cause of this is unknown, evidence suggests that it is caused by afferent neuronal muscle spindle activity that results from succinylcholine-induced muscle fasciculations. Indeed, in adults, pretreatment with a small dose of a nondepolarizing muscle relaxant may prevent this increase in ICP from succinylcholine. Since small children tend not to exhibit muscle fasciculations, this effect of succinylcholine may not be observed.

Nevertheless, unless succinylcholine is indicated based on the nature of the child's condition, it is best avoided during induction of general anesthesia.

When control of potential increases in ICP is of concern during induction of anesthesia, additional therapies are indicated. These include IV opioids, and lidocaine (1 mg/kg), both of which will blunt the hemodynamic response to laryngoscopy and tracheal intubation, and thus help prevent dangerous increases in ICP. In addition, scalp infiltration with a local anesthetic will limit the hemodynamic response to the surgical incision. Traditionally, the bulk of the opioid dose is given toward the beginning of the neurosurgical case, because tracheal intubation, positioning, and scalp incision are the most painful and stimulating events. Furthermore, residual opioid effect is undesirable at the end of the procedure when the goals are the rapid attainment of consciousness and tracheal extubation, to facilitate an immediate neurological exam. Fentanyl 4–6 µg/kg is commonly used during induction. Remifentanil is a reasonable alternative and can be used as a continuous infusion throughout the procedure. Some adult studies have suggested that alfentanil and sufentanil may increase ICP by either increasing CSF volume or increasing cerebral blood flow. A study in children examined the effect of alfentanil (10–40 µg/kg) on ICP in children with moderately elevated ICP presenting for revision of VP shunts. Alfentanil consistently produced a decrease in cerebral perfusion pressure that was largely accounted for by decreases in blood pressure. Increases in ICP were not observed. Ketamine is usually avoided in neuroanesthesia because of its propensity to increase ICP.

Any volatile agent can be used for maintenance of general anesthesia; in adults, this choice does not affect the outcome of neurosurgical procedures. All volatile general anesthetic agents can cause cerebral vasodilation and increase ICP by increasing cerebral blood flow and volume. Studies in children have used the transcranial Doppler technique to measure the blood flow velocity of the middle cerebral artery, which in turn may represent overall cerebral blood flow and volume. Halothane is generally considered to be the most potent cerebral vasodilator and is consequently not used during neurosurgery. In children, isoflurane appears to have minimal effects on cerebral blood flow and cerebrovascular reactivity to CO_2 between 0.5 and 1.5 MAC (minimum alveolar concentration). Furthermore, administration of a constant concentration of isoflurane over time does not affect cerebral hemodynamic variables. Sevoflurane appears to have similar effects as isoflurane, although it has not been well studied in children to date. Desflurane has been shown to increase ICP in adults despite application of hypocarbia, but has not been directly studied in children. Nitrous oxide increases cerebral blood flow when used alone, and in combination with propofol or sevoflurane.

However, it does not appear to increase cerebral blood flow when combined with desflurane. This lack of effect may be explained by the potent baseline cerebrovascular dilation effect of desflurane. Overall, the vasodilatory cerebrovascular effects of all inhalational anesthetics in children are similar to that of adults. With normal levels of ICP, there is probably no clinical difference between agents. In conditions of increased ICP, although effects on cerebral blood flow are believed to be mitigated by moderate hyperventilation for all volatile anesthetic agents, minimal concentrations of inhalational agents should be used with primary reliance on an opioid-based technique.

Normally, fentanyl 1–2 μg/kg/h is continued throughout the procedure, or remifentanil is targeted to desired hemodynamic parameters. In adults, studies that have examined the role of remifentanil as the primary anesthetic agent to facilitate early extubation have not demonstrated any differences in short- or long-term outcome. Similar studies have not been performed in children. Neuromuscular blockade throughout the procedure is encouraged to facilitate positioning, and to assure lack of patient movement during brain dissection. Children on chronic anticonvulsant therapy will require more frequent dosing of aminosteroidal muscle relaxants. If the child has a preexisting hemiparesis, the twitch monitor should be placed on the nonhemiparetic side.

Use of N_2O is controversial in neurosurgery because it raises cerebral metabolic oxygen consumption and may increase cerebral blood flow and, thus, ICP. No outcome studies exist that influence the decision to include it in the anesthetic management of children. However, since N_2O is not essential for any reason in neuroanesthesia, it should not be used when increased ICP is a possibility. In addition, N_2O is contraindicated in any child who returns for a repeat craniotomy within 1 month because of the possibility of development of pneumocephalus secondary to air remaining within the ventricles or cisternal system.

A general rule in pediatric neuroanesthesia is that if a child's trachea was not intubated on arrival to the OR, then he or she should be awakened at the completion of the procedure with the intent of tracheal extubation and immediate neurological evaluation. Exceptions include cases where adverse intraoperative events occurred that would likely cause postoperative cardiorespiratory depression or the inability of the child to protect their airway from obstruction or pulmonary aspiration of gastric contents. Children with acute head trauma who underwent tracheal intubation in the field or the emergency department are also candidates for tracheal extubation after a successful evacuation of a blood clot or hemorrhage, assuming all cardiorespiratory parameters have normalized. Children in whom life-threatening increased ICP is expected to persist into the postoperative period should receive continuous intravenous sedation and neuromuscular blockade, and should be managed postoperatively with mechanical ventilation.

POSITIONING CHILDREN FOR NEUROSURGERY

The positioning of pediatric patients for neurosurgery entails proactive attention to details that will prevent complications or problems during the procedure. This includes secure taping of the endotracheal tube, atraumatic placement of an orogastric tube and esophageal stethoscope, administration of petroleum-based eye lubrication, careful taping of arterial and intravenous catheters, and careful positioning of an indwelling urinary catheter. Most often the patient will be positioned supine with the head turned to the side, but many procedures require prone, lateral, or head-up (semi-sitting) positioning. All anesthetic monitors and access lines should be placed and their adequacy confirmed prior to draping. In addition, the anesthesiologist must plan his or her workspace so as to include adequate access to the patient during the surgery. Padding pressure points may help prevent compression injuries. If the patient is prone, free and easy abdominal movement with ventilatory movements should be confirmed by inspection of the abdomen and confirmation that ventilatory compliance is unchanged from baseline. Attention should also be paid to ensuring lack of compression of the eyes and other facial structures.

Though declining in frequency, the sitting position may occasionally be used in pediatric patients for surgical access to the posterior fossa; it entails the same monitoring and safety considerations as for adults in the sitting position. In children there is also the risk of venous air embolism from entrainment of air into open vessels. A recent retrospective audit of complications associated with the sitting position in children reported the incidence of venous air embolism to be 9.3%. All were detected and treated appropriately, and none directly caused morbidity or mortality. Other pediatric studies have reported an incidence of venous air embolism in the sitting position as high as 37%. Some evidence exists that children have higher dural sinus pressures than adults, and may account for the generally lower incidence of venous air embolism in children compared to adults. However, some studies suggest that venous air embolism is more likely to result in hypotension in pediatric patients because, in theory, the same-sized air bubble would be larger relative to the smaller blood volume of children, and therefore, cause greater hemodynamic instability. Overall, outcome studies in children in the sitting position do not show greater risk than in adults. If one is planning to use the sitting position in a child, it is strongly recommended to obtain preoperative echocardiography to rule out any interatrial or interventricular communications. Even when the standard sitting position is not used, the head of the table may be elevated to improve surgical access and cerebral venous drainage. Thus, venous air embolism may occur through open venous channels in the bone and dural sinuses.

When a child is positioned for neurosurgery in a head frame device, there is often flexion of the neck. This maneuver may result in downward displacement of the endotracheal tube within the trachea, and cause the endotracheal tube to enter the right main bronchus. Therefore, in anticipation of neck flexion, the endotracheal tube should be positioned "high" within the trachea, to compensate for its descent. Once positioning is finalized, bilateral breath sounds should be confirmed; in children with healthy lungs, any unexplained oxygen saturation below 96% should prompt an exploration for a right main bronchial intubation.

NEUROPHYSIOLOGIC MONITORING

Many neurosurgeons employ the use of neurophysiologic monitoring to detect intraoperative cerebral or spinal cord ischemia. This may include electrocorticography (ECoG), electroencephalography (EEG), somatosensory-evoked potentials, and motor-evoked potentials. When these modalities are used, the anesthesiologist should proactively discuss with the neurophysiologist the implications of anesthetic management on the accuracy of the monitoring. In most cases, clinically useful concentrations of volatile agents will interfere with neurologic signals. Therefore, an opioid-based technique is indicated, with either low-dose volatile agent or a continuous infusion of propofol to maintain unconsciousness and prevent intraoperative recall. Use of remifentanil is advantageous in these situations, as it will be rapidly eliminated at the end of the procedure. Muscle relaxants are contraindicated when motor-evoked potentials are used. In most instances, it is appropriate to use an intermediate-acting muscle relaxant such as vecuronium or rocuronium to facilitate tracheal intubation. In virtually all cases, preparation time is sufficiently long so that the effects of the relaxant have dissipated by the time monitoring is required.

FLUID MANAGEMENT DURING PEDIATRIC NEUROSURGERY

Except for neonates or other children who may be at risk for development of hypoglycemia, glucose-containing solutions are generally avoided during neurosurgical procedures. Though definitive outcome studies are lacking, hyperglycemia has been associated with worse outcomes during episodes of brain ischemia. Isotonic solutions such as normal saline are advocated during neurosurgery to lessen the risk of excess brain water. However, Lactated Ringers solution can also be used if ICP is not increased.

ANESTHETIC MANAGEMENT OF COMMON PEDIATRIC NEUROSURGICAL PROCEDURES

Ventriculoperitoneal Shunt Insertion or Revision

Ventriculoperitoneal (VP) shunt insertion or revision is probably the most commonly performed pediatric neurosurgical procedure. A shunt is initially placed to palliate disorders that cause hydrocephalus. The proximal end of the shunt is placed within the lateral ventricle of the brain, and the shunt is tunneled underneath the scalp and skin of the neck, chest, and abdomen, where it inserts into the peritoneal cavity to drain cerebrospinal fluid (CSF). Some children may have their shunts terminating into the atrium via one of the great veins of the neck or chest. Children with existing shunts will periodically require revisions because of a variety of reasons that include growth, obstruction, and infection, among others. Occasionally, these revisions will be performed on an emergent basis if the child exhibits signs or symptoms of acutely increased ICP.

There are a variety of causes of hydrocephalus. The most common cause of congenital hydrocephalus is narrowing of the Aqueduct of Sylvius. Acquired hydrocephalus is most commonly a result of intracranial hemorrhage in prematurely born infants. Other causes of hydrocephalus that require shunting include Arnold–Chiari compression associated with myelomeningocele, infections, tumors, and head injury.

Preoperative assessment consists of evaluation of comorbidities and the severity of increased ICP. Premedication with an anxiolytic such as midazolam is usually indicated, but when a child is deemed to have clinically important increased ICP, an intravenous catheter should be placed prior to surgery, and premedication is then carefully titrated under supervision of the anesthesiologist. There is no routine preoperative blood work except evaluation of electrolytes if protracted vomiting is present preoperatively.

Perioperative fluids should consist of normal saline solution or Lactated Ringers solution. Insensible losses usually range from 2 to 4 mL/kg/h. Standard monitors are appropriate. During VP shunts, one intravenous access line is usually sufficient.

In children with preoperative signs and symptoms of increased ICP, a modified rapid sequence IV induction is indicated. A moderate amount of opioid is used to facilitate induction and tracheal intubation, but should be tailored toward tracheal extubation at the completion of the procedure. Any of the volatile or IV anesthetic agents is appropriate for maintenance of general anesthesia. N_2O should be avoided if the child has had a craniotomy within the past month, because of the possibility of expanding an existing pneumocephalus. After tracheal intubation, the stomach should be suctioned with a large-diameter (14-French) orogastric tube, and an esophageal stethoscope and temperature probe are recommended.

The surgical procedure for initial insertion consists of two incisions – one on the lateral side of the head, and the other on the skin of the abdomen, with which to retrieve the tunneled shunt and insert it into the peritoneum. Ordinarily the entire unilateral area from the head to the abdomen is prepared and draped (Fig. 30-1). The child lies supine with the head turned away from the operative side. The OR table is ordinarily turned 90 degrees away from the anesthesiologist.

The most commonly used VP shunt is made of Silastic and contains a bubble reservoir with a one-way valve that allows passive flow of CSF out of the brain. With existing shunts that require revision because of malfunction and increasing hydrocephalus, the obstruction can be located either proximally, between the lateral ventricle and the valve, or distally between the valve and the tip of the shunt in the peritoneal cavity.

Postoperative concerns include observation for neurologic changes that may be a signal of impending shunt malfunction, or intracranial bleeding. Opioids are not usually required as pain associated with this procedure is relatively minor. Significant postoperative headache should initiate an investigation of an additional cause.

Anesthesia for CNS Tumor Resection

Most intracranial tumors in children are cerebellar and brainstem malignancies of the posterior fossa. Preoperative presentation includes vomiting, headache, and gait and balance abnormalities. Laboratory evaluation consists of hemoglobin, type and screen, and electrolytes, which may be altered by chronic vomiting or hormonal effects of tumors. Preoperative anxiolytic medications are tailored to the condition of the child.

A modified rapid sequence induction is most often chosen for induction of general anesthesia. Some children without preoperative signs and symptoms of increased

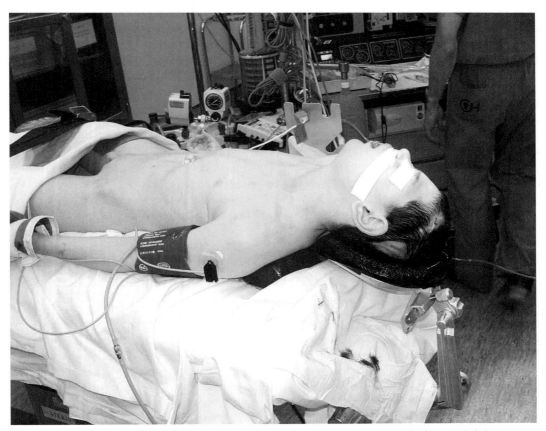

Figure 30-1   The patient is prepared for a VP shunt insertion. The head, neck, chest, and abdomen are prepped and draped. The OR table is turned 90 degrees away from the anesthesiologist.

ICP may be admitted to the hospital on the day of the surgery and can undergo mask induction of general anesthesia, with placement of cricoid pressure after consciousness is lost, and rapid placement of an intravenous cannula and administration of a neuromuscular blocker. After tracheal intubation, the stomach should be suctioned with an orogastric tube, and an esophageal stethoscope and temperature probe are recommended. An additional IV cannula is placed, and an arterial line is inserted to monitor blood pressure changes closely and facilitate access to blood for periodic measurement of hemoglobin, electrolytes, and acid–base status. Isotonic IV fluids (e.g., normal saline or plasmalyte) are recommended so as to be compatible with concomitant blood administration. Ventilation is adjusted to maintain the $P\text{CO}_2$ in the 35 ± 5 mmHg range.

The position of the child will depend on the nature and location of the tumor. It is not unusual for the child to be positioned in the lateral or prone position. Sitting positions are being used with decreasing frequency in children. The child's head is often secured with a Mayfield or Sugita head frame, or placed inside a horseshoe cushion (Fig. 30-2). Careful attention should be paid to securing the endotracheal tube, and ensuring that there is no excess pressure on the eye sockets or neck.

For virtually all major craniotomies, direct blood pressure measurement by arterial cannulation is recommended. Beat-to-beat arterial pressure is required when there is the possibility of rapid hemodynamic changes that may result from blood loss, venous air embolism, or unexpected effects from manipulation of the cranial nerves in the brainstem. An arterial catheter will also provide a method to easily obtain blood gas samples when using mild hyperventilation, or when the anesthesiologist needs rapid determination of hemoglobin.

Intraoperative risks include the possibility of unpredictable and sudden blood loss (from the area surrounding the tumor, or from a venous sinus tear), brain herniation,

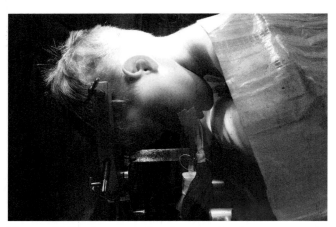

Figure 30-2 In preparation for posterior fossa surgery, the patient's head is stabilized in a Sugita head frame.

venous air embolism, and airway edema. Stimulation of brainstem structures in the posterior fossa may cause sudden hypertension, hypotension and/or bradycardia. Intraoperative adjuvant therapies include antibiotics, mannitol, and dexamethasone, depending on the preferences of the surgeon. Blood loss during tumor removal in small children and infants can be unexpected, rapid, and life-threatening. Prior to beginning a major craniotomy, two intravenous lines should be established in the extremities. Central access is unnecessary, unless dictated by the child's underlying medical condition. If adequate peripheral access is difficult, the femoral approach to venous cannulation is a feasible alternative, since it avoids the risk of pneumothorax associated with subclavian or internal jugular vein puncture, and will not interfere with cerebral venous return.

Mannitol is often administered during craniotomies at doses that range from 0.25 to 1.0 g/kg. It is almost always used in the setting of increased ICP, but many neurosurgeons will ask that it be administered during routine cases. By transiently raising serum osmolality, mannitol will draw fluid out of the brain and into the circulation. Because of its diuretic effect, urine output will increase for approximately one hour after its administration. It should be given no faster than 0.5 g/kg over 20–30 minutes because of the possibility of hypotension and decreased cerebral perfusion pressure if given at a faster rate. Furosemide (0.25–1 mg/kg) is also useful for decreasing cerebral edema, and has been shown *in vitro* to prevent rebound swelling due to mannitol. When diuretics are administered, urine output and electrolytes are rendered unreliable for diagnosing hypovolemia, and hormonal imbalances of sodium, such as diabetes insipidus, or syndrome of inappropriate antidiuretic hormone (SIADH) release. Dexamethasone is commonly administered to children to decrease brain swelling associated with intracranial masses, but does not possess acute effects.

Assuming there are no intraoperative events that would warrant postoperative ventilation, tracheal extubation at the completion of the procedure should be planned. The neurosurgeons will want to evaluate the child's neurological status as soon as possible after regaining consciousness. In fact, the child is often kept in the operating room until a superficial neurological exam is completed. Unexpected deficits may warrant reexploration or immediate head CT scan to detect unanticipated brain herniation or bleeding.

Postoperative considerations include frequent neurological assessments to detect intracranial events, and careful monitoring of cardiorespiratory parameters. Pain control is often easily accomplished as these children rarely have severe postoperative pain. Significant head pain should warrant an investigation for intracranial complications.

Myelomeningocele Repair

Myelomeningocele (also known as spina bifida) is the most common congenital defect of the central nervous system, with a prevalence rate of approximately 4 per 10,000 live births. A myelomeningocele is a fetal malformation involving a posterior protrusion of the spinal cord and meninges through a defect in the spinal column and back, usually at the lumbar level (Fig. 30-3). Because of the risk of meningitis, this is considered a surgical urgency and infants are almost always operated on within 24 hours of birth. Most infants born with myelomeningocele have an accompanying Arnold–Chiari malformation, resulting from downward displacement of the hindbrain into the foramen magnum, and thus receive a VP shunt prior to discharge home in the newborn period.

Preoperative assessment includes careful documentation of all neurologic deficits and a review of other organ systems to rule out additional congenital malformations. Blood work should include a hemoglobin and type and screen. Premedication is not indicated.

Positioning during induction of general anesthesia and tracheal intubation is challenging. A cushion is formed and placed under the back (Fig. 30-4) to prevent contact injury to the dural sac. Alternatively, the infant may be positioned in the lateral position during induction and intubation. The surgical repair is performed in the prone position, with appropriate cushioning that provides ample room for abdominal excursion during ventilation (Fig. 30-5). Avoidance of latex-containing products is begun at birth to prevent eventual development of sensitization.

Typically, two intravenous catheters are inserted for glucose maintenance solution and volume replacement with warmed normal saline or Lactated Ringers solution, up to

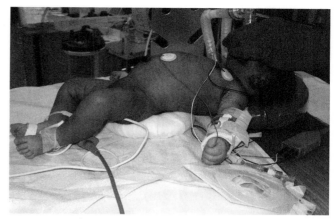

Figure 30-4   Supine positioning for myelomeningocele induction.

25 mL/kg in the first hour and 6–8 mL/kg/h thereafter. Blood loss is usually minimal, unless the skin is undermined and rotation of a myocutaneous flap is required. Therefore, packed red blood cells should be available for the procedure.

Standard monitors are indicated prior to turning the infant prone. The risk of intraoperative hypothermia is significant. A forced warm-air blanket should be placed underneath and around the infant, and all infused fluids should be warmed.

All standard intravenous and inhaled anesthetic agents are acceptable for use during induction and maintenance of general anesthesia, while planning for tracheal extubation at the completion of the procedure. Infants born with myelomeningocele have an increased incidence of an abnormally short trachea. Therefore, the endotracheal tube position and its relation to the carina should be precisely measured to determine the appropriate length of insertion. Regional anesthesia is usually not possible, although reports exist of the sole use of spinal anesthesia, administered by the surgeon throughout the procedure.

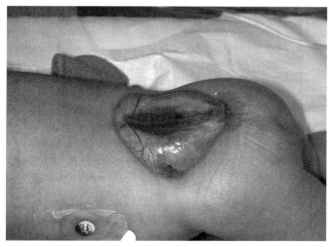

Figure 30-3   Myelomeningocele.

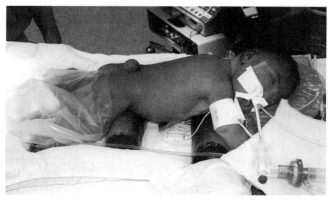

Figure 30-5   Prone positioning for myelomeningocele repair.

As with all neonates, postoperative monitoring for central apnea should be initiated for at least 24 hours following the procedure.

Latex Allergy

Latex allergy is the most frequent cause of intraoperative anaphylaxis in children. It occurs in children who have become sensitized to latex by virtue of their frequent exposure to latex-containing medical products, such as rubber gloves and urinary drainage equipment. The most common type of patient with latex allergy is the child with myelomeningocele because of the daily frequent bladder catheterizations. Up to 70% of children with myelomeningocele are reportedly allergic to latex, in contrast to approximately 1–5% in the general population of healthy children. Chronic exposure to latex early in life appears to be an important predecessor to the development of latex allergy.

An intraoperative reaction to latex usually occurs 30–60 minutes after the start of the surgical procedure. It may manifest as a spectrum of clinical findings that range from mild anaphylactoid reactions (e.g., rash) to severe anaphylaxis consisting of bronchospasm and hypotension. It is indistinguishable from other sources of anaphylaxis, and may be difficult to diagnose during a complicated surgical procedure, where these types of clinical findings may be due to any number of causes. Thus, it often becomes a diagnosis of exclusion.

Immediate treatment of anaphylaxis consists of epinephrine and volume replacement while removing the suspected latex-containing products. Histamine-1 and histamine-2 antagonists and steroids are administered as well. Bronchodilators may be included in the treatment regimen if bronchospasm persists.

Prevention of intraoperative latex reactions is accomplished by identifying susceptible patients and maintaining a completely latex-free OR environment. Children with myelomeningocele are automatically considered latex-sensitive from birth, so latex-containing products are not used in their care. Prophylactic medications prior to surgery are no longer used since their use does not necessarily protect against development of a reaction upon exposure. Furthermore, large case series have shown that children with latex allergy will not develop reactions when cared for in a latex-free environment.

CNS Trauma

Surgery for pediatric head trauma most often involves evacuation of a subdural or epidural hematoma, or evacuation of an intracerebral hemorrhage that is causing an increased mass effect and increased ICP. Other injuries of the head and neck should be strongly suspected. Cervical spine injuries are almost never ruled out when these children present for emergency surgery, so cervical spine precautions should be observed during induction of anesthesia and tracheal intubation. Clinically important head trauma is usually associated with hypertension and either obtundation or combativeness. When hypotension is present, other injuries causing major blood loss should be sought. The most common sites of significant blood loss in pediatric trauma are the intraabdominal organs, the pelvic bones, and the femur.

Preoperative assessment should include review of the child's medical history, physical exam with emphasis on airway anatomy and cardiorespiratory status, and review of laboratory tests. If time is available, blood tests should include hemoglobin, platelets, clotting factors, and a type-and-crossmatch. In the event of a severe acute event causing life-threatening increased ICP, these lab specimens can be sent from the operating room, and O-negative blood can be administered if necessary.

At least two large-bore venous cannulas should be placed, preferably in the upper extremities. Lower-extremity and femoral access is acceptable in the absence of intraabdominal trauma, which may include disruption of the inferior vena cava. An arterial line is preferable prior to induction of general anesthesia in cases where there is a reasonable threat of hemodynamic compromise or brain herniation. Otherwise, in most cases, it is inserted after induction of general anesthesia.

Intraoperative fluids should consist of isotonic crystalloid solutions such as normal saline or Plasmalyte, and blood products when indicated. An indwelling urinary catheter is almost always required, and can be removed at the end of the procedure if no longer necessary. Pediatric patients should be maintained normothermic. There is currently no indication for hypothermia in the acute management of pediatric head trauma.

A modified rapid sequence induction is most often performed, using propofol (2–4 mg/kg) or thiopental (4–6 mg/kg) as a hypnotic agent, rocuronium (1.2–1.6 mg/kg) or vecuronium (0.2–0.4 mg/kg) for neuromuscular blockade, lidocaine (1 mg/kg), and fentanyl (3–5 μg/kg) or remifentanil (bolus 1 μg/kg over 2 minutes, and followed by a continuous infusion at 0.25 μg/kg/min titrated to hemodynamic values). Unless the patient is severely hypovolemic, ketamine is avoided because of its propensity to increase ICP. If the child has a known full stomach and thus has a reasonable risk of pulmonary aspiration of gastric contents during induction, then a rapid sequence technique is indicated. Cervical spine precautions should be observed during tracheal intubation. This consists of manual in-line neck stabilization by an assistant, and maintenance of the head and neck in a neutral position during all subsequent procedures. During the approximately 1-minute latency period before the neuromuscular blocker takes effect, the child should be moderately hyperventilated with application of cricoid pressure.

Maintenance agents can include any volatile anesthetic agent, avoidance of N_2O if pneumothorax or pneumocephalus is considered, and titration of opioids with the intent of tracheal extubation at the completion of the procedure. In some cases, the neurosurgeon will request an immediate postoperative CT scan; the child should then remain anesthetized until the CT has been completed and the surgeon confirms that it is safe to awaken the patient.

Children with head trauma will almost always be transferred to an intensive care unit postoperatively. Analgesic requirements are relatively low. Bleeding and intracerebral swelling are possible postoperatively; children who manifest acute neurologic changes should receive an immediate head CT and possible reexploration.

Case

A 9-month-old male infant presents with a 3-week history of an enlarging head circumference, vomiting, and worsening irritability. Pregnancy, birth history, and family history are unremarkable. The infant's weight is 5.8 kg, and its hemoglobin is 38%. MRI reveals a large posterior fossa mass. Resection of the tumor is planned.

Is there anything else you need to know before going ahead with general anesthesia?

Chronic vomiting might lead to a sodium, chloride, or potassium imbalance, and should warrant preoperative electrolytes. If the child was sedated for the brain CT scan or MRI, I would like to know whether the sedation was well tolerated without airway or hemodynamic issues. Preoperative physical exam should be directed toward confirming normal airway anatomy and assessment of hydration status. Lastly, a type-and-cross should be obtained so that blood (red cells) will be immediately available during the surgery. This can be sent shortly after induction of anesthesia, provided the surgeon understands that tumor resection cannot proceed until red cells are immediately available.

What preoperative orders are appropriate for this infant?

Attention should be directed toward maintaining preoperative hydration status. An infant with this type of condition is usually admitted to the hospital prior to the day of surgery and will receive intravenous hydration. It is also possible that the infant is admitted from home on the day of surgery if the evaluation was performed as an outpatient. If he isn't vomiting, routine fasting orders are appropriate, including clear liquids 2 hours prior to the time of surgery. Premedication with an anxiolytic is usually not appropriate for this age group. Preoperative atropine is indicated if halothane is used for induction of anesthesia.

What monitors and intravenous access lines are appropriate for this case?

Since large blood loss is a possibility, direct arterial access allows monitoring of beat-to-beat changes in blood pressure and will facilitate blood collection for hemoglobin and blood gas values. Mean arterial blood pressure should be maintained within 20% of preoperative values. A central venous pressure monitor is not usually helpful. Two large-bore intravenous lines in any of the limbs are sufficient. If venous access is unobtainable in the extremities, a femoral venous cannula is a reasonable alternative. Normal saline is appropriate for fluid maintenance and replacement of deficits and insensible fluid losses, which typically average 5–10 mL/kg/h during the case. Esophageal or rectal temperature monitoring is required. Core body temperature should be kept reasonably close to normal using warmed IV fluids and a forced warm-air device underneath and around the child. Capnography should be utilized to keep the PCO_2 in the low- to-mid-30s throughout the case, unless the surgeon requests otherwise.

How would you induce and maintain general anesthesia?

Assuming the infant has a functioning intravenous catheter, any IV hypnotic agent, except ketamine, can be used for induction of general anesthesia. An opioid, such as fentanyl, is usually included, at a dose that will help prevent the hemodynamic changes (and subsequent rise in ICP) during laryngoscopy and tracheal intubation. Lidocaine can also be used for additional protection during airway stimulation. Any nondepolarizing neuromuscular blocker can be used. An assistant should apply cricoid pressure while the anesthesiologist ventilates the infant and intubates the trachea. The endotracheal tube should be well secured to the face, using benzoin if necessary. The surgeon should administer local anesthesia containing epinephrine into the scalp to attenuate acute rises in blood pressure during incision or pin placement, and to mitigate blood loss from the scalp. General anesthesia should be maintained with a moderate dose of volatile agent, with a moderate dose of opioid that can easily be eliminated by the end of the case, so as to facilitate tracheal extubation in the operating room and immediate neurological examination. N_2O is best avoided in these cases. Meticulous attention should be paid to fluid status; urine output should be monitored carefully and hemoglobin testing should occur at least hourly while surgical blood loss is occurring. Transfusion of red cells should occur when the hemoglobin decreases below 7 gm/dL.

Case   Cont'd

During an otherwise stable part of the tumor resection, the heart rate acutely decreases from 120/min to 60/min. What should you do?

There are several causes of sudden bradycardia in this setting. Hypoxemia should always be at the top of one's differential list and can be immediately ruled out by pulse oximetry. Even if hypoxemia isn't occurring, the oxygen concentration should be transiently increased to 100% until the bradycardia resolves to maximize oxygen delivery to the brain tissues. Severe hypotension should also be immediately ruled out. Venous air embolism is an important cause of sudden hemodynamic changes during a craniotomy in an infant, even while supine. If this is suspected, the surgeon should flood the field with saline, and carefully search for potentially open vessels through which air is being entrained. Bradycardia is a component of Cushing's triad and may be a sign of acutely increased ICP. Though possible, this is unlikely after the dura has been opened. The most probable cause of the bradycardia in this setting is the stimulation of the brainstem. The treatment is to temporarily discontinue the surgical stimulation, and administer intravenous atropine if the bradycardia continues or results in hypotension.

What are the important postoperative concerns in this infant?

Unexpected postoperative changes in neurologic exam or mental status are associated with life-threatening intracerebral bleeding or swelling. This is considered a neurosurgical emergency and warrants an immediate CT scan and possible reexploration. If mental status is declining, the patient should immediately receive tracheal intubation and mechanical ventilation; sedatives and paralytics should be administered as needed. Blood should be administered if hemoglobin testing reveals an acute decrease from baseline. Mannitol and furosemide should be considered if acute swelling is occurring.

ADDITIONAL ARTICLES TO KNOW

Adornato DC, Gildenberg PL, Ferrario CM et al: Pathophysiology of intravenous air embolism in dogs. *Anesthesiology* 49:120-127, 1978.

Artru AA, Cucchiara RF, Messick JM: Cardiorespiratory and cranial-nerve sequelae of surgical procedures involving the posterior fossa. *Anesthesiology* 52:83-86, 1980.

Bullock RM, Chesnut R, Clifton GL et al: Management and prognosis of severe traumatic brain injury: 1. Guidelines for the management of severe traumatic brain injury. *J Neurotrauma* 17:451-553, 2000.

Downard C, Hulka F, Mullins RJ et al: Relationship of cerebral perfusion pressure and survival in pediatric brain-injured patients. *J Trauma* 49:654-658, 2000.

Eker C, Asgeirsson B, Grande PO et al: Improved outcome after severe head injury with a new therapy based on principles for brain volume regulation and preserved microcirculation. *Crit Care Med* 26:1881-1886, 1998.

Harris MM, Yemen TA, Davidson A et al: Venous embolism during craniectomy in supine infants. *Anesthesiology* 67:816-819, 1987.

Harrison EA, Mackersie A, MEwan A et al: The sitting position for neurosurgery in children: a review of 16 years' experience. *Br J Anaesth* 88:12-17, 2002.

Hartley EJ, Bissonnette B, St-Louis P et al: Scalp infiltration with bupivacaine in pediatric brain surgery. *Anesth Analg* 73:29-32, 1991.

Markovitz BP, Duhaime A-C, Sutton L et al: Effects of alfentanil on intracranial pressure in children undergoing ventriculoperitoneal shunt revision. *Anesthesiology* 76:71-76, 1992.

Reasoner DK, Todd MM, Scamman FL et al: The incidence of pneumocephalus after supratentorial craniotomy: observations on the disappearance of intracranial air. *Anesthesiology* 80:1008-1012, 1994.

Rosner MJ, Rosner SD, Johnson AH: Cerebral perfusion pressure: management protocol and clinical results. *J Neurosurg* 83:949-962, 1995.

Viscomi CM, Abajian JC, Wald SL et al: Spinal anesthesia for repair of meningomyelocele in neonates. *Anesth Analg* 81:492-495, 1995.

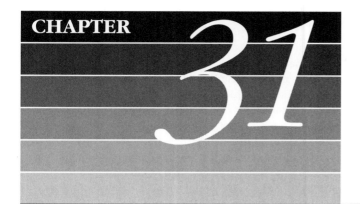

CHAPTER 31

Anesthesia for Pediatric Urologic Surgery

RONALD S. LITMAN

Urologic surgery is extremely common in children. Most procedures are simple surgical repairs in healthy children and are performed on an outpatient basis. This chapter reviews anesthetic management for these simple procedures, as well as some complex procedures with emphasis on those performed mainly in children.

CIRCUMCISION

Circumcision in the newborn period without general anesthesia remains one of the most common procedures performed in children. Older children may present for circumcision under general anesthesia as an elective procedure for cosmetic reasons, or as a treatment for recurrent phimosis. The vast majority of children are healthy without coexisting diseases.

Preoperative assessment is unremarkable. Premedication may include an anxiolytic, as well as an analgesic agent such as acetaminophen 15 mg/kg or ibuprofen 10 mg/kg. Induction and maintenance of general anesthesia are routine. Airway management is provided by facemask or laryngeal mask airway (LMA). Pain relief is provided by a penile block (see Chapter 20). Postoperative fever is very common after circumcision, especially in children with preexisting phimosis.

HYPOSPADIAS REPAIR

Hypospadias is a congenital defect that consists of an abnormal positioning of the penile meatus. It occurs in approximately one out of every 350 male births. It ranges from a very mild defect, in which the penile opening is located slightly more anterior than normal, to a severe defect where the opening is located on the underside of the scrotum. The severity of the lesion will determine the type of surgical procedure. Hypospadias is often associated with a chordee, which is a downward curve of the penis. There are usually no other congenital defects present in affected boys. Surgery is necessary to allow normal urination, to correct the deformation for cosmetic reasons, and to ensure normal sexual functioning in the case of a severe chordee. Repair is often performed during the first year of life.

There are several types of surgical procedures, depending on the severity of the lesion. In general, the more severe the lesion, the longer and more extensive the surgery. Preoperative assessment is routine and includes screening for other congenital anomalies, and optimizing coexisting medical conditions. Laboratory studies are not indicated. Anxiolytic premedication should be ordered if the child is older than 10 or 11 months. Induction and maintenance of general anesthesia is routine. Airway management consists of LMA placement or endotracheal intubation, and will depend on the length of the procedure. A penile block will provide analgesia to the distal two-thirds of the penis; if the repair involves the base of the penis, systemic analgesics should be administered.

TESTICULAR TORSION REPAIR

Testicular torsion is manifested by acute scrotal pain and results from a twisting of the spermatic cord with vascular compromise of the testicle. If the problem is not surgically corrected in a relatively short time (6–8 hours), testicular ischemia can result. This is generally considered a surgical emergency. Temporizing treatment involves manual detorsion; this may alleviate ischemia but orchidopexy is still required.

Preoperatively, the patient should be prepared for emergency surgery. This consists of a focused history and physical and optional administration of a prokinetic such as metoclopramide 0.1 mg/kg to facilitate gastric emptying. An intravenous catheter should be inserted to prevent dehydration and to prepare for a rapid sequence induction of general anesthesia. Adolescents may be offered spinal anesthesia with sedation. Intraoperative analgesia is provided by local infiltration at the surgical site and small doses of opioids. Postoperative concerns include pain and nausea/vomiting, which are treated by standard therapies.

ORCHIDOPEXY

Orchidopexy (also known as orchiopexy) is performed to repair cryptorchidism (also known as undescended testicles). During fetal development, the testicles develop in the abdomen and descend into the scrotum during the last trimester. In a small percentage of newborns (3%), one or both testicles fail to descend. Approximately half then descend within the first year of life. The remaining must undergo surgical intervention because of the increased risk of infertility and malignancy in testicles that remain undescended within the abdominal cavity.

Children with undescended testicles are usually healthy, although there is a higher incidence of prematurity.

Prune-belly syndrome consists of undescended testicles, absent anterior abdominal musculature, and dilatation of parts of the urinary tract. This rare syndrome may be accompanied by impaired renal function. A number of congenital syndromes are associated with undescended testicles and include Noonan's and Prader–Willi syndromes, among many others.

Preoperative assessment is routine and will depend on any coexisting medical conditions. Induction and maintenance of general anesthesia are routine. Airway management consists of LMA placement or endotracheal intubation. Regional analgesia is provided by a hernia block (see Chapter 20).

The procedure consists of two incisions – one in the lower groin to retrieve the testicle, and the other at the bottom of the scrotum to anchor the testicle. Infiltration of local anesthesia at the scrotal incision should be administered by the surgeon. Blood and insensible fluid losses are minimal. Postoperative concerns include pain and nausea/vomiting.

URETERAL REIMPLANTATION

Ureteral reimplantation is the surgical correction of vesicoureteral reflux (VUR), which is a congenital incompetence at the site where the distal ureter implants into the bladder. This results in the retrograde flow of urine from the bladder up into the ureter and kidneys during micturition. If undiagnosed or untreated, VUR may cause dilatation of the ureter and hydronephrosis. Long-term effects include pyelonephritis, hypertension, and progressive renal failure. Many children with severe

Article To Know

Park JM, Houck CS, Sethna NF et al: Ketorolac suppresses postoperative bladder spasms after pediatric ureteral reimplantation. Anesth Analg 91:11–15, 2000.

Painful bladder spasms commonly occur after bladder surgery in children. Furthermore, these spasms are not always relieved by standard parenteral opioid medications. Epidural analgesia is often successful in relieving the pain from spasms at the expense of a dense motor block. Other current treatment modalities include anticholinergics, musculotropic bladder smooth muscle relaxants, and local anesthetics, all of which have varying efficacy and are associated with their own side-effects. The authors of this study used ketorolac, an antiprostaglandin agent, to successfully prevent postoperative bladder spasms following ureteral reimplantation surgery in children.

This important study helped change the practice of pediatric anesthesia in two ways: (1) it established the efficacy of ketorolac for treatment postoperative bladder spasms after ureteral reimplantation; and (2) it contributed to the markedly decreased use of continuous epidural analgesia after this procedure.

Twenty-four children undergoing ureteral reimplantation were prospectively randomized to receive either intravenous ketorolac (0.5 mg/kg/dose every 6 hours for 48 hours) or placebo. All children also received an epidural infusion of bupivacaine (0.1%) with fentanyl (2 μg/mL) throughout the study. The parents recorded bladder spasm episodes using a standardized diary. Three patients (25%) in the ketorolac group experienced bladder spasms, compared with 10 patients (83%) in the placebo group ($p < 0.05$). In addition, bladder spasms were less severe in the ketorolac group. Although both groups received epidural analgesia in this study, the current clinical trend is to use a "one-shot" epidural analgesic administration for immediate postoperative surgical pain and rely on ketorolac to relieve the pain of bladder spasms for several days postoperatively.

VUR are diagnosed *in utero* by a fetal ultrasound that demonstrates hydronephrosis. More mild forms may manifest during childhood as recurrent urinary tract infections.

Preoperative assessment includes evaluation of renal function. Premedication and fasting guidelines are age-appropriate.

The procedure is performed in the supine position, with a low transverse incision. It involves reimplantation of the distal ureter into the bladder wall. Several surgical methods have been described to prevent VUR and are beyond the scope of this discussion. Less invasive injection of an antireflux material (Deflux) into the bladder wall is employed in selected cases. Intraoperative anesthetic considerations include maintenance of normothermia and administration of sufficient fluid to avoid stasis of blood within the bladder with subsequent formation of clots that may obstruct bladder outflow.

Induction and maintenance of general anesthesia are routine, with awakening occurring in the OR. Intraoperative and postoperative pain control can be accomplished using epidural analgesia. Typically, a "one-shot" caudal is performed using 0.25% bupivacaine (1 mL/kg) combined with epidural clonidine 2 μg/kg. Postoperative pain from bladder spasms can be troublesome. Treatment includes ongoing epidural analgesia, ketorolac, and anticholinergic agents.

PYELOPLASTY

A pyeloplasty is a procedure to repair ureteropelvic junction (UPJ) obstruction, the most common cause of congenital hydronephrosis. In most cases it is diagnosed by fetal ultrasonography. Older children may present with urosepsis, nausea/vomiting, failure to thrive, flank pain, abdominal mass, or hematuria. The most common surgical therapy is an open pyeloplasty, which involves excision of the narrowed segment of the UPJ and a reanastomosis of the ureter to the renal pelvis. It is usually performed through an extraperitoneal flank incision.

Preoperative assessment includes confirmation of normal renal function. Induction and maintenance of general anesthesia are standard with endotracheal intubation performed for the procedure. The infant may be placed in the semilateral position with flexion of the OR table. Blood loss should be minimal. Insensible fluid losses will average approximately 5-7 mL/kg/h due to a large flank incision. Routine monitors will suffice.

Intraoperative and postoperative analgesia can be accomplished with epidural analgesia or intercostal nerve blocks into the open incision. Systemic analgesia can include opioids and ketorolac. There are no unique postoperative anesthetic issues for these children.

WILM'S TUMOR

Wilm's tumor is the most common renal tumor in children. Most cases are sporadic but some are inherited. It is most commonly diagnosed in preschool children. Presenting signs and symptoms include a painless abdominal mass, abdominal pain, hypertension, fever, hematuria, and anemia. An associated, acquired Von Willebrand's disease has been reported in these children. In advanced disease, the tumor most commonly spreads to the liver and lungs, and may spread contiguously to the inferior vena cava and aorta. Treatment consists of a radical nephrectomy of the involved kidney, chemotherapy, and possibly radiation if there are pulmonary metastases. Anesthetic implications of chemotherapeutic agents are discussed in Chapter 8. The prognosis depends on the extent of spread and histology of the tumor.

Preoperative assessment should include a complete blood count, electrolytes, liver and renal function studies, coagulation studies, and a type-and-crossmatch. Radiological studies should assess the extent of spread of the tumor and presence of metastases. Cardiac function should be assessed in children who have received chemotherapy with anthracyclines (e.g., doxorubicin). Children with a large intraabdominal mass that impedes gastric emptying should have preoperative placement of an intravenous catheter for rehydration and to prepare for a rapid sequence induction of general anesthesia. Anxiolytics should be administered as appropriate. If delayed gastric emptying is suspected, administration of preoperative H_2-antagonists may be considered.

The procedure is performed with the child supine. Standard monitors are sufficient unless there is significant tumor involvement of the aorta or inferior vena cava (IVC). If this is the case, a central venous catheter may be inserted for monitoring central venous pressure and ease of large-volume infusions. In addition, an arterial catheter may be indicated for direct blood pressure measurement and facilitation of intraoperative blood tests. Two large-bore intravenous catheters should be placed in the upper extremities and red blood cells should be immediately available for transfusion if necessary. Intraoperative risks include sudden or massive blood loss, tumor embolism, or hypotension from IVC compression and loss of preload. Insensible fluid losses may exceed 10 mL/kg/h, depending on the extent of the surgical procedure. Hypothermia is common and should be prevented by warming the OR, use of a forced-air warming blanket, and warming of intravenous fluids and blood products.

Unless the tumor is small, and gastric emptying presumed normal, a rapid sequence induction of general anesthesia is indicated. Maintenance of general anesthesia should consist of a balanced technique using neuromuscular blockade to enhance surgical exposure. If coagulation studies are normal, an epidural catheter may be placed after induction to provide intraoperative and postoperative analgesia. Unless the surgical procedure involves large fluid shifts or clinically significant hemodynamic changes, these children are awakened in the OR.

Postoperative ICU admission is dependent on the medical condition of the patient and the extent of the surgery. Postoperative concerns include oliguria that may be caused by impaired renal function or hypovolemia if bleeding is continuing. Poor pain control may result in splinting, and cause atelectasis and hypoxemia.

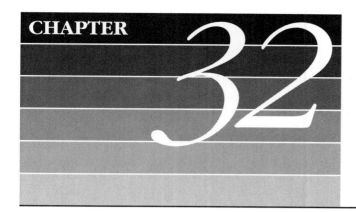

Anesthesia for Pediatric Ophthalmologic Surgery

RONALD S. LITMAN

This chapter covers general considerations for ophthalmologic procedures in children, specific anesthetic considerations for the more commonly performed pediatric ophthalmologic procedures, and several unique anesthetic complications that occur frequently in pediatric ophthalmologic procedures.

GENERAL CONSIDERATIONS

The vast majority of children presenting for surgery on the eye are healthy. However, there are a number of ophthalmologic conditions that are often accompanied by coexisting morbidities. The majority of infants presenting for cataract surgery in the newborn period do not have coexisting diseases, but a variety of pediatric syndromes include cataracts in the constellation of derangements. Some examples include intrauterine viral infection (e.g., rubella or toxoplasmosis) and metabolic disorders such as Lowe syndrome (mental retardation, hypotonia, and renal dysfunction) and hypocalcemic tetany. Infants with congenital glaucoma are less likely than those with cataracts to

have coexisting abnormalities. Infants with retinopathy of prematurity (ROP) who present for cryotherapy will often have multisystem abnormalities associated with extreme prematurity, and they should be thoroughly evaluated preoperatively. Finally, some children with strabismus may also have a myopathic disease (see Chapter 6).

Preoperative Considerations

For children without traumatic disorders of the eye, age-appropriate anxiolytic premedication is indicated. With ocular trauma, anxiety, pain, and crying must be controlled to prevent an increase in intraocular pressure (IOP) that may cause extrusion of the intraocular contents. If the child has had intravenous (IV) access established, a combination of midazolam and fentanyl should be titrated to the child's comfort while avoiding respiratory depression. In the absence of IV access, oral midazolam 0.5 mg/kg will provide anxiolysis and sedation prior to IV catheter placement.

Procedural Considerations

The major anesthetic implication for ophthalmologic procedures in children is the avoidance of factors that acutely increase intraocular pressure, especially in cases of ocular trauma where the integrity of the eye contents are at risk (Box 32-1). Normal IOP in children ranges from 10 to 21 mmHg. Acute increases of IOP during intraocular surgery can cause extrusion of the vitreous humor, lens prolapse, and/or hemorrhage into the eye.

Anesthesiologists should be familiar with the types of topical ophthalmic medications used in the perioperative period and the possible related systemic effects (Table 32-1).

Anesthetic Plan

Unless the child has significant comorbidities, routine monitors are sufficient for virtually all eye surgeries.

Box 32-1   Perioperative Factors that Potentially affect IOP

Factors Increasing IOP

Coughing, straining, bucking, crying, vomiting, head flexion, Valsalva maneuver
Succinylcholine administration
Ketamine (possibly)
Laryngoscopy and endotracheal intubation
Hypoxia, hypercarbia
External pressure on the eye
Acute hypertension
Contraction of the extraocular muscles or orbicularis oculi
Eyelid closure

Factors Decreasing IOP

IV lidocaine
Most sedative or general anesthetic agents
Hypothermia
Retrobulbar block
Head-up position
Diuretics
Systolic blood pressure <85 mmHg
Hypocarbia
Deep inspiration

Fluid and blood losses are minimal. Hypothermia is usually not a problem, except in the smallest infants. In fact, in most cases, since most of the child's body is covered with drapes, the child's body temperature tends to rise by the end of the procedure. Most intravenous and inhalational agents will tend to lower IOP (in a dose-dependent manner), so they can safely be used for induction and maintenance of general anesthesia. There are, however, some notable exceptions. Intravenous ketamine has been shown to acutely increase IOP in children. Administration of intramuscular (IM) ketamine is associated with both increased and decreased IOP, depending on the study one reads. Nevertheless, other associated effects of ketamine such as blepharospasm and nystagmus render it undesirable during eye procedures. If IM ketamine is required for an older uncooperative child who requires emergency eye surgery, then its advantages probably outweigh the risks; this decision should be made on a case-by-case basis. Administration of etomidate has been shown to reduce IOP, but in one case it was associated with loss of eye contents from a ruptured globe as a result of myoclonic movements that occurred after its administration. Lastly, N_2O should be avoided if the ophthalmologist plans to inject sulfur hexafluoride gas, since N_2O can then diffuse into the eye and increase IOP. This also applies if sulfur hexafluoride gas was injected into the eye in the previous 2 weeks.

Succinylcholine causes a 7- to 12-mmHg increase in IOP that lasts 5–6 minutes. The mechanism of this phenomenon is controversial: originally it was thought that succinylcholine uniquely caused contraction of the extraocular muscles, but a relatively recent study demonstrated an increase in IOP in an *in vitro* isolated eye model without extraocular muscles attached. Different induction regimens have been reported to attenuate the effects of succinylcholine prior to tracheal intubation, but none consistently decreases IOP. Therefore, most pediatric anesthesiologists prefer to avoid succinylcholine in open globe procedures, unless its beneficial effects (i.e., rapid paralysis) clearly outweigh its disadvantages. In other words, one would have to believe that the risk of pulmonary aspiration is sufficiently high so as to risk the loss of sight that would occur if succinylcholine caused extrusion of eye contents. On the other hand, proponents of succinylcholine cite the fact that there are no reported cases of succinylcholine-induced loss of sight, and an often-cited article described the use of succinylcholine in 71 patients with an open globe without a single instance of eye content extrusion. Fortunately, reasonable alternatives to succinylcholine exist, such as high-dose rocuronium or vecuronium (see Chapter 19). If a clinical situation arises whereby the anesthesiologist believes that succinylcholine is the

---

Table 32-1   Commonly Used Topical Ophthalmologic Medications

Medication	Concentration and Dose	Ocular Effects	Possible Systemic Effects
Phenylephrine HCl	2.5%; 1–2 drops in each eye	Preoperative mydriatic: dilates the pupil and constricts the blood vessels of the eye	Hypertension and reflex bradycardia
Cyclopentolate HCl	0.5% or 1%; 1 drop in each eye every 5 minutes (2 doses)	Preoperative cycloplegic: dilates the pupil and prevents lens accommodation	Usually none
Tropicamide	0.5% or 1%; 1 drop in each eye every 5 minutes (2 doses)	Preoperative cycloplegic: dilates the pupil and prevents lens accommodation	Usually none
Proparacaine, tetracaine	0.5%; 1 drop in each eye	Topical anesthetic	Usually none

most prudent method for relieving acute life-threatening airway obstruction, then it should be immediately used.

Lidocaine, in doses of 1 to 2 mg/kg, has been evaluated with regard to its ability to attenuate the increase in IOP seen after laryngoscopy and intubation during halothane/N$_2$O anesthesia, or after administration of succinylcholine. All doses of lidocaine were effective in decreasing, but not abolishing, the increase in IOP. Although there are no data evaluating the optimal timing of lidocaine administration, it is logical to administer it 1–3 minutes prior to intubation.

Unless specifically contraindicated, nondepolarizing neuromuscular blockers should be used during the maintenance phase of the anesthetic to ensure lack of movement that could endanger the contents of the eye. In the ASA closed claims analysis, lack of neuromuscular blockade and subsequent patient movement was commonly cited as the primary reason for vision loss. An additional safety procedure is the use of a skin-tight barrier across the bridge of the nose to prevent nasal secretions from entering the eye during an open procedure and introducing potential infectious organisms.

In many cases a deep extubation may be warranted to avoid acute increases in IOP during emergence, assuming there are no contraindications (e.g., full stomach, difficult airway). Lidocaine may attenuate the acute increase in IOP that may occur during emergence when the child reacts to the endotracheal tube, but no studies have specifically examined this issue.

Postoperative Considerations

Except for lacrimal duct probing, most children who undergo eye surgery either have their operative eye patched, or have some impairment of vision in the immediate postoperative period. This can cause a great deal of confusion and annoyance for the child. Parents should be allowed to comfort their children as soon as possible in the postoperative care unit. For hospitalized patients, mild sedatives and anxiolytics can be titrated to effect. Postoperative pain is often disabling. Eye surgery patients describe this feeling as having a foreign object stuck in their eye. Therefore, the child should be comforted and ongoing pain treated with oral or intravenous opioids and nonsteroidal anti-inflammatory drugs (NSAIDs) such as ketorolac.

ANESTHETIC MANAGEMENT OF COMMON PEDIATRIC OPHTHALMOLOGIC PROCEDURES

Lacrimal Duct Probing and Irrigation

Many infants are born with a blocked nasolacrimal (tear) duct, but more than 90% of cases resolve with conservative management (external massaging of the duct) by 1 year of age. Some families may choose to undergo this procedure earlier than 1 year of age because of constant eye irritation or recurrent infections. The procedure, which usually takes less than ten minutes to complete, involves the placement of a fine metal probe from the opening of the duct through to its exit in the nasal cavity, followed by irrigation to confirm that it is patent (Fig. 32-1). Occasionally, the probing includes moving a portion of the inferior turbinate, which can result in minor bleeding. In refractory cases, a silicone stent is placed into the duct, or balloon dilatation is performed.

The only anesthetic consideration for this procedure is the choice of airway management. (The oculocardiac reflex is possible but unlikely – see below.) Many anesthesiologists will be comfortable using a mask anesthetic throughout the procedure, with intermittent removal during the probing. However, it is possible that irrigation fluid or blood may enter the back of the pharynx and precipitate laryngospasm. A small suction probe is placed into the nasal canal to evacuate fluid and blood during the irrigation. It seems that a laryngeal mask would be ideal for this procedure, but some pediatric anesthesiologists may choose endotracheal tube placement instead. Postoperative pain from this procedure is usually not severe, and is easily treated with acetaminophen or ibuprofen.

Open Globe Injuries

A ruptured globe occurs from a blunt or penetrating injury into the eye and includes the potential loss of vitreous humor, which entails permanent blindness if severe. Therefore, it is usually a surgical emergency.

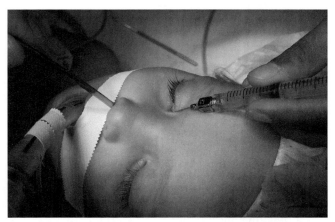

Figure 32-1 The technique of nasolacrimal duct probing and irrigation involves placement of a needle into the tear duct and through to the opening in the nasal cavity. The canal is then irrigated to ensure patency. In this picture a suction catheter is placed into the nasal canal to evacuate the irrigating solution.

Increases in IOP will potentially cause or exacerbate loss of the vitreous. The anesthesiologist should do everything possible to avoid acute increases in IOP (see Box 32-1). Preoperatively, the child's eye should be protected from further injury, and the child should be sedated to avoid crying or defiant behaviors. A full stomach should be assumed if the injury occurred within 6–8 hours following food ingestion. Preoperative sedation should not be so heavy as to compromise the child's airway reflexes that protect against pulmonary aspiration. Topical anesthetic cream placed over the dorsum of the hands may facilitate eventual placement of the intravenous catheter. No specific preoperative lab investigations are necessary unless clinically indicated. Intravenous metoclopramide 0.1 mg/kg may be administered to facilitate gastric emptying if time permits.

If the child is asleep on arrival in the OR suite, avoid awakening! Anesthetic induction is accomplished using cricoid pressure and a rapid sequence induction that is modified by avoiding succinylcholine and using a nondepolarizing muscle relaxant. An acceptable recipe is thiopental 4–6 mg/kg (thus avoiding propofol-induced pain) and rocuronium 1.2 mg/kg. Intravenous fentanyl 1–3 µg/kg (or other opioid of choice) and IV lidocaine 1.5 mg/kg will help prevent acute increases in IOP during laryngoscopy and tracheal intubation. Once the endotracheal tube is inserted, an orogastric tube should be placed to evacuate remaining gastric contents. Anesthetic maintenance can be accomplished with any technique that sufficiently controls hemodynamic responses to surgical stimulation. Mild hypocarbia may help keep IOP low. At the completion of the surgical procedure, arm restraints are often utilized to prevent the child from reaching up and disrupting the surgical repair.

During emergence, it will be important to avoid increases in IOP that may be caused by acute hypertension or coughing on the endotracheal tube. Strategies to avoid this include administration of IV lidocaine 1.5 mg/kg, or deep extubation. If deep extubation is preferred, endoscopic confirmation that the stomach is empty is strongly encouraged. In addition, antiemetic prophylaxis is indicated (ondansetron 0.05 mg/kg) to avoid emesis-induced increases in IOP postoperatively.

Strabismus Repair

The indications for strabismus repair include congenital esotropia or intermittent exotropia. The surgery, which is primarily performed for cosmetic reasons, consists of measuring and shortening the affected extraocular muscles (Fig. 32-2). There are various anesthetic considerations for strabismus repair. Its occurrence is associated with a variety of different pediatric medical disorders, the

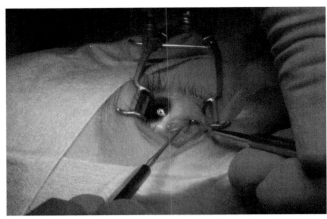

Figure 32-2   While the eyelids are retracted, the extraocular muscles are measured and shortened during strabismus repair.

most important of which are myopathies (see Chapter 6). Other common coexisting disorders include cerebral palsy, hydrocephalus, meningomyelocele, and a variety of congenital syndromes and chromosomal aberrations. There is also a possibility that children with strabismus may be at a higher risk than average for development of masseter muscle rigidity and malignant hyperthermia. Although there is no definitive data on the subject, it seems that if one examines the world's literature on cases of masseter muscle rigidity and malignant hyperthermia, children with strabismus seem to be overrepresented. This is probably merely an aberration, since strabismus is often associated with myopathies.

Aside from investigation of comorbidities, children presenting for strabismus repair require only routine preoperative assessment. Oral midazolam is the most common anxiolytic premedication used. Acetaminophen or ibuprofen syrup can be added to the premedication for their contribution to postoperative analgesia. Intraoperatively, fluid and blood losses are minimal, and active warming measures are usually unnecessary, as children tend to develop hyperthermia, not hypothermia. The unique aspects of the intraoperative anesthetic management for strabismus repair include occurrence of the oculocardiac reflex and postoperative nausea and vomiting (see section below). The oculocardiac reflex usually occurs during the initial stages of the repair (during pressure on the globe or traction on the extraocular muscles), and is easily treated with administration of intravenous atropine. Some pediatric anesthesiologists will choose to administer prophylactic atropine as part of the induction regimen. Postoperative nausea and vomiting is difficult to prevent. Induction and maintenance of general anesthesia with propofol may result in less postoperative nausea and vomiting than if an inhalational agent is used.

Article To Know

Carroll JB: Increased incidence of masseter spasm in children with strabismus anesthetized with halothane and succinylcholine. Anesthesiology 67:559-561, 1987.

This article represents one of the important links between strabismus repair, masseter muscle rigidity, and malignant hyperthermia (MH). Dr Carroll published a retrospective review of children who received mask induction with halothane and neuromuscular blockade for intubation with succinylcholine over an 18-month period at The Children's Hospital of Pittsburgh between 1983 and 1985. The incidence of masseter muscle rigidity was compared between children undergoing strabismus repair and all others. Masseter muscle spasm was defined as jaw tightness interfering with intubation that occurred despite adequate doses of succinylcholine. Dr Carroll found an overall incidence of 2.8% masseter muscle rigidity in children with strabismus, compared with 0.72% in children without strabismus, a fourfold difference. The overall results are presented in Table 32-2.

Table 32-2

Type of Surgery	Number of Cases	Cases with Masseter Muscle Rigidity
Strabismus	211	6[a]
Other	1257	9
Total	1468	15

[a] Fisher's exact test, $p < 0.05$.

Why are children with strabismus at higher risk of developing masseter muscle rigidity or malignant hyperthermia than the general population? The answer to this intriguing question remains speculative. In some children with strabismus, the muscular imbalance of the eye muscles may represent a manifestation of a subclinical muscle disorder, thereby causing an abnormal contracture response to administration of succinylcholine, and possibly causing susceptibility to malignant hyperthermia. The truth, however, remains unknown. Currently, succinylcholine is no longer used electively in most pediatric institutions, so masseter muscle rigidity rarely occurs.

This article was accompanied by an editorial entitled "Trismus is Not Trivial," written by Henry Rosenberg, a well-known malignant hyperthermia expert. In his editorial, Dr Rosenberg became one of the earliest advocates for abandoning elective use of succinylcholine in children.

Most pediatric anesthesiologists will attempt to prevent postoperative nausea and vomiting by administering a serotonin antagonist such as ondansetron (0.05 mg/kg, maximum 2 mg), plus dexamethasone (0.5 mg/kg, maximum 10 mg). The optimal timing and dose of administration of these antiemetics varies, depending on the study one reads.

Airway management for strabismus repair usually consists of a laryngeal mask airway (LMA), but some anesthesiologists prefer the security of an oral (RAE) endotracheal tube since access to the airway is limited during the procedure. Muscle relaxants should not be used if the surgeon plans to perform a forced duction test.

Postoperative pain can be significant. One should never withhold opioids in fear of precipitating nausea or vomiting. Administration of intraoperative IV ketorolac has been associated with postoperative pain relief for up to 5 hours following strabismus surgery. Intense pain that is unresponsive to opioids should prompt a reexamination by the ophthalmologist.

Cryotherapy for Retinopathy of Prematurity

Retinopathy of prematurity (ROP) is a vasoproliferative disorder of the retina that occurs in premature infants and is the leading cause of blindness in the United States. The disorder is primarily related to the immaturity of the retina and is exacerbated by oxygen therapy. These infants should be thoroughly screened for comorbidities associated with prematurity (see Chapter 10). The procedure is commonly performed in the first few months of life to the avascular part of the retina, and usually takes 30-60 minutes to perform. There are no other unique aspects to the anesthetic management. As with strabismus, an LMA is an acceptable alternative to an endotracheal tube. Anesthesiologists should never withhold oxygen for fear of causing or exacerbating ROP. On the other hand, in an otherwise healthy infant, there is no reason to maintain the oxyhemoglobin saturation greater than 97%. Postoperatively, residual pain is often not significant, but because of underlying prematurity, these infants are at risk of developing central apnea and should be monitored for at least 12 hours before discharge home (see Chapter 22).

UNIQUE COMPLICATIONS DURING ANESTHESIA FOR PEDIATRIC OPHTHALMOLOGIC PROCEDURES

Oculocardiac Reflex

The oculocardiac reflex (OCR) is defined as a decrease in pulse rate associated with traction on the extraocular muscles or compression of the eyeball. The bradycardia that ensues may be severe; asystole and ventricular dysrhythmias have been reported. The afferent arc of the reflex consists of the ophthalmic division of the trigeminal (V_1) nerve, whose constituents include the short and long ciliary nerves from the eye. The efferent arc consists of the vagus (X) nerve, which originates in the brainstem and terminates in the sinus node of the heart (Fig. 32-3).

The OCR can be prevented by prophylactic administration of IV atropine 0.02 mg/kg, or IV glycopyrrolate 0.01 mg/kg shortly before eye manipulation. Once the reflex occurs, and bradycardia results, immediate treatment consists of IV atropine 0.02 mg/kg. Other treatments that have been advocated include cessation of the offending stimulus and instillation of local anesthetic into the eye muscles. However, it is this author's opinion that the most practical treatment is administration of atropine, which reliably and rapidly increases the heart rate.

Studies have shown that OCR occurs less often when sevoflurane is used rather than halothane, and when pancuronium is used in comparison with other nondepolarizing neuromuscular blockers.

Postoperative Nausea and Vomiting

Postoperative nausea and vomiting (PONV) is a common complication after ophthalmic procedures, especially strabismus, with an incidence as high as 75% in some reported studies. A variety of regimens have been studied in an attempt to decrease its occurrence. In general, the incidence of PONV is decreased by using propofol instead of inhalational anesthetics for maintenance of general anesthesia, and decreasing the amount of opioids used intraoperatively. Prophylactic antiemetics

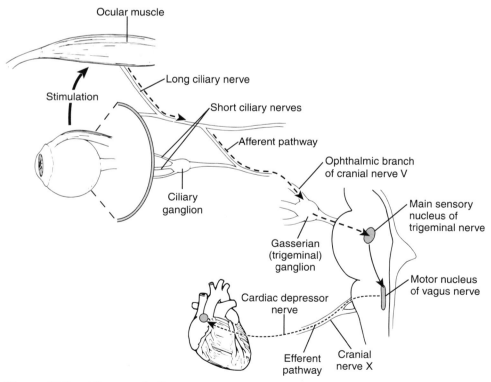

Figure 32-3   Afferent and efferent pathways of the oculocardiac reflex. (Reproduced with permission from Vassallo SA, Ferrari LR: Anesthesia for ophthalmology. In Cote CJ, Todres ID, Goudsouzian NG, Ryan JF eds: *A Practice of Anesthesia for Infants and Children*, 3rd edn, WB Saunders, Philadelphia, 2001.)

Case

A 3-year-old boy fell off a chair while eating dinner and now presents for emergency eye exploration and possible open globe repair. He is uncooperative with any physical exam and does not have an intravenous catheter placed. He is otherwise healthy, takes no medications, and has no allergies.

Is there anything else you need to know before going ahead with general anesthesia?

At this point, there's not a lot more to know. The most important things (e.g., last meal, general health, allergies) are known, and I would also make sure that no other injuries exist, especially to the head. I will make sure the child didn't lose consciousness from the fall. If he did, he probably needs a CT scan of the head prior to surgery to rule out an occult subdural or epidural hematoma. I'll also ask if anyone actually tried to get intravenous access in the emergency department. If not, I might look at potential sites and take an educated guess at whether or not I can easily procure access without too much of a fight.

What are the important anesthetic considerations for this case?

Assuming the physical exam indicates no difficulty with intubation or ventilation, the two most important considerations are avoidance of losing the eye contents (vitreous humor) by an acute increase in IOP, and avoidance of pulmonary aspiration of gastric contents during induction of anesthesia. I wouldn't worry too much about the child crying because he must have been crying after the injury. On the other hand, I wouldn't persist trying to get an IV line.

Is premedication necessary? If so, what will you use?

Premedication is definitely indicated here. There are several options. If the child will agree to take oral midazolam, it is a good way to allay his anxiety and allow for easy separation from his parents. (If I managed to procure IV access, then I would merely titrate midazolam by that route.) Another option is rectal methohexital, if the child is amenable. This is a nice way to induce unconsciousness smoothly but is probably riskier than midazolam in that it might compromise airway protective reflexes should the child vomit preoperatively. Intramuscular ketamine is an alternative but is not preferred because of crying associated with its administration, and some evidence that it may increase IOP.

How will you induce general anesthesia?

Assuming I didn't get intravenous access, I would bring the premedicated child into the OR, and again assess the child's veins for potential access. If I thought I could get an IV line quickly, I would administer a small amount of N_2O (perhaps 20–30%) and attempt IV insertion. I would also keep in mind that even low concentrations of N_2O can cause obtundation of airway protective reflexes, and if the child vomits from it, as many children do, I run the risk of pulmonary aspiration. Assuming I don't see any eligible veins, I would proceed with an inhalational anesthetic with sevoflurane. As soon at the child loses consciousness, an assistant would apply cricoid pressure, and other assistants would descend upon the child to procure IV access as soon as possible. Once access is assured, I would administer rocuronium 1.2 mg/kg, lidocaine 1.5 mg/kg, propofol 2 mg/kg, and fentanyl 2 μg/kg. This combination of medications will almost always allow easy intubation in 45–60 seconds. This is comparable to the intubating conditions attained after administration of succinylcholine but at the expense of the patient being paralyzed for at least 30–45 minutes.

One of the great debates of pediatric anesthesia is whether or not to administer succinylcholine to a patient with an open globe injury and full stomach. Proponents of succinylcholine cite its rapid onset and offset, and no good evidence that anyone's visual outcome ever worsened because of its administration. I prefer the route described above because it avoids the possible side-effects of succinylcholine, and I've never encountered an ophthalmologist who finished this type of surgery before the child's neuromuscular blockade was reversible. I would also make sure to empty the stomach with a large-bore orogastric tube once the endotracheal tube is placed.

How will you maintain general anesthesia?

Any agent (or combination) can be used for maintenance. I would talk to the surgeon to see whether he/she has a preference as to whether the child should undergo a deep extubation. I would want to know whether the surgeon felt that the integrity of the surgical repair would be compromised if the child awoke coughing on the endotracheal tube. If not, then I would probably administer desflurane for maintenance and extubate the child's trachea as awake as possible (without extremes of coughing). On the other hand, if the surgeon is worried about the integrity of the repair, then a classic deep extubation is in order, the details of which can be found in Chapter 19.

Would you do anything differently if the child had an aunt with malignant hyperthermia? How about a parent?

This is the classic examination question – with no right answer! I need to decide whether the child could be susceptible to malignant hyperthermia. Unless the child suffers from a disease that is associated with MH (i.e., myopathy), we only consider a child to be MH-susceptible if he or she had a proven or suspected episode of malignant hyperthermia, or if one of the

---

Case   Cont'd

first-degree relatives had a similar episode. So in the case of the aunt, unless the child had other risk factors, I wouldn't do anything different from the aforementioned technique.

With regard to the parent, that's a different story. If a first-degree relative is MH-susceptible, then the child should also be considered susceptible, and thus triggering agents need to be avoided. In cases like this, where no good choices exist, we usually invoke Alan Jay Schwartz's principle of prioritizing depending on the time course of death. To do so, you list the major issues, and rank them in the order in which, if the worst-case scenario occurs, death would ensue the soonest, then the next soonest, and so on. In almost all cases, airway management then becomes the first priority, since the worst-case scenario is immediate death upon loss of the airway. The next priority in this case is probably a toss-up between development of MH, loss of vision in one eye, and pulmonary aspiration (all low chances). Personally, I'll take the chance of vision loss and aspiration over the chance of MH. So I'd probably give the child IM ketamine 2-3 mg/kg, get IV access as soon as possible, and proceed with a modified rapid sequence intubation with rocuronium.

---

are routinely administered. This includes a combination of a serotonin antagonist and dexamethasone. Optimal doses and the time to administer the antiemetics have not been precisely determined, but differences in these factors probably do not alter the incidence significantly. PONV may also be decreased by intraoperative administration of intravenous lidocaine. Acupressure at the P6 point of the wrist appears to be effective in preventing or treating PONV after strabismus surgery, but it is not widely utilized in most institutions.

ADDITIONAL ARTICLES TO KNOW

Allison CE, De Lange JJ, Koole FD et al: A comparison of the incidence of the oculocardiac and oculorespiratory reflexes during sevoflurane or halothane anesthesia for strabismus surgery in children. *Anesth Analg* 90:306-310, 2000.

Berry JM, Merin G: Etomidate myoclonus and the open globe. *Anesth Analg* 69:256-259, 1989.

Kelly RE, Dinner M, Turner LS et al: Succinylcholine increases intraocular pressure in the human eye with the extraocular muscles detached. *Anesthesiology* 79:948-952, 1993.

Libonati MM, Leahy JJ, Ellison N: Use of succinylcholine in open eye surgery. *Anesthesiology* 62:637-640, 1985.

Mendel HG, Guarnieri KM, Sundt LM, Torjman MC: The effects of ketorolac and fentanyl on postoperative vomiting and analgesic requirements in children undergoing strabismus surgery. *Anesth Analg* 80:1129-1133, 1995.

Rose JB, Martin TM, Corddry DH, Zagnoev M, Kettrick RG: Ondansetron reduces the incidence and severity of poststrabismus repair vomiting in children. *Anesth Analg* 79:486-489, 1994.

Rosenberg H: Trismus is not trivial. *Anesthesiology* 67:453-454, 1987.

Tramer M, Moore A, McQuay H: Prevention of vomiting after paediatric strabismus surgery: a systematic review using the numbers-needed-to-treat method. *Br J Anaesth* 75:556-561, 1995.

Watcha MF, Simeon RM, White PF, Stevens JL: Effect of propofol on the incidence of postoperative vomiting after strabismus surgery in pediatric outpatients. *Anesthesiology* 75:204-209, 1991.

Woods AM, Berry FA, Carter BJ: Strabismus surgery and postoperative vomiting: clinical observations and review of the current literature; a medical opinion. *Paediatr Anaesth* 2:223-229, 1992.

CHAPTER 33

Anesthesia for Pediatric Orthopedic Surgery

MARY C. THEROUX

Orthopedic surgery is common in pediatric patients because of the wide variety of bone and muscle injury or disease during childhood. These entities range from simple fractures in healthy children to complex spinal fusions in children with debilitating neuromuscular disorders.

FRACTURE REDUCTION PROCEDURES

Fractures occur commonly in children: boys have a 40% risk and girls a 25% risk of incurring a fracture before the age of 16 years, and roughly 20% of these will require surgical intervention. Anesthetic management of pediatric fracture reduction is straightforward in healthy children, but it is challenging in children with widespread skeletal disorders such as osteogenesis imperfecta.

The majority of fracture reduction procedures are scheduled electively. The children will have adhered to standard fasting guidelines and will pose little risk for pulmonary aspiration of gastric contents, unless there are other reasons for delayed gastric emptying such as recent opioid administration. Therefore, any anesthetic or airway management technique is feasible. Children who require emergent surgical reduction are considered to have "full stomach" status and should be managed accordingly with a rapid sequence induction and tracheal intubation. Pelvic and lower-extremity fractures may be associated with a significant amount of blood loss.

The supracondylar fracture at the elbow is one of the most common fractures requiring surgery in children.

Accompanying vascular and nerve injury may occur. Nerve injuries (neuropraxia) occur in 15% of cases and resolve spontaneously in most. Primary closed reduction and pinning is the preferred mode of treatment for displaced fractures. The major anesthetic concern is the full stomach. Succinylcholine can be used as a component of a rapid sequence induction, but for most situations a modified rapid sequence induction using rocuronium and propofol will allow for rapid induction of general anesthesia and tracheal intubation.

SLIPPED CAPITAL FEMORAL EPIPHYSIS

Slipped capital femoral epiphysis (SCFE), a common hip disorder that occurs during adolescence, is characterized by a displacement of the femoral neck anteriorly, while the femoral head is held within the acetabulum. African–American and Polynesian populations are affected most frequently. SCFE usually affects adolescents aged between 10 and 16 years and has a strong association with obesity. The operative procedure involves percutaneous placement of a femoral head pin within 1–2 days following the diagnosis. The major anesthetic concern is the obesity of these children. Regional anesthesia is possible but is not usually used in children and is not necessary for control of postoperative pain.

CONGENITAL DYSPLASIA OR DISLOCATION OF THE HIP

The term CDH (congenital dysplasia or dislocation of the hip) is being replaced by the term DDH (developmental dysplasia/dislocation of the hip). This includes all cases of dysplasia, subluxation, or dislocation of the hip joint. CDH is more common among female infants and infants born in the breech presentation.

CDH is best treated as early in infancy as possible with bracing techniques that immobilize the affected hip. Severely affected infants may require surgical intervention consisting of an open reduction with a femoral or pelvic osteotomy. Adductor muscle release may also be performed. There are no important surgical considerations for the anesthesiologist. Regional anesthesia for postoperative pain control is not necessary if reduction of the hip has been accomplished without invasive surgery. If a minimal amount of surgery was performed, postoperative analgesia can be accomplished by intraoperative infiltration of a local anesthetic or administration of an epidural local anesthetic. If the procedure is more involved and prolonged postoperative pain is expected, insertion of an epidural catheter is recommended. At the completion of the procedure, a spica cast or other immobilization device is applied. Anesthetic implications for spica cast placement are discussed in the next section.

SPICA CAST PLACEMENT

A spica cast immobilizes both lower extremities and part of the lower trunk for a variety of hip and upper-leg orthopedic procedures (Fig. 33-1). Many infants will present for replacement or revision of a spica cast following its initial placement. This procedure is performed under general anesthesia. Endotracheal tube placement is recommended for optimal ventilation during movement of the child to an elevated platform which is routinely used for spica cast placement. Anesthetic agents normally include a potent agent without analgesics. Muscle relaxation may aid in reduction of the hip joint in some cases.

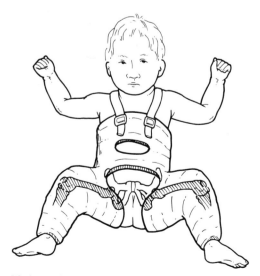

Figure 33-1   Schematic drawing of a spica cast that immobilizes both lower extremities and lower torso.

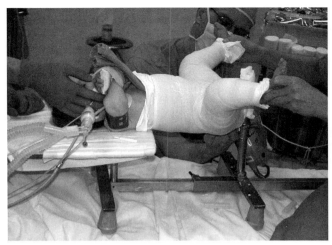

Figure 33-2   A child is placed on an elevated platform while a spica cast is being applied. A folded towel is placed beneath the upper part of the cast to create room for respiratory movements.

As the surgeon begins to apply the spica cast, a folded towel is placed under the upper portion of the cast to ensure that it is not too tight on the abdomen (Fig. 33-2). The towel is removed once the cast is set, allowing some space between the anterior abdominal wall and the cast. Upon emergence from general anesthesia, crying infants may swallow air and appear to have much less room between the spica cast and the abdominal wall. If the infant is inconsolable and appears to be in distress, even after pain has been treated, a tight cast may be considered. The surgeon should recheck the cast and, if necessary, cut a "window" over the abdomen.

SCOLIOSIS

Scoliosis is defined as a deviation of the spine in the frontal plane. A scoliotic spine also rotates maximally at the apex of the curve. The etiology of scoliosis remains unknown, and the term "idiopathic" remains appropriate when otherwise healthy children develop this condition. For descriptive purposes, the curve locations in children with scoliosis are classified into separate anatomical locations (Table 33-1).

Most cases of idiopathic scoliosis occur in healthy adolescent females. The most important preoperative medical concern in these patients is determination of the severity of restrictive lung disease. In most cases, especially when the scoliosis is idiopathic, there are only mild abnormalities that do not impact on intraoperative ventilation or interfere with successful extubation in the immediate postoperative period. Preoperative pulmonary function testing (PFT) is indicated for curves >80 degrees, or >60 degrees if the child also exhibits reactive airway

Table 33-1	Classification of Scoliosis by Anatomic Location
Description	**Spinal Level**
Cervical	C2-C6
Cervicothoracic	C7-T1
Thoracic	T2-T11
Thoracolumbar	T12-L1
Lumbar	L2-L4
Lumbosacral	L5 or below

disease or if an anteroposterior fusion is being performed. A vital capacity less than 30% of predicted may indicate the need for postoperative mechanical ventilation. Severely affected patients may also suffer from cardiovascular dysfunction and will require echocardiography and cardiology consultation.

A thorough discussion should take place with family and patient about the nature and risks of the anesthetic and the surgical procedure. Neurophysiologic monitoring should be explained, especially if it begins in the preoperative period when the patient is conscious. If an intraoperative "wake-up" test is planned, the procedure is discussed in detail with the patient – this will facilitate intraoperative success. The patient and family should also be told that it is common for their face to be extremely swollen postoperatively, and that it will subside over the first two postoperative days. Adolescents may elect to have preoperative intravenous catheter placement, and/or preoperative anxiolysis with oral midazolam.

Preoperative assessment includes hemoglobin and coagulation function testing, and a type-and-crossmatch. Autologous or directed-donor blood donation is performed for most patients. A 1997 study reported that of 168 patients scheduled for idiopathic scoliosis repair, 144 participated in autologous predonation. More than 90% of these patients successfully avoided allogeneic red cell transfusion. Other useful techniques are intraoperative blood salvaging and preoperative erythropoietin administration, especially in cases of Jehovah's Witness patients. Intraoperatively, normovolemic hemodilution can be useful especially when preoperative autologous blood donation was not performed.

Induction of general anesthesia is performed with standard intravenous or inhalational agents on the patient's bed or gurney to facilitate turning to the prone position on the OR table. Administration of a moderate dose of a nondepolarizing muscle relaxant to facilitate endotracheal intubation will allow return of neuromuscular function to obtain baseline motor-evoked potentials (MEP) before surgery begins. Following induction of general anesthesia and tracheal intubation, and prior to

turning the patient prone, all the necessary monitors and lines are inserted. This includes a urinary catheter, nasogastric tube, and two peripheral intravenous lines, one of which should be large enough for rapid fluid and blood administration. The larger-caliber line should be dedicated to the use of warmed fluids. The smaller-caliber line is usually used for infusion of medications.

An arterial line is obtained, usually by cannulating the radial artery. The presence of both an ulnar and radial artery should be checked before cannulating either one. The ulnar artery should not be cannulated if the radial artery on the same side was punctured but not cannulated or if a hematoma of the radial arterial site develops. Early decision to abandon a failed site due to spasm of the artery or hematoma of the site and to move on to the contralateral side will save time and avoid injury.

Maintenance of intraoperative normothermia is essential for avoiding hypothermia-induced coagulation abnormalities and delayed awakening. Hypothermia can be minimized by using a forced warm-air blanket and warming the intravenous fluids and blood products.

Following tracheal intubation and placement of monitors and lines, the patient is placed in the prone position for the procedure. A variety of different types of prone stabilizing devices are utilized, depending on the preference of the surgeon and the institution. All pressure points are well-padded; the anesthesiologist must ensure that the abdomen moves freely with each breath between the pads, and that all skin surfaces are adequately protected, with special attention to the face around the eyes (Fig. 33-3). An increase in intraabdominal pressure may increase bleeding in the epidural venous plexus.

The most important factor that influences the choice of anesthetic agents is the use of evoked potentials to assess spinal cord integrity. Only minimal concentrations of volatile agents are used. Nitrous oxide may or may not be included, depending on the preference of the neurophysiologist. Maintenance of general anesthesia usually consists of a continuous propofol infusion with an opioid (Table 33-2). A remifentanil infusion will allow for easy intraoperative titration tailored to the hemodynamic status. Remifentanil may also preserve integrity of evoked potentials better than intravenous anesthetic agents. If evoked-potential monitoring is not performed, any anesthetic technique can be used.

A variety of neurophysiologic techniques will be used during spinal fusion procedures, depending on the preference of the surgeon and the neurophysiologist. Most commonly, somatosensory evoked potentials (SSEP) and motor evoked potentials (MEP) are used. Their complete description is beyond the scope of this discussion.

A sudden loss of evoked potentials (loss of MEP, or 50% decrease in SSEP) has the same effect as a red traffic light (Fig. 33-4). All surgical momentum stops and, if necessary, the last instrumentation is reversed (e.g., loosening

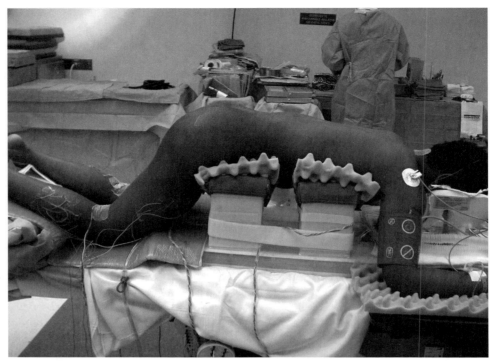

Figure 33-3 Prone position with all pressure points padded. Electrodes for evoked potential monitoring are in place.

of a pedicle screw or sublaminar wire). The anesthesiologist should increase the mean arterial pressure to at least 90 mmHg. If improvement in the evoked potentials is not observed, the patient is treated with steroids (30 mg/kg bolus of methylprednisolone followed by an infusion at 5.4 mg/kg/h for 23 hours). The instrumentation may be removed and the patient awakened.

Some surgeons still prefer using a Stagnara wake-up test, in which the patient is transiently awakened immediately following spinal cord distraction and asked to wiggle their toes to demonstrate spinal cord integrity. Preparation of their patient is the key to its success.

A useful approach is to practice with the child as he or she is being anesthetized by simply asking the child to wiggle their toes several times just before losing consciousness. Even if the wake-up test is not performed, a child who was prepared for it will emerge from anesthesia and wiggle their toes on command thus expediting tracheal extubation. It is common practice not to extubate the patient's trachea until the patient has moved his or her toes, which is the best assurance of spinal cord integrity.

The most common surgical instrumentation used for idiopathic scoliosis is a double-rod technique with hooks or pedicle screws to secure the rods, which are then distracted to straighten the spine (Fig. 33-5). Intraoperatively, at the time when the surgeon is straightening the spine maximally, the spinal cord is vulnerable to ischemia from compression of the arterial supply and from direct damage from insertion of the wires or screws. The anesthesiologist must ensure that the patient is neither anemic nor hypotensive at this point to prevent any decline in oxygen delivery to the spinal cord. Mean arterial pressures are maintained above 70 mmHg and the hemoglobin is raised to over 9 g/dL. During and following the distraction, the neurophysiologist continually monitors the patient's evoked potential signals to detect any abnormalities that indicate spinal cord compression.

When the surgeon has completed the rod insertion and distraction of the spine and the neurophysiologist

Table 33-2	Intravenous Anesthetic Agents during Scoliosis Repair

Agent	Dose
Propofol	150–250 µg/kg/min
Sufentanil	0.2–0.3 µg/kg/h
Remifentanil	0.1–1.0 µg/kg/min (usually varies greatly during case)
Fentanyl	2–4 µg/kg/h
Ketamine[a]	2–4 µg/kg/h

[a] The ketamine dose will vary, especially when it is used as the main anesthetic in a neuromuscular scoliosis patient.

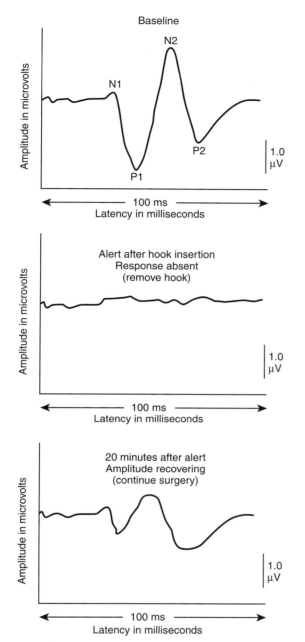

Figure 33-4 The top trace shows a representation of a normal evoked-potential waveform. The second curve depicts loss of the evoked-potential wave following insertion of a hook. The bottom shows eventual recovery of the evoked-potential wave.

is satisfied that the evoked potential signals are intact, the surgeon will begin to close the wound. The anesthesiologist may elect to discontinue all intravenous anesthetic agents and begin administration of N_2O with a small concentration of an inhaled agent, to facilitate rapid awakening at the completion of the procedure. Tracheal extubation is performed after the patient has been turned supine and has demonstrated the ability

to move his or her legs and toes to reconfirm spinal cord integrity.

An important aspect of the anesthetic management of these patients is planning for postoperative analgesia. For healthy adolescents, patient-controlled analgesia (PCA) with opioids is the preferred technique. Additional pain control can be gained from administration of intrathecal opioids. Preservative-free morphine (2.5 µg/kg) is injected into the cerebrospinal fluid (CSF) by the surgeon under direct vision when exposure is obtained. Intrathecal morphine provides prolonged postoperative analgesia and decreased parenteral opioid requirements for the first 24 hours, and may decrease intraoperative blood loss. Placement of an intrathecal opioid requires the child to be admitted to the intensive care unit or another appropriately monitored ward.

NEUROMUSCULAR SCOLIOSIS

Commonly encountered neuromuscular diseases include cerebral palsy and various types of myopathies. The primary reason for repairing the spines of these debilitated children is to allow them to sit upright without assistance, thus decreasing the incidence of chronic pulmonary aspiration and extending life-expectancy. The surgical instrumentation used for correction of neuromuscular scoliosis differs from that used for idiopathic repair, and can vary between institutions. The most involved surgical procedure performed in these children is when the spine is instrumented from C7 to the sacrum using a unit rod (Fig. 33-6). These procedures typically involve much greater blood loss than for idiopathic repair, up to 1–3 times the patient's blood volume. The reason for this increased blood loss in these patients is unclear and is often attributed to their poor nutritional status or lifelong inability to ambulate.

In a study at the author's institution, when we measured clotting indices in these children, we found abnormally decreased factor levels before and during surgery. Of five patients with severe, spastic cerebral palsy, two had abnormally low factor levels before surgery. All five had at least one factor below normal by the time they lost 25% of their estimated blood volume. Therefore, early use of blood and fresh frozen plasma is recommended. Platelet quantity and quality are often impaired in these children from prolonged use of anticonvulsants. Therefore, if intraoperative bleeding does not abate, or when there is an absence of a clot in the wound despite administration of fresh frozen plasma, administration of platelets is indicated. Procoagulants such as desmopressin (DDAVP), tranexamic acid, and aprotinin have been studied in an attempt to reduce operative blood loss in these patients, but definitive results are lacking.

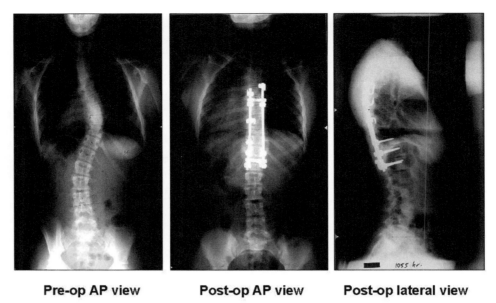

Pre-op AP view   **Post-op AP view**   **Post-op lateral view**

Figure 33-5   Radiographic views before and after correction of idiopathic scoliosis with a double rod technique. Also shown is a lateral view after correction is included, showing the pedicle screws.

ANTERIOR SPINAL FUSION

Both idiopathic and neuromuscular scoliosis patients may require a combined anterior and posterior spinal fusion. The indications for combined fusion include: (1) a curve >75 degrees, (2) a rigid curve, and (3) patients at risk for crankshaft deformity. A crankshaft deformity is a condition where anterior spinal growth continues despite successful posterior spinal fusion, causing a rotational deformity. This occurs in skeletally immature patients who have potential for further spinal bone growth.

Anterior spinal fusion consists of anterior disk excision, release of the anterior longitudinal ligament, removal of the annulus fibrosis and nucleus pulposus, and excision of the vertebral endplate cartilage through a thoracic approach with the patient positioned laterally. A thoracoscopic approach is preferred by some surgeons, particularly when the number of disks to be released is minimal. This approach will require initial placement of an endotracheal

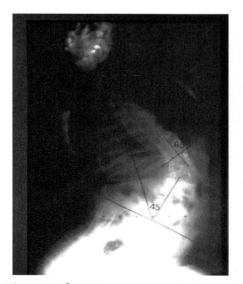
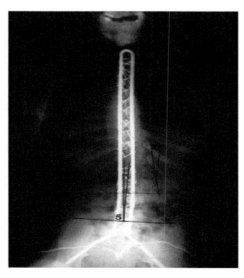

Figure 33-6   Radiographic views before and after correction with a unit rod technique in a child with neuromuscular scoliosis. The spine is fused from T1 to the sacrum.

Case

A 13-year-old, 55-kg adolescent with idiopathic scoliosis is scheduled for posterior spinal fusion. The preoperative history is positive for reactive airway disease for which she takes albuterol inhaler when needed. Two autologous units of predonated blood are available for intraoperative use.

Is there anything else you would like to know?

I would like more details of her reactive airway disease to get a better idea of its severity and frequency. I'll estimate this by finding out if she's ever been admitted to the hospital for asthma, and if so, if she required mechanical ventilation. I'll also find out how often she requires steroid treatment as an indication of the overall severity.

Should this patient receive premedication?

An anxiolytic is desirable in this patient. This can consist of oral midazolam 15 mg or oral diazepam 15 mg.

How will you maintain general anesthesia for this case?

The neurophysiologist will be monitoring both somatosensory evoked potentials as well as motor evoked potentials, and, therefore, requests TIVA (total intravenous anesthesia). A continuous propofol infusion can be combined with any opioid. Remifentanil is the easiest to use and titrate to hemodynamic status intraoperatively.

After spine exposure and during hook placement, the patient begins to have difficulty maintaining an adequate mean arterial pressure, which is drifting down into the 50s. What would you do?

An occasional bolus of ephedrine 5–10 mg will allow time to adjust the infusion rates and bring up the mean arterial pressure (MAP), but I need to make sure I don't lower the propofol too much and risk intraoperative awareness. A bispectral index (BIS) monitor may be helpful here. This situation is almost always amenable to infusion of crystalloid and blood products when appropriate. I will try to keep the urine output steady at 1–2 mL/kg/h, and obtain a blood gas and hemoglobin level to determine the extent of tissue hypoperfusion that is reflected in the severity of metabolic acidosis. The results of these tests will guide further management.

During placement of the second rod, the neurophysiologist states that the motor evoked potential (MEP) on the right side has disappeared. What will you do?

Several things should happen simultaneously. The surgeon should stop whatever he or she is doing and, if possible, loosen the hook. The anesthesiologist should increase the blood pressure by decreasing anesthetic infusions, giving fluids and administering ephedrine or epinephrine. If there is no improvement in the MEP signal by 15–20 minutes, there should be a consideration of administration of steroids. A wake-up test may be indicated at this point, and if still negative, the surgeon should consider reversing all previous spinal instrumentation.

How would you perform a "wake-up" test?

A wake-up test requires a minimum of 20–30 minutes of lead time to prepare the patient for awakening. The anesthetic infusions are discontinued, a 20-mL syringe of propofol is on standby and ready to be injected, an endotracheal tube with a stylet is immediately available, and the patient's bed should be in the OR or just outside, in the event that patient needs to be urgently placed in the supine position to secure the airway. As the heart rate and blood pressure begin to rise and the patient starts to breathe spontaneously, a nurse or surgical resident should look under the drapes at the end of the bed to visualize toe movements. When the anesthesiologist believes the patient may be able to follow commands, he or she speaks directly and close to the patient's ear and asks them to wiggle or move their toes. When the patient has been prepared preoperatively, they will often wiggle their toes when they are seemingly under a fair amount of anesthetic agents. When the surgical team is satisfied, propofol and opioid are reinfused rapidly, and the infusions are continued. Very few, if any, children will remember this sequence of intraoperative events.

tube that allows single lung ventilation. Most surgeons, however, will employ an open approach which may not intrude within the thoracic cavity. The procedure is often done in combination with a posterior fusion on the same day. Some surgeons may schedule them as separate procedures with several days in between.

Acknowledgments

The author thanks Drs Shanmuga Jayakumar, Freeman Miller, Kirk Dabney, and Suken Shah in the Department of Orthopaedics and at the Alfred I. duPont Hospital for Children and Lawrence R. Wierzbowski, Au.D., of Surgical Monitoring Associates for their assistance with this chapter.

Article To Know

Fontana JL, Welborn L, Mongan P et al: Oxygen consumption and cardiovascular function in normovolemic hemodilution. Anesth Analg 80:219-225, 1995.

This study demonstrates how one should use caution and exercise common sense and good judgment when reading the experimental literature. Eight adolescents undergoing idiopathic scoliosis correction were enrolled in a study in which they predonated blood immediately prior to their surgery to achieve a hemoglobin level of 7 g/dL. This predonation was in addition to the more conventional autologous predonation of 2-4 units of packed red cells 3-30 days prior to surgery. Normovolemia was maintained by infusing 5% albumin. The goal of the study was to determine the safety of hemodilution based on acid–base status and hemodynamic parameters. Further fluid administration during surgery lowered the patients' hemoglobin to an average of 3.0 ± 1.6 g/dL. One of eight patients had transient ST segment depression that resolved upon reinfusion of autologous blood. In another patient, the mixed venous saturation decreased below 60%, which also triggered retransfusion of autologous blood. Thus, two of eight patients demonstrated limits of cellular oxygen delivery. In spite of these adverse effects, the study concluded that profound hemodilution to a mean hemoglobin level of 3.0 g/dL is safe.

This article is noteworthy because the authors radically lowered these patients' hemoglobin levels far below a presumed safe level, yet few patients demonstrated physiologic derangements and no patient was harmed in any obvious way. The authors attribute their success to the maintenance of normovolemia with colloid administration, and the healthy baseline status of the patients. Despite publication of this report, the practice of allowing hemoglobin levels to decrease below 7 g/dL has not been adopted in most centers.

ADDITIONAL ARTICLES TO KNOW

Boezaart AP, Eksteen J, Spuy GVD, Rossouw P, Knipe M: Intrathecal morphine: double-blind evaluation of optimal dosage for analgesia after major lumbar spinal surgery. *Spine* 24:1131-1137, 1999.

Bracken MB, Shepard MJ, Collins WF et al: A randomized, controlled trial of methylprednisolone or naloxone in the treatment of acute spinal-cord injury: results of the Second National Acute Spinal Cord Injury Study. *N Engl J Med* 322:1405-1411, 1990.

Dias RC, Miller F, Dabney K, Lipton G, Temple T: Surgical correction of spinal deformity using a unit rod in children with cerebral palsy. *J Pediatr Orthop* 16:734-740, 1996.

Murray DJ, Forbes RB, Titone MB, Weinstein SL: Transfusion management in pediatric and adolescent scoliosis surgery: efficacy of autologous blood. *Spine* 22, 2735-2740, 1997.

Padberg AM, Wilson-Holden TJ, Lenke LG, Bridwell KH: Somatosensory and motor-evoked potential monitoring without a wake-up test during idiopathic scoliosis surgery: an accepted standard of care. *Spine* 23:1392-1400, 1998.

Peterson DO, Drummond JC, Todd MM: Effects of halothane, enflurane, isoflurane, and nitrous oxide on somatosensory evoked potentials in humans. *Anesthesiology* 65:35-40, 1986.

Samra SK, Dy EA, Welch K, Lovely LK, Graziano GP: Remifentanil and fentanyl-based anesthesia for intraoperative monitoring of somatosensory evoked potentials. *Anesth Analg* 92:1510-1515, 2001.

Scheufler K, Zentner J: Total intravenous anesthesia for intraoperative monitoring of the motor pathways: an integral view combining clinical and experimental data. *J Neurosurg* 96:571-579, 2002.

Theroux MC, Corddry DH, Tietz A et al: Effect of preoperative desmopressin on blood loss during spinal fusion for neuromuscular scoliosis: a randomized, controlled and double blinded study. *Anesthesiology* 87:260-267, 1997.

Anesthesia for Pediatric Plastic Surgery

RONALD S. LITMAN

The anesthetic management of plastic surgical procedures in the pediatric population is often challenging because of the variety of congenital syndromes that require cosmetic repair. These syndromes are associated with altered airway anatomy, as well as complex coexisting medical conditions. This chapter reviews anesthetic management of the more commonly performed plastic surgery procedures – cleft lip and palate, and craniosynostosis repair. In addition, considerations for subcutaneous administration of epinephrine are reviewed.

CLEFT LIP REPAIR

A cleft lip is a unilateral or bilateral split of the upper lip between the mouth and nose (Fig. 34-1). It can range from a slight notch to a complete separation of one or both sides of the lip extending up and into the nose, and is often accompanied by a cleft palate. The overall incidence of cleft lip is approximately 1 in 800 live births; Asians are most commonly affected and African-Americans least commonly affected. While the majority of cleft lips are not associated with any predisposing factors, a history of maternal smoking or phenytoin use increases the risk. Associated congenital defects such as congenital heart disease occur in approximately 10% of affected children, and these are often combined as one of the velocardiofacial syndromes. Feeding difficulties in the newborn period may lead to poor growth and anemia. Surgical repair is usually performed within the first several months of life; some centers are correcting these lesions in the neonatal period. Older children may return for subsequent cosmetic repairs of the lip or nasal tip.

If the infant is otherwise healthy, there are no unique preoperative considerations. A hemoglobin level is indicated if the infant has exhibited poor growth, or to satisfy institutional requirements for routine preoperative testing in the first year of life. A mask induction of general anesthesia is most often performed, followed by endotracheal intubation with an oral RAE endotracheal tube (Fig. 34-2). The patient's eyes are protected using a petroleum-based lubricant, which is covered by a transparent adhesive covering to preserve visible surgical landmarks. The OR table is turned 90 degrees away from the anesthesiologist to facilitate the surgical repair from the head or side of the table. A small amount (usually <1 mL) of local anesthetic with epinephrine is injected into the surgical field to control hemostasis at the incision site. Blood and fluid losses are minimal. Therefore, maintenance and preoperative deficit fluid replacement is sufficient. Small amounts of opioid may be administered intraoperatively or held until the infant demonstrates signs of postoperative pain. Rectal administration of acetaminophen may also be helpful. Soft arm restraints are often used to keep the infant from handling the repair postoperatively.

Many pediatric anesthesiologists advocate regional anesthesia for cleft lip repair. An infraorbital nerve block with a long-acting local anesthetic can provide up to 18 hours of pain relief and decrease the frequency of postoperative administration of opioids.

CLEFT PALATE REPAIR

A cleft palate occurs when the roof of the mouth (i.e., hard and/or soft palate) has not joined completely during fetal development. A cleft palate can range from a

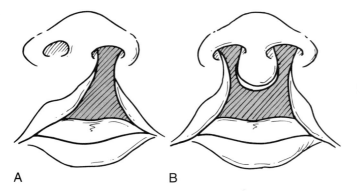

Figure 34-1 **A**, Unilateral cleft lip. **B**, Bilateral cleft lip.

small bifid uvula to a complete separation of both the soft and hard palate. The incidence of cleft palate is approximately the same as that of cleft lip, with a similar racial distribution. Associated congenital defects occur in up to 50% of infants born with a cleft palate. Cleft palate can exist as a component of the Pierre–Robin sequence (cleft palate, glossoptosis, and micrognathia). Early concerns in the newborn period relate to feeding difficulties and airway compromise. Mild forms of this disease are managed adequately by prone positioning. Severe forms, however, manifest as life-threatening upper-airway obstruction in the newborn period, necessitating placement of an oral or nasal airway, or tracheostomy (see Chapter 18).

Surgical correction of cleft palate is usually performed by 12 months of age. Older children may present for subsequent procedures such as correction of velopharyngeal incompetence, or repair of bony palatal defects with a bone graft. If a child is born with both cleft lip and cleft

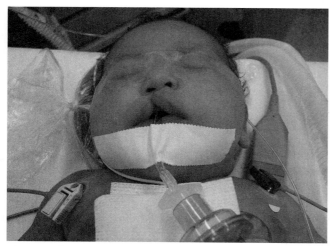

Figure 34-2 Infant with a right-sided cleft lip. An oral RAE endotracheal tube is inserted and the OR table is turned 90 degrees away from the anesthesiologist.

palate, the lip repair is performed first because the repaired lip helps to decrease the width of the palatal defect.

Preoperative considerations for children presenting for cleft palate repair are focused on delineation of coexisting medical problems and assessment of airway patency. Infants older than 6 months of age and without airway compromise are candidates for anxiolytic premedication. Unless intravenous access is previously established, inhalational induction of general anesthesia is performed. Upper-airway obstruction during this phase is common and is almost always relieved by placement of an oral airway device to prevent the tongue from becoming lodged in the cleft. Endotracheal intubation may be complicated by the presence of micrognathia or unintentional placement of the laryngoscope blade into the cleft during laryngoscopy. Some pediatric anesthesiologists prefer to place gauze material into the cleft prior to laryngoscopy attempts. An oral RAE tube is inserted and the OR table turned 90 degrees to facilitate surgical repair from behind the head of the infant.

The cleft palate is exposed by placement of a mouth-opening device (usually a Dingman mouth gag) and extending the child's head and neck, in a similar position as that for a tonsillectomy. Bilateral breath sounds should be reconfirmed after these maneuvers because they may cause caudad movement of the endotracheal tube and a right main bronchial placement. A small amount of local anesthetic with epinephrine is injected into the palate. Blood and fluid losses are minimal but somewhat greater than for cleft lip repair, and may not always be readily apparent. A throat pack is often helpful to prevent the passage of blood into the larynx or esophagus.

The choice of anesthetic agent for maintenance of general anesthesia is unimportant. Most pediatric anesthesiologists will administer a moderate amount of opioid intraoperatively while recognizing that airway obstruction may occur following tracheal extubation at the completion of the procedure. Prior to tracheal extubation, the oropharynx should be gently suctioned to remove retained blood and secretions while taking care not to disrupt the delicate suture lines. Many surgeons will place a loop suture through the anterior portion of the tongue which can be pulled anteriorly if the tongue is causing postoperative upper-airway obstruction. This suture is then usually removed within several hours after the procedure when the child has demonstrated the ability to maintain airway patency without assistance.

The primary postoperative concerns following cleft palate repair are airway assessment and pain control. Prone or lateral positioning is often helpful to alleviate obstruction by the tongue. If indicated, small doses of morphine are administered while monitoring upper-airway patency. Placement of a nasal or oral airway is relatively contraindicated (unless absolutely necessary) because it may disrupt the surgical repair. A nasal airway is also relatively contraindicated in any future anesthetic if a posterior pharyngeal flap was used to repair the cleft.

CRANIOSYNOSTOSIS REPAIR

Types of Craniosynostosis

At birth, the skull consists of distinct cranial bones separated by malleable strips of connective tissue that are known as "sutures" (see Fig. 2-5). During the first 2 years of life, the sutures serve as growth sites for the deposition of additional cranial bone with eventual formation of the adult-like skull. *Primary* craniosynostosis, which occurs in approximately 1 in 2000 live births, results when one these sutures closes prematurely, thus restricting growth of the adjacent cranial bones in a perpendicular direction. The remaining cranial bones that are adjacent to normal sutures continue to grow

unchecked, producing a misshapen head that may affect facial anatomy, as well as brain structure and function. *Secondary* craniosynostosis results from an abnormal progression of brain growth and expansion. Most forms of craniosynostosis are diagnosed in the first several months of life, after the completion of normal cranial molding that is attributed to the birth process.

A large number of craniosynostosis syndromes are possible, depending on the specific bones involved, and the underlying genetic syndrome. In most infants with craniosynostosis that involves only a single suture, the primary concern is cosmetic: surgery will prevent a permanent craniofacial deformity. More severe forms of craniosynostosis, especially when seen as part of a genetic syndrome, are associated with increased intracranial pressure, neurologic deficits, and ophthalmologic problems. Surgical correction of craniosynostosis is usually performed as early as 3-6 months of age to prevent permanent craniofacial deformities and secondary brain abnormalities.

Scaphocephaly (dolichocephaly) is the most common type of craniosynostosis (50%) and results from premature closure of the sagittal suture. The cranial bones continue to grow in an anteroposterior direction and produce an elongated skull with frontal bossing and occipital protrusion (Fig. 34-3). Although the transverse dimension of the head is narrow, head volume is normal; therefore, increased intracranial pressure and neurologic deficits are not usually observed.

A number of surgical procedures have been developed to correct scaphocephaly, the simplest of which is a strip craniectomy, in which the fused sagittal suture is removed and the remainder of the skull is allowed to remodel itself through normal growth. More often, however, complete reconstruction of the infant skull is required to achieve satisfactory cosmetic results.

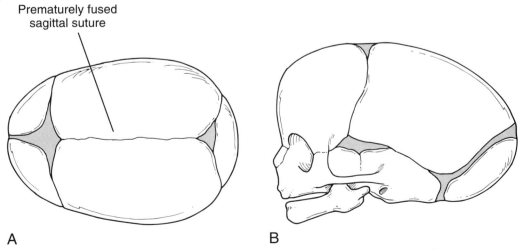

Figure 34-3 **A,** Premature fusion of the sagittal suture produces scaphocephaly. **B,** The result is a misshape head that is narrow and long.

The frontal, parietal, and occipital bones are excised and then trimmed, reshaped, relocated, and affixed with biodegradable plates and screws with the objective of restoring a normal biparietal diameter and reducing the severity of frontal bossing and occipital protrusion.

Plagiocephaly (18%) results from a unilateral synostosis of a coronal suture, producing a unilateral "tilting" forehead and orbital anomalies. *Brachycephaly* (9%) results from a bilateral coronal synostosis and causes a broadened skull and midface hypoplasia. Brachycephaly occurs in Apert's and Crouzon's syndromes. Brachycephaly is associated with a higher incidence of neurologic complications, including increased intracranial pressure, optic atrophy, and mental retardation. These deformities are corrected surgically by advancement of the frontal bone and orbital segments of the skull.

Trigonocephaly (9%) is the result of premature closure of the metopic suture, resulting in a triangular-shaped head and hypotelorism, with an increased risk for associated anomalies of the forebrain. It is often accompanied by additional congenital deformities including cleft palate and urinary tract anomalies. Trigonocephaly is surgically corrected by incision, reconstruction, and replacement of the frontal bone.

Anesthetic Management for Craniosynostosis Repair

Preoperative assessment of the infant presenting for craniosynostosis repair should include a thorough investigation of all comorbidities, congenital anomalies, and the possibility of increased intracranial pressure. In particular, examination of the facial structure and upper airway may reveal the possibility of a difficult intubation. A complete blood count, coagulation studies, and a type-and-crossmatch should be obtained. A preoperative anxiolytic may be indicated in some infants older than 6 months. These infants are usually admitted from home on the day of surgery.

Most infants with craniosynostosis receive an inhalational induction of general anesthesia. A muscle relaxant is administered in the absence of suspicion of a difficult airway. Direct visualization of the larynx may not be possible in infants with syndromic midface hypoplasia. In these cases, fiberoptic bronchoscopy or a lighted stylet is often required to achieve endotracheal intubation via the nasal or oral route, depending on the site of the surgery and the preferences of the surgeon. The endotracheal tube should be carefully taped (or even sutured) in place so as not to become dislodged during critical portions of the surgical procedure.

Maintenance of general anesthesia can be accomplished with any inhalational agent supplemented with opioids and a neuromuscular blocker. Intraoperative nitrous oxide is avoided because of the risk of venous air embolism (see below). Two large-bore (at least 20-gauge) intravenous catheters and an arterial catheter are inserted once the child is anesthetized. The arterial catheter provides continuous assessment of blood pressure and facilitates frequent sampling of blood for hemoglobin and blood gas determinations. In addition, intraoperative examination of the arterial tracing can aid in predicting hypovolemia by noting the presence of respiratory variation as well as a "thinning" of each pulsation. Some centers utilize central venous access for these procedures. A rectal temperature probe is inserted since exposure of the infant and a large amount of administered crystalloid and blood can result in hypothermia. Hypothermia is minimized by using fluid- and blood-warming devices, a forced warm-air blanket over the unexposed portions of the infant, a heating mattress between the infant and the OR table, a heated, humidified breathing circuit, and when necessary, heating the OR environment. An indwelling urinary catheter is inserted and maintained postoperatively.

During the craniotomy portions of the surgical procedure, rapid and significant blood loss is expected as a result of bleeding from the scalp incisions, osteotomy sites, and the dural venous sinuses. Life-threatening hypovolemia may occur because of the small total blood volume of these infants. All attempts should be made to prepare for this eventuality by keeping pace with blood loss, maintaining a hemoglobin level >7.5 mg/dL, and using large amounts of crystalloid to maintain end-organ perfusion. During a large craniofacial reconstruction over several hours, crystalloid amounts exceeding 125 mL/kg are common. Platelets and fresh frozen plasma administration are often necessary after one blood volume of red blood cells has been lost and replaced. Measures to reduce intraoperative blood loss include infiltration of the scalp with local anesthetic containing epinephrine, and preoperative administration of erythropoietin.

Venous air embolism (VAE) has been reported to occur in up to 83% of infants undergoing craniosynostosis repair because the noncollapsible veins of the skull at the operative site are often above the level of the heart and are exposed to air. VAE is reported to be responsible for life-threatening hemodynamic instability and death intraoperatively. Some centers routinely use a precordial Doppler ultrasonic probe to detect the occurrence of a VAE, and will attempt to aspirate air using an inserted central venous catheter. However, this intervention has not been shown to influence outcome during this complication. Although undocumented, at The Children's Hospital of Philadelphia it is believed that continuous and vigilant expansion of the intravascular space using ample crystalloid and blood replacement leads to a clinically low incidence of VAE.

Following craniosynostosis repair, virtually all children are awakened and their tracheas extubated in the OR.

All children are routinely admitted to the intensive care unit because of concerns for ongoing blood loss and hemodynamic instability, and for careful monitoring for upper-airway obstruction which may occur as a consequence of the large amount of swelling that occurs in the facial region. Postoperative mechanical ventilation is not often required.

SUBCUTANEOUS EPINEPHRINE USE IN CHILDREN

Subcutaneous administration of a local anesthetic containing epinephrine is common in pediatric plastic surgical procedures with the goal of attaining epinephrine-mediated vasoconstriction and minimization of blood loss. In anesthetized patients this poses a potential danger because the ability of epinephrine to induce ventricular dysrhythmias is exacerbated in the presence of an inhalational anesthetic agent. The alkane anesthetic agents (i.e., halothane) are characterized by their propensity to "sensitize" the myocardium to endogenous or exogenously administered catecholamines. The ethers (i.e., isoflurane, sevoflurane, desflurane) do not sensitize the myocardium to the same extent as that for the alkane anesthetics.

The maximum amount of epinephrine that may be safely administered is unknown. However, a retrospective study that examined subcutaneous administration of epinephrine in children in the presence of halothane reported that doses up to 15.7 µg/kg did not cause ventricular arrhythmias. Maintenance of general anesthesia with an agent other than halothane would be expected to carry an even greater margin of safety.

ARTICLES TO KNOW

Bosenberg AT, Kimble FW: Infraorbital nerve block in neonates for cleft lip repair: anatomical study and clinical application. *Br J Anaesth* 74:506–508, 1995.

Faberowski LW, Black S, Mickle JP: Craniosynostosis: an overview. *Am J Anesthesiol* 27:76–82, 2000.

Gunawardana RH: Difficult laryngoscopy in cleft lip and palate surgery. *Br J Anaesth* 76:757–759, 1996.

Karl HW, Swedlow DB, Lee KW, Downes JJ: Epinephrine-halothane interactions in children. *Anesthesiology* 58:142–145, 1983.

Meyer P, Renier D, Arnaud E et al: Blood loss during repair of craniosynostosis. *Br J Anaesth* 71:854–857, 1993.

Nicodemus HF, Ferrer MJ, Cristobal VC, de Castro L: Bilateral infraorbital block with 0.5% bupivacaine as postoperative analgesia following cheiloplasty in children. *Scand J Plast Reconstr Surg Hand Surg* 25:253–257, 1991.

Tobias JD, Johnson JO, Jimenez DF, Barone CM, McBride DS: Venous air embolism during endoscopic strip craniectomy for repair of craniosynostosis in infants. *Anesthesiology* 95:340–342, 2001.

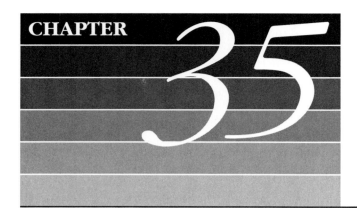

CHAPTER 35

Anesthesia for Pediatric Thoracic Surgery

JOSEPH D. TOBIAS

LYNNE G. MAXWELL

Anesthetic care for pediatric thoracic surgery covers a wide range of ages, concomitant disease processes, and surgical pathology. The clinical scenario ranges from an elective, outpatient procedure on an otherwise healthy patient to an emergent procedure in a neonate with a severe underlying illness or associated congenital heart disease. The surgical pathology may have limited physiological impact on the patient; or in the case of an anterior mediastinal mass, a cystic adenomatoid malformation, or a tracheoesophageal fistula, it may result in significant patient compromise. Newer surgical techniques such as thoracoscopy carry additional anesthetic implications.

This chapter covers general considerations for thoracic surgical procedures in infants and children and anesthetic considerations for common thoracic surgical techniques including thoracoscopy. Unique considerations for the most common neonatal thoracic surgical procedures are discussed, as well as techniques for facilitation of one-lung ventilation.

PREOPERATIVE CONSIDERATIONS FOR THORACIC SURGERY

There exists a spectrum of diseases for which thoracic surgery is required. For example, a child undergoing a thoracotomy and resection of a pulmonary nodule may have no other associated conditions, or may have received large doses of chemotherapy, or may have associated pulmonary parenchymal disease that impacts on the anesthetic management. Therefore, the preoperative history and physical exam should identify acute problems, underlying medical conditions, and previously undiagnosed problems that may impact on perioperative management. Preoperative laboratory evaluation depends more on the clinical status of the patient than the procedure itself. Blood loss is usually minimal during most thoracic procedures; however, because of the proximity to the great vessels and the risk of unintentional damage to these structures, blood should be immediately available in the perioperative period. A blood sample for type-and-crossmatch can be obtained after the induction of anesthesia and the placement of intravascular catheters, provided the blood bank can expedite processing of the specimen. Other preoperative studies, such as pulmonary function tests (PFTs) or an electrocardiogram, are not routinely indicated; rather, they are obtained on the basis of the patient's medical history and the reason for the surgical procedure.

In patients with compromised respiratory function, preoperative PFTs may help to estimate the potential risk for intraoperative or postoperative respiratory complications and to ensure that there has been optimization of preoperative therapy, such as antibiotics for pulmonary infections, and bronchodilators in patients with reactive airway disease. Preoperative PFTs will also help categorize the type of respiratory disease (obstructive or restrictive) and document the response to bronchodilator therapy.

Cognitively normal children are usually able to cooperate with pulmonary function testing when they are older than 6 years. However, there are limited data regarding the ability of PFTs in pediatric patients to guide anesthetic management and postoperative care decisions. For example, in the adult population, a reduction of the forced vital capacity (FVC) or the forced expiratory volume in 1 second (FEV_1) to less than 60% of predicted is associated with postoperative complications such as the need for postoperative mechanical ventilation. However, these same criteria cannot necessarily be applied to pediatric patients, as there are generally fewer comorbidities in children, such as associated cardiac disease, when compared with adults. In a study in pediatric thoracotomy patients, most children had only small decreases in PFTs after thoracotomy. Children with mild to moderate decreases in pulmonary function preoperatively and a small group with severe postoperative impairment of PFTs had no postoperative mortality and no need for prolonged mechanical ventilation. Preoperative PFTs may not identify all patients at risk for post-thoracotomy complications, but they can identify some high-risk patients, which can direct preoperative teaching and optimization of respiratory function. All children undergoing thoracotomy, if old enough, should receive preoperative teaching regarding the use of incentive spirometry and high-flow nebulization therapy.

Systemic disease processes are less frequently encountered in children than adults presenting for thoracic surgery. In oncology patients, however, there may be concerns such as previous chemotherapy or the presence of an anterior mediastinal mass (see Chapter 8). When evaluating the pediatric oncology patient, careful attention should be directed toward his or her disease process and previous chemotherapeutic regimen and the impact these may have on end-organ functioning.

Patients with an anterior mediastinal mass require a meticulous preoperative assessment to evaluate the location and severity of intrathoracic airway obstruction or interference with cardiovascular function before any surgical procedure requiring general anesthesia or sedation. Depending on the location of the mass and the degree of tracheal compression, administration of anesthetic or sedative agents may impair spontaneous ventilation, which may lead to total tracheal or bronchial occlusion and an inability to provide ventilation by facemask or endotracheal tube.

Computed tomography (CT) of the chest may be helpful in planning the anesthetic technique and in evaluating the potential for airway compromise during anesthetic care. Compression of more than 50% of the cross-sectional area of the trachea on CT imaging has been suggested to identify a population at risk of airway collapse during induction of general anesthesia. In patients with this degree of tracheal compression, preoperative therapeutic options include radiotherapy, and/or administration of steroids or chemotherapy to shrink the mass and decrease the severity of the tracheal obstruction. Except in situations in which the size and/or location of the mass is truly life-threatening, many oncologists would prefer to refrain from the use of such preoperative treatments because of their effect on the histopathology or tumor markers in the specimen. However, in patients in whom an anterior mediastinal mass causes a high degree of airway compromise (frequently expressed as an inability to lie supine because of shortness of breath, which is relieved by lying on the side or sitting up), administration of a general anesthetic may be contraindicated. In patients who have additional tissue sites from which to obtain a biopsy (e.g., cervical, axillary, or inguinal lymph nodes), it may be safer to proceed with the patient in a semisitting position using local anesthesia and carefully titrating sedation so that spontaneous ventilation is preserved. If general anesthesia is necessary for biopsy of the chest mass, patients with a significant degree of upper-airway obstruction require an induction technique which preserves spontaneous ventilation. In severe cases, it may be necessary to arrange for standby extracorporeal membrane oxygenation (ECMO) or cardiopulmonary bypass.

With a large mediastinal mass, there may not be airway compromise, but rather obstruction of blood flow from the right or left ventricle. This may be responsible for the cardiorespiratory collapse that has been described during anesthetic induction and loss of spontaneous ventilation. Preoperative echocardiography is suggested to rule out compression of the heart or great vessels by the tumor mass.

In the otherwise healthy patient without signs of airway compromise, several options are available for preoperative anxiolysis. Midazolam, the most commonly administered pediatric premedication, is given orally (0.5 mg/kg up to 10 mg) 15–20 minutes before anesthetic induction. This provides anxiolysis, allowing for easy separation from parents, acceptance of the anesthesia facemask, and facilitates a "gentle" inhalational induction. Additional agents that may be included as part of the premedication process include:

- High-flow nebulization of albuterol and an anticholinergic agent such as ipratropium in children with reactive airway disease
- Corticosteroids for patients with airway reactivity or those having airway procedures that may result in postoperative airway edema
- Gastrointestinal prophylaxis with an H_2-antagonist such as ranitidine and/or a promotility agent such as metoclopramide for patients at risk for pulmonary aspiration
- An antisialagogue such as glycopyrrolate to decrease secretions and blunt cholinergic-mediated airway reactivity.

The last agent is indicated if a ketamine anesthetic is being used to preserve spontaneous ventilation.

ANESTHETIC TECHNIQUES FOR THORACIC SURGERY

Anesthetic induction for thoracic surgery in children can include inhalation with sevoflurane or halothane in nitrous oxide and oxygen, or one of the various intravenous anesthetic agents. Some practitioners prefer halothane because it may preserve spontaneous ventilation better than sevoflurane, which is associated with a high incidence of apnea at moderate concentrations. Halothane should be avoided in patients with known myocardial dysfunction, whether due to mechanical compression or prior chemotherapy. For patients with obstructive airway lesions (tracheal compression from subglottic stenosis or vascular rings), sevoflurane or halothane can be administered with a mixture of oxygen and helium. As helium is less dense than nitrogen, it decreases resistance to turbulent airflow. Once adequate bag–mask ventilation has been demonstrated, either technique can be followed by the administration of a nondepolarizing neuromuscular blocking agent to facilitate tracheal intubation and provide ongoing neuromuscular blockade during the surgical procedure, unless contraindicated by the presence of an anterior mediastinal mass compressing the distal trachea.

Following loss of consciousness, adequate venous access and intraarterial monitoring (when indicated) are secured before the start of the procedure. Since thoracic surgical procedures are performed in the lateral decubitus position, access to the extremities to obtain additional venous sites may be limited once the procedure begins. In patients with normal cardiovascular function, the monitoring of central venous or arterial pressure may offer little additional information to improve or influence anesthetic care. Central venous access is generally reserved for cases in which adequate peripheral intravenous access is unavailable. If central venous access is necessary, internal jugular or subclavian vein cannulation on the side of the procedure is recommended. This avoids the possibility of bilateral pneumothoraces (the surgical pneumothorax induced on the side of the thoracotomy and the unintentional pneumothorax as a complication of the venous access procedure). Invasive hemodynamic monitoring of arterial blood pressure is guided by the clinical status of the child and the specific surgical procedure, and the need for postoperative blood pressure monitoring or blood gas sampling requirements. As many of these procedures use one-lung ventilation (OLV), arterial access may be needed to allow for intermittent sampling of arterial blood gases. Standard intraoperative monitoring as suggested by the American Society of Anesthesiologists includes continuous electrocardiogram, automated noninvasive blood pressure monitoring, pulse oximetry, continuous monitoring of temperature, and end-tidal carbon dioxide ($P_{ET}CO_2$) measurement. As $P_{ET}CO_2$ monitoring may be inaccurate during thoracic procedures because of alterations in deadspace and shunt fraction, especially during OLV, transcutaneous carbon dioxide (TC-CO_2) monitoring may be considered if the continuous monitoring of carbon dioxide is indicated. However, TC-CO_2 technology may not be available in most centers.

ONE-LUNG VENTILATION TECHNIQUES FOR PEDIATRIC PATIENTS

Many thoracic procedures require lung deflation and minimal movement on the operative side while ventilating the nonoperative lung. Even during thoracoscopy, where insufflation of gas may help to collapse the operative lung, OLV should be considered if the surgeon requires additional exposure. In the pediatric patient, there are several options for attaining unilateral lung isolation (Table 35-1).

Double-lumen Endotracheal Tube

A double-lumen endotracheal tube (DLT) is the most common method for attaining lung separation in adult patients. However, the smallest, commercially available DLT is size 26-French, which precludes its placement in children weighing less than 30–35 kg or younger than 8–10 years of age. A DLT provides several advantages over other techniques:
1. Rapid and easy separation of the lungs
2. Access to both lungs to facilitate suctioning
3. The ability to rapidly switch to two-lung ventilation if needed
4. The ability to administer continuous positive airway pressure (CPAP) or oxygen insufflation to the operative lung, when necessary.

Table 35-1   Techniques of One-lung Ventilation in Children

Double-lumen endotracheal tube (DLT)
Univent™ tube (Fuji Systems, Tokyo, Japan)
Selective unilateral bronchial intubation
Bronchial blocker
    Fogarty embolectomy catheter
    Arndt bronchial blocker (Cook Critical Care, Bloomington, IN)
    Pulmonary artery catheter
    Atrial septostomy balloon catheter

Left-sided DLTs are used almost exclusively as they are relatively easy to insert into the appropriate position and their use eliminates the possibility of obstruction of the right upper lobe bronchus given its short distance from the carina. Following placement into the trachea and a 90-degree counterclockwise rotation, the DLT is advanced until resistance is encountered, and the tracheal and bronchial cuffs are inflated. Inflation of the bronchial cuff with 1–2 mL of air prior to advancement may help guide the DLT into the correct position, which is verified by auscultation and direct visualization using flexible bronchoscopy. After attempting placement of a DLT, there are four possible sites where the tube may be incorrectly located, one of which is in the esophagus. The remaining three possibilities are:

1. If the tube has not been advanced far enough, both tracheal and bronchial lumens will open into the trachea.
2. If the tube has been advanced too far, both tracheal and bronchial lumens will open into the left main bronchus.
3. If the tube was unintentionally advanced into the right main bronchus, the bronchial (and possibly the tracheal) lumen will open into the right main bronchus.

The correct position is with the tracheal lumen opening into the trachea above the carina and the bronchial lumen opening in the proximal left main bronchus. After turning the child to the lateral decubitus position, correct DLT positioning should be reconfirmed using auscultation and flexible bronchoscopy. With the smallest DLT (26-Fr), pediatric-sized bronchoscopes with outside diameters of 3.5–3.7 mm or more are too large to fit within the lumen, mandating the use of an ultrathin bronchoscope.

Univent™ Endotracheal Tube

The Univent™ tube (Fuji Systems Corporation, Tokyo, Japan) is a single-lumen endotracheal tube with a moveable bronchial blocker built into its sidewall (Fig. 35-1). The bronchial blocker has a central channel used for suctioning the blocked lung and insufflation of oxygen. After the Univent tube is placed into the trachea, the bronchial blocker is advanced into the main bronchus of the operative lung using flexible bronchoscopy. Advantages of the Univent tube include ease of placement, the ability to easily change from OLV to two-lung ventilation, and (unlike the standard DLT) the ability to pull the bronchial blocker back into its channel and to leave the Univent tube in place for postoperative ventilation.

Univent tubes are available with internal diameters of 3.5 (uncuffed), 4.5, 6.0, 6.5, 7.5, 8.0, 8.5, and 9.0 mm. The outer diameter is larger than that of a conventional endotracheal tube of the same internal diameter (Table 35-2). The internal diameters of the 3.5- and 4.0-mm Univent tubes limit the passage of a standard pediatric bronchoscope with an outside diameter ≥3.5 mm, thereby requiring an ultrathin pediatric bronchoscope to visualize the bronchial blocker.

Selective Endobronchial Intubation

In infants and young children whose small size precludes placement of a DLT or Univent, there are two additional options for OLV: selective endobronchial intubation with a standard endotracheal tube, or placement of a separate bronchial blocker. The major disadvantage of selective endobronchial intubation is that it is

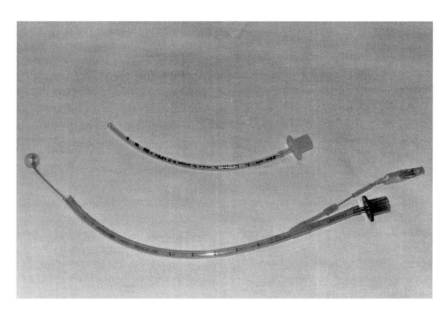

Figure 35-1 A standard 3.5-mm endotracheal tube (top) and a 3.5-mm Univent tube (Fuji Systems, Tokyo, Japan). The Univent is a single-lumen endotracheal tube with a moveable bronchial blocker that is incorporated into a channel alongside the tube. When compared with a standard 3.5-mm endotracheal tube, the 3.5-mm Univent has an outside diameter of 7.5–8.0 mm, making it equivalent to a standard 5.5 to 6.0-mm endotracheal tube.

Table 35-2	Inner and Outer Diameters of Standard and Pediatric Univent™ Endotracheal Tubes	
Inner Diameter (mm)	Outer Diameter of Standard Tube (mm)	Maximum Outer Diameter of Univent (mm)
3.5	4.9	8.0[a]
4.5	6.2	9.0[b]
6.0	8.2	11.5[c]

[a] Corresponds to a 6.0-mm internal diameter standard endotracheal tube.
[b] Corresponds to a 6.5-mm internal diameter standard endotracheal tube.
[c] Corresponds to a 8.5-mm internal diameter standard endotracheal tube.

not possible to quickly change from OLV to two-lung ventilation since it requires repositioning of the endotracheal tube from the bronchus into the trachea and vice versa. Furthermore, with unintentional movement of the endotracheal tube, bronchial extubation may occur. Our practice is to achieve standard endotracheal tube placement in the mid-portion of the trachea and note the depth of insertion at the teeth. The tube is then advanced into the bronchus and the depth of position is again noted. This allows for a measure of the depth of insertion when manipulating the tube during the surgical procedure.

Right-sided endobronchial intubation is easily accomplished blindly because of the anatomic orientation of the right main bronchus at a less acute angle to the trachea. A cuffed endotracheal tube is recommended in children older than 2 years so that an effective seal can be achieved without the need to advance the endotracheal tube deeply into the bronchus, which may occlude the opening to the right upper lobe. Use of a cuff also

facilitates total isolation of the lung, which will help prevent spread of an infectious process to the opposite side. The cuffed endotracheal tube size chosen for endobronchial intubation of either side should be one-half to one size smaller than usual, based on the patient's age. This is suggested because the cuff adds to the outer diameter of the tube, and the diameter of the bronchus is smaller than the trachea.

Blind placement into the left main bronchus is not as straightforward as for the right main bronchus. The usual orientation of the distal bevel of the tube should be reversed (using a stylet) so that the concave segment becomes convex. When this is done, the angle of the bevel will face the patient's right side with the Murphy eye along the left lateral wall of the trachea. Once the endotracheal tube is positioned in the mid-portion of the trachea, the stylet is removed and the tube advanced. Other maneuvers suggested to aid the successful left main bronchus placement include elevating the contralateral shoulder or turning the head to the contralateral side. The authors' preference, and perhaps the easiest technique, is to use bronchoscopic guidance by placement of the flexible bronchoscope through the endotracheal tube and into the left main bronchus, followed by advancement of the tube over the bronchoscope.

Bronchial Blockers

When a DLT or a Univent tube cannot be used because of the patient's size or technical difficulty, a bronchial blocker should be considered. Several different devices can be used as bronchial blockers, including a Fogarty embolectomy catheter and the Arndt (Cook Critical Care, Bloomington, IN) endobronchial blocker (Fig. 35-2). Atrioseptostomy and pulmonary artery catheters have also

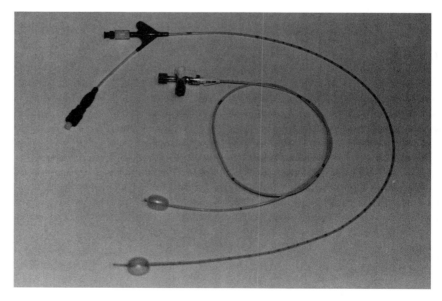

Figure 35-2 A 7-French Fogarty embolectomy catheter (inside) with the 7-French Arndt endobronchial blocker. The Arndt system has a hollow central channel and a wire loop for fiberoptic bronchoscope-guided placement. The Fogarty catheter does not have a central channel, but does have a removable, malleable wire inside which allows for bending or angling the distal end to help with placement.

been used, but they have no advantage over the others and are more expensive. All these devices have a balloon at the distal end that when inflated will occlude the bronchus of the operative lung. Those devices with a central channel provide the advantage of allowing suctioning and application of oxygen and CPAP. Because of the small size of the channel, suctioning will not clear the lung of secretions but it is used to deflate the operative lung and improve surgical visualization. Without the central channel, air or gas cannot exit from the lung once the balloon is inflated; therefore, the lung may not completely deflate and may obscure surgical visualization. In these cases, the lung can be manually compressed by the surgeon during a brief period of apnea and the balloon then inflated prior to the provision of positive-pressure ventilation. Alternatively, the lungs can be ventilated with a mixture of air and oxygen (the concentration of nitrogen up to 70% as tolerated by the patient) and the balloon inflated at the end of exhalation followed by an immediate switch to ventilation with 100% oxygen. By doing this, the lung is filled with an oxygen/nitrogen mixture which allows for the absorption of the nitrogen into the bloodstream. When the patient is ventilated with 100% oxygen the lung will collapse as a result of absorption atelectasis of the blocked lung.

The bronchial blocker can be placed either alongside or through a standard endotracheal tube. When placed through the tube, there will be a decrease in the internal cross-sectional area, thereby increasing the resistance to airflow. The degree to which this occurs depends on the outer diameter of the bronchial blocker and the inner diameter of the endotracheal tube. When placed inside the endotracheal tube, the blocker may be secured easily as it exits the proximal end of the tube. This can be accomplished using a T-piece bronchoscopic airway adaptor with a self-sealing diaphragm (Fig. 35-3). An additional option is to make a small hole in the wall of the proximal endotracheal tube; the bronchial blocker is then passed from the outside to the inside of the tube (Fig. 35-4). The bronchial blocker can then be positioned and secured in place by taping it to the outside of the endotracheal tube, but subsequent manipulation may be more difficult.

The bronchial blocker can be positioned in the main bronchus of the operative side blindly, using fluoroscopic guidance, or most easily and safely under direct vision using flexible bronchoscopy. If bronchoscopy is used, and the bronchial blocker is passed into the lumen of the endotracheal tube, the bronchoscope and bronchial blocker must be small enough so both can pass through the endotracheal tube. The ease with which these instruments can be passed through the tube is greatly enhanced by prior application of a silicone spray. The proper fit of these instruments should be checked before induction of the anesthesia.

If a flexible device such as a pulmonary artery catheter is used, given its flexibility, it may be more difficult to direct it into the bronchus of the operative side. In such a case, the bronchus of the operative lung can be selectively intubated and the catheter passed through the endotracheal tube into the bronchus. The tube is then withdrawn into the mid-portion of the trachea. Alternatively, a wire can be placed through the endotracheal tube in the main bronchus and used as a guide for the catheter as the endotracheal tube is withdrawn back into the trachea. One advantage of the Fogarty catheter is that it contains a wire stylet which allows the catheter to be bent at the tip to facilitate proper angulation into the desired bronchus.

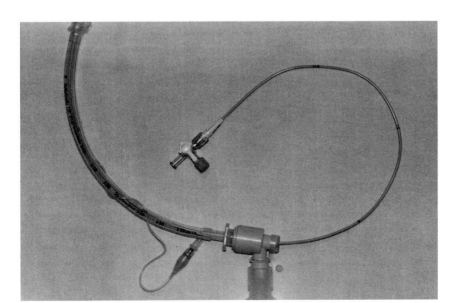

Figure 35-3 Fogarty embolectomy catheter placed through a bronchoscopy adaptor and into an endotracheal tube.

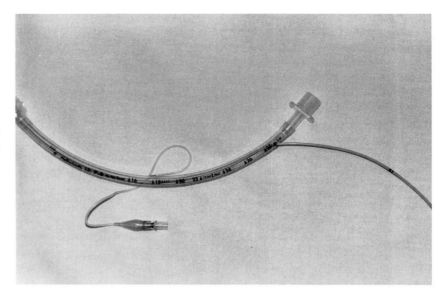

Figure 35-4 Fogarty embolectomy catheter placed through a hole in the side of a standard endotracheal tube.

The Arndt bronchial blocker has an inflatable cuff and a central lumen, through which a wire with a looped end can be passed. The bronchial blocker is passed through a specialized adaptor that is placed at the proximal end of the endotracheal tube. This adaptor contains four ports (Fig. 35-5). The bronchial blocker is passed through the appropriate port and placed at the entrance of the endotracheal tube. The bronchoscope is passed through the port and then through the wire loop at the end of the bronchial blocker. The bronchoscope and bronchial blocker are passed under direct vision as a single unit into the main bronchus of the operative side. The bronchoscope is withdrawn into the trachea and the balloon inflated under direct visualization. When correct placement has been confirmed, the wire loop is removed from the central channel. Once the wire guide is removed from the channel, it cannot be replaced. The Arndt blocker is currently available in three sizes, with the 9-French recommended for endotracheal tubes of internal diameter ≥7.5 mm, the 7-French for 6.0- to 7.0-mm tubes, and the 5-French for 4.5- to 5.5-mm tubes. When the 5-French blocker is placed in an endotracheal tube smaller than 6.0 mm, or a 7-French placed in an endotracheal tube smaller than 7.0 mm, airway pressures will be increased by 3–5 cmH$_2$O.

If a child requires an endotracheal tube smaller than 4.5 mm, it may be necessary to place the bronchial blocker alongside the endotracheal tube if the bronchoscope and

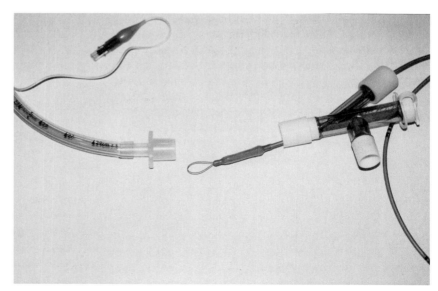

Figure 35-5 Arndt adaptor (Cook Critical Care, Birmingham, IN) with four ports: (1) the top (angled) port for the Arndt endobronchial blocker, (2) the right port for the fiberoptic bronchoscope, (3) the bottom port with a standard 15-mm adaptor to connect to the anesthesia circuit, and (4) the left port for attachment to the endotracheal tube.

bronchial blocker will not fit through its lumen. In such cases, the bronchial blocker can be placed directly into the bronchus on the operative side using direct laryngoscopy, through a rigid bronchoscope or under fluoroscopy. Alternatively, the bronchus on the operative side can be intubated, the bronchial blocker passed through the endotracheal tube, which is then withdrawn and the trachea reintubated, so that the bronchial blocker lies on the outside of the endotracheal tube. The authors' preference is to perform direct laryngoscopy, place the bronchial blocker through the glottic opening and into the tracheal lumen followed by tracheal intubation with the endotracheal tube. A flexible bronchoscope is then placed through the endotracheal tube and the bronchial blocker advanced into the bronchus of the operative lung under direct vision.

Regardless of which catheter or placement technique is chosen, there remains a risk of displacement of the bronchial blocker during the surgical procedure or with repositioning of the patient. If this occurs, the bronchial blocker may occlude the tracheal lumen just beyond the endotracheal tube, resulting in inadequate ventilation. Continuous auscultation of breath sounds on the nonoperative side and monitoring of inflating pressures, respiratory compliance, and end-tidal CO_2 should help to identify this problem rapidly. Clinical experience suggests that inflating the balloon of the bronchial blocker with saline as opposed to air may limit movement and dislodgement during surgical manipulation. Additionally, with any change in the patient's position, correct placement of the bronchial blocker should be confirmed using flexible bronchoscopy.

Anesthetic Management during One-lung Ventilation

After separation of the lungs using one of the techniques described above, general anesthesia is maintained with a combination of intravenous and inhalational anesthetic agents. Hypoxic pulmonary vasoconstriction (HPV) maintains oxygenation during OLV by restricting pulmonary blood flow to the unventilated lung. Therefore, a nonspecific vasodilator (e.g., terbutaline, albuterol, isoproterenol, dobutamine, nicardipine, nitroglycerin, sodium nitroprusside, and inhalational anesthetic agents) may impair HPV and decrease oxygenation. Isoflurane has been shown to have less of an effect on HPV than either halothane or enflurane. The effects of isoflurane, sevoflurane, and desflurane (at minimum alveolar concentrations of 1 MAC) on oxygenation during OLV are similar. Regardless of which inhalational agent is chosen, its expired concentration should be limited to 0.5–1.0 MAC to limit the effect on HPV.

With normal preoperative respiratory function, 100% oxygen may not be required to maintain an adequate arterial oxygen saturation during OLV. Therefore, the fraction of inspired oxygen (F_iO_2) can be decreased as needed by utilization of an air–oxygen mixture. Anesthesia is supplemented as needed with intravenous agents such as fentanyl (3–10 µg/kg), ketamine, benzodiazepines, propofol, and barbiturates, all of which will not affect HPV. Ketamine preserves HPV whereas propofol potentiates pulmonary vasoconstriction during hypoxia.

During OLV, ventilation is maintained with tidal volumes of 8–10 mL/kg and the respiratory rate adjusted as needed to maintain normocarbia. Hypocarbia should be avoided as it may interfere with HPV. The use of OLV may precipitate hypoxemia in children with preexisting lung disease or an alteration of pulmonary function. Treatment of this may require the intermittent provision of two-lung ventilation or a modification of OLV such as oxygen insufflation or application of CPAP to the operative lung. If adequate oxygenation cannot be maintained during OLV using 100% oxygen to the nonoperative side, CPAP of 4–5 cm H_2O can be applied to the operative lung provided that a DLT, Univent, or bronchial blocker with a central channel has been used. Although this will improve oxygenation, it may also distend the operative lung to some degree and impair surgical visualization. The other option to improve oxygenation is the application of positive end-expiratory pressure (PEEP) to the nonoperative side. Applying excessive PEEP to the dependent or nonoperative side may impair oxygenation by decreasing blood flow in the nonoperative lung and shunting blood to the unventilated, operative side. If the above measures fail, it may be necessary to provide intermittent two-lung ventilation.

ANESTHETIC MANAGEMENT FOR THORACOSCOPY

The reports of successes in the adult population combined with ongoing refinements in the technique and equipment have led to the application of thoracoscopy in infants and children. Although initially used to biopsy intrathoracic neoplasms, thoracoscopy has now been applied to more involved surgical procedures including the treatment of empyema, ligation of a patent ductus arteriosus, and anterior spinal fusion. Various anesthetic techniques have been described in the adult population for thoracoscopy, including local anesthetic infiltration and regional anesthetic techniques; however, in the pediatric population, general anesthesia is required.

The anesthetic technique for thoracoscopy in children is straightforward. After the induction of general anesthesia, OLV is established using one of the techniques previously described. The patient is then positioned in either the supine or lateral decubitus position.

After repositioning, the efficacy of OLV is again demonstrated and the endotracheal tube or bronchial blocker repositioned as needed. A needle is inserted through an intercostal space into the interpleural space and an artificial pneumothorax created to allow for better surgical visualization. In some centers, the addition of a low-flow (1 L/min) and low-pressure (4–6 mmHg) CO_2 insufflation into the operative hemithorax is used to prevent overdistention of the lung on the operative side and facilitate surgical visualization. The latter technique is particularly useful if there is inadequate isolation of the two lungs with overflow ventilation into the operative side.

There are a number of possible complications related to the thoracoscopic technique. The hemidiaphragm on the operative side, which has been isolated by the technique of OLV, will move cephalad, so trocar entry below the third or fourth intercostal space may result in hepatic or splenic injury. The artificial pneumothorax may decrease blood pressure and cardiac output by altering preload and/or afterload. In addition, inadvertent gas embolism may occur with the use of CO_2 insufflation. Carbon dioxide embolism can occur from direct injection during insufflation or from the entry of the gas, which is under pressure in the hemithorax, into an internal vessel that has been damaged during the procedure. The physiologic effects and clinical manifestations of gas embolism are dependent on the type and volume of embolized gas, the rate of injection; and the patient's baseline cardiovascular function.

Treatment of inadvertent gas embolism begins with the immediate cessation of insufflation or release of the artificial pneumothorax. Because CO_2 is rapidly absorbed from the bloodstream, the cardiovascular changes usually reverse rapidly. Additional treatment, determined by the severity of the cardiovascular changes, includes the administration of fluids to increase preload and inotropic agents to augment cardiac contractility. With severe cardiovascular compromise, placement of the patient in the head-down, left lateral decubitus position (Durant's maneuver) may displace the gas into the apical portion of the right ventricle, alleviate the air block, and restore cardiovascular function. Aspiration from a central venous catheter should be attempted if one is present.

At the completion of the procedure, the pneumothorax is evacuated and two-lung ventilation is reinstituted. Several large-volume breaths are delivered to ensure reexpansion of the lung on the operative side. In most cases, residual neuromuscular blockade is reversed and the patient's trachea is extubated. A long-acting local anesthetic solution should be infiltrated into the trocar insertion sites. Additional postoperative pain is usually adequately controlled using a combination of oral opioids and nonsteroidal anti-inflammatory agents.

NEONATAL THORACIC SURGERY

Thoracic surgery in neonates is primarily performed to correct congenital lung anomalies. These include congenital cystic adenomatoid malformation (CCAM), congenital lobar emphysema (CLE), pulmonary sequestration, and tracheoesophageal fistula (TEF) with or without esophageal atresia. All except pulmonary sequestration have an association with additional congenital anomalies, including congenital heart disease. TEF is often found as part of the VATER (or VACTERL) syndrome (Table 35-3). These associations necessitate a thorough preoperative evaluation to identify associated congenital anomalies, including echocardiography to rule out congenital heart disease.

When anesthetizing infants with congenital lung lesions, one of the most important preoperative assessments is whether or not positive-pressure ventilation will cause cardiopulmonary deterioration. This could occur in a lesion that contains a bronchial connection to a segment of lung with abnormal parenchyma, such as CLE. In this condition, positive-pressure ventilation results in progressive distention of the abnormal lobe with compression of normal lung due to a ball-valve effect, leading to hypoxemia. Mediastinal shift may torque the great vessels, causing decreased cardiac output and leading to cardiac arrest. If it is not known whether the lesion connects to a bronchus, spontaneous ventilation is indicated until one-lung ventilation of the contralateral lung is achieved or until the chest is opened. Maintenance of spontaneous ventilation is achieved by carefully titrating a combination of intravenous (e.g., propofol, ketamine) and inhalational (e.g., sevoflurane) induction agents, and performing endotracheal intubation without

Table 35-3   VATER and VACTERL Syndromes

VATER
Vertebral anomalies (hemivertebra)
Anal anomalies (imperforate anus)
Tracheoesophageal fistula
Esophageal atresia
Renal anomalies (single, horseshoe, or pelvic kidney) or
    Radial aplasia

VACTERL
Vertebral anomalies (hemivertebra)
Anal anomalies (imperforate anus)
Congenital heart disease (ventricular septal defect, Tetralogy
    of Fallot)
Tracheoesophageal fistula
Esophageal atresia
Renal anomalies (single, horseshoe, or pelvic kidney)
Limb anomalies (radial aplasia, club feet)

muscle relaxation. Placement of a rostrally advanced caudal catheter or thoracic epidural catheter will provide thoracic analgesia and aid in the preservation of spontaneous ventilation.

If the application of positive pressure is not of concern, routine intravenous induction of general anesthesia followed by administration of a neuromuscular blocking agent may be performed. Induction of general anesthesia in neonates is preceded by preoxygenation and administration of intravenous atropine 0.02 mg/kg. Maintenance of general anesthesia is provided by a combination of an inhaled agent, and an opioid or regional anesthetic technique. Nitrous oxide is avoided because of the risk of increasing the size of an air-filled mass.

Postoperative analgesia following neonatal thoracic surgery is best accomplished using an epidural catheter that has been advanced to the thoracic level via the caudal canal (see Chapter 20). Infants who remain on mechanical ventilation can receive a continuous opioid infusion.

Congenital Cystic Adenomatoid Malformation

A congenital cystic adenomatoid malformation (CCAM) is a cystic, solid, or mixed intrapulmonary mass that communicates with the normal tracheobronchial tree. A CCAM may grow large *in utero*, causing hydrops fetalis and even fetal demise. Fetal surgery is now available in some centers for such lesions. More commonly, a CCAM is detected by prenatal ultrasound, does not compromise the fetus, and is surgically excised in the neonatal period. CCAM may be associated with a mediastinal shift and respiratory distress, which necessitates emergent resection. Most cases, however, are asymptomatic and resection is performed as an elective procedure.

There are few unique anesthetic considerations for CCAM resection. Since most are of the solid variety, positive-pressure ventilation can be accomplished without cardiopulmonary compromise. The CCAM is usually "delivered" out of the chest for resection. Therefore, one-lung ventilation is not usually required, but this decision should be made in consultation with the surgeon prior to the case.

Congenital Lobar Emphysema

Congenital lobar emphysema (CLE) consists of an abnormally emphysematous lobe that communicates with the bronchial tree. It occurs, in order of frequency, in the left upper, right middle, or left lower lobes of the lung. Unless the lesion is large or has been expanded by bag–valve–mask ventilation at birth, the infant is usually asymptomatic initially, but may develop wheezing or respiratory distress soon after birth. In the presence of a bronchial connection and abnormal inelastic

parenchyma within the lesion, positive-pressure ventilation may lead to rapid expansion due to a ball-valve effect, with compromise of subsequent ventilation and/or cardiac output. Preservation of spontaneous ventilation or minimizing the inflating pressure prior to establishment of one-lung ventilation will help prevent this complication. If cardiopulmonary deterioration occurs, immediate thoracotomy with delivery of the lobe from the thoracic cavity may be life-saving.

Reinstitution of two-lung ventilation will be necessary prior to closure of the chest wall to ensure the absence of an air leak at the site of the bronchial resection and suture ligature. At the completion of the surgical procedure, the infant's trachea should be extubated to avoid the development of an air leak at the bronchial suture/staple line as a result of positive-pressure ventilation. Continuation of epidural analgesia into the postoperative period will help maintain spontaneous ventilation and avoid opioid administration.

Pulmonary Sequestration

A pulmonary sequestration is a portion of nonfunctioning lung tissue that does not contain a bronchial connection. Its blood supply is derived from anomalous vessels (usually bronchial or aortic) with azygous venous drainage, sometimes below the diaphragm. Pulmonary sequestrations may be intralobar (within the pleura of a lobe) or extralobar (within its own pleura). Both types occur mainly in the lower lobes. Intralobar sequestration may be confused with a CCAM, which may also have aberrant subdiaphragmatic venous drainage. Although frequently diagnosed *in utero*, these lesions are usually asymptomatic at birth, unless the lesion is large and compressing normal lung, or the lesion's blood supply is large and results in high-output cardiac failure. More often, however, these lesions remain asymptomatic until they become infected and present as a pneumonia that is resistant to conservative therapy. Magnetic resonance imaging or angiography may be required to delineate the blood supply and drainage of the lesion prior to surgery. Since a pulmonary sequestration has no bronchial connection, there is no risk of overexpansion of the lesion during positive-pressure ventilation, but one-lung ventilation is usually required to allow the surgeon to carefully identify and ligate the arterial supply and venous draining vessels.

Tracheoesophageal Fistula with or without Esophageal Atresia

Tracheoesophageal fistula (TEF) occurs in approximately 1 in 3000 births, and can exist in five different forms (the sixth is isolated esophageal atresia without a TEF) (Fig. 35-6). Esophageal atresia with a distal TEF

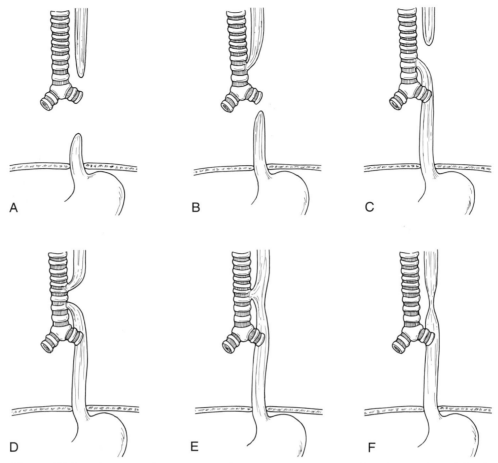

Figure 35-6   The Gross classification of the most common types of tracheoesophageal fistula with esophageal atresia.

(type C) is the most common form (85%). The fistula is usually located slightly above the carina, but may also be found as a "trifurcation" at the carina. Any type of esophageal atresia with or without a TEF is usually diagnosed immediately after birth by the inability to pass an orogastric tube into the stomach. Infants with a TEF are distinguished from those with isolated esophageal atresia by the presence of a gastric air bubble on a radiograph. Since TEF is a component of the VATER or VACTERL syndrome (see Table 35-3), additional congenital abnormalities may be present, including congenital heart disease. Thus, an echocardiogram is indicated in the early newborn period as well as an abdominal ultrasound to detect renal abnormalities. Prior to surgery, these infants are maintained in a head-up position with a suction tube draining the esophageal pouch, to minimize the possibility of aspiration of gastric and nasopharyngeal contents.

TEF is usually repaired within the first several days of life. A thoracotomy incision is performed on the side opposite the aortic arch (since the vast majority of these children have a left-sided arch, a right thoracotomy is performed). The first and most important part of the procedure is ligation of the TEF. The second portion of the procedure involves repair of the esophageal atresia. In most cases, the proximal and distal segments of the esophagus are joined using a primary anastomosis. However, occasionally the two ends are too far apart, and need to be connected by a section of the infant's colon at a later date. In premature infants smaller than 1800 g, the esophageal atresia repair may be deferred until the infant grows larger, because of technical difficulties in these small infants, and nutritional deficiencies that may impair proper healing. In these cases, a gastrostomy tube will be placed after the thoracotomy is closed.

An important consideration during induction of general anesthesia for TEF repair is the avoidance of positive-pressure ventilation. Some of this airflow may exit the trachea through the fistula and cause gastric distention, which may impair subsequent ventilation and lead to the reflux of gastric contents through the fistula into the lungs. Cases of massive gastric distention resulting in respiratory compromise, cardiovascular collapse, and emergency gastrostomy have been reported. Therefore, maintenance of spontaneous ventilation has been recommended until the fistula has been surgically ligated. A combination of intravenous or inhaled anesthetic agents can be administered and titrated to a sufficient depth of anesthesia to allow endotracheal intubation while maintaining spontaneous ventilation. However, because of loss of functional residual capacity and high oxygen consumption in newborn infants, it is unusual to be able to preserve spontaneous ventilation while avoiding hypoxemia. Therefore, many pediatric anesthesiologists will gently provide assisted or controlled positive-pressure ventilation prior to endotracheal intubation, and may even administer a neuromuscular blocker if required. Others recommend a rapid sequence induction of general anesthesia as a first-line approach to minimize possible pulmonary aspiration of secretions retained within the proximal esophageal pouch while avoiding positive-pressure ventilation until the endotracheal tube is advanced distal to the fistula. Awake endotracheal intubation in these infants (and other newborns) is no longer considered to be the standard of care, unless the infant is critically ill.

To minimize gastric inflation following tracheal intubation, the tip of the endotracheal tube should be placed between the fistula and the carina. In most cases, this can be easily accomplished by initially advancing the endotracheal tube into the right main bronchus and gradually pulling it back while auscultating over the left thorax. The endotracheal tube is kept at the position where breath sounds are first heard on the left side, indicating that the tip of the tube is above the carina and probably below the take-off of the fistula. To further minimize the possibility of gastric inflation through the fistula, the bevel of the endotracheal tube is turned anteriorly because the fistula always exits on the posterior surface of the trachea. If the fistula exits the trachea close to the carina, it may be necessary to position the endotracheal tube in the bronchus of the nonoperative lung until the fistula is ligated, at which time the tube is withdrawn above the carina.

In rare cases, when the fistula is large, and high inspiratory pressures are required for lung ventilation (due to the presence of aspiration pneumonia or lung disease of prematurity), adequate ventilation cannot be accomplished until the fistula is obstructed prior to surgical ligation. Several methods have been described to accomplish blockage of the fistula, including insertion of an embolectomy catheter balloon from a cephalad tracheal approach or from a caudad gastric approach if a gastrostomy has been performed (Fig. 35-7). Both approaches require bronchoscopic guidance, and substantial expertise and training.

Intraoperatively, if neuromuscular blockers have not been administered, spontaneous ventilation can be continued until surgical ligation of the fistula, at which time the infant may be safely paralyzed and given positive-pressure ventilation. There are many instances when, during spontaneous ventilation, hypoxemia intervenes because of surgical lung compression on the operative side. It then becomes necessary to begin controlled ventilation to improve ventilatory function and alleviate hypoxemia.

Article To Know

Iannoli ED, Litman RS: Tension pneumothorax during flexible fiberoptic bronchoscopy in a newborn. Anesth Analg 94:512-513, 2002.

Drs Iannoli and Litman reported a near-tragic complication that occurred while performing flexible bronchoscopy in a full-term, 2.1-kg neonate presenting for repair of a tracheoesophageal fistula. After successfully placing an endotracheal tube alongside a balloon-tipped embolectomy catheter they inserted an ultrathin (2.8-mm) bronchoscope into the endotracheal tube with the intent of localizing the TEF. Because of limitations in visualization due to secretions, the authors attempted to displace the secretions by insufflating oxygen (3 L/min) by short bursts through the suction port of the bronchoscope. Shortly after beginning the insufflation, the infant developed a tension pneumothorax, characterized by a tense expansion of the chest and abdomen, inability to deliver positive-pressure ventilation, and bradycardia to 40 beats/min. Upon insertion of an 18-gauge IV catheter into the right chest cavity (at the midaxillary line), there was an audible release of air, after which positive-pressure ventilation was immediately restored and the heart rate increased above 180 beats/min. Once cardiorespiratory stability was ensured, the surgical team performed a percutaneous gastrostomy, ligation of the TEF, primary repair of the esophageal atresia, and placement of bilateral chest tubes. The patient had no further complications, with tracheal extubation occurring on postoperative day 4 and discharge to home in good condition on day 12 of life.

Tension pneumothorax can occur when oxygen is administered under pressure into the respiratory tract. The smaller the cross-sectional area of the endotracheal tube, and/or the larger the external diameter of the bronchoscope, the higher will be the resistance to exhalation. When air entry exceeds air exit, lung hyperinflation, tension pneumothorax, pneumomediastinum, and subcutaneous emphysema can occur. This complication has also been reported during the exchange of an endotracheal tube using a tube exchanger with a central lumen for oxygen insufflation. Oxygen insufflation through a flexible bronchoscope may be safe when introduced into the trachea of a neonate without the presence of an endotracheal tube, but it should not be performed inside a small endotracheal tube that may not allow sufficient egress of the insufflated gas since the maximum pressure achievable within the closed system (i.e., the airways distal to the tip of the bronchoscope) is that proximal to the flow regulator (i.e., 45–50 psi).

Case

A 2-day-old, 2.8-kg, full-term, male infant presents for repair of esophageal atresia and TEF. He has been admitted to the neonatal intensive care unit (NICU) and is breathing spontaneously without oxygen supplementation. He has an oral suction tube draining the proximal esophageal pouch. A 24-gauge intravenous catheter has been inserted into the hand and is running dextrose 10% in water (D10W), with sodium and potassium at a maintenance rate.

Is there anything else you want to know before proceeding with general anesthesia?

Given the association of tracheoesophageal fistula with congenital anomalies, including the VACTER/VACTERL associations, a preoperative echocardiogram is necessary to rule out associated congenital heart disease and a renal ultrasound should be obtained to rule out anatomic abnormalities of the genitourinary system. The chest radiograph should be reviewed looking for signs of hyaline membrane disease and the presence of a stomach bubble which will help define the type of TEF that is present.

What preoperative lab studies are indicated? Are blood products required?

During the first few hours of birth, the infant's electrolytes, and blood urea nitrogen and creatinine levels are reflective of maternal levels; however, most centers will send a preoperative electrolyte panel as well as a complete blood count. Although the administration of blood products is seldom necessary, a type-and-screen should be sent, and blood should be available within a reasonable period of time.

What premedication will you order?

In most cases, no specific premedication is necessary other than atropine to prevent bradycardia associated with laryngoscopy and endotracheal intubation.

How will you induce and maintain general anesthesia?

With a type C TEF, positive-pressure ventilation can result in gastric distention and compromise of cardiorespiratory function. Therefore, if possible, spontaneous ventilation is maintained until the trachea is intubated and the endotracheal tube is positioned below the fistula. This is accomplished by administered general anesthesia with sevoflurane in 100% oxygen. After achieving an adequate depth of anesthesia, intravenous lidocaine 1–2 mg/kg is administered or applied topically to the trachea to blunt any response to placement of the endotracheal tube. Alternatively, a small dose of propofol (1 mg/kg) can be administered prior to laryngoscopy. Once the endotracheal tube is inserted, it is advanced into the main bronchus and then withdrawn until breath sounds are heard in the left axilla. At this point, it is assumed that the tip of the endotracheal tube is just above the carina and distal to the fistula. General anesthesia is maintained with short-acting anesthetic agents (remifentanil and desflurane) with anticipation of extubation after completion of the procedure.

During ligation of the fistula, the infant's oxygen saturation decreases to 86%. What will you do?

The infant's lungs should be ventilated by hand with 100% oxygen and bilateral breath sounds confirmed. It is possible that, during surgical manipulation, the tip of the endotracheal tube has passed into the right main bronchus. It is also possible that the hypoxemia is caused by right lung compression during the surgical technique. Intermittent reexpansion of the lung is then warranted.

Will you extubate the trachea at the end of the case? Why/Why not?

If there is no associated prematurity or lung disease, tracheal extubation should be attempted because it eliminates the concerns regarding positive-pressure ventilation on the suture line. However, the need for reintubation can be equally hazardous as bag–valve–mask ventilation and/or neck extension and laryngoscopy can also disrupt the suture line.

How will you accomplish postoperative pain management?

In many cases, a regional anesthetic technique (epidural or intrathecal opioids) can be supplemented with acetaminophen to provide effective postoperative analgesia and to eliminate the concerns regarding the respiratory depressant effects of intravenous opioids.

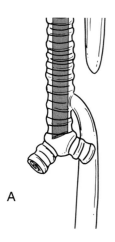
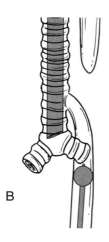
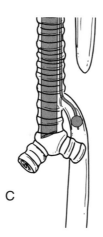

A   B   C

Figure 35-7   Methods for minimizing gastric insufflation in infants with a tracheoesophageal fistula. The tip of the endotracheal tube may be placed distal to the fistula in many cases (**A**). Alternatively, a balloon-tipped catheter may be placed in the fistula via a gastrostomy (**B**) or the trachea (**C**). (Redrawn with permission from Hammer GB: Pediatric thoracic anesthesia. *Anesth Analg* 92:1449-1464, 2001.)

Prior to chest wall closure, the lung on the operative side should be reexpanded under direct vision to minimize the risk of postoperative atelectasis.

Most otherwise healthy infants after TEF repair are awakened and extubated in the operating room at the completion of the procedure. Since manipulation and suture ligation of the fistula may result in the presence of blood in the tracheobronchial tree, the endotracheal tube should be gently suctioned prior to tracheal extubation. On occasion, a small volume of saline irrigation is required to clear the blood and secretions. A theoretical risk in infants that have been extubated is disruption of the esophageal repair from bag-mask ventilation and head extension or laryngoscopy should tracheal reintubation be necessary in the postoperative period. Additional complications of early extubation include hypoxemia and hypoventilation due to airway plugging from secretions, blood, and atelectasis, or inability of smaller infants to maintain increased work of breathing due to decreased compliance related to parenchymal disease.

Infants with evidence of pulmonary aspiration prior to surgery, or those with parenchymal lung disease due to prematurity, may require postoperative mechanical ventilation. In these cases, the endotracheal tube should be positioned in the upper trachea, 1 cm or more away from the fistula site to allow healing of the fistula repair. In addition, the length between the patient's lips and the site of the esophageal repair should be determined to use as a guide for the uppermost limit to which to advance a suction catheter postoperatively to avoid disruption of the esophageal anastomosis.

ADDITIONAL ARTICLES TO KNOW

Baraka AS: Tension pneumothorax complicating jet ventilation via a Cook airway exchange catheter. *Anesthesiology* 91: 557-558, 1999.

Benumof JF, Augustine SD, Gibbons JA: Halothane and isoflurane only slightly impair arterial oxygenation during one-lung ventilation in patients undergoing thoracotomy. *Anesthesiology* 67:910-914, 1987.

Filston HC, Chitwood WR, Schkolne B, Blackmon LR: The Fogarty balloon catheter as an aid to management of the infant with esophageal atresia and tracheoesophageal fistula complicated by severe RDS or pneumonia. *J Pediatr Surg* 17:149-151, 1982.

Hamaya H, Krishna PR: New endotracheal tube (Univent) for selective blockade of one lung. *Anesthesiology* 63:342-344, 1985.

Jones TB, Kirchner SG, Lee FA, Heller RM: Stomach rupture associated with esophageal atresia, tracheoesophageal fistula, and ventilatory assistance. *Am J Roentgenol* 134:675-677, 1980.

Kosloske AM, Jewell PF, Cartwright KC: Crucial bronchoscopic findings in esophageal atresia and tracheoesophageal fistula. *J Pediatr Surg* 23:466-470, 1988.

Pullertis J, Holzman R: Anesthesia for patients with mediastinal masses. *Can J Anaesth* 36:681-688, 1989.

Salem MR, Wong AY, Lin YH, Firor HV, Bennett EJ: Prevention of gastric distention during anesthesia for newborns with tracheoesophageal fistulas. *Anesthesiology* 38:82-83, 1973.

Schwartz N, Eisenkraft JB: Positioning the endotracheal tube in an infant with tracheoesophageal fistula. *Anesthesiology* 69:289-290, 1988.

Shamberger RC, Holzman RS, Griscom NT et al: CT quantification of tracheal cross-sectional area as a guide to the surgical and anesthetic management of children with anterior mediastinal masses. *J Pediatr Surg* 26;138-142, 1991.

Tobias JD, Bozeman PM, Mackert PW, Rao BN: Postoperative outcome following thoracotomy in the pediatric oncology patient with diminished pulmonary function. *J Surg Oncol* 52: 105-109, 1993.

Wang JYY, Russell GN, Page RD et al: A comparison of the effects of desflurane and isoflurane on arterial oxygenation during one-lung ventilation. *Anesthesia* 55:163-183, 2000.

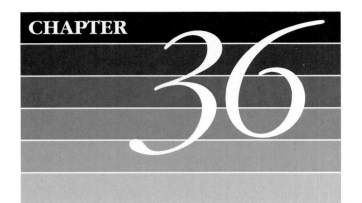

Pediatric Trauma and Burn Management

MONICA S. VAVILALA

Trauma is the leading cause of death in children over 1 year of age and a significant source of morbidity in the pediatric population. The most common cause of pediatric trauma is motor vehicle accidents (MVA), and the most common organ injured is the brain. However, most brain injuries below 4 years of age are attributed to falls or child abuse. Of children who die from the trauma, approximately 50% will succumb at the scene as a result of brain injury, spinal cord injury, or hemorrhage. Some will die within a few hours after the injury from pulmonary aspiration, internal hemorrhage, or central nervous system (CNS) injury. The remainder will die within several weeks of the injury from sepsis, acute respiratory distress syndrome (ARDS), or multisystem organ failure.

BRAIN INJURY

Severe brain injury is the most common cause of death in injured children. An acceleration or deceleration injury can result in a cerebral contusion, which may be located on the same side as the impact, on the opposite side of the impact (contra-coup injury), or both. Blunt or penetrating trauma may cause an intracranial hemorrhage. A tear of the middle meningeal artery produces an epidural hematoma, and trauma that causes rupture of bridging veins results in a subdural hematoma. Any of these aforementioned injuries may produce a condition known as diffuse axonal injury (DAI), which is associated with permanent disability. Children are more susceptible to brain injury because of less CNS myelination, thinner and more compliant cranial bones, and a larger head-to-body ratio than adults.

Contusions and intracranial bleeds are diagnosed by computed tomography (CT). Patients with DAI and abnormal neurologic exams may initially have a normal CT scan. Cerebral edema may be evident on a subsequent scan.

Brain injury should be suspected in children with head trauma despite an absence of neurologic abnormalities. Indicators of occult brain injury include loss of consciousness any time after the event, and multiple episodes of emesis. The multiply injured and sedated child who has undergone tracheal intubation should be considered to have brain injury because of the inability to perform a reliable neurologic exam.

Child Abuse

Brain injury resulting from child abuse is the leading cause of death in children under 1 year of age. This diagnosis should be considered when the child's injuries are out of proportion to the history or the child's developmental level. Common presenting signs include irritability, emesis, depressed consciousness, seizures, and coma. Injuries may be severe and include subdural hematoma, subarachnoid hemorrhage, skull fracture or DAI with or without cerebral edema. While state law varies, all physicians must report suspected child abuse to the proper authorities, or confirm that it was reported in an expedient manner. Careful documentation of intraoperative findings and events is helpful if legal testimony is required at a later date.

Cervical Spine Injury

The incidence of spinal cord injury (SCI) in pediatric trauma is estimated to be 1%. This lower incidence than is normally found in adults may be attributable to the greater flexibility of the pediatric cervical spine. Any child with an unknown mechanism of injury, multisystem trauma, brain injury, or a known injury above the clavicle should be suspected to also have SCI. Approximately 50% of children with SCI have concomitant brain injury. Conversely, the presence of brain injury substantially increases the risk of SCI.

The age of the child will influence the level at which SCI occurs. In younger children, maximal movement occurs between the first and third cervical vertebrae. In children over 12 years of age, this point moves caudad to the C5 or C6 level. Thus, SCI in younger children will usually occur at a more cephalad level than in older children.

Spinal cord injury in children is diagnosed and managed in a similar manner to adults. Radiographs of the cervical spine should include anteroposterior (AP) and lateral views that include the cervicothoracic junction ("swimmer's view"), and views of the odontoid process of C2. However, the cervical spine cannot be "cleared" by radiographic examination without a normal neurologic exam. Therefore, children with normal cervical spine radiographs should be kept immobilized until thoroughly examined because spinal cord instability and neurologic deficits may occur without a fracture. A neurologic deficit without a fracture is called SCIWORA (spinal cord injury without radiologic abnormalities). The term was coined in the pre-MRI era. We now know that most of these children will have demonstrable abnormalities on MRI. SCIWORA can occur in the cervical or thoracic spinal cord. The onset of the neurological deficit is delayed in about one-quarter of children with SCIWORA. These children will initially have minor sensory or motor deficits that progress over time. The majority of SCIWORA injuries are caused by severe flexion or extension injuries of the neck that cause ligamentous stretching or disruption without bony injury. Continued immobilization and cervical spine precautions are necessary because of the possibility of evolving injury.

Other Common Injuries

The majority of thoracic trauma in children consists of blunt injuries caused by motor vehicle accidents. They are the second leading cause of death despite accounting for less than 5% of pediatric trauma. Pulmonary contusion is the most common type of thoracic injury; rib fractures are less common than in adults. As in adults, pneumothorax, hemothorax, and lung laceration are important sequelae of penetrating thoracic trauma.

Blunt abdominal trauma is primarily associated with injuries to the spleen and liver, but renal, pancreatic, and hollow viscous injuries can also occur. A child who was restrained by a lap belt who presents with abdominal or flank ecchymosis (lap belt sign) is likely to have an abdominal injury or a horizontal fracture of a lumbar vertebral body (Chance fracture). Management of solid organ injury is largely expectant unless the child demonstrates hypotension or anemia that does not respond favorably to medical management. Penetrating abdominal injuries usually result in intestinal injury and require surgical intervention. Extremity injuries with or without underlying vascular tears are common in children, as are complex lacerations and growth plate injuries. Simple scalp lacerations may be the cause of a significant amount of blood loss in children.

Attention to the quantity and quality of the urine output is important. Head trauma is associated with development of diabetes insipidus or the syndrome of inappropriate antidiuretic hormone (SIADH) secretion. Direct muscle injury may result in rhabdomyolysis, which may cause myoglobinuria and lead to renal damage.

ANESTHETIC CONSIDERATIONS IN PEDIATRIC TRAUMA

Principles of anesthetic management of pediatric trauma are largely extrapolated from adult data. As a result, there are no standards that are specifically described for pediatric trauma patients. However, the quality of anesthetic management can be maximized by appreciating the physiological and anatomical differences between children and adults. Differences in body size, airway anatomy, normal hemodynamic values, and types of anesthetic equipment will influence pediatric trauma management.

Management

Emergency Management

The initial management period (the "golden hour") after an injury is focused on cardiorespiratory resuscitation and transport to an appropriate facility. As with adult trauma, there is controversy concerning the most appropriate care facility for pediatric trauma victims; outcome studies that provide a definitive answer are lacking. Management during this period is guided by the principles of "advanced trauma life support" (ATLS). The initial approach involves primary and secondary surveys, followed by definitive care of all injuries. The primary survey consists of optimizing oxygenation and ventilation, and stabilizing the cervical spine. All life-threatening conditions are identified and managed simultaneously. Once the primary survey is completed, a thorough head-to-toe examination (secondary survey) is performed to identify all injuries.

Ventilatory Management

The most important initial consideration is assuring the child's oxygenation and ventilation. The lucid and hemodynamically stable child can be managed conservatively; oxygen can be delivered by face mask as required. In the child with depressed consciousness, chin-lift and jaw-thrust maneuvers may be required to maintain upper-airway patency while simultaneously stabilizing the child's neck in the neutral position. Additional interventions may include oropharyngeal suctioning, insertion of an oral airway, cricoid pressure, and positive pressure ventilation using a bag–mask device or following insertion of a laryngeal mask airway (LMA). Poor ventilatory effort despite airway management techniques suggests brainstem or spinal cord dysfunction.

Injured children with a decreasing level of consciousness (Glasgow Coma Scale <9; see below), marked respiratory distress, or hemodynamic instability require endotracheal intubation to maintain a patent airway, to protect against pulmonary aspiration of gastric contents, and to facilitate hyperventilation during management of increased intracranial pressure. Endotracheal intubation is not possible in conscious or even semiconscious children. Unless consciousness is severely depressed, endotracheal intubation is accomplished by induction of general anesthesia using a modified rapid sequence technique with application of cricoid pressure and hyperventilation with 100% oxygen.

There are no universal recommendations regarding the most appropriate approach to maintain cervical spine stabilization during tracheal intubation. As in adults, manual in-line stabilization by an assistant is used most often, with care taken to keep the cervical spine in as neutral a position as possible during direct laryngoscopy or fiberoptic-guided tracheal intubation. Flexible fiberoptic bronchoscopy is possible in pediatric trauma patients but pediatric-sized bronchoscopes are not available in all facilities and often have poor optical resolution and limited suctioning capabilities. Nasotracheal intubation may be easier using fiberoptic bronchoscopy but is contraindicated in patients with basilar skull fractures. Characteristics of a basilar skull fracture include periorbital (raccoon's eyes) and mastoid (Battle's sign) ecchymosis, and CSF drainage from the nose or ear canals.

Additional precautions during airway manipulation are warranted for the pediatric trauma patient with possible head or neck injury. These include Trendelenburg positioning, and keeping the neck in the neutral position at all times to avoid jugular kinking. In infants under 6 months of age, the head and cervical spine should be immobilized using a spine board with tape across the infant's forehead, and blankets or towels around the neck. In older infants and children, the head should

---

Article To Know

Gausche M, Lewis RJ, Stratton SJ et al: Effect of out-of-hospital pediatric endotracheal intubation on survival and neurological outcome: a controlled clinical trial. JAMA 283:783–790, 2000.

Tracheal intubation (TI) of children is commonly performed in the field by emergency medical technicians. The advantage of TI over bag–mask ventilation (BMV) was not studied until this randomized, controlled, prospective trial in children requiring prehospital airway management (including trauma). The investigators compared survival and neurological outcomes of pediatric patients randomized to BVM or BVM + TI in two large, urban, rapid-transport emergency medical services (EMS) systems. The investigators enrolled 830 children under 12 years of age, or estimated to weigh less than 40 kg, who required airway management; 820 were available for follow-up. Outcome variables included survival to hospital discharge and neurological status at discharge from the acute care hospital. There was no significant difference in survival between the BVM group (123/404; 30%) and the TI group (110/416; 26%) (odds ratio [OR], 0.82; 95% confidence interval [CI], 0.61–1.11) or in the rate of achieving a good neurological outcome (BVM, 92/404 [23%] vs TI, 85/416 [20%]) (OR, 0.87; 95% CI, 0.62–1.22). Thus, prehospital TI did not improve survival or neurological outcome of pediatric patients when compared to BMV in an urban EMS system.

be immobilized in the manner described above or by using a small rigid cervical collar. Children over 8 years of age require a medium-sized cervical collar. In infants with a prominent occiput, a roll placed under the shoulders provides neutral alignment of the spine and avoids excessive flexion that often occurs in the supine position. These maneuvers will help prevent further cervical spine injury. A rigid collar will effectively prevent cervical spine distraction. A soft collar will permit a 5- to 7-mm distraction of the cervical spine during laryngoscopy.

Cardiovascular Management

Primary cardiac arrest is unusual in pediatric trauma unless the child has suffered direct cardiothoracic trauma. Commotio cordis is the term given to the development of ventricular fibrillation after a sudden, intense, nonpenetrating impact on the chest wall over the anatomic location of the left ventricle. Animal studies demonstrate that the timing of this impact in relation to the cardiac cycle (between the QRS complex and the T wave) is crucial for development of this fatal complication.

Pediatric trauma more commonly causes shock, which is usually classified as hypovolemic, cardiogenic, neurogenic, or septic. The traumatized, hypovolemic child presents unique physiologic patterns, in that children tend to compensate for blood loss and may retain normal vital signs until 30–40% of their blood volume has been lost. In other words, blood pressure may remain normal during clinically significant anemia and hypovolemia. The systolic and diastolic blood pressures may be maintained by vasoconstriction and the pulse pressure may be narrow, rather than wide, as observed during general anesthesia and neurogenic shock (owing to loss of arterial and venous peripheral tone). Hypotension occurs when shock becomes uncompensated. Bradycardia in this setting is an ominous sign as heart rate is a major component of cardiac output in small children.

Brain injury in pediatric trauma patients may directly cause hypotension. The hypertensive component of Cushing's triad may not be present and cerebral perfusion pressure (CPP; mean arterial pressure minus ICP or CVP, whichever is higher) may not be maintained. The minimum CPP necessary to meet metabolic demands in infants and children has not been established and is largely extrapolated from adults. In children under 6 years of age, cerebral blood flow averages 106 mL per 100 g of brain tissue, and cerebral metabolic rate averages 5.2 mL/min per 100 g of brain tissue. This is in contrast to 58 mL and 3.3 mL per 100 g of brain, respectively, in the adult, and indicates greater cerebral blood flow and metabolic requirements in children. As cerebral autoregulation can also be impaired in children with brain injury, systemic blood pressure should be maintained above normal in the absence of ICP monitoring.

With increased ICP (>20 mmHg), CPP less than 50 mmHg is associated with a poor outcome. Additional risk factors in brain-injured children include $Pa_{O_2} < 60$ mmHg, $Pa_{CO_2} < 25$ mmHg or >45 mmHg, and a systolic blood pressure <90 mmHg.

Vascular access is an important and challenging component of pediatric trauma management. A 22-gauge or larger peripheral intravenous catheter will suffice for induction of general anesthesia but may not be adequate for resuscitation of the child with major trauma. In the latter scenario, at least two large-bore intravenous catheters are recommended. Saphenous veins are larger than the peripheral veins of distal extremities and thus are commonly used to secure vascular access, either percutaneously or by surgical exposure. In an emergent situation, if peripheral access is unobtainable after two rapid attempts, an intraosseous (IO) line should be inserted using any large-bore or bone marrow needle (Fig. 36-1). Any nontraumatized long bone may be used. The preferred site is the anteromedial surface of the proximal tibia, 2 cm below and 1–2 cm medial to the tibial tuberosity on the flat part of the bone. Other possible sites of insertion include the distal femur 3 cm above the lateral condyle in the midline, and the medial surface of the distal tibia 1–2 cm above the medial malleolus. The insertion technique entails the advancement of a large-bore needle until the periosteum of the bone is contacted. With a twisting, boring motion the needle is advanced until it is felt to penetrate into the marrow

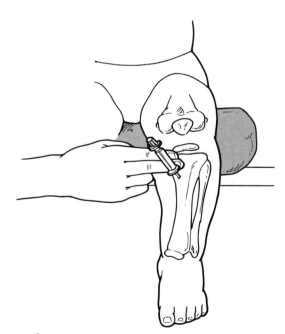

Figure 36-1 Intraosseous vascular access using the anteromedial portion of the proximal tibia. (Reproduced with permission from Siberry GK, Iannone R, Childs B: *Harriet Lane Handbook*, 15th edn, Mosby, Philadelphia, 2000.)

cavity by a loss of resistance. Negative aspiration of marrow does not preclude use of the intraosseous line provided that infused fluids do not extravasate into the subcutaneous tissues. If marrow is obtained, it may be sent for routine lab investigation and type-and-crossmatch. Any type of crystalloid or colloid solution may be infused into the marrow, and higher than normal infusion pressures may be required. This route of access is temporary until more definitive access can be secured.

Central venous catheters are acceptable routes of venous access in children (see Chapter 38). The femoral vein is preferred in children with head or neck injuries but should not be used when inferior vena cava injury is suspected as a result of abdominal trauma.

Resuscitation fluids for pediatric trauma patients consist of isotonic crystalloids and blood products as necessary. Hypotonic dextrose-containing crystalloid solutions should be avoided. The role of colloid administration is controversial. Hydroxyethyl starch administration is discouraged because it may exacerbate a coexisting coagulopathy when administered in amounts greater than 20 mL/kg. Hypertonic saline lowers intracranial pressure and improves cerebral blood flow in patients with brain injury: further study is ongoing to determine its role in pediatric trauma resuscitation.

Neurologic Assessment

In infants, levels of consciousness are described by a Glasgow Coma Score with a modified verbal component to allow a developmentally appropriate evaluation (Table 36-1). The trend in this score is more important than the absolute number. Pupillary examination is also an important component of the neurologic assessment. For example, pinpoint pupils indicate pontine herniation and dilated pupils suggest uncal herniation.

Exposure

In the final phase of the primary survey, the entire body must be examined while maintaining normal body temperature. The child's immediate environment should be warmed by increasing the room temperature, using overhead warming lights and forced warm-air blankets.

Preoperative Considerations

Anesthesiologists should be acquainted with their institution's trauma evaluation protocol. In most centers, the following tests are obtained immediately upon arrival or shortly thereafter: radiographs of the cervical, thoracic, lumbar and sacral spine, chest, abdomen and pelvis, and ultrasound of the abdomen. CT of the head and abdomen are performed shortly after initial stabilization. Serial complete blood counts, coagulation studies, electrolytes, and urinalysis are also obtained. If possible, the results of these tests should be known prior to proceeding with surgery. A type-and-crossmatch is obtained in all children with major trauma or those with

Table 36-1   Glasgow Coma Scale Modified for Infants

Glasgow Coma Scale		Infant's Coma Scale	
Response	Score	Response	Score
Eye opening		*Eye opening*	
Spontaneous	4	Spontaneous	4
To speech	3	To speech	3
To pain	2	To pain	2
None	1	None	1
Best motor response		*Best motor response*	
Obeys verbal command	6	Normal spontaneous movements	6
Localizes pain	5	Withdraws to touch	5
Withdraws in response to pain	4	Withdraws to pain	4
Abnormal flexion	3	Abnormal flexion	3
Extension posturing	2	Extension posturing	2
None	1	None	1
Best verbal response		*Best verbal response*	
Oriented and converses	5	Coos, babbles, interacts	5
Confused	4	Irritable	4
Inappropriate words	3	Cries to pain	3
Incomprehensible sounds	2	Moans to pain	2
None	1	None	1

Glasgow Coma Scale scores of 13–15, <13, and <9 represent, respectively, mild, moderate and severe neurologic insult.
Reproduced with permission from Siberry GK, Iannone R, Childs B: *Harriet Lane Handbook*, 15th edn, Mosby, Philadelphia, 2000.

minor trauma who are expected to have significant blood loss during surgery.

A focused preanesthetic history should elicit information regarding allergies, medications, time of the last meal, and events (AMPLE) surrounding the injury. A general principle is that the true fasting interval is the time between the most recent meal and the traumatic event. Patients who have fasted for at least 8 hours from the time of the injury are still considered to be at risk of pulmonary aspiration of gastric contents during induction of general anesthesia because gastric emptying may be delayed by a variety of factors that include catecholamine release, opioid administration, and direct abdominal trauma.

Children experience pain and anxiety following trauma. For many years, these two aspects of medical care were neglected because of fear of the adverse effects of sedatives and opioids in the pediatric population, but hemodynamically stable children should receive sedation and analgesia in the emergency department. Unstable children who receive only muscle relaxants to facilitate tracheal intubation may have recall of the event.

Anesthesia Techniques

In pediatric trauma, general principles of airway management are followed, with the focus on the possibility of a difficult ventilation or intubation (see Chapter 18). Preoxygenation may be difficult to achieve in the frightened or agitated child. One has to weigh the risks and benefits of forcing preoxygenation in this setting. As in adult trauma, an intravenous induction technique is preferred. The choice of induction agent will depend largely on the child's clinical condition. For example, ketamine should not be used in a child with brain injury and increased intracranial pressure. Etomidate 0.3 mg/kg may be preferable for a child who is suspected to be hypovolemic. Intravenous lidocaine 1.5 mg/kg, used in addition to a sedative hypnotic agent, may help achieve sufficient anesthetic depth without compromising cerebral perfusion pressure. Succinylcholine is the neuromuscular blocker of choice to rapidly obtain endotracheal intubation. In children under 1 year of age, its use is preceded by administration of atropine to prevent bradycardia. In children over 1 year, atropine may be administered if decreased cardiac output is anticipated. Succinylcholine causes an increase in intracranial pressure that is transient and can be attenuated by hyperventilation, intravenous lidocaine, and mannitol administration. Rocuronium 1.2–1.6 mg/kg is an alternative to succinylcholine but will entail a greater duration of action.

The clinical condition of the child will determine the choice of agents for maintenance of general anesthesia. A balanced anesthetic technique is most often selected. Nitrous oxide is avoided because of concern of its diffusion into closed spaces and exacerbation of pneumocephalus, pneumothorax, or bowel distention, and the possibility that it may increase intracranial pressure. Isoflurane and sevoflurane have a favorable cerebrovascular profile (less cerebrovascular dilation, and preserved cerebral autoregulatory capacity) compared to halothane. Intravenous fentanyl 2–20 µg/kg, or morphine 0.1–0.2 mg/kg, may be administered as a bolus during induction of general anesthesia, or in divided doses or as a continuous infusion (fentanyl 0.02–0.04 µg/kg/h; morphine 10–40 µg/kg/h) during maintenance. Remifentanil has the advantage of being more easily titratable during periods of hemodynamic instability. Neuromuscular blockade can be achieved with any nondepolarizing neuromuscular blocker. In pediatric trauma, it is important to consider possible awareness as the child's depth of anesthesia is balanced with his or her hemodynamic status.

Monitoring

Direct arterial access is recommended for continuous monitoring of blood pressure and facilitation of blood sampling, and central venous pressure monitoring can be used to detect trends in intravascular volume status. Urine volume and content is continuously monitored. Continuous intracranial pressure monitoring has not been subjected to a randomized controlled trial, but it can be useful for detecting and monitoring increased intracranial pressure. Retrograde jugular venous bulb monitoring can estimate global cerebral oxygenation and may be used as a guide to hyperventilation therapy in children with increased intracranial pressure. However, this modality is used in only a few centers in the United States. Continuous temperature monitoring is essential because of the high likelihood of hypothermia in trauma patients. Intentional hypothermia as a brain protection strategy is not currently advocated in children.

Glucose

When cerebral ischemia occurs in the presence of hyperglycemia, anaerobic metabolism produces accumulation of excess lactic acid, which can worsen neurologic injury. In a retrospective study of the relationship between serum glucose on admission and outcome following brain injuries in children, hyperglycemia (glucose >250 mg/100 mL) was associated with worse outcomes. There are no prospective controlled trials that have determined the relationship between serum glucose and outcome in pediatric trauma patients. However, sustained hyperglycemia should be treated aggressively.

PEDIATRIC BURN MANAGEMENT

Burns are the leading cause of in-home fatalities during childhood. The type of burn depends on the child's developmental status. For example, infants too young to walk are burned when they are placed in contact with hot surfaces, or as a result of a hot liquid spill. A mobile toddler, on the other hand, can pull a cup containing hot liquid off a table, chew on an electrical cord, and accidentally step on hot coals. Adolescents may experiment with gasoline and fire. Overall, 70% of pediatric burns are associated with hot liquids.

Classification

Burns are classified according to percentage body surface area (BSA) and depth. The total percentage BSA derives from the "Rule of Nines," which is different in children than in adults since the pediatric head accounts for a larger percentage of BSA (Fig. 36-2). The depth of the burn is classified as first-, second-, or third-degree

Table 36-2 Classification of Burns by Depth	
Classification	**Depth and Description**
First-degree	Only epidermis involved; painful and erythematous
Second-degree	Epidermis and dermis involved, but dermal appendages spared
	Superficial 2nd-degree burn is blistered and painful
	Any blistering qualifies
	Deep 2nd-degree burn may be white and painless, require grafting, and progress to full-thickness burn with wound infection
Third-degree	Full-thickness burn involving epidermis and all of the dermis, including dermal appendages
	Leathery and painless
	Requires grafting

Reproduced with permission from Siberry GK, Iannone R, Childs B: *Harriet Lane Handbook*, 15th edn, Mosby, Philadelphia, 2000.

(Table 36-2). Morbidity and mortality increase with increasing size and depth of the burn. Inhalational smoke injury and early shock are additional risk factors for death from burns. The prognosis of patients with a greater than 50% burn is poor, yet patients with a 90% burn have survived. Severely burned patients may survive the initial insult, only to die later of infection or other complications. In pediatric patients, survival increases with increasing age.

A "major burn" is defined as: (1) a second-degree burn >10% BSA (20% for children over 10 years); or (2) a third-degree burn >5% BSA; or (3) a second- or third-degree burn of the hands, feet, perineum, or major joints, electrical or chemical burns, inhalational injury, or burns in patients with preexisting medical conditions. Following initial resuscitation, children with major burns should be transferred to a regional burn center for further management (Box 36-1).

Acute Management of Pediatric Burns

Respiration

The burned child is immediately treated by ensuring adequate oxygenation, ventilation, and circulatory stability. Wound care is deferred until after the acute resuscitation. Endotracheal intubation is indicated if there is evidence of inadequate ventilation, singed nasal hair, facial or upper airway edema, hoarseness, or stridor. Early tracheal intubation is advocated prior to development of significant facial and airway edema. In adults, awake intubation is preferred if upper airway edema or injury is suspected, but children will require tracheal intubation following induction of general anesthesia.

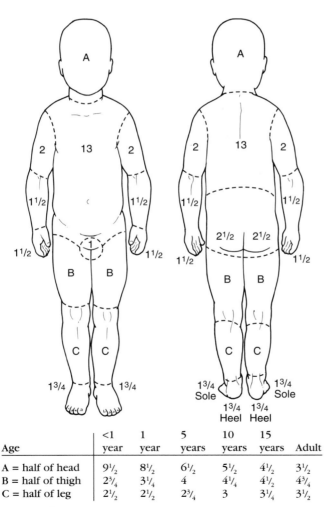

Age	<1 year	1 year	5 years	10 years	15 years	Adult
A = half of head	$9\frac{1}{2}$	$8\frac{1}{2}$	$6\frac{1}{2}$	$5\frac{1}{2}$	$4\frac{1}{2}$	$3\frac{1}{2}$
B = half of thigh	$2\frac{3}{4}$	$3\frac{1}{4}$	4	$4\frac{1}{4}$	$4\frac{1}{2}$	$4\frac{3}{4}$
C = half of leg	$2\frac{1}{2}$	$2\frac{1}{2}$	$2\frac{3}{4}$	3	$3\frac{1}{4}$	$3\frac{1}{2}$

Figure 36-2 Body surface area percentage distribution of burns in the pediatric population. (Reproduced with permission from Siberry GK, Iannone R, Childs B: *Harriet Lane Handbook*, 15th edn, Mosby, Philadelphia, 2000.)

Box 36-1 American Burn Association (ABA) Criteria for Transferring a Burned Child to a Regional Burn Center

Partial-thickness burns >10% total BSA

Burns involving the hands, feet, face, perineum, genitalia, or major joints

Electrical, chemical, or inhalation burns or injuries

Any third-degree burn

Any indication that the injury was deliberately inflicted or if there is any question as to the ability of at-home care provision

Significant concomitant injuries, such as smoke inhalation, fractures, or head trauma

Any child with a preexisting medical disorder that will affect burn treatment

Burned children in hospitals without qualified personnel or equipment for the care of children

Reproduced from the website of the American Burn Association: www.ameriburn.org/pub/guidelinesops.pdf

Respiratory failure and asphyxia may result from inhalation of toxic fumes, chemical injury from smoke, upper-airway edema and, in the later stages, eschar formation on the chest wall. Inhalation of toxic chemicals can cause airway hypersecretion, irritability, capillary leaking, and pulmonary edema. Clinical manifestations include hypoxia, hypercapnia, dyspnea, bronchospasm, cough, rhonchi, and stridor. Circumferential burns of the chest wall can cause restrictive respiratory failure for which an escharotomy may be required.

Carbon monoxide (CO), which is a prominent byproduct of combustion, and present in smoke, is thought to be responsible for up to 80% of deaths from smoke inhalation. CO has a 250 times greater affinity for hemoglobin than oxygen, displaces oxygen from hemoglobin binding sites, and shifts the oxygen dissociation curve to the left. Although the arterial partial pressure and saturation of oxygen is read as normal, the oxygen content of the blood is decreased. Thus, carboxyhemoglobin must be specifically measured as a component of blood gas analysis. Clinical symptoms are directly proportional to CO levels (Table 36-3). Low CO levels cause mild CNS symptoms; high CO levels cause coma. The 4-hour half-life of CO can be decreased to 40 minutes with 100% oxygen therapy. Severe CO intoxication can be treated with hyperbaric oxygen therapy; however, there is little evidence that it prevents permanent neurological deficits.

Smoke from the burning of plastic materials with elevated nitrogen content may contain large amounts of hydrogen cyanide. Children who sustain cyanide poisoning as a result of inhalational injury may succumb from

Table 36-3 Carbon Monoxide Levels and Clinical Symptoms

CO Level	Symptoms
<20%	Headache
30–50%	Irritability, confusion, visual disturbances, emesis, fainting
50–80%	Convulsions, respiratory failure, coma, death

asphyxiation and should be treated with sodium thiosulfate or sodium nitrite if seizures, cardiopulmonary failure, or persistent lactic acidosis occurs.

Circulation, Hemodynamics, and Intravascular Volume Resuscitation

Intravenous fluids are indicated with a burn >10% BSA. Several formulas have been proposed to estimate fluid requirements in children. In one example, the Parkland formula, Lactated Ringers solution is administered at the child's maintenance rate plus 4 mL/kg per 1% total BSA burn for the initial 24 hours. At some institutions, half the total fluid is given over the first 8 hours and the remainder is given over the next 16 hours; however, it is safe and perhaps preferable to accelerate this resuscitation. Regardless of the formula used, it is important to remember that fluid requirements are greatest during the first 24 hours after injury and that formulas provide only estimates of need. The rate of urine output should be maintained at a minimum of 0.5–1.0 mL/kg/h. Oliguria in burned patients is usually the result of inadequate fluid resuscitation and not renal insufficiency.

After the first day, fluid losses occur by evaporation through denuded skin and as a component of the burn exudate. Maximum weight gain due to edema occurs on the second or third day and is followed by a diuresis and return to normal weight by day 14. Protein loss through the burn exudate occurs until all wounds are grafted and healed. During graft harvesting, the surgeon may infuse crystalloid solution under the donor skin to facilitate harvesting. The amount infused can sometimes be large and should be accounted for in the total volume of fluids given. The use of colloids as a component of fluid resuscitation is controversial. In children, albumin administration increases the serum albumin level, but no data exist to support its routine administration.

Other Organ Systems

During the acute phase of injury, the child with a major burn is at high risk of renal failure secondary to rhabdomyolysis, myoglobinuria, and hypotension. Neurologic dysfunction can result from hypoxia, hyperthermia, electrolyte imbalance, and hypertension.

Hematologic abnormalities may include anemia from red cell hemolysis and decreased red cell survival, thrombocytopenia, development of a hypercoagulable state, and disseminated intravascular coagulation. The burned child is susceptible to development of sepsis secondary to the loss of skin and intestinal mucosal barriers, and an impaired immune response. Liberal application of topical antibiotic ointment has decreased the mortality from infection. Children with major burns are at risk of hypothermia from evaporative losses through large areas of exposed skin. Duodenal and gastric stress ulcers may cause chronic occult bleeding, so H_2-antagonists are routinely administered. Nearly all patients will develop an ileus and will require gastric decompression with a nasogastric tube.

Electrical Burns

Patients with electrical burns may sustain deep tissue injuries despite a superficial point of current entry on the skin. Seemingly superficial and small injuries may overlie devitalized muscle. Electrical burns can also cause dysrhythmias and brain or spinal cord injury.

Hypermetabolism: Stress Response and Major Organ Effects

After the acute phase of the burn injury, a hypermetabolic state develops and lasts until all wounds are healed (possibly many months). The degree of hypermetabolism depends on the severity of the burn. The mechanisms involved in this response are complex and may include increased adrenergic output, gut-induced endotoxemia, and endogenous resetting of energy production. The hypermetabolic state manifests as increased catabolism, nitrogen wasting, hyperthermia, hyperglycemia, increased CO_2 production, and increased oxygen utilization. Approximately 8 hours after the burn the hypothalamic-pituitary thermoregulatory set point resets to a higher than normal body temperature. During the hypermetabolic phase, high caloric nutritional support will help prevent protein breakdown and promote wound healing. Since hypermetabolism increases oxygen consumption and CO_2 production, minute ventilation should be increased, and a warm ambient temperature ($\geq 30°C$) should be maintained to help prevent catabolism due to hypothermia.

ANESTHETIC MANAGEMENT OF THE BURNED CHILD

Burns >30% BSA should be excised and grafted early after injury. Following initial grafting, extremely painful dressing changes are required once or twice daily. Split-thickness skin grafts and scar revisions may occur weeks or months after the initial injury. The most important anesthetic implications include airway management, vascular access, blood loss, and provision of adequate analgesia.

Preoperative Evaluation

The preoperative evaluation involves assessment of the degree and location of the burns, physiologic abnormalities, and analgesic requirements. A thorough examination of the face, neck, and oral airway must be performed to estimate the likelihood of a difficult airway, and the presence of other injuries must be recognized. Premedication with a benzodiazepine should be given prior to transporting a child to the operating room. Tolerance to anxiolytics and sedatives develops soon after burn injury. Because these patients need increased nutritional support, fasting intervals for nasogastric feeds can be shortened to 3–4 hours prior to surgery if the trachea is not intubated and 1 hour if the trachea is intubated.

For patients requiring extensive excision and grafting, early tracheal intubation is preferred because of the potential for fluid shifts and blood loss, and the need for controlled ventilation due to the hypermetabolic state. Fiberoptic intubation may be necessary for children with face and neck contractures who present weeks or months after the initial burn. If the contractures limit tracheal intubation, these should be surgically released during anesthesia with mask ventilation. If the patient has been previously ventilated, and has developed acute respiratory distress syndrome, the ventilator on the anesthesia machine may not be capable of delivering adequate tidal volumes, inspiratory pressures, or positive end-expiratory pressure (PEEP). Thus, a more sophisticated ventilator may be necessary in the OR.

Monitoring

Depending on the extent and location of the burn, it may be necessary to place the blood pressure cuff over a burned area, and use needle electrodes for electrocardiographic monitoring. In addition to standard monitoring, including urine output, the use of an arterial catheter and/or central venous access can facilitate management of these children. Measurement and maintenance of temperature is essential since burned children are susceptible to hypothermia. The operating room should be warmed to at least 25°C, all preparatory and intravenous solutions should be warmed, inspired gases should be heated and humidified, and all exposed body surfaces covered.

Anesthetic Technique

The choice of anesthetic induction agent will depend on the clinical condition of the child. Thiopental or propofol are acceptable if the child is normovolemic. Ketamine or etomidate are suitable alternatives if the child is hypovolemic. The choice of neuromuscular blocker used to intubate the trachea in burned patients depends on the time from the injury and concern for a difficult airway. Following the initial 24-hour post-burn period, administration of succinylcholine can cause significant hyperkalemia secondary to up-regulation of extrajunctional acetylcholine receptors on injured or burned muscle. This risk peaks between 5 days and 3 months and may persist for up to 2 years after the initial injury or until the patient has regained adequate muscle function. Patients with burns exhibit resistance to the nondepolarizing neuromuscular blockers, so relatively larger doses are required to achieve relaxation. This effect is usually seen in patients with >30% of their body surface area burned, and is most prominent 1–2 months after the burn. This resistance is thought to be caused by changes in postjunctional acetylcholine receptors. One exception to this is mivacurium, where normal doses result in adequate relaxation. This is thought to be caused by a decrease in circulating plasma cholinesterase in burned children, which increases the effective concentration of mivacurium that reaches the muscle receptors. Maintenance of general anesthesia can be accomplished using a balanced technique with no preference for any inhalational agent. Titration of opioid should be based on the expectation of rapidly acquired tolerance. Anesthesiologists should anticipate large opioid needs during the intraoperative and postoperative periods. For example, it is not unusual for children to require intravenous morphine doses ≥ 0.5 mg/kg/h.

The debridement procedure commonly causes extensive blood loss because of the relatively large surface area of denuded skin from both the donor and graft sites. Once the burn eschar is excised and the large capillary bed is exposed, bandages soaked in epinephrine are often placed over the wound to decrease bleeding. Nevertheless, blood loss is frequently underestimated during these procedures. Hence, blood transfusions are usually necessary during surgical excision of the burn and may even need to be started prior to surgery.

Red blood cell transfusion is indicated when oxygen-carrying capacity is inadequate to meet the metabolic demands of the tissues. The maximum allowable blood loss is determined using the estimated blood volume (EBV) of the child, which varies with age (see Chapter 16). Prior to the start of surgery, the maximum allowable blood loss (MABL) is calculated as follows:

$$\mathrm{MABL} = \left[\frac{(\mathrm{hematocrit}_{initial} - \mathrm{hematocrit}_{target})}{\mathrm{hematocrit}_{average}} \right] \times \mathrm{EBV}$$

Most centers use a target hematocrit of 30%. However, there is no absolute hematocrit below which all patients require blood transfusion. Most previously healthy children will tolerate a hematocrit lower than 30% without adverse sequelae. The lowest acceptable hematocrit in premature infants may be 35% or higher, whereas in the full-term newborn an acceptable hematocrit may be 30–35%. Over 3 months of age, a hematocrit between 20% and 25% is acceptable in the normovolemic state. In the trauma setting, the hematocrit is often unknown and estimates of EBV, blood loss, and blood needs are empiric. In life-threatening emergencies, immediate transfusion with type-O blood is warranted. There are no national standards as to whether children should receive O-negative or O-positive blood. Some centers administer O-positive blood to boys and O-negative to girls (to avoid alloimmunization), while more conservative centers administer O-negative blood to all children. Group-specific blood, when available, is always preferred to type O-blood. Administration of large amounts of blood to small children entails risks that include hyperkalemia from lysis of stored red cells, hypocalcemia from citrate toxicity, hypothermia, and coagulopathy that results from dilution of platelets and clotting factors.

Anesthesia for Wound Care

The adequate provision of anxiolysis and analgesia for daily wound care can be exceptionally challenging for these patients. An opioid-based technique is most commonly used. The route of administration depends on the availability of intravascular access and the expected number of dressing changes over time. Benzodiazepines are used to relieve anxiety. Inhaled N_2O is a suitable alternative for mildly painful procedures. Oral or intravenous ketamine in conjunction with a benzodiazepine can also be used. The role of epidural analgesia is limited to repeated wound care of the lower extremities. However, the long-term use of this modality is usually not feasible because of the increased risk of infection as well as coagulation abnormalities that often accompany burns. Hypnosis, distraction therapy, child life specialists, presence of parents, and topical anesthesia on the wound should all be incorporated into the overall therapeutic plan and can be coordinated by physicians with expertise in pediatric pain. Frequently, general anesthesia by mask or LMA is required to facilitate wound care or dressing changes. Using the same medical and nursing personnel for repeated wound care will increase the child's comfort level.

Postoperative Considerations

Most children with major trauma or burns will remain intubated while transported to an intensive care unit (ICU). Adequate analgesia and sedation must be administered for the transport from the operating room to the

Case

A 14-month old boy presented to the emergency ward after accidentally being placed into a scalding hot water bath. He sustained an approximate 35% BSA burn that consists of second- and third-degree burns to the lower extremity and perineum. He is conscious and crying inconsolably with otherwise stable vital signs. Anesthesiology consultation is requested for evaluation of airway management.

What will you recommend?

My primary concerns are optimization of ventilation and circulation. I will assess upper airway patency and adequacy of ventilation by auscultating the lungs and noting the oxyhemoglobin saturation. I will then turn to less critical yet clinically important issues, the most important of which at this juncture is pain control. With such a large surface area burn, this child will require surgical intervention with continuous intravenous opioid analgesia, and he is expected to mount a systemic inflammatory reaction as a result of mediators released from the burned tissue and invading pathogens. This child will require immediate placement of large-bore venous access lines, a urinary catheter, a nasogastric tube in the anticipation of an ileus, and possibly an arterial line. Therefore, I will recommend induction of general anesthesia, endotracheal intubation, and institution of mechanical ventilation prior to any painful or invasive procedures.

Is there anything else you should know before proceeding with induction of general anesthesia?

Additional information that I would elicit would include the immediate and past medical history including allergies, and family history of medical and anesthetic problems. I would also perform a brief and focused physical examination of the airway and acquire the results of any laboratory evaluations.

How will you induce general anesthesia?

I would perform a modified rapid-sequence induction using fentanyl 2 µg/kg, lidocaine 1 mg/kg, thiopentothal 5 mg/kg, and rocuronium 1.2 mg/kg. An assistant will apply cricoid pressure during manual positive pressure ventilation prior to tracheal intubation. The child will need continuous maintenance of deep sedation using any combination of propofol, opioids, and benzodiazepines. Once the airway is secured and the child well-sedated, invasive procedures can be performed.

The following day, the child is scheduled for an excision of the burn tissue and a split thickness skin graft. What are the important anesthetic concerns?

The two most important anesthetic concerns are blood loss and hypothermia. This procedure entails a large amount of obvious blood loss from the donor site and occult blood loss beneath the sponges at the excision site. During these procedures, the volume of blood lost is typically underestimated and hypovolemic shock can occur rapidly. Urine output must be monitored closely to detect impending hypoperfusion. Arterial blood gases should be obtained at least hourly to monitor ventilatory and acid–base status. Packed red blood cells should be immediately available for rapid transfusion if necessary. Additional personnel must also be immediately available to assist with volume resuscitation.

Hypothermia results from the large amount of exposed tissue surfaces and the rapid infusion of blood products or crystalloid solutions. The OR should be maximally warmed, a forced warm-air heating blanket should be placed over nonsurgical surfaces, and a fluid-warming device should be used to warm all intravenous fluids and blood products.

Is there any role for regional anesthesia?

Based on the pattern of this child's burns, a lumbar epidural catheter would seem ideal for providing analgesia of the perineum and lower extremity, especially postoperatively when daily painful dressing changes are necessary. However, this child is expected to become bacteremic, if not outright septic, and an epidural catheter would provide an additional nidus for infection in the central nervous system. In addition, donor sites are expected to come from the trunk above the potential analgesic level that an epidural catheter would provide. Lastly, this child is expected to require at least several more days of sedation and mechanical ventilation. Under these circumstances, liberal titration of opioid analgesia can be administered without fear of ventilatory depression. Epidural analgesia would be advantageous and more feasible in an unventilated child with isolated lower-extremity burns.

ICU or other location where further diagnostic evaluation is performed. The decision to extubate the trachea will depend on clinical circumstances, including preoperative findings, intraoperative events, and the expected postoperative course. Prior to leaving the OR, an assessment to rule out physiologic derangements must be performed. Resuscitation medications and intubation equipment should be carried on transport along with a full tank of oxygen. In general, it is advisable to anticipate the child's anesthetic needs for the hour following surgery since transport of the patient and handing over care to the primary medical service takes some time. On arrival at the ICU, a hematocrit, arterial blood gas, and electrolytes should be obtained as well as a chest radiograph to exclude pathophysiologic changes that might have occurred during transport.

ADDITIONAL ARTICLES TO KNOW

Kokoska ER, Keller MS, Rallo MC et al: Characteristics of pediatric cervical spine injuries. *J Pediatr Surg* 36:100-105, 2001.

Martyn JA, Chang Y, Goudsouzian NG, Patel SS: Pharmacodynamics of mivacurium chloride in 13- to 18-yr-old adolescents with thermal injury. *Br J Anaesth* 89:580-585, 2002.

Michaud, LJ, Rivara FP, Longstreth WT, Grady MS: Elevated initial blood glucose levels and poor outcome following severe brain injuries in children. *J Trauma* 31:1356-1362, 1991.

Mills AK, Martyn JA: Evaluation of atracurium neuromuscular blockade in paediatric patients with burn injury. *Br J Anaesth* 60:450-455, 1988.

Mills AK, Martyn JA: Neuromuscular blockade with vecuronium in paediatric patients with burn injury. *Br J Clin Pharmacol* 28:155-159, 1989.

Muizelaar JP, Ward JD, Marmarou A, Newlon PG, Wachi A: Cerebral blood flow and metabolism in severely head-injured children. 2: Autoregulation. *J Neurosurg* 71:72-76, 1989.

Puffinbarger NK, Tuggle DW, Smith EI: Rapid isotonic fluid resuscitation in pediatric thermal injury. *J Pediatr Surg* 29:339-342, 1994.

Sheridan RL: Comprehensive treatment of burns. *Curr Probl Surg* 38:657-756, 2001.

Stoddard FJ, Sheridan RL, Saxe GN et al: Treatment of pain in acutely burned children. *J Burn Care Rehabil* 23:135-156, 2002.

White JR, Dalton HJ: Pediatric trauma: postinjury care in the pediatric intensive care unit. *Crit Care Med* 30(11 Suppl): S478-488, 2002.

Pediatric Anesthesia in Nonoperating Room Locations

RONALD S. LITMAN

OVERVIEW

A large percentage of pediatric anesthesia practice takes place outside the traditional operating room (OR) environment. This practice presents unique challenges because of unfamiliar surroundings, lack of sufficient space, and ancillary personnel who are not familiar with anesthetic procedures and techniques. Furthermore, we are often scheduled in multiple locations throughout the institution on the same day. Therefore, equipment is transported and set up multiple times. This increases the risk of equipment-related problems.

Although the physical locations differ, the anesthesiologist who provides care outside the OR must abide by the same safety and monitoring standards that are followed inside the OR (Box 37-1). It is not necessary to always have an anesthesia machine at the off-site anesthetizing location. Its presence will depend on the comfort of the anesthesiologist and the anticipated use of inhalational anesthetic agents. When one anticipates the use of capnography, it is often easier to transport the entire anesthesia machine that stores the capnograph device. Children who are expected to present a difficult airway should undergo induction of general anesthesia and full airway management in the OR environment, where personnel and equipment are readily available. Once tracheal intubation is safely accomplished, the child is then transported, while anesthetized, to the procedural area.

There are numerous anesthetic techniques that are acceptable in off-site locations – the choice will primarily depend on the preference of the anesthesiologist and the type of procedure being performed. Children undergoing radiological procedures that are not painful are best managed by a hypnotic agent without analgesic properties, such as propofol or a barbiturate. Painful procedures are best managed using analgesics or inhalational anesthetics. It is possible to use high doses of a hypnotic agent during a painful procedure. However, for a severely painful procedure (e.g., bone marrow biopsy), few anesthetic agents will provide adequate analgesia and immobility without respiratory depression and the need for assisted ventilation (ketamine being a possible exception). Whatever the choice, the anesthesiologist should always have immediately available three syringes during and following each procedure: succinylcholine, atropine, and an induction agent of choice.

Transport of the child to the postanesthesia care unit (PACU) at the completion of the procedure is a consideration that should be addressed proactively. If there are recovery facilities in the anesthetizing area, emergence and tracheal extubation can occur at that location, and standard discharge criteria then apply. When the PACU is a considerable distance from the anesthetizing location, the anesthesiologist can choose to either: (1) keep the child anesthetized during transport, with emergence and extubation occurring in the PACU; or (2) transport a child who is emerging from anesthesia. Ultimately, the personal preference of the anesthesiologist is the most important determinant. Either way, it is essential to have at least a pulse oximeter, reliable oxygen source, and a positive-pressure ventilation device en route.

The cost efficiency of remote anesthesia presents an additional challenge. The daily schedule should reflect transport times between the anesthetizing location and the PACU, as well as between remote locations. The most common obstacle is delay, either because the remote

Box 37-1   American Society of Anesthesiologists Guidelines for Nonoperating Room Anesthetizing Locations[a]

These guidelines apply to all anesthesia care involving anesthesiology personnel for procedures intended to be performed in locations outside an operating room. These are minimal guidelines which may be exceeded at any time based on the judgment of the involved anesthesia personnel. These guidelines encourage quality patient care but observing them cannot guarantee any specific patient outcome. These guidelines are subject to revision from time to time, as warranted by the evolution of technology and practice.

- There should be, in each location, a reliable source of oxygen adequate for the length of the procedure. There should also be a backup supply. Prior to administering any anesthetic, the anesthesiologist should consider the capabilities, limitations, and accessibility of both the primary and backup oxygen sources. Oxygen piped from a central source, meeting applicable codes, is strongly encouraged. The backup system should include the equivalent of at least a full E cylinder.
- There should be, in each location, an adequate and reliable source of suction. Suction apparatus that meets operating room standards is strongly encouraged.
- In any location in which inhalation anesthetics are administered, there should be an adequate and reliable system for scavenging waste anesthetic gases.
- There should be in each location: (a) a self-inflating hand resuscitator bag capable of administering at least 90% oxygen as a means to deliver positive-pressure ventilation; (b) adequate anesthesia drugs, supplies, and equipment for the intended anesthesia care; and (c) adequate monitoring equipment to allow adherence to the "Standards for Basic Anesthetic Monitoring." In any location in which inhalation anesthesia is to be administered, there should be an anesthesia machine equivalent in function to that employed in operating rooms and maintained to current operating room standards.
- There should be, in each location, sufficient electrical outlets to satisfy anesthesia machine and monitoring equipment requirements, including clearly labeled outlets connected to an emergency power supply. In any anesthetizing location determined by the healthcare facility to be a "wet location" (e.g., for cystoscopy or arthroscopy or a birthing room in labor and delivery), either isolated electric power or electric circuits with ground fault circuit interrupters should be provided.
- There should be, in each location, provision for adequate illumination of the patient, anesthesia machine (when present), and monitoring equipment. In addition, a form of battery-powered illumination other than a laryngoscope should be immediately available.
- There should be, in each location, sufficient space to accommodate necessary equipment and personnel and to allow expeditious access to the patient, anesthesia machine (when present), and monitoring equipment.
- There should be immediately available, in each location, an emergency cart with a defibrillator, emergency drugs, and other equipment adequate to provide cardiopulmonary resuscitation.
- There should be immediately available, in each location, a reliable means of two-way communication to request assistance.
- For each location, all applicable building and safety codes and facility standards, where they exist, should be observed.

[a] Approved by the House of Delegates on October 19, 1994.

location is not properly prepared to begin on time or because of an unexpected delay during the previous case. When a significant delay occurs, the anesthesiologist must decide whether to move on to the following scheduled case, or delay the entire schedule. The solutions to these problems are to develop a fluid working relationship with the staff in each remote location, enabling them to understand the economic pressures, and to administer anesthesia in a cost-efficient manner with rapid induction and emergence times. An on-site recovery facility with staff trained in the recovery of anesthetized patients also enhances efficiency. Flexibility is essential on the part of the anesthesiologist but the anesthesiologist shouldn't expect staff in remote areas to be flexible as well. In fact, from their standpoint, the most important ingredient for success is consistency. At first these statements may seem paradoxical. However, with

experience, the anesthesiologist will become familiar with the remote location's surroundings and staff and will develop a consistent procedure for taking care of their patients. This is especially true in the hematology/ oncology or radiation oncology departments where the same patients require many procedures over time. Ideally, in any given institution a small cadre of anesthesiologists will make up the "off-site team" so that differences in preferences and techniques will be minimized and a trusting relationship can develop between members of the team and non-anesthesiology staff in these areas.

MAGNETIC RESONANCE IMAGING

The number of infants and small children requiring magnetic resonance imaging (MRI) has increased substantially in recent years because MRI is superior to CT for demonstrating most central nervous system lesions (except acute subarachnoid hemorrhage, skull fractures, and various craniofacial and sinus-related disorders), without the risk of ionizing radiation or iodinated contrast agents. Increasing numbers of newborns and small infants are being referred for MRI because of sacral dimples, developmental delay, apnea, seizures, and stridor (for evaluation of a possible vascular ring). This has presented anesthesiologists with an enormous challenge, especially during times of staffing shortages and decreasing reimbursement from third-party payers for these services.

The overriding concern during MRI anesthesia is that the powerful magnetic field precludes the use of metallic devices in the area around the scanner, whether or not a scan is in progress. This includes virtually all our monitors and safety equipment, as well as credit cards, identification badges, and expensive pens. Thus, the challenge is to safely conduct general anesthesia from a distance.

The performance of general anesthesia on children for MRI has been facilitated by the availability of MRI-compatible anesthesia machines, MRI-compatible monitoring stations, and MRI-compatible electronic infusion pumps. Therefore, it is fairly easy to comply with all monitoring standards during anesthesia for MRI. The one exception is that a precordial stethoscope (plastic type) is useful only intermittently because of the noise from the scanner that interferes with auscultation. Temperature measurement is difficult inside the scanner and, because of the cool environment and the scanner fan, neonates and small infants are susceptible to hypothermia. These patients should be covered with several layers of blankets and the scanner fan should be turned off. Hypothermia can also be minimized by limiting the volume of administered intravenous fluids.

Most children anesthetized for MRI are outpatients, and are processed along with all other ambulatory surgical patients. There are no unique preoperative considerations. One of several different anesthetic techniques may be used. At The Children's Hospital of Philadelphia, children for MRI undergo induction of general anesthesia by sevoflurane inhalation in an area separate from the scanner, to optimize the use of ferromagnetic equipment that cannot be used in the immediate scanner vicinity. We utilize three separate MRI scanners, and thus it is most practical to maintain one anesthesia machine in a central anesthetic induction area. Maintenance of general anesthesia is most often accomplished using a continuous infusion of propofol at 200 µg/kg/min. This infusion dose is occasionally titrated upward, especially for neonates and small infants. With this technique, most children will not exhibit upper-airway obstruction during spontaneous ventilation. Adequate oxygenation is easily maintained using a nasal cannula with a capnograph attachment.

Occasionally, when upper-airway obstruction occurs, insertion of a nasal or oral airway will provide a patent airway and relieve the rocking motion of the head and neck that interferes with acquisition of artifact-free images. Use of a laryngeal mask airway (LMA) or endotracheal intubation is infrequent, although preferred by some anesthesiologists. Intubated children who require scans of the head or neck will benefit from the use of an oral RAE tube, which is more convenient when using a head coil.

The most important anesthetic consideration is the avoidance of a tragic accident by a ferromagnetic object that, in the presence of a strong magnetic field, is transformed into a dangerous projectile missile that can easily injure the patient or nearby personnel. This includes all types of anesthesia equipment, oxygen tanks, IV poles, gurneys, etc. Anesthesiologists should ensure that all spare oxygen tanks in the MRI facility are made of aluminum. Each scanning facility must enforce strict safety precautions that limit the number and types of personnel within the scanner area, and a protocol should be established for detecting metallic objects that are transported into the scanner facility. Additional equipment hazards involve the use of MRI-compatible monitors, as burns have occurred when coiled electrocardiograph and pulse oximeter cables are allowed to rest on the patient's skin.

COMPUTERIZED TOMOGRAPHY

With improvements in CT scan technology, the need for sedation or anesthesia in children has decreased considerably. Multisection helical CT is three to five times faster than standard helical CT. Thus, more children are able to remain calm and lie still long enough to obtain good images. Yet, anesthesiologists are still called upon for children with severe anxiety, or significant medical disease. As opposed to MRI, there are far fewer anesthetic implications for the child who requires general anesthesia for a CT scan. Standard anesthesia machines and monitoring devices can be used in close proximity to the child. The anesthesiologist wears lead protection and may remain near the child during the scan, the duration of which is usually less than 20 minutes. The preoperative considerations and anesthetic technique options are the same as for MRI.

The recent literature has focused on two important issues with respect to sedation or general anesthesia for CT. The first is the timing of the administration of oral contrast prior to abdominal CT. This oral contrast is diatrizoate meglumine (Gastrografin, Gastroview, Hypaque, etc.), a water-soluble iodinated substance with an osmolality of 1900 mmol/L. From the radiologist's perspective, better diagnostic scans are obtained when the contrast is administered within an hour or so of the time of the scan.

Article To Know

Kanal E, Borgstede JP, Barkovich AJ et al: American College of Radiology White Paper on MR Safety. Am J Roentgenol 178: 1335-1347, 2002.

This important paper should be studied by all anesthesiologists who take part in MRI anesthesia. It is intended to be used as a template for MRI facilities when developing a safety program, in response to the growing number of reports of injuries from ferromagnetic objects inside the scanner area.

The authors of this paper (American College of Radiology Blue Ribbon Panel, which included a representative from the Anesthesia Patient Safety Foundation) begin to establish guidelines and standards for MRI facilities to maximize safety. These include important recommendations for:

- Establishing, implementing, and maintaining safety policies and procedures.
- Establishing separate safety zones in and around the scanner, that include restrictions on personnel allowed in each of these areas.
- Screening procedures for patients, staff, and possible ferromagnetic objects.
- A variety of other technical issues related to scanner safety.

Of note, the panel does not recommend metal detectors because of their inconsistent efficacy.

Case

A 4-year-old boy requires MRI of the brain to further elucidate a suspected brain tumor. His history includes intermittent headaches for 2 months, vomiting for 1 week, and occasional loss of balance. Two days prior, CT scanning using chloral hydrate sedation demonstrated a posterior fossa mass. He is otherwise healthy. His vital signs on admission to the day-surgery unit are: temperature 36.6°C, heart rate 120/min, respiratory rate 24/min, blood pressure 98/38 mmHg.

Is there anything else you would like to know before proceeding with general anesthesia?

My main concern in this child is his increased intracranial pressure, which is manifested clinically as headaches and vomiting. We can assume that the CT scan did not reveal evidence of impending herniation (e.g., midline shift of the brain), which would be unlikely in a posterior fossa mass. Since the child did not exhibit worsening of his condition following chloral hydrate sedation, I will assume that his increased intracranial pressure is not at a critically high level.

Is premedication indicated in this child?

I would consider premedication with an anxiolytic such as oral midazolam, but this will depend on his behavior at the time of the scan. Ideally, I would like to avoid premedication, because of the possible respiratory depressant effect that could worsen his increased intracranial pressure. I would have the child's parents accompany him into the MRI scanner (or induction area), and attempt to induce general anesthesia without much of a struggle using imagery techniques and magic tricks. The theoretical risk of a "stormy" induction in this setting is acutely increasing the intracranial pressure. On the other hand, if I think that this child will be difficult to calm, even in the presence of his parents and by using behavioral techniques, I would administer oral midazolam premedication.

How will you induce general anesthesia in this child?

Since this child has preexisting increased intracranial pressure, the technique of choice would be a modified rapid sequence induction, as described in Chapter 30. However, this child is arriving from home, and does not yet have existing intravenous access. I now have to choose between an inhalational induction by mask with placement of intravenous access after loss of consciousness, or placement of intravenous access while the child is awake. Personally, I'll choose the inhalation induction, knowing that not all pediatric anesthesiologists may agree with this approach. In this child, who appears to have marginally increased intracranial pressure, I don't feel there is any more of a risk of increasing it further by the effects of sevoflurane on the cerebral vasculature or the hypercapnia that might result from respiratory depression caused by the inhalational agent. If I observe a marked decrease in ventilatory effort after loss of consciousness, I will augment ventilation using a bag–mask technique. In addition, as long as the child has followed normal fasting guidelines (see Chapter 12), I don't believe he is at risk of having an increased amount of gastric contents that would predispose to pulmonary aspiration.

Placing an intravenous catheter in a conscious child will almost always result in a substantial amount of pain, crying, and restraint. Some argue that this process may cause greater increases in intracranial pressure than would be observed during an inhalational induction. Furthermore, those who prefer preanesthetic placement of the intravenous catheter presumably are doing so because they want to utilize the modified rapid sequence induction technique, perform endotracheal intubation, and

Case *Cont'd*

continue with controlled mechanical ventilation for the duration of the MRI. If I choose not to control ventilation, then the induction technique is irrelevant.

How will you maintain anesthesia?

As with induction, I must choose between a controlled ventilation technique following endotracheal intubation, or a spontaneously breathing technique in a nonintubated child using deep sedation with a propofol infusion. Some anesthesiologists feel it is most prudent to control ventilation to avoid increasing the intracranial pressure further. However, my preference is the spontaneous ventilation technique. The first response from the astute clinician would be that a spontaneous ventilation technique should not be used in any patient with increased intracranial pressure for fear of causing hypercapnia, increased cerebral blood flow, and thus, increasing intracranial pressure. However, the controlled ventilation technique can also be associated with dangerous increases in intracranial pressure from the sympathetic response generated during tracheal intubation and emergence. This child tolerated chloral hydrate sedation without any apparent worsening of his clinical status, and although I don't know for sure, I will assume that ventilatory parameters between chloral hydrate and propofol deep sedation are somewhat similar. If, on the other hand, this child demonstrated clear evidence of critically increased intracranial pressure (e.g., Cushing's triad, midline shift on the CT scan), a controlled-ventilation technique is indicated.

After obtaining several scans, the MRI technologist informs you that there is motion artifact caused by movement of the child's head during respiration, and they cannot proceed further. What will you do?

Movement of the child's head during respiration is almost always caused by partial upper-airway obstruction, which, other than interfering with adequate MRI, can cause hypercapnia and exacerbate increased intracranial pressure. One possible therapeutic maneuver is deepening the level of unconsciousness by administering a propofol bolus and then increasing the infusion dose. However, I don't want to depress consciousness to the point of further ventilatory depression. Therefore, I will initially attempt to alleviate the head motion by adjusting the head and neck position, usually in more extension, to increase patency of the upper airway. My next choice would be placement of an oral or nasal airway. This will alleviate any upper-airway obstruction in the majority of cases. In the event that these devices continue to be ineffective, I will insert an LMA, or perform endotracheal intubation as a last resort.

Approximately 10 minutes after alleviating the upper-airway obstruction with a nasal airway, the MRI technologist says alarmingly "Yipes! He's trying to crawl out of the scanner!" What will you do?

This is a common problem in MRI and almost always results from a lack of sufficient anesthesia because of technical errors. As the ongoing scan is aborted, I will go into the scanner room and immediately administer a bolus of propofol (approximately 2 mg/kg) as the MRI technologist simultaneously brings the MRI table out from the scanner. This bolus of propofol may cause apnea so my immediate attention will turn to ensuring adequate ventilation. Once the patient has lost consciousness, and after I have repositioned the head and neck, I will attempt to investigate the cause of the awakening. Most likely, it was a failure to deliver the propofol in a sufficient amount. This can be caused by an infiltrated or blocked intravenous site, an accidental disconnection of the intravenous tubing, a faulty infusion pump, or simply that I didn't remember to actuate the "Deliver" button on the infusion pump after the previous dose change. If one performs enough anesthetics for MRI, one or some of these mishaps will eventually occur.

However, anesthesiologists are concerned with this practice because it violates generally accepted fasting guidelines. The gastric emptying time of diatrizoate has not been evaluated but there is no ingredient (fat or protein) that should cause it to empty slower than a clear liquid. However, should pulmonary aspiration of this agent occur, its high osmolality renders it potentially toxic to the lung. Therefore, many pediatric anesthesiologists choose to perform rapid sequence induction of general anesthesia with tracheal intubation after contrast administration, instead of "deep sedation" without airway protection. Alternatively, the contrast material can be administered via an orogastric tube following routine administration of general anesthesia and endotracheal intubation.

The second issue concerns children with cancer undergoing chest CT for detection of primary or metastatic lesions. Radiologists are concerned that the development of atelectasis that accompanies induction of general anesthesia may mask underlying abnormalities (Fig. 37-1). Because of this, many radiologists request routine performance of tracheal intubation to provide positive-pressure ventilation prior to chest CT. A recent study demonstrated that the addition of 5 cmH$_2$O of positive end-expiratory pressure (PEEP) attenuated

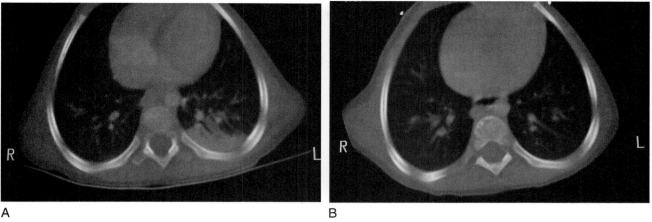

A   B

Figure 37-1   **A**, CT scan of the chest in a child prior to instituting positive pressure. Note the atelectasis at the base of the left lung, which may obscure an abnormality. **B**, CT scan of the chest of the same child following several positive-pressure breaths with several seconds of inspiratory hold to alleviate any existing atelectasis.

anesthesia-related atelectasis in children undergoing CT of the chest. An alternate method is to provide transient PEEP and positive-pressure ventilation using a bag–mask technique in unintubated children under deep sedation.

RADIATION THERAPY

Located in the bowels of the hospital, far from civilization, there exists no more daunting environment for the anesthesiologist than radiation oncology. There are several considerations that make this environment different from other remote locations. The first is the anesthetic considerations surrounding the patient's underlying illness; these are reviewed in Chapter 8. The second is that the child must lie completely motionless for a procedure that normally takes less than 10 minutes, with all personnel, including the anesthesiologist, outside the room. Typically, two video cameras are used: one is positioned to view the patient and the other to view the screen of the patient monitor, which displays values for oxyhemoglobin saturation, electrocardiography, capnography, and blood pressure. The anesthesiologist observes the patient on video monitors located immediately outside the treatment room (Fig. 37-2).

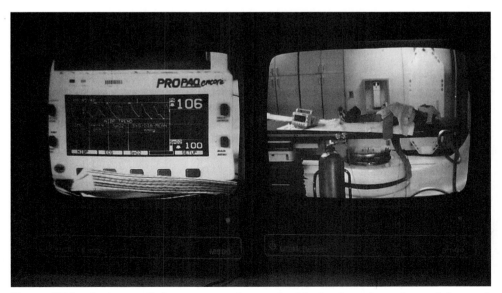

Figure 37-2   During a radiation treatment, the anesthesiologist views the patient and the monitor in an observation area immediately outside the treatment room.

Various successful anesthetic techniques exist. However, we have found that the most practical method for rapid induction and recovery of general anesthesia is a propofol-based technique, with the child breathing spontaneously. Supplemental oxygen is provided via a nasal cannula with a capnograph attachment. This can even be accomplished in most children who are required to lie prone for each treatment (Fig. 37-3). Propofol maintenance is provided by continuous infusion or intermittent boluses throughout the procedure. Once the adequacy of ventilation is confirmed, without airway obstruction or oxyhemoglobin desaturation, all staff immediately leave the room and observe the video monitors during the treatment. The tones of the pulse oximeter should be heard via a microphone inside the treatment room that is transmitted to speakers located in the observation area. Acceptable alternative airway methods include use of oral or nasal airways, LMA, or tracheal intubation, if necessary.

Logistical issues should be proactively addressed at the outset of the treatments, which are usually performed once or twice daily for 2–6 weeks. Most children have indwelling tunneled central venous catheters (e.g., Broviac). If not, every attempt is made at the first visit to place a long intravenous catheter that can remain for the duration of the treatment (i.e., PIC line). This enables the child to become anesthetized each day without the emotional trauma of a mask inhalation induction or the need for premedication. Parents should be counseled about proper fasting guidelines and encouraged to offer their child clear liquids on the morning of each treatment. Since it is quite a burden for the child (and parents!) to remain fasted each day, these treatments should be scheduled as early in the day as possible.

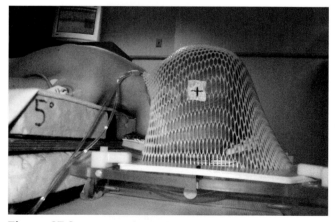

Figure 37-3 An anesthetized child is lying prone in a head molding with his chin resting on a soft cushion. Oxygen is provided via a nasal cannula attached to a capnograph to monitor ventilation.

Some anesthesiologists prefer to have these children awaken at the end of the treatment, whereas others will maintain propofol anesthesia until they arrive in the PACU to avoid awakening during transport.

ONCOLOGY CLINIC

The most common procedures that require general anesthesia in the oncology clinic are bone marrow biopsy and lumbar puncture for administration of intrathecal chemotherapy. These procedures are performed with the child lying prone or in the lateral position, depending on the preference of the practitioner performing the procedure. Most children who are currently receiving chemotherapy will have an indwelling central venous catheter, so oral premedication may not be necessary. Others may be undergoing routine surveillance following remission, so will have had their intravenous access removed.

Different anesthetic techniques can be successfully utilized for these procedures, which involve a brief, severe painful stimulus. Some anesthesiologists prefer a "deep sedation" technique using a combination of a benzodiazepine (e.g., midazolam) and an opioid (e.g., fentanyl). The use of remifentanil will facilitate a rapid recovery and discharge from the unit. This technique will rarely ensure complete loss of consciousness and immobility, and is preferred by some older children and adolescents. Postanesthetic emesis is common and may be a result of the opioid or intrathecal chemotherapy. Therefore, antiemetic prophylaxis is indicated.

Other anesthesiologists prefer to use a propofol-based general anesthetic technique. Clinic staff and parents tend to prefer this technique because the child is rendered unconscious. However, propofol is not an analgesic agent, and in most children it will cause central apnea at lower doses than are required for adequate analgesia and immobility during the procedure. Therefore, if one chooses a general anesthetic technique with propofol, and the practitioner performing the procedure requests immobility, the child will likely require assisted ventilation.

ENDOSCOPY SUITE

Esophagogastroduodenoscopy (EGD) and colonoscopy are commonly performed in children in a specially designated endoscopy suite, and require some form of sedation or general anesthesia. Common indications for EGD in children include evaluation of reflux disease, chronic abdominal pain, evaluation and treatment of esophageal varices in chronic liver disease (see Chapter 2), chronic nausea/vomiting, hematemesis, melena, peptic ulcer disease, and weight loss, among others. Upper endoscopy is usually performed in the lateral position, while colonoscopy is usually performed with the child supine. The most important consideration for anesthesia during upper endoscopy is airway protection. Unless the child is an adolescent, and a sedative technique chosen, tracheal intubation is preferred for all children undergoing this procedure. The anesthetic technique reflects the fact that these procedures tend to end abruptly with little advance warning. Therefore, short-acting muscle relaxants (e.g., mivacurium) and maintenance of general anesthesia with desflurane are preferred. Opioids are rarely used because pain is not a prominent concern during and following upper endoscopy and their administration may delay awakening.

Common indications for colonoscopy in children include evaluation of chronic diarrhea, inflammatory bowel disease, and familial polyposis. Colonoscopy is more painful than it appears; opioids are often used as a component of the anesthetic technique. These children rarely require tracheal intubation unless they are susceptible to pulmonary aspiration of gastric contents due to preexisting medical conditions. Following induction of general anesthesia with sevoflurane, a propofol-based anesthetic technique is used most commonly, with opioid supplementation as needed. The length of the procedure varies depending on the number of biopsies required and the gastroenterologist's ability to reach the cecum, which can occasionally be quite challenging.

ADDITIONAL ARTICLES TO KNOW

Federle MP, Peitzman A, Krugh J: Use of oral contrast material in abdominal trauma CT scans: is it dangerous? *J Trauma* 38: 51-53, 1995.

Lam WW, Chen PP, So NM, Metreweli C: Sedation versus general anaesthesia in paediatric patients undergoing chest CT. *Acta Radiol* 39:298-300, 1998.

Lim-Dunham JE, Narra J, Benya EC, Donaldson JS: Aspiration after administration of oral contrast material in children undergoing abdominal CT for trauma. *Am J Roentgenol* 169: 1015-1018, 1997.

Litman RS: Conscious sedation with remifentanil and midazolam during brief painful procedures in children. *Arch Pediatr Adolesc Med* 153:1085-1088, 1999.

Long FR, Castile RG: Technique and clinical applications of full-inflation and end-exhalation controlled-ventilation chest CT in infants and young children. *Pediatr Radiol* 31:413-422, 2001.

Malviya S, Voepel-Lewis T, Eldevik OP et al: Sedation and general anaesthesia in children undergoing MRI and CT: adverse events and outcomes. *Br J Anaesth* 84:743-748, 2000.

Sargent MA, Jamieson DH, McEachern AM, Blackstock D: Increased inspiratory pressure for reduction of atelectasis in children anesthetized for CT scan. *Pediatr Radiol* 32:344-347, 2002.

Sargent MA, McEachern AM, Jamieson DH, Kahwaji R: Atelectasis on pediatric chest CT: comparison of sedation techniques. *Pediatr Radiol* 29:509-513, 1999.

Ziegler MA, Fricke BL, Donnelly LF: Is administration of enteric contrast material safe before abdominal CT in children who require sedation? Experience with chloral hydrate and pentobarbital. *Am J Roentgenol* 180:13-15, 2003.

PEDIATRIC CRITICAL CARE

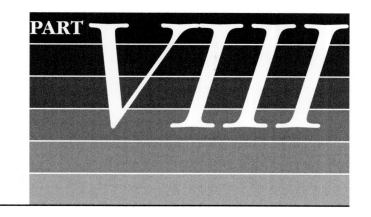

CHAPTER 38

Pediatric Critical Care

MARGARET A. PRIESTLEY

JAMES W. HUH

ATHENA F. ZUPPA

Anesthesiologists are frequently required to deliver pediatric critical care in the perioperative setting. Familiarity with life-threatening pediatric medical conditions, invasive access and monitoring techniques, and pharmacology of medications that affect the cardiovascular system is essential. This chapter provides an overview of the most important aspects of pediatric critical care for the general anesthesiologist.

PEDIATRIC ADVANCED LIFE SUPPORT (PALS)

Pediatric patients with cardiopulmonary compromise require immediate and effective therapy to prevent hypoxic–ischemic organ damage. Treatment should be in accordance with the guidelines of the American Academy of Pediatrics and the American Heart Association. One of the most important priorities during cardiopulmonary resuscitation (CPR) is to have an identified "leader" with the most experience with critically ill children. The leader's role is to direct the resuscitation and assign specific roles to the members of the resuscitation team. The initial approach to pediatric CPR is the "ABCDE" system (Box 38-1). This provides a systematic way to approach the patient. During the resuscitation, it is often helpful to occasionally restart at "A" to assess the effects of prior interventions.

A (Airway) and B (Breathing)

Proper airway positioning is important to maximize oxygenation and ventilation. In suspected cervical spine injury, a chin lift or jaw thrust maneuver (without distracting the neck) may help relieve upper-airway obstruction caused by oropharyngeal tissues. A nasopharyngeal airway may provide a patent airway in conscious and unconscious patients but is relatively contraindicated in facial or head trauma. An oropharyngeal airway is usually tolerated only by unconscious patients. Suction equipment should always be available in order to remove secretions, vomitus, or other foreign debris that contribute to airway obstruction. Tracheal intubation is

Box 38-1 The ABCDE Approach to Pediatric CPR

A

Airway

B

Breathing

C

Circulation
Cervical spine immobilization if trauma

D

Disability
Drugs such as epinephrine, antibiotics, and dextrose, if indicated

E

Exposure
Environment (such as temperature)
Electrical activity of the heart
Extracorporeal membrane oxygenation, if necessary or available as a last resort

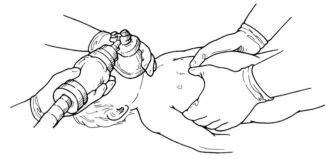

Figure 38-1 In the two-thumb-encircling hand technique for chest compression in infants, the thumbs should be located one finger width below the intermammary line. The sternum should be depressed one-third to one-half the depth of the infant's chest at a rate of at least 100 times per minute.

indicated for respiratory failure and protection against pulmonary aspiration.

C (Circulation and Cervical Spine)

Cardiac arrest is the absence of pulses and a perfusing rhythm in the area of the large arteries (brachial, carotid, or femoral). Chest compressions should immediately be initiated. In infants under 12 months old, the hands encircle the chest, and the thumbs are placed one finger-width below the intermammary line to compress the chest evenly over the mid-sternum (Fig. 38-1). The sternum should be depressed one-third to one-half the depth of the infant's chest at a rate of at least 100 times per minute. Chest compressions should not be administered over the lower third of the infant's sternum to avoid abdominal trauma. For children aged between 1 and 8 years, the heel of the hand is placed two-finger breaths above the lower end of the sternum. The chest compression to ventilation ratio should be 5:1 (a compression rate of 100 times per minute). *Maintaining the frequency and depth of the compressions are the most important elements for the provision of life-sustaining circulation.*

Vascular access is critical in pediatric CPR. Peripheral venous access should be attempted, but if unsuccessful after three attempts or 90 seconds, whichever comes

first, intraosseous (IO) vascular access is recommended and now includes all children regardless of age (see Chapter 36 for methods of securing IO access). Once vascular access is established, isotonic fluids such as Ringer's lactate or normal saline 10–20 mL/kg should be rapidly administered in every pediatric arrest unless caused by myocardial dysfunction (e.g., myocarditis). Children with hemorrhagic shock should immediately receive un-crossmatched type O Rh-negative packed red blood cells or whole blood. Type-specific blood is recommended if the patient's blood type is known. Medications that can be administered through the endotracheal tube include lidocaine, atropine, naloxone, and epinephrine (mnemonic = LANE).

Pulseless electrical activity (PEA) is most commonly caused by mechanical obstruction to blood flow; however, the differential diagnosis should be reviewed quickly. Remember the 4Hs and 4Ts:

Hypoxemia
Hypovolemia
Hypothermia
Hyper/Hypokalemia

and

pericardial Tamponade
Tension pneumothorax
Thromboembolism
Toxins.

Specific therapies should be directed at these causes if spontaneous circulation does not return.

In addition to *Circulation*, the "C" in "ABCDE" reminds us of cervical spine immobilization, especially if there is a suspected traumatic mechanism of injury. Cervical spinal cord trauma may cause neurologic deficits and neurogenic circulatory shock, which is characterized by hypotension without tachycardia.

D (Disability and Drugs)

Disability

This reminds us to quickly assess the child's neurologic status. This involves calculating a Glasgow Coma Scale score (see Chapter 36), assessing focal neurologic injury, and examining for pupillary responses that suggest impending cerebral herniation (e.g., unilateral dilated pupil). Glucose measurement should always be checked during a pediatric arrest since hypoglycemia can lead to additional neurologic injury. Hypoglycemia is treated using any immediately available intravenous glucose solution.

Drugs

The most important drug in a pediatric arrest is epinephrine. The recommended initial resuscitation dose of epinephrine for pediatric CPR is 0.01 mg/kg via the intravenous (IV) or IO route, or 0.1 mg/kg by the tracheal route. Repeated doses are recommended every 3–5 minutes for ongoing arrest. The same dose of epinephrine is recommended for subsequent doses, but higher doses (0.1–0.2 mg/kg) may be beneficial.

E (Exposure, Environment, Electrical Activity of the Heart, and Extracorporeal Membrane Oxygenation)

Exposure and Environment

The patient should be fully exposed to identify all injuries and to remove potentially contaminated clothing (e.g., toxic chemicals). Temperature should be closely observed (environment). Hyperthermia should be aggressively treated, especially in patients with head injury or reduced cardiac output.

Electrical Activity of the Heart

This should also be assessed during *Circulation* of the "ABCDE" system. Anesthesiologists should be familiar with, or have immediate access to, the published algorithms for treating pediatric arrhythmias.

Extracorporeal Membrane Oxygenation

In certain tertiary-care pediatric institutions, some patients who sustained a witnessed cardiopulmonary arrest have been successfully resuscitated with extracorporeal membrane oxygenation (ECMO) when traditional treatments have been unsuccessful. However, ECMO has its own potential complications and further evaluation of its utility for pediatric arrest is ongoing.

COMMON PEDIATRIC CRITICAL ILLNESSES

Status Asthmaticus

Status asthmaticus is a state of severe, persistent, life-threatening bronchospasm that is resistant to standard bronchodilator therapies. Clinical features include cyanosis, absent breath sounds, poor respiratory effort, fatigue, agitation, and depressed consciousness. As airway obstruction worsens, work of breathing increases. The combination of small and large airway collapse leads to air trapping and hyperinflation. In turn, hyperinflation leads to decreased lung and chest wall compliance and impaired diaphragmatic contraction since flattening places it at a mechanically disadvantageous fiber length. As the volume of the lungs increases, the vital capacity decreases and the work of breathing increases further. The increased airway resistance causes the respiratory muscles to perform increased pressure/volume work, which leads to increased CO_2 production, further stressing the respiratory system.

Air trapping is accompanied by ventilation/perfusion mismatch that contributes to increased deadspace and a compensatory increase in minute ventilation. Hypocapnia, respiratory alkalosis, and hypoxemia are seen early in uncomplicated acute asthma. A normal or elevated Pa_{CO_2} raises concern of respiratory muscle fatigue and the inability to maintain adequate ventilation. Hypercapnia normally occurs when the forced expiratory volume at 1 second (FEV_1) falls below 20% of the predicted value, signifying severe obstructive disease.

Cardiovascular effects of severe asthma relate to the dramatic swings in intrathoracic pressure during respiration. Pulsus paradoxus, defined as a >10–12 mmHg difference in systolic blood pressure between inspiration and expiration, is a marker for severity of airway obstruction and increased respiratory muscle work. Assuming pleural pressures are transmitted to the pericardial space, large negative intrathoracic pressures during inspiration increase ventricular afterload, and decrease systemic blood pressure. This is exacerbated by intravascular depletion caused by decreased fluid intake, increased insensible respiratory losses, and an increased metabolic rate.

Treatment of status asthmaticus consists of reducing airway obstruction while maximizing oxygenation and ventilation. Beta-adrenergic agonists reverse bronchiolar smooth muscle contraction and remain the primary treatment modality, but they are associated with adverse effects (Box 38-2). Long-acting β-agonists (e.g., salmeterol) are not indicated during status asthmaticus, and orally administered β-agonists are also ineffective.

In the past, initial therapy for severe bronchospasm consisted of subcutaneous injections of epinephrine. This has been replaced with equally effective inhaled bronchodilators (Table 38-1). Albuterol is most commonly used and can be administered continuously to a child in status asthmaticus. Parenteral β-agonists (e.g., terbutaline) are administered when there is no improvement with continuous nebulized therapy. Subcutaneous administration, as a first-line therapy, is reserved for children with minimal air entry or depressed mental status.

Box 38-2 Effects of Beta-receptor Stimulation for the Treatment of Status Asthmaticus

Beneficial Actions

Increases cyclic AMP[a] concentration, leading to smooth muscle relaxation

Prevents and reverses the effect of bronchoconstrictor substances on small- and large-airway smooth muscle cells

Enhances mucociliary clearance

Inhibits cholinergic transmission

Inhibits mediator release

Adverse Actions

Tremors secondary to skeletal muscle β_2 stimulation

Tachycardia secondary to β_1 (cardiac) and β_2 (vasodilation) stimulation

Dysrhythmias

Hypertension or hypotension

Ventilation/perfusion mismatch with reversal of hypoxic pulmonary vasoconstriction

Metabolic: hyperglycemia, hypokalemia, hypomagnesemia

Downregulation of β receptors

[a]AMP, adenosine monophosphate.

Combination therapy using additional bronchodilators is also available (Table 38-2). Anticholinergic agents (e.g., ipratropium bromide) block the vagal tone of airway smooth muscle with an effect predominantly on M3 receptors; this leads to bronchodilation and may decrease mucous secretion. These drugs have a slow onset of action and do not possess anti-inflammatory action. In severe exacerbations of asthma, the combination of an anticholinergic agent with a β-agonist is significantly more effective than either drug alone; the anticholinergic agent will have a longer duration of action.

Corticosteroids should be started early in any asthma exacerbation. They decrease inflammation, decrease microvascular permeability, and potentiate the response of β_2 receptors to β-agonists. Intravenous corticosteroids are more effective than inhaled steroids.

Magnesium sulfate is increasingly used to treat moderate to severe asthma exacerbations. It is thought to relax bronchiolar smooth muscle by antagonizing calcium or interfering with acetylcholine release at the neuromuscular junction. Dose-related side-effects of magnesium therapy include hypotension, flushing, hyporeflexia, and sedation.

Other therapies exist that are used infrequently or remain unproven. Theophylline has become a thirdline therapy. Its mechanism of action is uncertain; it is thought to weakly decrease airway smooth muscle tone, increase central respiratory drive, and enhance diaphragmatic contractility, and it may possess anti-inflammatory or immunomodulator properties. Theophylline possesses a narrow therapeutic range and its use is complicated by a variety of drug interactions. Its side-effects include nausea, vomiting, tachycardia, arrhythmias, and seizures.

Tracheal intubation and mechanical ventilation is reserved for the child with status asthmaticus who develops life-threatening respiratory failure. The absolute indications for instituting mechanical ventilation are a respiratory or circulatory arrest. The relative indications include acidemia, hypercapnia, silent chest, or decreased level of consciousness. The goals of mechanical ventilation are to avoid barotrauma, maximize the expiratory time, and limit the static (plateau) airway pressure to $<35\,cmH_2O$. Eucapnia is not an appropriate objective; the present authors' utilize a strategy of permissive hypercapnia while maintaining a serum pH above 7.25. Tracheal intubation may aggravate bronchospasm, and positive-pressure ventilation increases the risk of air leak and circulatory collapse. With the institution of mechanical ventilation, the addition of an inhalational anesthetic agent may decrease bronchospasm.

Table 38-1 Beta-adrenergic Therapies for Status Asthmaticus

Drug	Route	Dose	Interval
Albuterol 0.5% solution	Aerosolized	0.03 mL/kg (= 0.15 mg/kg) Maximum 1 mL (5 mg)	Every 20 minutes × 3, but can be given continuously
Terbutaline 0.05%	Subcutaneous	0.01 mg/kg/dose (= 10 µg/kg) Maximum 0.25 mg	Every 15–20 minutes × 3
Epinephrine 1:1000	Subcutaneous	0.01 mL/kg/dose (= 10 µg/kg) Maximum 0.3 mL	Every 15 minutes × 3
Terbutaline 0.05%	Intravenous	2–10 µg/kg loading dose, then 0.08–6 µg/kg/min	Continuous infusion

Table 38-2   Additional Therapies for Status Asthmaticus

Drug	Dosing Regimen	Notable Effects
Atropine	0.03–0.05 mg/kg aerosolized every 1 h or more frequently as needed	Anticholinergic: dry mouth, blurred vision, tachycardia
Ipratropium bromide (Atrovent)	*Infants:* 0.25 mg aerosolized. *Children >7 years:* 0.5 mg aerosolized	Peak effect: 30 minutes. *Frequency:* Every 4–6 h
Methylprednisolone	*Loading dose:* 2 mg/kg IV. *Maintenance:* 0.5–1 mg/kg IV every 6 h	Hyperglycemia, hypertension, acute psychosis
Hydrocortisone	2–4 mg/kg IV every 4–6 h	
Magnesium sulfate	25–50 mg/kg IV (Maximum 1–2 gm/dose)	Hypotension, flushing

Status Epilepticus

Status epilepticus is continuous seizure activity lasting for more than approximately 30 minutes. Pediatric status epilepticus is caused by epilepsy, head trauma, hypoxic-ischemic encephalopathy, infection (e.g., meningitis, encephalitis), medication toxicity, genetic or metabolic disease, or electrolyte imbalance (e.g., hypoglycemia, hyponatremia). However, the etiology is unknown in approximately 50% of cases.

Status epilepticus is a medical emergency, because if left untreated it entails a risk of permanent neurologic damage or death. Hypoventilation and pulmonary aspiration may occur during the seizure or post-ictal period, or as a result of the sedating effects of the treatment drugs. Management priorities include preventing secondary organ damage (especially to the brain), terminating seizure activity, and determining the etiology. Immediate treatment consists of ensuring upper-airway patency, administration of supplemental oxygen, and possibly endotracheal intubation. Use of a neuromuscular blocker to facilitate endotracheal intubation will temporarily mask recognition of continued seizure activity, so only short- or intermediate-acting agents should be used. Hypotension from prolonged seizure activity or cardiodepressant effects of anticonvulsant drugs should be aggressively treated with volume expansion and vasopressors, if necessary. Persistent hypoxemia, hypotension, hypoglycemia, and metabolic acidosis all contribute to additional neuronal damage. Dextrose should be administered if the serum glucose is below 60 mg/dL. Fever should be aggressively treated since an elevated temperature will lower the seizure threshold and increase cerebral oxygen consumption.

Pharmacologic management is aimed at stopping the seizure and preventing recurrence (Fig. 38-2). The longer status epilepticus persists, the harder it is to control. The most common anticonvulsants used during initial treatment are benzodiazepines, phenytoin, and phenobarbital.

Intravenous lorazepam, midazolam, and diazepam are the first-line anticonvulsants in status epilepticus because of their efficacy and rapid onset of action. Lorazepam is usually preferred because of its relatively long duration of action. If vascular or intraosseous access is not rapidly obtained, intramuscular, sublingual, or rectal administration is also effective. Midazolam is preferred for intramuscular or rectal treatment. Benzodiazepines are not suited for long-term seizure control, but midazolam infusions have been used as a temporizing measure in the pediatric intensive care unit.

Phenytoin (Dilantin) is a second-line anticonvulsant because of its slower onset of action (peak effect 10–30 minutes) owing to its low lipid solubility. Phenytoin is associated with less sedation and respiratory depression than phenobarbital (see below). An intravenous loading dose of 15–20 mg/kg should be administered slowly (0.5–1 mg/kg/min for children and up to 50 mg/min for adults) because of potential adverse cardiovascular effects such as bradycardia, conduction abnormalities, and hypotension. It should be infused in saline since it is incompatible with dextrose-containing fluids. Close monitoring of the electrocardiograph (ECG) and blood pressure should be performed during administration. Because of the cardiovascular effects, phenytoin should be avoided in children with congenital heart disease or arrhythmias. Manifestations of phenytoin toxicity include diplopia, nystagmus, ataxia, and slurred speech.

Phenobarbital is a third-line anticonvulsant because of its delayed onset of action. The intravenous loading dose is 20 mg/kg infused slowly. Side-effects include respiratory depression (especially when used in combination with benzodiazepines), hypotension, and prolonged sedation.

Status epilepticus that remains unresponsive to conventional therapies should be aggressively managed with adjunct therapies. Pentobarbital, a long-acting barbiturate, can be administered using a loading dose of 5–15 mg/kg, followed by an infusion of 1–2 mg/kg/h. The goal is to obtain burst suppression on electroencephalography (EEG). Side-effects include cardiorespiratory depression

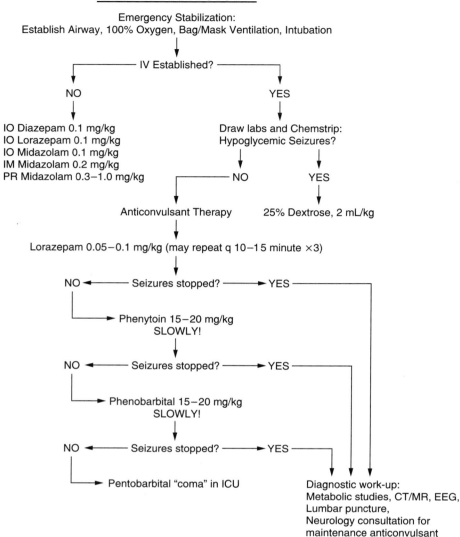

Figure 38-2 Algorithm for treatment of status epilepticus. (Redrawn with permission from Nichols et al: *Golden Hour: The Handbook of Advanced Pediatric Life Support,* 2nd edn, Mosby, Philadelphia, 1996.)

(that often requires inotropic therapy) and granulocytopenia. As a last resort, inhalational general anesthetics may be required for neuronal suppression.

Following control of seizures, attention is turned toward determining the etiology. This evaluation includes investigation of metabolic, infectious, and toxic causes. Hyponatremia should be ruled out. A lumbar puncture with an opening pressure measurement may be indicated to rule out meningitis or meningoencephalitis. However, a lumbar puncture should be delayed in the presence of focal neurologic signs, increased intracranial pressure, cardiorespiratory depression, or coagulopathy. The delay in performing a lumbar puncture should not delay administration of broad-spectrum antibiotics or antiviral therapy if an infection is suspected. Head CT imaging should be obtained if there is a history of trauma, signs

of elevated intracranial pressure, or presence of focal neurologic signs.

Shock

Shock occurs when there is insufficient delivery of oxygen and nutrients to meet the metabolic demands of the body. *Shock can exist even if the blood pressure is normal.* It is helpful to consider three progressive stages of shock: compensated, uncompensated, and irreversible.

Early compensated shock is notable for the activation of mechanisms that maintain a normal blood pressure and organ perfusion. This is usually accomplished by increasing the heart rate and the systemic vascular resistance (SVR). Neonates and young infants are unable to significantly increase their stroke volume, so tachycardia is the only way to augment cardiac output (cardiac output = stroke volume × heart rate). Peripheral vasoconstriction increases the diastolic pressure and narrows the pulse pressure (systolic BP − diastolic BP). The physical exam will reveal cool, pale extremities with delayed capillary refill (>4 seconds), and decreased urine output. In the uncompensated stage, circulatory compensation fails and leads to cellular dysfunction, ischemia, and endothelial injury. Hypoperfusion of the brain leads to an altered level of consciousness and renal hypoperfusion leads to anuria. The child develops tachypnea to compensate for the metabolic acidosis caused by hypoperfusion and decreased oxygen delivery. Bradycardia is a worrisome sign in an infant because it significantly decreases cardiac output. Hypotension is a late finding in pediatric shock and places the patient at risk for multiorgan system failure (Table 38-3). Irreversible shock occurs when there is unrecoverable end-organ damage.

Shock is classified into four major categories: hypovolemic, septic, distributive, and cardiogenic. *Hypovolemic shock* is the most common cause of shock in children. It results from decreased intravascular volume, which leads to decreased venous return and preload. This can be caused by water and electrolyte loss (e.g., vomiting, diarrhea, renal losses, or heat stroke), blood loss, or plasma losses (e.g., burns, nephrotic syndrome). Initial management is focused on airway, breathing, and circulation (Fig. 38-3). Fluid resuscitation is guided by heart rate, peripheral perfusion, and urine output. Isotonic fluids such as Lactated Ringers or normal saline are used during the initial volume replacement. With blood loss, the "3 to 1 rule" applies: for every 1 mL of blood loss, 3 mL of isotonic fluids should be administered since only one-third of the volume remains in the intravascular space. Patients with severe liver disease may be unable to metabolize the lactate in Lactated Ringers solution. Development of a hyperchloremic metabolic acidosis from excessive normal saline administration is also possible. Patients with severe renal disease may not be able to excrete the potassium contained in Lactated Ringers solution.

If blood loss continues, hemorrhagic shock develops and can be classified into four categories based on the

Fluid Volume Resuscitation in Hypovolemic Shock

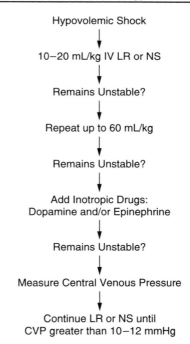

Figure 38-3   Algorithm for treatment of hypovolemic shock. (Redrawn with permission from Nichols et al: *Golden Hour: The Handbook of Advanced Pediatric Life Support*, 2nd edn, Mosby, Philadelphia, 1996.)

estimated blood volume deficit (Table 38-4). When available, fresh whole blood (<48 hours old) is the blood product of choice since it contains red blood cells, platelets, and clotting factors. This is rarely available, so packed red blood cells are used. If blood is needed immediately, type O, Rh-negative blood is the "universal donor." Also, type-specific blood without a full crossmatch can be obtained quickly. A dilutional coagulopathy is often present in massively transfused patients. Abnormalities can start when a 1.5–2 blood volume loss is replaced with crystalloid and packed red blood cells alone.

Septic shock occurs due to overwhelming infection. It is a combination of hypovolemia, altered vascular tone, cardiac pump failure, and cellular metabolic derangements that result in metabolic acidosis. In the initial stages, the extremities can be warm and well perfused or cold with delayed capillary refill. Vasodilation is caused by inflammatory mediators (e.g., endotoxin, tumor necrosis factor, and interleukin-1), and is manifested clinically as diastolic hypotension and a wide pulse pressure. If untreated, persistent shock will lead to multiorgan system failure. These patients may require massive administration of isotonic fluids (>60 mL/kg) and vasopressors. Further management includes continuous assessment and treatment of end-organ perfusion abnormalities: oliguria, mental status changes, metabolic acidosis, decreased

Table 38-3 Hypotension in Infants and Children	
Age	**Minimum Systolic Blood Pressure (mmHg)**
<1 month	60
1–12 months	70
>1 year	70 + (2 × age in years)
>10 years	90

Table 38-4 Classification of Hemorrhagic Shock				
	I	**II**	**III**	**IV**
Estimated blood volume deficit	10–15%	20–25%	30–35%	>40%
Pulse (beats/min)	>100	>150	>150	>150
Respiratory rate	Normal	Increased	Increased	Increased or apnea
Capillary refill	<5 s	5–10 s	10–15 s	>20 s
Blood pressure	Normal	Decreased pulse pressure	Decreased	Severely decreased
Mental status	Normal	Anxious	Confused	Unconscious
Orthostatic hypotension	+	++	+++	+++
Urine output	1–3 mL/kg	0.5–1 mL/kg	<0.5 mL/kg	None

Reproduced with permission from Nichols et al: *Golden Hour: The Handbook of Advanced Life Support*, 2nd edn, Mosby, Philadelphia, 1996.

cardiac output, coagulopathy, and disseminated intravascular coagulation (DIC).

Distributive shock is caused by abnormalities in vasomotor tone. Vasodilatation and peripheral intravascular pooling cause relative hypovolemia. Neurogenic shock caused by spinal cord injury, usually at the cervicothoracic area, is a classic example. Loss of sympathetic vascular tone causes bradycardia, vasodilation, and hypotension. Another example is anaphylaxis. In distributive shock, Trendelenburg positioning (head down with cervical spine immobilized if indicated) and administration of isotonic fluids can be helpful to restore circulatory stability. Vasopressor drugs with direct α_1-adrenergic activity may be necessary.

Cardiogenic shock can result from congenital heart disease, trauma, prolonged arrhythmias (e.g., supraventricular tachycardia), cardiac tamponade, infection (e.g., myocarditis), acquired cardiomyopathies (Kawasaki's disease with coronary aneurysms), and drug intoxications. Central venous pressure monitoring and physical examination will guide cautious fluid administration. These patients will usually benefit from inotropic support and afterload reduction.

Special consideration should be given to neonates presenting in shock. They may have undiagnosed congenital heart disease that has ductal-dependent systemic circulation. These babies are asymptomatic at birth because aortic blood flow is provided by the patent ductus arteriosus (PDA). However, when the PDA closes, shock develops from inadequate systemic output. These patients usually have left-sided obstructive lesions, for example hypoplastic left heart syndrome (HLHS), aortic valve stenosis, interrupted aortic arch, or coarctation of the aorta. Prostaglandin E_1 (0.05–0.1 µg/kg/min) should be started in an attempt to open the ductus arteriosus until a definitive surgical procedure can be performed.

Inotropic Agents

Dopamine

Dopamine is the metabolic precursor of norepinephrine and epinephrine. It is a central neurotransmitter that is also found peripherally in the sympathetic nervous system and in the adrenal medulla. Depending on the local concentration, dopamine produces vascular dilatation or constriction by stimulation of dopaminergic, α, and β receptors in the brain and peripheral vascular beds.

Dopamine is used to treat hypotension and oliguria in children with distributive, septic, or cardiogenic shock when volume resuscitation has been ineffective. Low infusion rates (1–5 µg/kg/min) stimulate dopamine receptors and are associated with increased glomerular filtration and renal blood flow. Intermediate doses (5–10 µg/kg/min) are associated with increased heart rate and improved myocardial contractility via β-receptor stimulation and release of norepinephrine from nerve terminals. Administration of dopamine in the intermediate dosing range usually results in an increase in systolic blood pressure and minimal change in diastolic pressure. SVR is unchanged; however, a higher infusion dose (>10 µg/kg/min) is associated with an increase in SVR secondary to α-receptor stimulation.

Adverse effects of dopamine include tachycardia, hypertension, dysrhythmias, and increased myocardial oxygen consumption. Administration of dopamine is associated with decreases in Pao_2 by inhibition of hypoxic pulmonary vasoconstriction. Dopamine depresses the ventilatory response to hypoxemia by as much as 60%.

The clearance of dopamine decreases with age throughout childhood. During the first 20 months of life, dopamine clearance decreases by almost 50%. All studies of dopamine pharmacokinetics in seriously ill children show substantial interindividual variation in pharmacokinetic parameters. This is especially true for clearance, which appears to be not only age- but also concentration-dependent. This causes a large variation in the dose requirements required to achieve a desired clinical response.

Dobutamine

Dobutamine resembles dopamine structurally but has greater selectivity for β_1 and β_2 receptors. When administered in a dose range of 5–20 µg/kg/min, it primarily enhances myocardial contractility and increases stroke volume, with less increase in heart rate than dopamine. Its administration is associated with decreases in SVR and PVR, such that hypotension may occur from vasodilatation in children who are volume depleted or who have an elevated baseline sympathetic imbalance.

Dobutamine is indicated in the treatment of cardiac decompensation, as may occur after surgery for congenital heart disease, or in children with congestive heart failure or myocarditis. Dobutamine may be used to treat myocardial dysfunction associated with sepsis, but it is rarely the sole inotropic agent. Because of its inotropic properties, dobutamine increases myocardial oxygen demand, and may predispose to arrhythmias.

Ephedrine

Ephedrine possesses α- and β-agonist activity but primarily acts indirectly by enhancing the release of norepinephrine from sympathetic neurons. Heart rate and cardiac output are increased with a variable increase in SVR. Ephedrine is used intraoperatively (0.2–0.3 mg/kg/dose) to treat hypotension related to administration of general or regional anesthesia.

Epinephrine

Epinephrine is the principal hormone involved in the normal stress response and produces widespread metabolic and hemodynamic effects. It activates α, β_1, and β_2 receptors, and is useful in treating shock associated with myocardial dysfunction and hypotension. During epinephrine infusions, hepatic and splanchnic blood flow increases, while renal blood flow may be reduced. In addition, administration of epinephrine results in bronchial and gastrointestinal smooth muscle relaxation.

At relatively low doses (0.05–0.1 µg/kg/min), epinephrine stimulates β_1 receptors. Therefore, one of the earliest effects is an increase in heart rate and inotropy. At these doses, stimulation of β_2 receptors promotes relaxation of resistance arterioles, promoting a decrease in SVR and a decreased diastolic blood pressure. Higher plasma concentrations activate α receptors, with a subsequent increase in SVR. High infusion doses (1–2 µg/kg/min) are associated with significant vasoconstriction, and possible compromise of blood flow to

individual organs. Plasma concentrations of epinephrine correlate with the infusion rate, suggesting linear pharmacokinetics. Epinephrine clearance rates in critically ill children appear to be lower than the reported clearance rates in healthy adults.

In the pediatric critical care environment, the most frequent indications for intravenous epinephrine are cardiogenic shock and septic shock with reduced stroke volume. The septic patient who does not improve after aggressive volume repletion and treatment with dopamine and/or dobutamine may benefit from epinephrine. Epinephrine boluses are used to treat asystole and other dysrhythmias that cause hypotension. The recommended dose is 0.01 mg/kg (0.1 mL/kg of the 1:10,000 preparation). Epinephrine is the treatment of choice for signs and symptoms of anaphylaxis and may occasionally be used in the treatment of severe bronchospasm.

Adverse effects of epinephrine administration include enhanced automaticity and increased oxygen consumption. An imbalance of myocardial oxygen delivery and consumption can produce ECG changes consistent with ischemia. Additional adverse effects include hypokalemia secondary to β_2-adrenergic stimulation, and hyperglycemia secondary to α-adrenergic mediated insulin suppression.

Isoproterenol

Isoproterenol, a synthetic derivative of norepinephrine, is a potent, nonselective β-adrenergic agonist with very low affinity for α-adrenergic receptors. Isoproterenol increases heart rate and enhances myocardial contractility. Peripheral vasodilatation produces a decrease in systemic vascular resistance. The increase in inotropy and chronotropy in the face of decreased SVR results in an increase in cardiac output. Pulmonary bronchial and vascular bed β_2-adrenergic receptor agonism results in bronchodilation and pulmonary vasodilation.

Isoproterenol currently has limited clinical applicability in children. It may be used to treat hemodynamically significant bradycardia, and has been used in infants after cardiac surgery to improve cardiac index. Isoproterenol has also been used as an adjunct to therapy for children with status asthmaticus, but it is being replaced with continuous nebulized albuterol and intravenous terbutaline.

Norepinephrine

Norepinephrine is an endogenous catecholamine with potent α and β_1 activity and little β_2 activity. Infusions in normal subjects result in elevations of SVR because α effects are not opposed by β_2 stimulation. Reflex vagal activity reduces the rate of sinus node discharge, blunting the expected chronotropic effect of β_1 stimulation. Stroke volume increases, but there is minimal change in cardiac output. Resistance increases in most vascular beds, including the kidney, liver, and skeletal muscle. Glomerular filtration is maintained unless renal blood flow is decreased substantially. Coronary blood flow increases, due to direct coronary dilation and an increase in blood pressure.

Norepinephrine improves perfusion in children with hypotension and a normal or elevated cardiac index that has not responded favorably to volume resuscitation. Treatment with norepinephrine is beneficial in the setting of tachycardia, because it can increase SVR, arterial blood pressure, and urine flow without an increase in heart rate. The usual starting infusion dose is 0.05–0.1 µg/kg/min, which is then titrated to the desired effect. Norepinephrine administration may improve blood pressure without improving perfusion. This is most commonly seen in children with a low cardiac index and stroke volume.

Phenylephrine

Phenylephrine is predominantly an α-adrenergic agonist and is used to treat hypotension when SVR is low. By vasoconstricting arteriolar beds, phenylephrine increases blood pressure and causes a vagally mediated sinus bradycardia. There are few data available on its use in pediatric patients and it is rarely used intraoperatively because children do not usually exhibit hypotension related to regional anesthesia.

Milrinone

Milrinone is a phosphodiesterase inhibitor that produces inotropy (without tachycardia) and vasodilatation by increasing concentrations of intracellular cyclic AMP. Milrinone has been used in children for the treatment of low-output states following cardiac surgery and in the management of shock when catecholamine infusions alone are unsuccessful. Pharmacokinetic parameters of milrinone are different in children from in adults, reflecting a higher volume of distribution and more rapid clearance rate. An initial intravenous loading dose of 50–75 µg/kg over 15–60 minutes is followed by a continuous infusion of 0.375–0.75 µg/kg/min, which is then titrated to effect. Administration of milrinone may be associated with atrial or ventricular arrhythmias.

Intracranial Hypertension

Intracranial hypertension, defined as an intracranial pressure (ICP) above 20 mmHg persisting for more than 5 minutes, is most commonly due to pediatric traumatic brain injury. No intervention can reverse the primary brain injury; supportive measures are aimed at preventing secondary injury or damage to surrounding neurons.

The components of the rigid cranial vault include brain tissue, cerebrospinal fluid (CSF), and blood. For the ICP to remain normal, alterations in the volume of one compartment must be compensated for by opposite changes in another compartment (the Monro-Kellie doctrine). For example, an epidural blood collection can initially increase without affecting ICP because of a compensatory decrease in CSF volume. However, once these compensatory measures have been maximized, the ICP will rise dramatically with a small increase in blood volume (Fig. 38-4). Clinically, this causes a Cushing's reflex that consists of hypertension, bradycardia, and abnormal respirations.

Autoregulation refers to the brain's ability to maintain cerebral blood flow (CBF) despite changes in blood pressure. In the uninjured brain, CBF remains relatively constant within mean arterial pressures between 50 and 150 mmHg. In the traumatized brain, this ability may be lost and CBF may increase or decrease as the blood pressure increases or decreases, respectively. CBF remains constant when the Pao_2 is above 60 mmHg, but increases dramatically with hypoxemia. A linear relationship exists between CBF and $Paco_2$ – blood flow increases as carbon dioxide increases (Fig. 38-5). Furthermore, CBF is closely linked to the cerebral metabolic rate of oxygen consumption ($CMRO_2$); it will increase if $CMRO_2$ increases due to seizures, pain, or agitation, and decrease as $CMRO_2$ decreases due to hypothermia or sedation.

The major goal in the management of intracranial hypertension is to ensure adequate oxygen and substrate delivery to the brain. This is achieved by ensuring adequate oxygenation and ventilation, lowering the intracranial pressure, and maintaining an adequate cerebral perfusion pressure (Fig. 38-6). The cerebral perfusion pressure (CPP) is the difference between mean arterial pressure (MAP) and ICP (or central venous pressure (CVP), whichever is greater). In adolescents and adults, CPP greater than 70 mmHg suggests adequate CBF, while in infants, an acceptable CPP is one greater

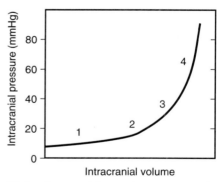

Figure 38-4   Intracranial compliance curve. When the intracranial volume increases from points 1 to 2, the ICP slightly increases. However, from points 3 to 4, a small increase in volume will cause a dramatic increase in ICP (Monro-Kellie principle). (Redrawn with permission from Nichols et al: *Golden Hour: The Handbook of Advanced Pediatric Life Support*, 2nd edn, Mosby, Philadelphia, 1996.)

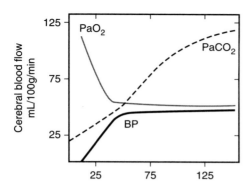

Figure 38-5   Relationship between cerebral blood flow and mean arterial pressure, arterial oxygen tension, and arterial carbon dioxide tension. (Redrawn with permission from Nichols et al: *Golden Hour: The Handbook of Advanced Pediatric Life Support*, 2nd edn, Mosby, Philadelphia, 1996.)

than 50 mmHg. Intracranial pressure can be monitored using extradural, intraparenchymal, or intraventricular catheters. Intraventricular catheters have the additional benefit of providing a therapeutic option of CSF drainage to lower ICP.

Tracheal intubation is indicated if airway protective reflexes are absent or if there is a depressed level of consciousness (Glasgow Coma Scale ≤8). Short-term hyperventilation is one of the most potent therapies to lower elevated ICP. However, prolonged hyperventilation is associated with worsening of cerebral ischemia and therefore is not recommended. Recent studies indicate that positive end-expiratory pressure (PEEP) does not increase intracranial pressure. Therefore, PEEP should be used to maintain adequate oxygenation and prevent alveolar collapse. The current cardiovascular management strategy consists of volume resuscitation and transient

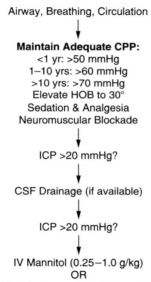

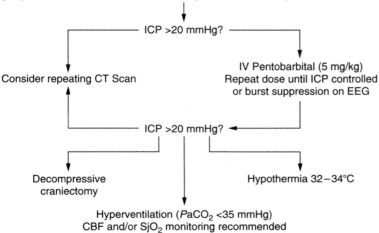

Figure 38-6   Algorithm for treatment of increased intracranial pressure. (Redrawn with permission from Nichols et al: *Golden Hour: The Handbook of Advanced Pediatric Life Support*, 2nd edn, Mosby, Philadelphia, 1996.)

periods of hypertension to maintain CPP. Hypotonic solutions will exacerbate cerebral edema.

Additional principles of ICP management include avoidance of hyperthermia, prevention of venous outflow obstruction, normoglycemia, and seizure prophylaxis if indicated. Hyperthermia increases $CMRO_2$ and may cause a mismatch between demand and supply. The head should be elevated and maintained in the midline position to avoid jugular venous compression. Cervical collars and endotracheal tube ties should not be too tight. Hyperglycemia will exacerbate neuronal injury and therefore should be aggressively treated with insulin. If an intraventricular catheter is in place, CSF drainage can be therapeutic.

Hyperosmolar therapy continues to be an important component of ICP management. Mannitol (0.25–1 g/kg IV infused over 10–30 minutes) creates an osmotic gradient that draws extracellular brain water across the blood–brain barrier into the intravascular space. It is also thought to decrease blood viscosity, thereby enhancing oxygen delivery. The prophylactic use of mannitol is not recommended owing to its volume-depleting diuretic effect. It should be used in patients demonstrating signs of transtentorial herniation. Hypertonic saline (3% NaCl) is being used more frequently to control ICP. It is thought to reduce cerebral swelling by producing an osmolar gradient to decrease cerebral water content. Continuous infusion of 3% NaCl through a central line will prevent swings in osmolality and maintain intravascular volume. It is not unusual to have serum sodium concentrations between 150 and 160 mEq/L. Side-effects of hyperosmolar therapy include renal failure (especially if the serum osmolality is >320 mEq/L), hemolysis, and subarachnoid hemorrhage related to tearing of bridging vessels due to rapid brain shrinkage. Rapid increases in serum sodium are also associated with development of central pontine myelinolysis.

Barbiturate coma (burst suppression on EEG) is indicated when intracranial hypertension is not controlled with conventional therapies. It lowers ICP by lowering $CMRO_2$, which then results in cerebral vasoconstriction and a reduction in cerebral blood flow and volume. Barbiturates produce respiratory depression and a dose-dependent decrease in arterial blood pressure and cardiac output that often requires significant volume resuscitation and inotropic therapy. When the above measures fail, a measure of last resort is a decompressive craniectomy.

Hepatic Failure

Acute or fulminant hepatic failure is a clinical syndrome that results from massive necrosis of liver cells leading to the development of hepatic encephalopathy and severe impairment of hepatic function. Hepatic failure can occur as a primary process in a healthy person, as an exacerbation of a chronic liver disease, or as part of multiorgan system failure. Several authors have suggested redefining the syndrome into three categories based on the time interval between the onset of jaundice and encephalopathy: hyperacute (0–7 days), acute (1–4 weeks), and subacute (4–12 weeks). Causes of fulminant hepatic failure in children include viral hepatitis, drug-induced liver injury, and inherited metabolic diseases, among others.

The diagnosis of acute hepatic failure is based on clinical findings (jaundice, enlarged liver, and encephalopathy) in conjunction with abnormal biochemical data (low serum albumin, hyperbilirubinemia, and prolongation of the prothrombin time). There is no specific therapy for acute hepatic injury, except early administration of N-acetylcysteine in acetaminophen toxicity.

Fulminant hepatic failure can adversely affect all organ systems. Hepatic encephalopathy may result from diminished hepatic synthesis of an unknown substance(s) needed for normal brain function or diminished hepatic metabolism of an unknown substance(s) that possesses neurotoxicity or promote neural inhibition. As liver function deteriorates, hepatic encephalopathy worsens (Table 38-5). Serum ammonia levels do not correlate with the severity of encephalopathy. Advanced encephalopathy is associated with severe cerebral edema and life-threatening cerebral herniation.

Acute renal failure develops in 30–50% of patients with acute liver failure (hepatorenal syndrome). Contributing factors include intravascular volume depletion caused by excessive diuresis or untreated gastrointestinal hemorrhage, and nephrotoxic drug administration.

Hemorrhagic complications in liver failure result from inadequate synthesis of clotting factors, thrombocytopenia from DIC, and splenic sequestration of platelets. Blood loss may occur from stress-induced gastritis or from esophageal or gastric varices that develop secondary to portal hypertension. Vitamin K administration augments production of factors II, VII, IX, and X. Fresh frozen plasma and/or cryoprecipitate is

Table 38-5	Clinical Staging of Hepatic Encephalopathy
Grade	**Description**
0	No disease
1	Periods of lethargy, altered personality, altered spatial orientation
2	Inappropriate behavior or drowsiness, confusion, asterixis, hyperreflexia
3	Stuporous but arousable, sleeps most of the time, agitated, incoherent speech
4	Coma: 4a = responds to painful stimuli; 4b = unresponsive to painful stimuli

administered when patients are bleeding or prior to an invasive procedure.

Hypoxemia can develop in acute liver failure for several reasons. Failure of the damaged liver to clear vasodilating humoral substances can cause intrapulmonary shunting and ventilation/perfusion mismatch. Pulmonary edema results from low oncotic pressure and fluid overload associated with antidiuretic-like activity. Atelectasis can develop from massive ascites that impedes full respiratory excursion or hypoventilation caused by encephalopathy. Ascites develops as a result of increased hepatic vascular resistance, decreased oncotic pressure, and altered aldosterone secretion.

Patients with chronic liver failure develop a high cardiac output in conjunction with a low SVR. Oxygen delivery is increased, but oxygen consumption is decreased due to microcirculatory disturbances that lead to tissue hypoxia.

Orthotopic liver transplantation is the most important advance in the therapy of acute liver failure. There is no clear set of indications for liver transplantation in pediatric patients, but without hepatic transplantation, acute hepatic failure carries a grim prognosis with an 80–85% mortality rate. Death is usually caused by cerebral herniation from intracranial hypertension.

Renal Failure

Acute renal failure is the sudden inability of the kidney to regulate fluid, electrolyte, and solute balance; this can occur with or without a change in urine volume. Causes of acute renal failure can be categorized into three major categories: prerenal, intrinsic renal parenchymal damage, and postrenal (Table 38-6).

Prerenal renal failure is caused by inadequate renal perfusion from systemic hypovolemia, poor cardiac output, or vascular obstruction. Drugs can also have an adverse effect on renal perfusion: nonsteroidal anti-inflammatory drugs (NSAIDs) promote renal vasoconstriction, and angiotensin-converting (ACE) inhibitors reduce glomerular filtration pressure. Intrinsic renal parenchymal damage affects the structures of the nephron. Most intrinsic renal failure is caused by ischemia, nephron damage from toxins, or inflammation. Acute tubular necrosis (ATN) is the most common form of intrinsic renal failure. Postrenal renal failure is due to mechanical obstruction in the urinary collecting system. When the obstruction occurs at the level of the bladder or urethra, renal function is more likely to be severely affected since both kidneys will be injured. Unilateral obstruction does not result in renal failure if the other kidney is healthy.

The diagnosis of acute renal failure requires a stepwise approach. The patient's history and physical exam can yield important clues in the evaluation. Analysis of urinary sediment can be helpful: white cell casts suggest

Table 38-6 Causes of Acute Renal Failure

Pathogenesis	Clinical Scenario
Prerenal	
Hypovolemia	Vomiting, diarrhea, hemorrhage
Hypoperfusion	Myocardial dysfunction, sepsis, hypoxia
Drugs	NSAIDs, ACE inhibitors
Renal	
Vascular occlusion	Bilateral renal artery or vein thrombosis
Glomerular injury	Hemolytic uremic syndrome, glomerulonephritis
Tubular injury	Acute tubular necrosis, nephrotoxins (aminoglycosides)
Tubular obstruction	Tumor lysis syndrome, rhabdomyolysis
Postrenal	
Obstruction	Urinary tract anomalies: posterior urethral valves
	Renal stones
	Neurogenic bladder

ACE, angiotensin-converting enzyme; NSAID, nonsteroidal anti-inflammatory drug.

interstitial nephritis; red cell casts are found in glomerulonephritis; and heme-positive urine without red blood cells suggest myoglobinuria or hemoglobinuria. Analysis of urine osmolality, urine creatinine (Cr) and electrolytes can also aid diagnosis. Calculation of the fractional excretion of sodium (FE_{Na}) will help distinguish prerenal from renal causes:

$$FE_{Na} = \left(\frac{Urine_{(Na)}}{Plasma_{(Na)}} \right) \times \left(\frac{Plasma_{(Cr)}}{Urine_{(Cr)}} \right) \times 100$$

In general, patients with hypovolemia will have concentrated urine: urine osmolality >500 mOsm/kg, urine sodium content <20 mEq/L, and FE_{Na} <1. In patients with tubular necrosis, the urine is dilute: urine osmolality <350 mOsm/kg, urine sodium content usually >40 mEq/L, and FE_{Na} usually >1.

The management of acute renal failure is aimed at treating the underlying disorder or causative mechanism. Restoring effective circulating volume is one of the most important management issues, especially if volume depletion causes hemodynamic instability. If the patient is euvolemic with oliguria, then replacement of fluid losses is indicated. This includes insensible losses calculated at 300 mL/m^2/day in addition to measuring and replacing other losses such as urine output, nasogastric tube drainage and diarrhea. If significant volume overload exists, then fluid restriction to insensible losses or even smaller quantities may be necessary.

Electrolyte and acid–base abnormalities are frequently encountered in renal failure. Hyponatremia is usually caused by water retention. In hospitalized patients with oliguria, the administration of excessive amounts of

Table 38-7   Treatment of Hyperkalemia

Drug	Dose	Mechanism of Action	Complication
Calcium gluconate (10%)	50–100 mg/kg IV	Stabilizes myocyte membrane potential	Bradyarrhythmias
Calcium chloride (10%)	10–20 mg/kg IV	Stabilizes myocyte membrane potential	Bradyarrhythmias
Sodium Bicarbonate	1–2 mEq/kg IV over 10–30 minutes	Shifts extracellular K^+ into cells	Hypernatremia, alkalosis, tetany (decreases ionized calcium)
Insulin	0.1 units/kg IV	Stimulates cellular uptake of K^+	Hypoglycemia; administer IV glucose 0.5 g/kg
Albuterol (0.5%)	0.03 mL/kg nebulized in normal saline	Stimulates uptake of intracellular K^+	Tachycardia; arrhythmias
Sodium polystyrene sulfonate (Kayexalate)	1 g/kg by mouth or per rectum	Exchange of Na^+ for K^+ across gut mucosa	Hypernatremia, diarrhea

hypotonic fluids can contribute or worsen hyponatremia. Restriction of free water is indicated if the patient is volume overloaded. When hyponatremia is symptomatic (i.e., seizures and obtundation), it is appropriate to administer hypertonic saline (approx. 4 mL/kg) to raise the serum sodium to 125 mEq/L. Rapid correction of serum sodium to normal (140 mEq/L) can lead to central pontine myelinolysis and cerebral injury. Hyperphosphatemia develops because of decreased renal phosphate clearance. This is treated with dietary restriction and agents that bind phosphate enterally (e.g., calcium carbonate). A metabolic acidosis develops because of impaired renal excretion of acids and alterations in renal bicarbonate reabsorption and regeneration. In the case of acidosis and severe hypocalcemia, calcium must be replaced first since alkalinization will decrease the ionized calcium levels further and may exacerbate symptoms of hypocalcemia such as tetany or cardiovascular electrical abnormalities.

Hyperkalemia (potassium >6.0 mEq/L) is the major life-threatening electrolyte abnormality in acute renal failure and must be aggressively treated. ECG abnormalities include tall, peaked T waves initially, followed by prolongation of the P-R interval and widening of the QRS complex, leading to ventricular fibrillation and cardiac arrest. Therapy involves stabilizing the myocardium, redistributing potassium from the extracellular to intracellular space to decrease serum potassium levels, and enhancing potassium elimination from the body (Table 38-7).

The absolute indications for dialysis in renal failure are: intractable acidosis; hyperkalemia; symptomatic uremia such as pericarditis, bleeding or encephalopathy; volume overload with congestive heart failure, pulmonary edema, or hypertension; and toxins that are dialyzable (e.g., ammonia, salicylates, methanol, ethylene glycol). A relative indication is to provide better nutrition or multiple blood products during periods of oliguria.

Peritoneal dialysis, intermittent hemodialysis, or continuous hemofiltration are all viable options, determined in consultation with a pediatric nephrologist.

Chronic renal failure (Box 38-3) is the irreversible deterioration in the glomerular filtration rate (GFR) to a point that renal replacement therapy is necessary to sustain life. This usually occurs with a GFR below 10–20 mL/min/1.73 m².

Box 38-3   Common Features in Chronic Renal Failure

Electrolyte Disorders

Hyperkalemia
Hyperphosphatemia
Hypocalcemia
Hypermagnesemia
Hyponatremia
Metabolic acidosis

Gastrointestinal

Delayed gastric emptying
Nausea and vomiting

Hematologic

Anemia
Platelet dysfunction secondary to uremia

Cardiovascular

Hypertension
Volume overload

Endocrine

Growth failure

Respiratory Failure

Respiratory failure is the inability to maintain normal exchange of oxygen and carbon dioxide between the atmosphere and blood. It occurs more frequently in infants and children because of a developmentally immature respiratory system, greater oxygen consumption and carbon dioxide excretion demands, and a higher frequency of disease processes with primary or secondary respiratory complications.

One schematic used to identify the etiology for respiratory failure divides the respiratory system into three parts: the extrathoracic airway, the lung, and the respiratory pump. Maturational changes in the structure and function of these parts during infancy and early childhood influence the susceptibility to respiratory failure (see Chapter 2). Respiratory failure can be classified into two main patterns based on blood gas abnormalities (Table 38-8). Type I (hypoxemic) respiratory failure results from poor matching of pulmonary ventilation to perfusion, leading to noncardiac mixing of venous blood with arterial blood. It is characterized by arterial hypoxemia with normal or low arterial carbon dioxide. Type II (hypercarbic) respiratory failure results from inadequate alveolar ventilation in relation to physiologic needs and is characterized by hypoxemia and arterial hypercarbia. This occurs when a disease or injury leads to an imbalance between the power available to do the respiratory work and the load on the respiratory system. In general, diseases that affect the anatomic components of the lung will result in regions of low or absent ventilation/perfusion ratios, leading initially to type I respiratory failure. Diseases of the extrathoracic airway and respiratory pump result in a respiratory power/load imbalance and type II respiratory failure.

Arterial hypoxemia is caused by several mechanisms: hypoventilation; ventilation/perfusion (V/Q) mismatch; shunting of systemic venous blood to the systemic arterial circuit; impaired alveolar diffusion of oxygen; inhalation of a hypoxic gas mixture; and abnormal desaturation of systemic venous blood in the presence of other mechanisms for hypoxemia.

Initial treatment of hypoxemia is supplemental oxygen. When lung disease results in significant oxygenation abnormalities ($F_IO_2 \geq 0.60$ required to maintain $Pao_2 \geq 60$ mmHg), continuous positive airway pressure (CPAP) may be helpful. CPAP, ranging from 3 to 10 cmH$_2$O, increases lung volume, and enhances ventilation to areas with low V/Q ratios and improves respiratory mechanics. CPAP is often applied using a tight-fitting mask or nasal cannula. If CPAP ≥ 10 cmH$_2$O does not relieve severe hypoxemia, decrease work of breathing, or fails to resolve hypercarbia with a pH ≤ 7.25, treatment with mechanical ventilation is indicated.

Diseases of the respiratory pump (central nervous system, respiratory muscle, or chest wall) cause type II respiratory failure. Noninvasive and invasive modes of mechanical ventilation can be instituted to decrease the work of breathing and provide adequate gas exchange. Noninvasive mechanical ventilation refers to nasal prongs or facemask. During the last decade, the widespread availability of inspiratory pressure support has made noninvasive mechanical ventilation more successful than in previous eras. Inspiratory pressure support is a ventilator modality where the patient's effort is boosted by increased circuited pressure during inspiration. This allows the patient to initiate his or her own breaths and regulate inspiratory time and tidal volume. The pressure support strategy promotes patient synchrony and comfort with mechanical support. Disease severity limits the use of this technique if periodic relief from the interface is unavailable for days. A tracheal tube is necessary and safer under these circumstances.

Conventional modes of mechanical ventilation are designed to assist physiologic respiratory pump function and improve lung volumes. Positive pressure is used to inflate the lungs. The clinician monitors the $Paco_2$ to evaluate therapeutic adjustments in the minute ventilation. The minute ventilation is adjusted by modifying the frequency or the tidal volume. In turn, tidal volume is adjusted by controlling either the delivered volume (volume-controlled ventilation) or the inspiratory pressure (pressure-controlled ventilation). The duration of inspiration is adjustable but this parameter only indirectly effects minute ventilation through its effect on expiratory time or when high airway resistance is present. Inspiratory time adjustments have a more direct influence on mean airway pressure (MAP), and therefore oxygenation.

Principles of Pediatric Mechanical Ventilation

The goals of mechanical ventilation are to improve alveolar ventilation, reduce ventilation/perfusion (V/Q) mismatch, reexpand collapsed lung segments, reduce work of breathing, and eliminate respiratory muscle fatigue. Indications for institution of mechanical ventilation in children include:

1. Hypoxemic respiratory failure, defined as inadequate arterial oxygenation with $Pao_2 < 50$ mmHg

Table 38-8	Classification of Respiratory Failure	
Arterial Pressure	**Type I (Hypoxemic)**	**Type II (Hypercarbic)**
Pao_2	Low	Low
$Paco_2$	Normal or low	High

at $F_{I}O_2$ >0.50. The most common causes include alveolar diseases such as pneumonia, acute respiratory distress syndrome, or pulmonary edema.

2. Type II or hypercarbic respiratory failure, defined as inadequate ventilation with $Paco_2$ > 50 mmHg and an arterial pH <7.30. It can develop with or without hypoxemia. It is caused by respiratory pump failure, which includes abnormalities in the central nervous system, respiratory muscles, or chest wall. Examples include a child with a neuromuscular disease (e.g., spinal muscular atrophy) or hypoventilation (e.g., accidental narcotic overdose).

3. Circulatory failure such as shock or congestive heart failure. In this setting, mechanical ventilation can cause a reduction in metabolic expenditure, decrease respiratory muscle dysfunction caused by hypoxia, or decrease respiratory dysfunction associated with shock (i.e., ARDS).

4. Neurologic injury. Tracheal intubation and mechanical ventilation ensures a stable airway in patients with an acute neurologic injury. Mechanical ventilation can control arterial $Paco_2$, which influences cerebral blood volume and intracranial pressure.

5. Postoperative surgical conditions that require sedation and/or immobility.

Mechanical ventilation is accomplished using pressure-controlled or volume-controlled ventilation. The fundamental difference between the two modes is the targeted goal; pressure ventilation modes guarantee a certain peak inspired airway pressure at the expense of a variable tidal volume, while volume ventilation guarantees flow and the set volume at the expense of inspiratory pressures.

With pressure-controlled ventilation, the physician determines the targeted inspiratory pressure and the inspiratory time. After the breath is initiated, the targeted pressure is attained early during the breath and is maintained at the airway opening during inspiration. Pressure ventilation has an almost unlimited ability to deliver flow and possesses a decelerating flow profile that tends to improve the distribution of ventilation in a lung with heterogeneous disease. With comparable settings in volume control, pressure-control ventilation will maintain a higher mean airway pressure. A potential disadvantage with this type of ventilation is that tidal volume, and therefore minute ventilation, is variable. The tidal volume generated will depend on the compliance and resistance of the respiratory system. As lung compliance improves, the tidal volume will increase with the same inspiratory pressure. This type of ventilation will compensate for an air leak around an uncuffed endotracheal tube.

With volume-controlled ventilation, a preset tidal volume (the volume of gas to be moved in and out of the lungs) is delivered unless a pressure limit is exceeded. Tidal volume is controlled by a constant inspiratory flow rate and a set inspiratory time. A decrease in lung compliance or increase in airway resistance will be reflected by an increase in peak inspiratory pressures. For example, if an endotracheal tube becomes occluded, the airway resistance will increase, and the same tidal volume will now generate a higher inspiratory pressure. For healthy individuals, a normal tidal volume breath is 6–8 mL/kg. But when initiating volume control ventilation, the prescribed tidal volume is usually 8–10 mL/kg since "extra" volume is needed to compensate for the compressible volume lost in the ventilator circuit. This volume is adjusted based on adequacy of chest rise in each patient.

In children with severe lung disease, such as acute respiratory distress syndrome (ARDS), closing volume is increased above that of the functional residual capacity, causing diffuse atelectasis. By increasing mean airway pressure, lung volumes may be increased above that of the closing volume, leading to alveolar recruitment. This is why some clinicians prefer the use of pressure-controlled ventilation, which maintains a higher mean airway pressure. Others will use volume-controlled ventilation and increase the mean airway pressure by optimizing positive end-expiratory pressure (PEEP).

PEEP increases the functional residual capacity of the lung (the volume of gas in the lung after normal exhalation) above the closing volume (the volume of gas in the lung after maximal exhalation at which the airways close). PEEP maintains alveolar volume, prevents atelectasis, and improves oxygenation by increasing the mean airway pressure (MAP). PEEP is set in either volume- or pressure-controlled ventilation; it is the lowest *expiratory* pressure reached during mechanical ventilation. However, excess PEEP may cause lung hyperinflation, air trapping, or air leaks. PEEP has a double effect on the cardiovascular system: it will increase intrathoracic pressure and may decrease systemic venous return to the heart (preload). On the other hand, PEEP improves cardiac output by decreasing afterload of the left ventricle. One of the major goals in mechanical ventilation is to find a balance between the good and bad effects of PEEP in each patient.

Inverse-ratio ventilation and high-frequency ventilation are unconventional modes of mechanical ventilation used in pediatric patients. Inverse-ratio ventilation prolongs the inspiratory phase in excess of the expiratory phase during positive-pressure ventilation; this increases mean airway pressure and oxygenation during severe acute lung disease. It is a nonphysiologic pattern for breathing and therefore these patients are administered heavy sedation and paralysis. Airway pressure-release ventilation (APRV) is a newer form of inverse-ratio ventilation that utilizes a continuous gas flow circuit to allow the patient to breathe spontaneously throughout the ventilatory cycle. This is more comfortable for the patient. Less sedation is needed, so patients can contribute to their ventilation. High-frequency jet ventilation and high-frequency oscillatory ventilation both combine small tidal volumes (smaller than calculated airway deadspace) with increased frequencies (>1 Hz) in order to minimize the effects of elevated peak and mean airway pressures. High-frequency ventilation reduces the occurrence and treatment of air-leak syndromes associated with neonatal and pediatric acute lung injury.

INVASIVE LINE PLACEMENT AND MONITORING

Arterial Catheter Insertion

Arterial catheters are indicated when there is a need for precise beat-to-beat blood pressure monitoring or determination of acid–base status using arterial blood gases. There are no absolute contraindications to placing an arterial catheter, but a risk/benefit analysis should be performed in patients with a hypercoaguable state or bleeding disorder.

The radial artery is a favored site for arterial cannulation because the vessel is superficial and easily accessible. Other anatomic sites frequently used are the ulnar, dorsalis pedis, posterior tibial, and femoral arteries. In general, the brachial artery should be avoided because of the risk of median nerve damage.

After palpating and localizing the artery with the non-dominant hand, the selected artery can be cannulated either by inserting the catheter directly into the artery using a catheter-over-needle device or by using the Seldinger technique. The Seldinger technique involves entering the vessel with a needle, placing a guidewire through the needle after the vessel is entered, removing the needle, and then placing the catheter over the wire into the vessel. This can be performed for arterial and venous cannulations. When cannulating a peripheral artery, it is helpful to immobilize the extremity with a board. Aseptic technique should always be followed when placing an arterial line.

All arterial lines must be clearly identified to avoid accidental infusion of hypertonic solutions and sclerosing medications that would injure the artery. Arterial catheters are at risk for infection, disconnection causing significant blood loss, and arterial thrombus formation. Also, ischemic distal necrosis can occur from arteriolar spasm or emboli from air or clot.

Central Venous Catheter Insertion

Central venous catheters are used in pediatric patients for several reasons. They provide cardiac filling pressure measurements. They are also a secure route for:

- Administration of fluids and drugs to the central circulation
- Rapid infusion of large volumes of fluids and blood products
- Administration of high-concentration parenteral alimentation that would be sclerosing to peripheral veins
- Administration of parenteral fluid and drugs when peripheral venous access is poor
- Access for hemodialysis, plasmapheresis, right heart catheterization and placement of a temporary transvenous pacemaker.

The common sites for central venous cannulation are the femoral, internal jugular, and subclavian veins. There are no absolute contraindications to place a central venous catheter, but each site has potential risks. All sites share the common complications of infection (site cellulitis, bacteremia), venous thrombosis with potential emboli, air embolism, catheter malfunction (occlusion, dislodgement, fractures), dysrhythmias (when the catheter tip is in the heart), and bleeding. Universal precautions and sterile technique should be used when placing a central venous catheter.

Femoral Vein Cannulation

Femoral venous catheterization is the central venous access route used most commonly in infants and children in emergency situations because it lies adjacent to the easily palpable femoral artery. Furthermore, femoral anatomy is easily learned, and hemostasis can be obtained quickly in the event of an accidental arterial puncture. Disadvantages of this approach include the possibility of unintentional femoral artery puncture and subsequent limited ability to flex the hip. Numerous studies have shown no higher incidence of complications from femoral cannulation compared to the subclavian or internal jugular routes. If the patient has abdominal wounds or a significant intraabdominal process, central venous access should be obtained above the diaphragm.

At the level of the inguinal ligament, the femoral vein is the most medial structure in the femoral sheath, which also contains the femoral nerve and artery. To optimize successful femoral cannulation, the patient's leg should be slightly rotated externally. In infants and small children, a towel under the buttocks flattens the inguinal area and makes the angle less acute to enter the femoral vein. The femoral artery is identified approximately 1 cm below the inguinal crease where the needle is inserted in a medial direction towards the umbilicus, and advanced at a 45-degree angle until free flow of blood is obtained in the syringe. After successful venous puncture, the Seldinger technique is used to complete the cannulation.

If the femoral pulse cannot be palpated, it is usually located at the midpoint between the anterior superior iliac spine and the symphysis pubis.

Internal Jugular Vein Cannulation

The internal jugular vein is located under the sternocleidomastoid muscle in the neck and follows an oblique course as it runs down the neck in the carotid sheath. It drains into the subclavian vein to form the brachiocephalic (innominate) vein behind the head of the clavicle. The right side is preferred because the vessel runs a straighter course to the right atrium and the dome of the right lung is lower compared to the left side, reducing the risk of pneumothorax. The patient is placed in the Trendelenburg position, with the head turned to the opposite side. Turning the head straightens the vein from the pinna of the ear to the sternoclavicular joint. There are three common approaches for cannulation:

1. The *anterior* approach introduces the needle at the midpoint of the anterior border of the sternocleidomastoid muscle. The needle is directed toward the ipsilateral nipple.

2. The *middle* approach is through the triangular region created by the two heads of the sternocleidomastoid muscle and the clavicle. The carotid artery is palpated and retracted medially. The needle is inserted at the apex of the triangle, lateral to the carotid artery. While continuously aspirating, the needle is advanced at a 30-degree angle towards the ipsilateral nipple.

3. The *posterior* approach identifies the posterior aspect of the lateral edge of the sternocleidomastoid muscle and the needle is inserted superior to the point where the external jugular vein crosses over the muscle. The needle is inserted and advanced along the underbelly of the muscle towards the suprasternal notch.

Once the venipuncture is accomplished, the syringe is removed and the end of the needle occluded to prevent air embolism. The Seldinger technique is used to complete the cannulation; the location of the catheter tip should be confirmed radiographically. The most ideal position for the tip of the catheter is at the junction of the superior vena cava and the right atrium. Using the middle insertion approach, the proper length can be estimated from the patient's weight (Table 38-9).

Successful cannulation of the internal jugular vein can be improved by using ultrasound guidance. Additional maneuvers that improve cannulation success are to enlarge the internal jugular vein by a Valsalva maneuver or external compression over the liver.

Complications of internal jugular vein cannulation include carotid artery puncture, and thoracic duct injury with left-sided attempts. If a previous attempt led to a

Table 38-9 Recommended Length of Central Venous Catheter Insertion Using the Middle Approach to the IJV	
Patient Weight (kg)	Length of CVC Insertion (cm)
2– 2.9	4
3– 4.9	5
5– 6.9	6
7– 9.9	7
10–12.9	8
13–19.9	9
20–29.9	10
30–39.9	11
40–49.9	12
50–59.9	13
60–69.9	14
70–79.9	15
≥80	16

Reproduced with permission from Andropoulos DB, Bent ST, Skjonsby B, Stayer SA: The optimal length of insertion of central venous catheters for pediatric patients. *Anesth Analg* 93:883–886, 2001.

hematoma, the other side should not be attempted because bilateral hematomas may lead to upper-airway compromise. Also, placing an internal jugular venous catheter is relatively contraindicated in patients at risk for intracranial hypertension because venous occlusion may increase intracranial pressure. Some drawbacks of a catheter in this position are that conscious patients have limited neck mobility, there is a higher risk of thrombotic occlusion from neck flexion, and it is difficult to keep the area clean, especially in patients with a tracheostomy.

Subclavian Vein Cannulation

The subclavian vein is a continuation of the axillary vein as it passes over the first rib and lies posterior to the medial third of the clavicle. At the thoracic inlet, it meets the internal jugular vein to form the brachiocephalic (innominate) vein. The left subclavian vein is longer and follows a straighter path, making it easier to insert a catheter. The technique is used less frequently in children because the vessel is smaller and more cephalad under the clavicle. The advantages of this approach are its fixed landmarks and patient comfort once secured. The risks of pneumothorax and hemothorax appear to be slightly higher with the subclavian approach than with the internal jugular approach. These risks are increased if there is a chest wall deformity.

To catheterize the subclavian vein, the patient is placed in the Trendelenburg position with the head turned away from the insertion site (if there is no cervical spine injury).

With the infraclavicular approach, the needle is inserted at a point one-half to two-thirds its length away from the sternoclavicular junction. If the patient is receiving mechanical ventilation, temporary disruption of ventilation during insertion of the needle keeps the apex of the lung away from the needle. While continuously aspirating, the needle is advanced under the clavicle toward the suprasternal notch. Once a free flow of blood is obtained in the syringe, the syringe is disconnected and a finger is placed over the hub of the needle to prevent entrainment of air. During a positive-pressure breath or exhalation, the guidewire is advanced into the right atrium. The needle is removed, the tract is dilated, and the catheter is inserted using the Seldinger technique. Blood should be easily aspirated from all ports of the catheter. A chest radiograph should be obtained to verify the position of the catheter tip and to rule out pneumothorax.

ARTICLES TO KNOW

Bayir H, Clark RSB, Kochanek PM: Promising strategies to minimize secondary brain injury after head injury. *Crit Care Med* 31:S112-117, 2003.

Bengur AR, Meliones JN: Cardiogenic shock. *New Horizons* 6:139-149, 1998.

Carcillo JA, Fields AI: Clinical practice parameters for hemodynamic support of pediatric and neonatal patients in septic shock. *Crit Care Med* 30:1365-1378, 2002.

Kirkham FJ: Non-traumatic coma in children. *Arch Dis Child* 85:303-312, 2001.

Morgan WM, O'Neill JA: Hemorrhagic and obstructive shock in pediatric patients. *New Horizons* 6:150-154, 1998.

Qureshi AI, Suarez JI: Use of hypertonic saline solutions in treatment of cerebral edema and intracranial hypertension. *Crit Care Med* 28:3301-3313, 2000.

Scott RC, Surtees RA, Neville BG: Status epilepticus: pathophysiology, epidemiology, and outcomes. *Arch Dis Child* 79:73-77, 1998.

Treem WR: Fulminant hepatic failure in children. *J Pediatr Gastroent Nutr* 35(Suppl 1):S33-38, 2002.

Werner HA: Status asthmaticus in children: a review. *Chest* 119:1913-1929, 2001.

Williams DM, Sreedhar SS, Mickell JJ, Chan JC: Acute kidney failure: a pediatric experience over 20 years. *Arch Pediatr Adolesc Med* 156:893-900, 2002.

Wood RA: Pediatric asthma. *JAMA* 288:745-747, 2002.

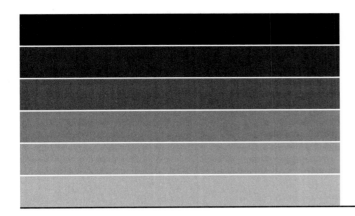

Index

As pediatric anesthesia is the subject of the book, all index entries refer to anesthesia in pediatric medicine unless otherwise indicated.
Abbreviations: CHD - congenital heart disease